M. Isabel García Real

ATLAS OF RADIOGRAPHIC INTERPRETATION in small animals

SECOND EDITION

edra
PUBLISHING

This book was originally published in Spanish under the title:
Atlas de interpretación radiológica en pequeños animales (2.ª edición)

ISBN Spanish edition: 978-84-18339-54-7

Atlas of Radiographic Interpretation in Small Animals (2nd edition)
M. Isabel García Real

Cover picture of the Multivet X-ray machine courtesy of Sedecal.

ISBN: 978-1-957260-29-7
eISBN: 978-1-957260-36-5

Book Publishing Manager: Costanza Smeraldi, Edra S.p.A.
Paper, Printing and Binding Manager: Paolo Ficicchia, Edra S.p.A.
Cover, Layout, and Copyediting: Grupo Asís Biomedia SL, Zaragoza, Spain
Translation: Chef du Monde, Grupo Asís Biomedia SL, Zaragoza, Spain
Project Manager: María Menéndez Carreño, Grupo Asís Biomedia SL, Zaragoza, Spain
Illustrator: Jacob Gragera Artal

Edra Publishing US LLC
3309 Northlake Boulevard, Suite 203
Palm Beach Gardens, FL, 33403
EIN: 844113980
info@edrapublishing.com
www.edrapublishing.com

edra
PUBLISHING

Printed by Etiquetas Alhambra, S.L., Granada, Spain, October 2023

"Radiographic interpretation: a balance between science and art"

Clifford R. Berry, Donald E. Thrall

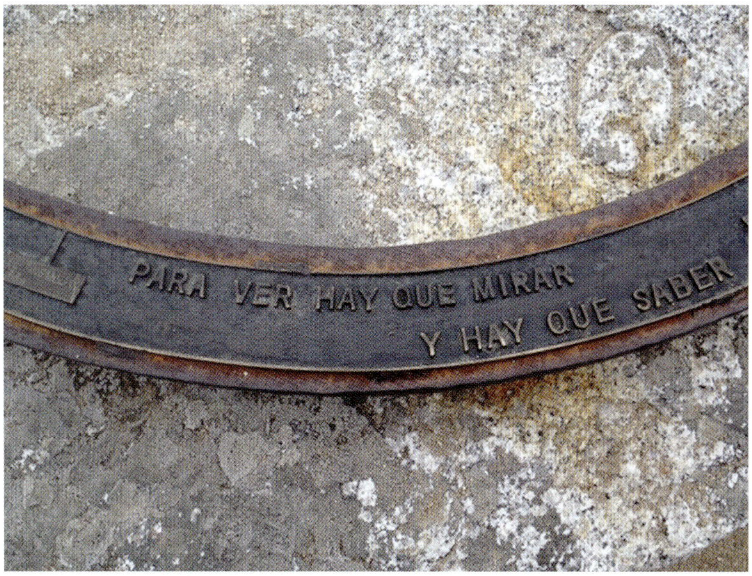

To see, you must look, and you must know.
Mirador de los Robledos, Sierra de Guadarrama, Madrid

To my family

To all those who have learned with me in the past
or will learn with me in the future

Acknowledgements

My colleagues at the Diagnostic Imaging Service of the Complutense Veterinary Teaching Hospital, including those no longer with us, because they have all contributed in some way to this book. Several people deserve special mention in this second edition: Pilar Llorens Pena, with whom I have shared 28 years of teaching, María José Ruiz Fernández, who is following in my footsteps in this fascinating discipline of radiology, and Carmen Osorno, Isabel García Nieto and Sonia Pavón, "my professional family". Not forgetting those who have sadly left us, like Miguel Rodríguez Castaño.

The clinicians at the Complutense Veterinary Teaching Hospital, with whom the Diagnostic Imaging Service makes an "almost" perfect team.

The owners and their pets who come to our Hospital, because they are the real source of, and reason for, our work.

Veterinary students, who keep demanding a constant effort of self-improvement from us, so that their training as future vets is increasingly better.

The staff at the San Carlos Teaching Hospital (especially Dr Antonio Casado) and Severo Ochoa Hospital for their contribution to making this project possible.

Finally, I would like to especially thank my family and friends for their immense patience while I worked on this book instead of spending time with them.

Author

M. ISABEL GARCÍA REAL

She is a Doctor in Veterinary Medicine. She graduated from the Complutense University of Madrid in 1993 and obtained her Ph.D. in 2000. She joined the Department of Animal Medicine and Surgery of the Faculty of Veterinary Medicine of the Complutense University of Madrid in 1993, where she now continues to lecture on Radiology and Diagnostic Imaging.

She has been the Head of the Diagnostic Imaging Service at the Complutense Veterinary Teaching Hospital since 2005 and Director of the Magnetic Resonance Unit of the hospital since its opening in December 2008. Her teaching and research work focuses on radiology, abdominal ultrasounds, CT scans and MRI.

She has been a visiting scholar at the Universities of California (Davis, USA) and Cambridge (United Kingdom) and has completed internships at the Animal Medical Center in New York and the Animal Health Trust (Newmarket, United Kingdom).

She is the author of several national and international publications, and has participated as a speaker in various courses and national and international conferences.

She is the main author and academic supervisor of the online course of Radiographic interpretation in small animals which she has taught each year since 2016 in collaboration with the Official College of Veterinarians of Madrid.

Prologue

Radiography still is the diagnostic imaging technique most frequently used in small animal clinical medicine. That is why those graduate and postgraduate students and professionals who wish to practice clinical medicine need a reference book to use as a guide to radiographic interpretation.

The first edition of this book fulfilled this purpose impeccably. Now, with the second edition, further information on radiographic positioning and anatomy is added to assist readers when taking and interpreting radiographs. Some of the content of the chapters has been updated and new or updated high-quality images and videos have been added. The number of images (about 1000) represents and conveys the author's extensive professional experience and they encompass the most prominent diseases so that veterinary students and clinicians may become familiar with the most important and most common radiographic signs. In addition, some images are accompanied by diagrams that illustrate the position of the organs, as well as by images obtained with other diagnostic imaging techniques such as ultrasonography, computed tomography and magnetic resonance imaging. It also includes complementary material which can be accessed on the Internet, as well as a section with self-assessment case studies.

I would like to congratulate the author for this atlas which is sure to prove invaluable to veterinary students and clinicians.

Amalia Agut Giménez, Diplomate ECVDI
Professor at the Faculty of Animal Medicine and Surgery (Diagnostic Imaging)
University of Murcia

Preface

In these times when veterinarians have access to advanced diagnostic imaging techniques (such as computed tomography and magnetic resonance imaging), the enormous value that radiography still has as an essential diagnostic tool in small animal clinical medicine is sometimes underestimated.

In my years of experience as a lecturer in the field of Diagnostic Imaging (29 years this year, in 2022), I have noted a general tendency among small animal clinical veterinarians to try to advance their training in the use of other techniques, such as ultrasound or even computed tomography, assuming that a very basic knowledge of radiology is sufficient for the correct development of their professional activity. My greatest satisfaction when teaching continuing education courses for professionals is helping them understand that radiology can provide them with "way more" than what they expect from it *a priori*. The more they learn, the more they grasp both the complexity and the usefulness of learning to correctly interpret the radiograms they see every day in their clinics. This book also aims to convey this idea to you, confident that it will be of benefit to you in your daily diagnostic tasks.

A section on the basic principles of radiological interpretation was not included in the first edition but which I now consider essential for this second edition. Readers must understand how a radiograph is obtained and on what principles the creation of the image is based before they can evaluate it. Reviewing these principles in a straightforward manner will, I believe, help lay more solid foundations for a good diagnostic interpretation.

Another improvement in this second edition is that the Atlas of Radiographic Anatomy of the Dog is included (this was available with the previous edition on the publisher's website) within the book and is complemented by an atlas of radiographic positioning. On each page of this section in Chapter 1, there is an image of the patient's positioning and the normal X-ray image, together with clear identification of the most relevant anatomical structures. These images can be easily and rapidly consulted directly in the book or may also be consulted on the online version of the Atlas of Radiographic Anatomy, available via a password included in each copy of the book.

QR codes are available with this second edition that allow access to the Atlas of Radiographic Anatomy of the Dog on the publisher's website and to self-assessments at the end of each chapter, except Chapter 1. Another change introduced with this edition is how the self-assessments can be conducted. Initially the reader has access only to the patient's clinical data and images with the first QR code. Then with a second code, access is given to a video explanation of the radiographic findings and the final diagnosis. We have also added material on videofluoroscopy and dynamic digital radiographic imaging throughout the text. This can also be accessed via QR codes.

Finally, an enormous thanks to my publisher for agreeing to let me expand the number of images per chapter. Most of these were obtained with the latest direct digital radiology equipment and will, undoubtedly, be much appreciated by readers familiar with the first edition.

I sincerely hope that the efforts that went into updating and expanding the first edition will meet the expectations of all readers who purchase this book. My intention was to improve the book to the best of my ability and to help veterinarians and veterinary students learn more about this discipline that I am so passionate about.

María Isabel García Real
February 2022

Table of contents

CHAPTER 1 BASIC PRINCIPLES OF RADIOGRAPHY

CHAPTER 2 ABDOMEN

CHAPTER 3 NECK AND THORAX

CHAPTER 4 APPENDICULAR SKELETON

CHAPTER 5 SPINE

CHAPTER 6 HEAD

ATLAS OF RADIOGRAPHIC INTERPRETATION
in small animals

Basic principles of radiography

1

Fundamentals of radiography

X-rays were discovered in 1895 by the German physicist Wilhelm Conrad Röntgen. Their discovery revolutionised the diagnosis and treatment of an immense spectrum of diseases in both human and veterinary medicine. In 1901, Röntgen was awarded the first Nobel Prize in Physics for this breakthrough. While radiography is an extremely valuable technique in medicine, the X-rays involved interact with the body's tissues, causing **ionisation**, which can result in significant biological damage. As such, it is important to understand a number of basic principles about the generation and action of X-rays in order to use them correctly in a clinical setting.

Definition of X-rays

X-rays are a type of **electromagnetic radiation**, as are radio waves, radar waves and visible light. Electromagnetic radiation is a type of energy that can propagate through space without the need for a medium. It can be thought of as a considering two components - a vibrating electric field and a vibrating magnetic field.

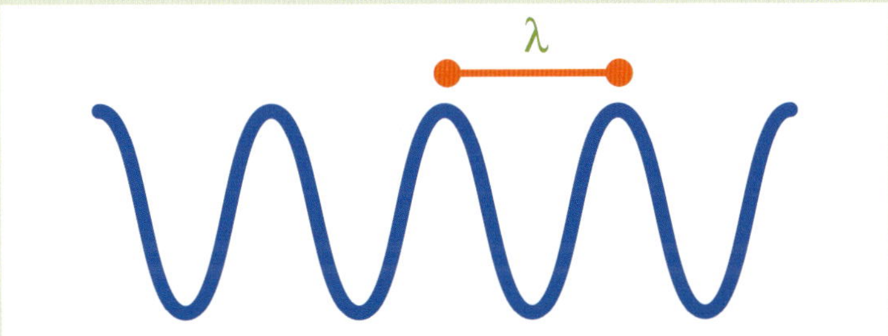

FIGURE 1.1. Illustration of an electromagnetic wave. λ: wavelength.

Electromagnetic waves, like any other type of wave, are characterised by their frequency (v) and wavelength (λ) (fig. 1.1). The frequency of an electromagnetic wave is the number of oscillations (cycles) completed by the electromagnetic field per unit time and is expressed as cycles per second or hertz (Hz). The wavelength is the shortest distance between two points in the wave that are in the same state of oscillation at any given moment (e.g. peak to peak). This is measured in units of length (metres, centimetres, microns, etc.).

The relantioship between frequency and wavelength is given by the equation:

$$\lambda = c/v$$

where "c" equals the propagation speed of the electromagnetic wave. The propagation speed is always the same in a vacuum and often referred to as the speed of light (approx. 300,000 km/s). Thus, the frequency and wavelength are inversely proportional to each other, so the higher the frequency, the shorter the wavelength.

The electromagnetic spectrum covers a wide range of frequencies (or wavelengths) which are classified according to their main source of generation (fig. 1.2).

X-rays span the range of wavelengths from 10^{-8} to 10^{-12} m, corresponding to frequencies from 3×10^{16} to 6×10^{19} Hz. They are invisible because these wavelengths fall outside the visible light spectrum.

The energy associated with a source of electromagnetic radiation is directly proportional to its frequency (and inversely proportional to wavelength); in other words, the higher the frequency (and therefore the shorter the wavelength), then the higher the level of electromagnetic radiation energy.

X-rays are a high-frequency, high-energy electromagnetic radiation with a short wavelength.

X-ray production

X-rays are emitted when high-speed electrons strike a metal. In an X-ray tube, electrons are accelerated down the tube until they bombard a metal target.

X-ray tubes contain two electrodes, the negatively charged **cathode** and the positively charged **anode**.

The cathode contains a coiled filament, similar to that found in a light bulb. When an electric current is passed through the filament, it heats up and emits the electrons (which always carry a negative charge) that remain stationary around the filament. A potential difference is then applied between the two electrodes to accelerate the electrons towards the anode. The high-speed electrons collide with the anode and release 99 % of their kinetic energy in the form of heat, while just is emitted 1 % as X-rays (fig. 1.3).

If the current passed through the cathode is increased, then the filament reaches higher temperatures, so more electrons are emitted and collide with the anode and to produce more X-rays. The current intensity is measured in milliamperes (mA) and determines the number of electrons flowing from the cathode to the anode per second. In most equipment, the X-ray' current tube cannot usually be modified under an unbroken range, rather just a few discrete milliamperes values can be selected (e.g. 50, 100, 200, 400, etc). The total number of X-rays produced in each burst depends on the strength of the current selected and the exposure time in seconds (mAs).

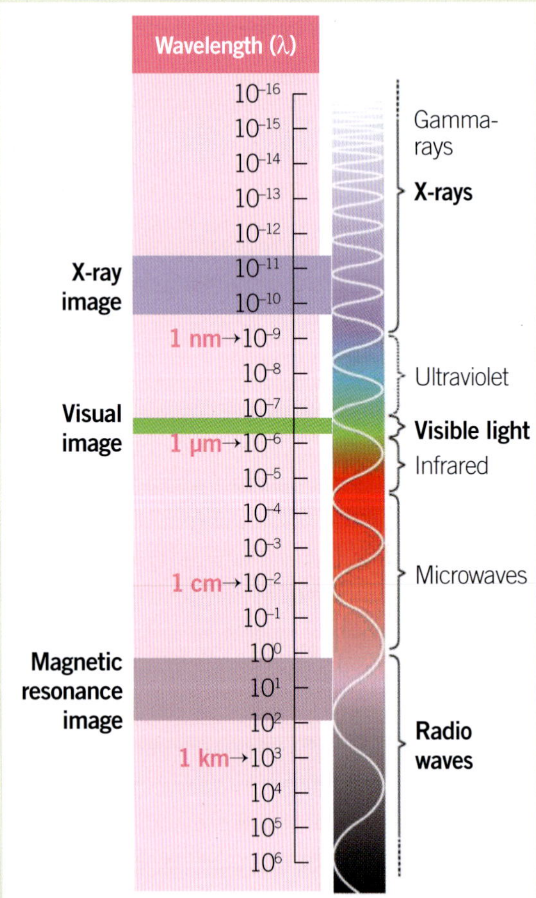

FIGURE 1.2. The electromagnetic radiation spectrum.

FIGURE 1.3. Schematic diagram of the production of X-rays. When an electrical current passes through the cathode filament (red spiral), electrons (e⁻) are released which, after applying a potential difference, flow from the cathode towards the anode to reach the target area of the anode (blue band). The kinetic energy of the electrons is then transformed into 99 % heat and 1 % X-rays (grey waves).

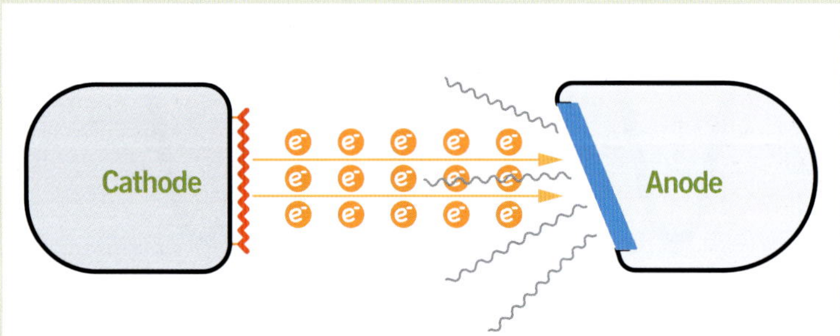

The higher the milliamperage (mA) and the longer the exposure time (s), then more number of X-rays are generated.

The greater the potential difference, or voltage, applied between the cathode and anode, then the faster the electrons will flow to the anode. When the electrons carry more kinetic energy at the time of the collision, they produce more heat and therefore higher energy X-rays which are more penetrating. The potential difference is adjusted using the X-ray equipment's kilovoltage selector (in kV), so the penetration strength of the resulting X-ray depends directly on the voltage.

At higher voltage, the X-rays have more energy.

When the electrons collide with the metal target, X-rays are produced through either a collision or braking interaction. Atoms are made up of tiny particles called protons, neutrons and electrons. The nucleus of an atom consists of protons (positively charged) and neutrons (no electric charge). Electrons (which have a negative charge) revolve around the nucleus in specific orbits called energy levels or shells.

In **collision interactions**, a high-speed electron (emitted from the cathode and accelerated by the potential difference) collides with an atom in the anode and forcing the expulsion an electron orbiting the atom. As a result, an outer-shell electron (higher energy) moves in to fill the vacancy left by the ejected electron with the release of energy in the form of X-ray photons. X-rays produced via this mechanism are called characteristic X-rays because they have specific energies (equal to the energy needed to expel the electron from its shell). These X-rays represent only a fraction of the full beam produced by a diagnostic X-ray tube.

In **braking or** *bremsstrahlung* **interactions,** a high-speed electron passes close to the nucleus of an atom without expelling any electrons from its orbit. The positively charged nucleus attracts the electron which deflects it from its path and reduces its velocity. This leads to a loss of kinetic energy released in the form of X-ray photons. The X-rays produced by this mechanism are called **braking radiation** and have a wide spectrum of energies, depending on the degree to which the nucleus decelerates each electron. Most electrons are deflected like this by multiple nuclei, gradually losing their kinetic energy.

The parts of an X-ray machine

The basic components of X-ray machines (fig. 1.4) commonly used in diagnostic imaging suites are:

- X-ray tube: emits the radiation that creates the radiographic image. Only the protective lead housing is visible from the outside.
- Generator: the X-ray tube is powered a high-voltage generator, which consists of various elements such as transformers, current rectifiers, etc.
- Control panel: used to select exposure parameters.
- Examination table with a radiolucent material top surface, under which there should be trays to house cassette or digital receiver system.
- Collimator: a device attached to the X-ray tube consisting of parallel pairs of lead plates that are used to alter the shape and size of the X-ray beam depending on the anatomical region being examined.

Portable X-ray machines are also used in veterinary medicine and can be used outside the clinic, on farms or in the field.

The cathode and the anode are both located in the **X-ray tube**. The tube is made from heat-resistant glass (Pyrex®) constructed to form a hermetically sealed enclosure where a vacuum is created to prevent electrons from interacting with air molecules before they reach the anode (fig. 1.5). There is a small area in the tube where the glass is much thinner, called the window, through which the X-ray beam is emitted. Given the high temperatures reached inside the tube, the window is enclosed within an oil-or water-based cooling system. Together, the tube and cooling system are surrounded by a protective lead lining to prevent unwanted X-rays from leaking out, given that radiation is emitted in all directions inside the tube, but only the X-rays scaping through the window are of interest. On the other hand, the rays in the beam have a wide spectrum of frequencies and wavelengths, that is, the beam includes X-rays with different energies (some more penetrating than others). Low-energy X-rays do not have any value for diagnostic purposes because they are absorbed by the patient and do not contribute to the image formation. As such, X-ray tubes are designed with internal filters to attenuate these low-energy (soft) rays.

Both the anode and cathode reach very high temperatures when producing X-rays, so they are always built using high-melting point materials, such as tungsten. This material also has a high atomic number, which is the number of protons held in the atom's nucleus, as well as corresponding to the number of electrons orbiting each atom. The higher the atomic number, therefore, the greater the availability of electrons, which increases the efficiency of X-ray production.

There are two types of anodes, stationary or rotating. Stationary anodes are used for small, portable or dental X-ray equipment. Rotating anodes are preferable, however, as the rotation increases the effective surface area bombarded by the electrons, thereby reducing anode deterioration.

The focal spot is the region of the anode bombarded by the electrons and therefore where X-rays are produced. The smaller the focal spot, the sharper the detail in the resulting X-ray. By adjusting the anode angle, the focal spot can be made to appear smaller than it actually is (effective focal spot), while maintaining a large area of electron bombardment (fig. 1.6). Some machines have two focal spots of different sizes that can be selected by the operator. The small focal spot is selected when sharper, more detailed images are required. However, it should only be used at low milliamperages (e.g. when talking X-ray of limbs) as high values can cause radiation burns. When high milliamperages are required (e.g. X-rays of the chest, abdomen, hip, etc.), the larger focal spot should be selected despite the slight loss of image sharpness.

The **generator** (fig. 1.7) supplies the tube with the correct current and high voltage needed to produce an X-ray beam with the appropriate characteristics. The voltage of the power supply hospitals receive from the main grid can vary by up to 5 %. This variation could significantly affect X-ray production, so the generator incorporates a line compensator that adjusts the voltage to exactly 220 V. The transformers increasee the input voltage from a conventional power source by a factor of 500 to 1,000, as X-ray production requires potential differences of 40,000 to 120,000 V (40-120 kV). The apparatus also includes current rectifier, which converts alternating current to direct current, so electron flow can be driven in just one direction, from the cathode to the anode.

The controls for the main settings used to determine the quantity and quality of X-rays produced in the tube are found on the **control panel** (fig. 1.8):

- Voltage selector.
- Milliamperage selector (current intensity).
- Exposure time selector.
- Milliampere second selector.
- Fine and coarse focus selector.

A **variable-aperture collimator** (fig. 1.9) is a light source that illuminates the X-ray field at the selected beam size. The illuminated area usually has a cross-shaped shadow marking the exact centre of the X-ray beam. This is important as the resulting image will have maximum sharpness at this point. The beam should be adjusted to the minimum size required, to reduce the amount of useless primary and secondary radiation that is harmful to both the operator and patient, so beam collimation is an essential step in radiation protection. It also improves image quality.

Beam collimation is an essential radiation protection measure and improves image quality.

How X-rays interact with matter

To understand how X-ray images are produced, it is important to understand how they interact with matter. X-rays can penetrate matter, where they either totally or partially release their energy by interacting with the atoms making up the matter.

X-rays are composed of photons or quanta of energy ("packets" of energy), which photons have no mass or electrical charge.

Photons can interact with matter in five different ways:

1. Coherent scattering
2. Photoelectric effect
3. Compton scattering
4. Pair production
5. Photodisintegration

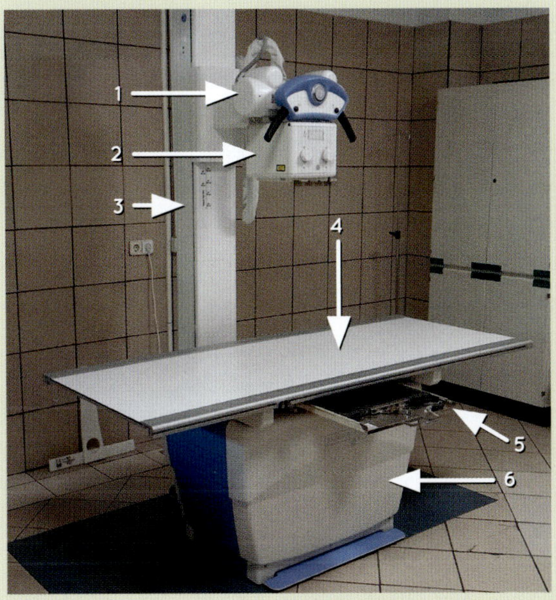

FIGURE 1.4. X-ray machine for veterinary use. 1: X-ray tube with protective lead housing; 2: Variable aperture collimator; 3: Tube sliding column; 4: Patient table; 5: Cassette tray/ detector panel; 6: Generator cabinet.

FIGURE 1.5. X-ray tube removed from its protective housing.

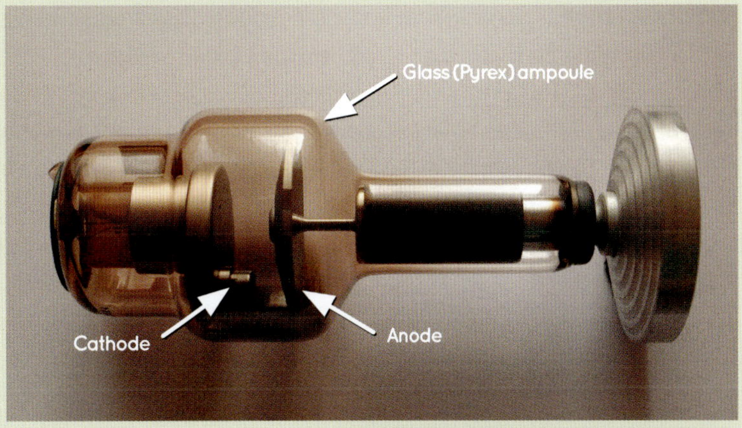

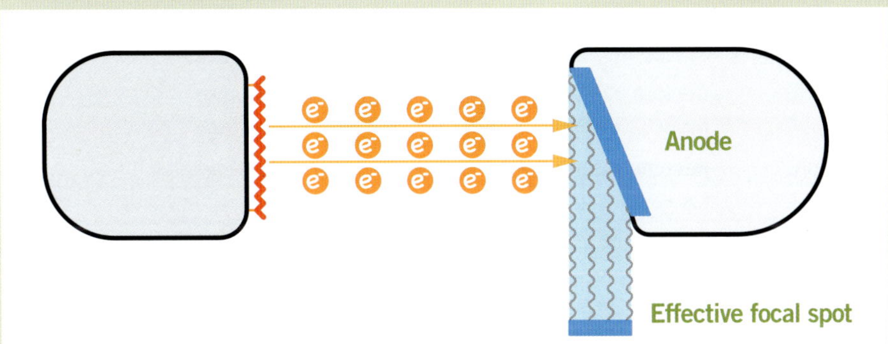

FIGURE 1.6. Schematic diagram of the effective focal point, resulting from the angled collision area of the electrons at the anode (target zone).

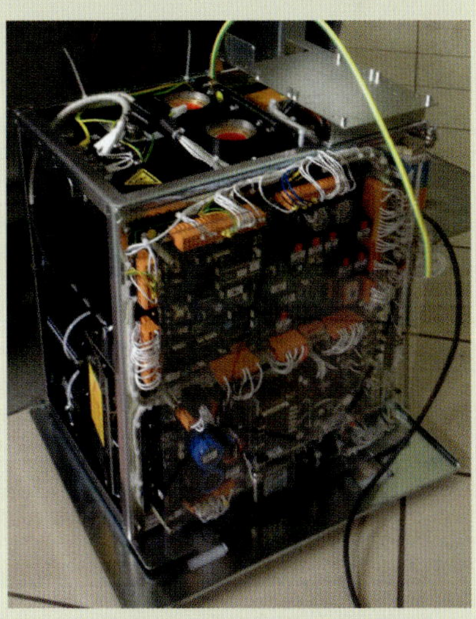

FIGURE 1.7. Image of an X-ray machine generator at time of installation.

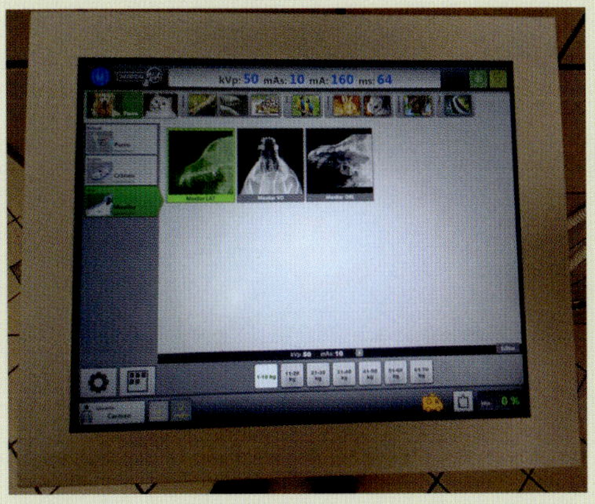

FIGURE 1.8. Digital control panel where exposure parameters are selected using a computer program and a touch screen monitor.

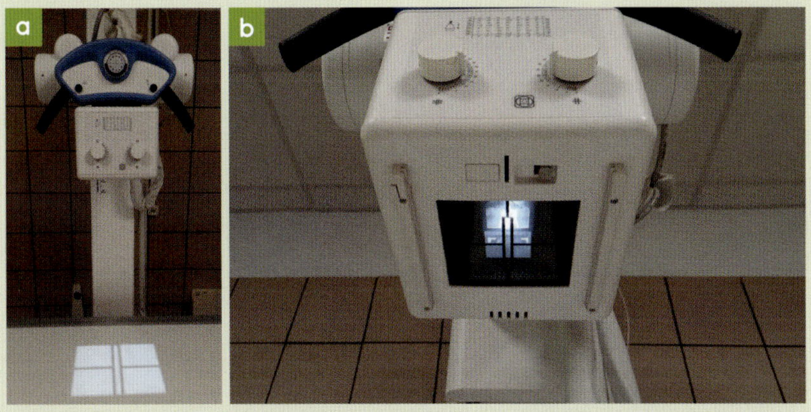

FIGURE 1.9. Variable aperture collimator. Front of the collimator attached to the X-ray tube and the table area illuminated by the light source inside it, corresponding to the selected X-ray beam size (A). Underneath the collimator, with the light source and the two/two parallel lead strips that allow the beam size to be adjusted (b).

Of these five mechanisms, the photoelectric effect and Compton scattering are the most important for diagnostic purposes.

The **photoelectric effect** (fig. 1.10) occurs when photons interact and are absorbed by an object. The photons strike the material's atoms and eject electrons from their orbit around the atoms. The ejected electrons are called photoelectrons. As outer-shell electrons transition to fill the vacancy left by the ejected electron, they release energy in the form of new photons, which are known as characteristic X-rays. The same process occurs at the anode of and the X-ray tube. But the characteristic X-rays when accelerated electrons collide with the tungsten atoms have a much higher energy than those released by the interaction of the X-ray beam's photons with the atoms in the patient's tissues, which are low energy and absorbed by the patient. As they do not reach the radiographic film, they neither contribute to image formation, nor affect staff in the room, but they add to the patient's dose of radiation.

Compton scattering (fig 1.11) occurs when photons interact with atoms in the patient, expelling an electron from the outer layer (called a Compton or recoil electron), while the incident photons are scattered at a different angle. Scattered photons or X-rays have less energy than original photons. Almost all the scatter radiation produced during diagnostic X-rays comes from Compton scattering. This scattering is harmful to the operator holding or close to the patient as they may be exposed. It also reduces image quality by printing in the wrong location on the X-ray film, resulting in a hazy, loss of sharpness.

Image formation

X-rays can pass through matter. They can also interact with photographic emulsions to create an image, which is the basis of conventional radiography (non-digital radiography). In digital radiography, however, the image captured using photostimulable phosphor screens or electronic detector panels. The first part of the chapter looks at conventional radiography systems and later describes the evolution to digital radiography.

When an object (or patient) is placed between an X-ray tube and a sheet of photographic film, the X-ray beam produced by the tube passes through the object and strikes the film creating a radiographic image of the internal structure of that object, that is, an "X-ray".

When an X-ray beam is directed onto a patient, the following occurs (fig. 1.12):

- Some of the beam's rays pass through the different tissues and reach the film, thus determining the formation of the radiographic image. These rays lose some of their energy along the way, that is, they **become attenuated**. The degree of attenuation varies depending on the tissues they pass through.
- Some rays change direction (**scatter**) and do not reach the X-ray film or, if they do, they affect areas that do not correspond to their initial pathway. Deflected or scattered rays are called scatter or diffuse radiation. Scatter radiation is harmful to operators and diminishes the image quality.
- The lower energy rays are **absorbed** by the tissues and do not reach the film, so they do not contribute to image formation.

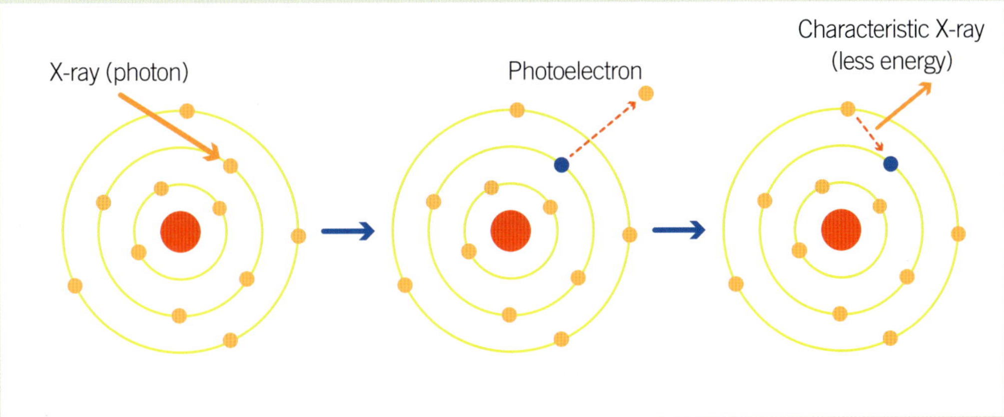

FIGURE 1.10. Schematic diagram of the photoelectric effect.

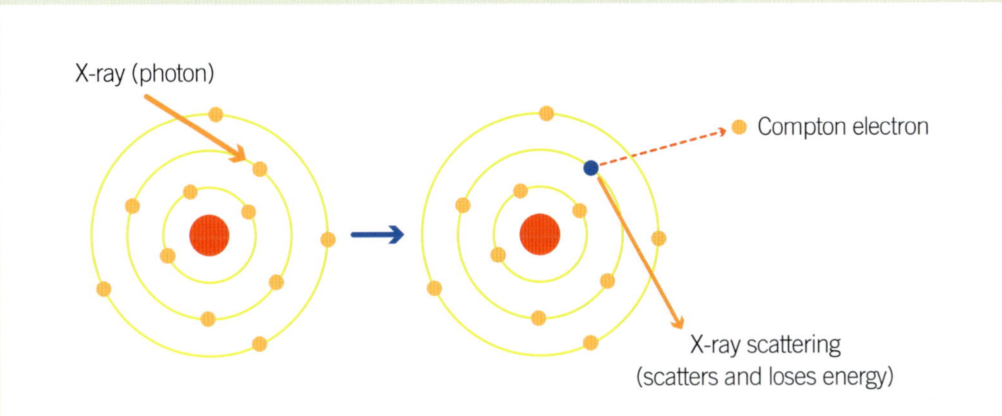

FIGURE 1.11. Schematic diagram of Compton scattering.

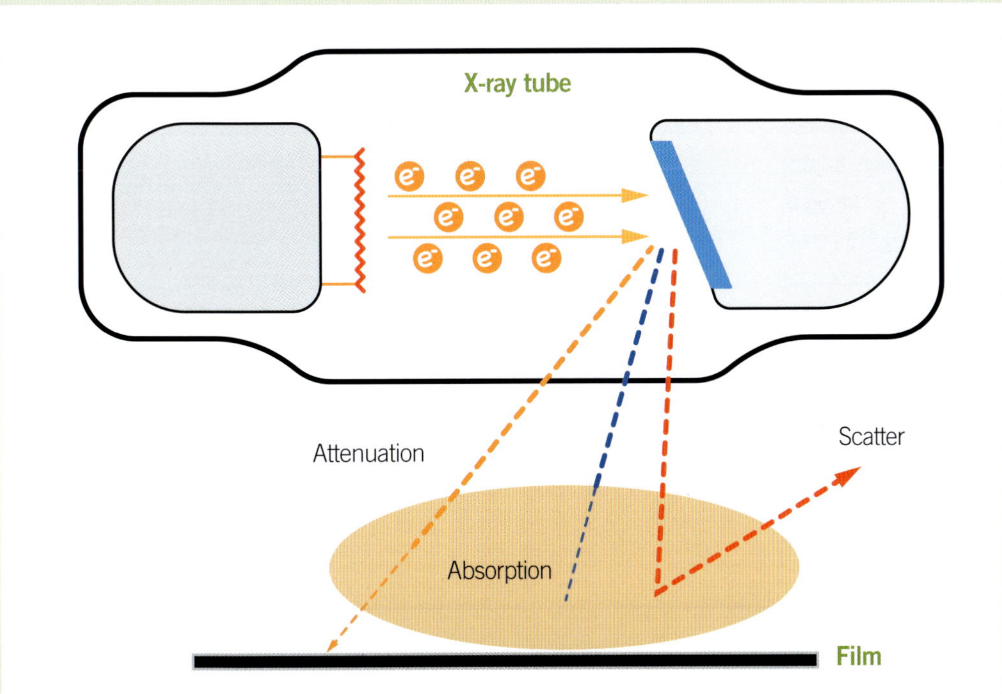

FIGURE 1.12. Schematic diagram of the X-ray attenuation, absorption and scattering that occurs when the beam passes through an object.

The extent to which X-rays are attenuated and absorbed as they pass through an object or tissue depends on two factors, the atomic number and thickness of the matter.

- The higher the atomic number of an object or tissue, the greater the degree of attenuation and absorption of X-rays (fig 1.13).
- The thicker an object or tissue, the greater the degree of X-ray attenuation and absorption. In other words, if we compare two objects or tissues with the same composition and different thickness, the thicker one will absorb more X-rays and those that do not pass through will be more attenuated (lost more energy) (fig 1.14).

X-ray film is basically a film coated on one side with a light-sensitive emulsion, containing silver halide crystals. After being exposed to light or X-rays and subsequently developed, the silver halide crystals precipitate out of the emulsion as neutral silver ions, which form a black deposit. Unexposed crystals are washed away during the fixating process, which leaves light-coloured areas on the film. The areas of the film that are highly exposed to light or X-rays appear totally black or dark grey depending on the quantity and energy of the incident X-rays. Areas of the film that receive very little light or few X-rays produce much lighter shades of grey or white.

Objects with a high atomic number absorb more rays, so the film is bombarded by fewer X-rays with less energy. Therefore, objects or substances with a high atomic number appear much lighter on X-ray images. Materials with a very high atomic number, such as metals, appear white on the image, whereas substances with a low atomic number, for example gases, create black areas on the X-ray image.

Given that tissues are made up of very different molecules with different atomic numbers, radiographers use an average value called the **effective atomic number**. Depending on its effective atomic number, a given tissue appears as a lighter or darker shade of grey on the resulting X-ray image: higher effective atomic numbers result in lighter grey areas, while lower values produce darker regions.

There are five basic radiographic densities (fig 1.15):

- **Air:** appears black on X-rays images.
- **Fat:** appears as a darker grey than soft tissue/fluid as its effective atomic number is lower.
- **Soft tissue (water):** soft tissue and fluids have very similar effective atomic numbers, so they all produce the same intermediate grey tone.
- **Mineral (bone):** bone and mineralised structures have a very high effective atomic number, resulting in a very light grey (almost white).
- **Metal:** metals appear white on X-ray films.

Contrast media used in radiography are classified as either positive or negative. Substances used as positive contrast agents (e.g. barium, iodine) have a high atomic number, so they appear white on X-rays. Negative contrast agents are gases (e.g. air, nitrous oxide or carbon dioxide).

The term radiographic density refers to how much darkening a particular material or tissue causes on the X-ray film. The property is also called opacity or radiopacity.

The terms radiopaque or radiodense are generally used to describe materials or tissues that absorb most of the incident X-rays, thus appearing light grey on the

X-ray images. Radiolucent or radiotransparent refers to material or tissues that absorb a small quantity of X-rays and therefore produce darker shades of grey on the X-ray. These terms can also be used to compare the radiographic densities of different materials or tissues (e.g. bone is more radiopaque/radiodense than soft tissue, fat is more radiolucent/radiotransparent than soft tissue).

On the other hand, the **thicker** a material or tissue, the greater the X-ray attenuation and absorption and fewer rays with less energy reach the film, hence the higher that material's or tissue's final radiopacity in the image. For example, the liver and kidneys have the same generic radiographic density (soft tissue/water), but the liver usually appears lighter grey than the kidney because the liver is thicker and so the X-rays lose more energy (fig. 1.16).

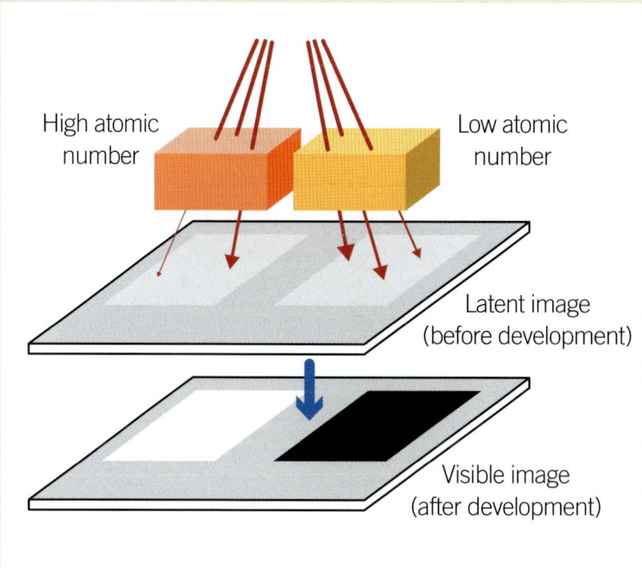

FIGURE 1.13. Schematic diagram of the effect of the atomic number of objects on X-ray penetration. The higher the atomic number, the greater the attenuation and absorption of X-rays by the object.

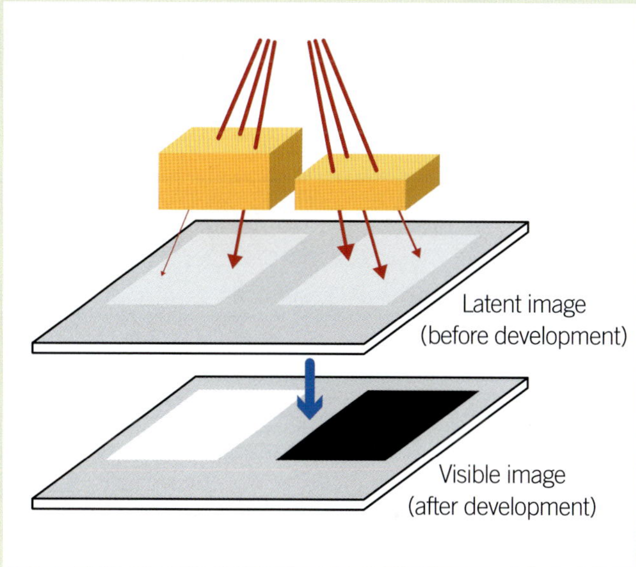

FIGURE 1.14. Schematic diagram of the effect of the thickness of the object on X-ray penetration. With the same atomic number, the thicker an object, the greater the attenuation and absorption of the X-rays.

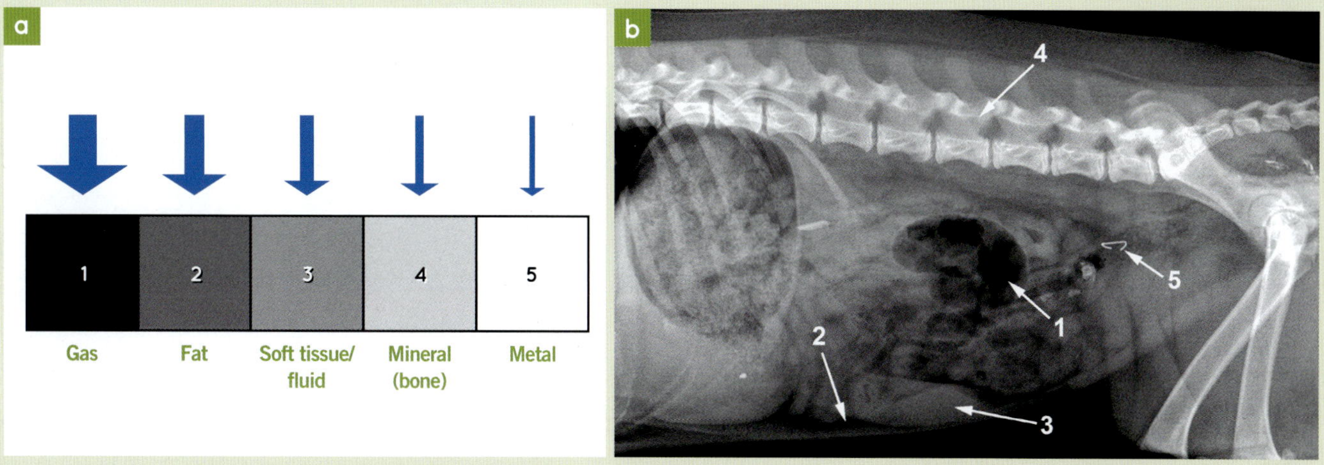

FIGURE 1.15. Schematic diagram of the five X-ray densities, also called opacities or radiopacities (a) and X-ray of a dog's abdomen where all five densities can be identified (b).

In conventional X-rays, anatomical structures appear as overlapping shadows and **their radiographic densities,** both positive and negative, are acumulative (fig. 1.17). Thus, in an X-ray with partially overlapping of the two kidneys, the area of overlap will appear lighter grey than the non-overlapping areas (fig. 1.18). Conversely, if part of the kidney silhouette overlaps a gas-filled segment of the intestines, the area of overlap will appear darker than the rest of the kidney (fig. 1.19).

When two adjacent structures have the same radiographic density, it is impossible to discern the borders

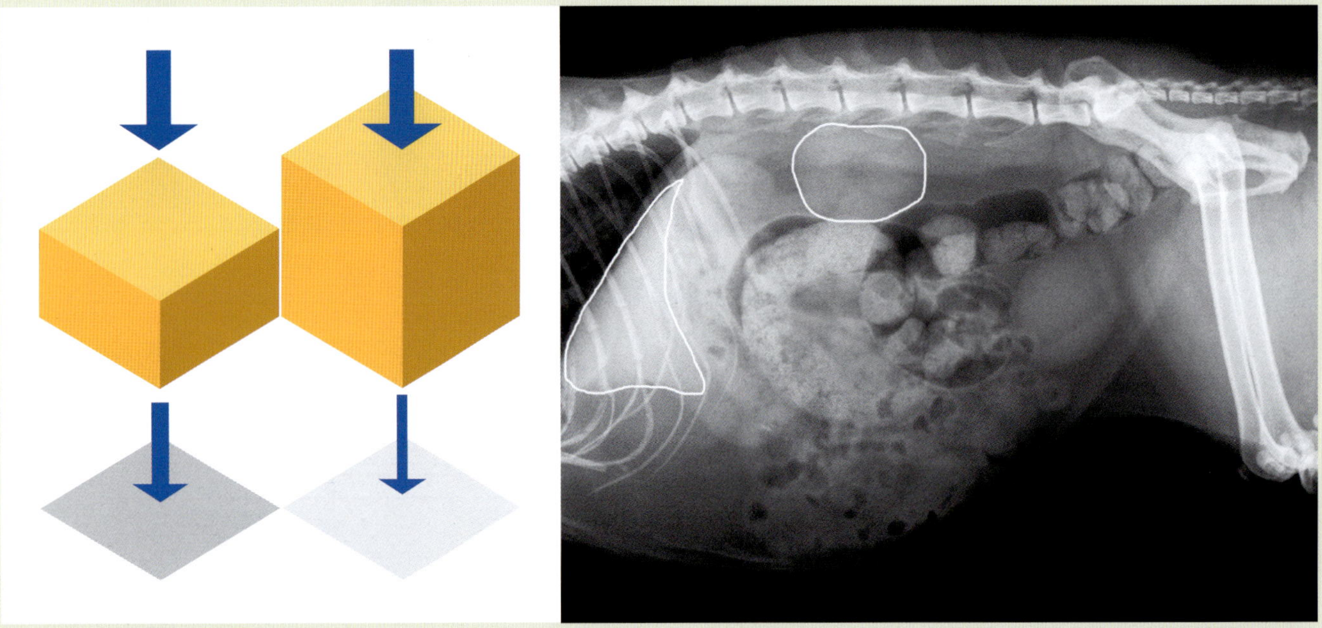

FIGURE 1.16. Schematic diagram of the difference in grey tones of two objects with equal radiographic density but of different thickness (a) and X-ray of a cat's abdomen where the different grey shades of the liver and kidney can be seen, even though both organs have soft tissue density (b).

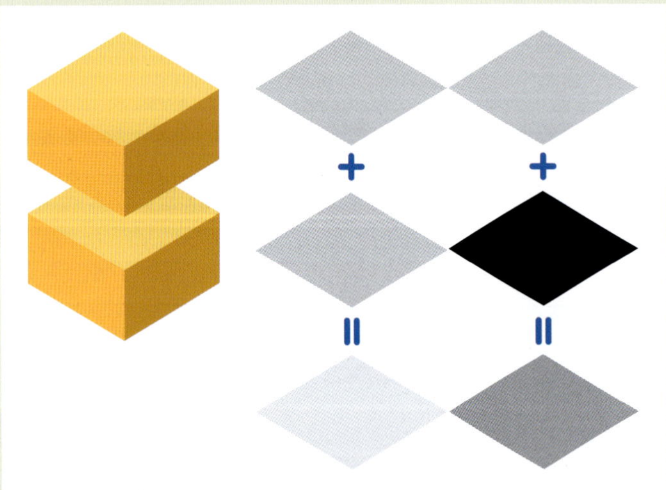

FIGURE 1.17. Schematic diagram of the sum, positive and negative, of the radiographic densities of overlapping silhouettes.

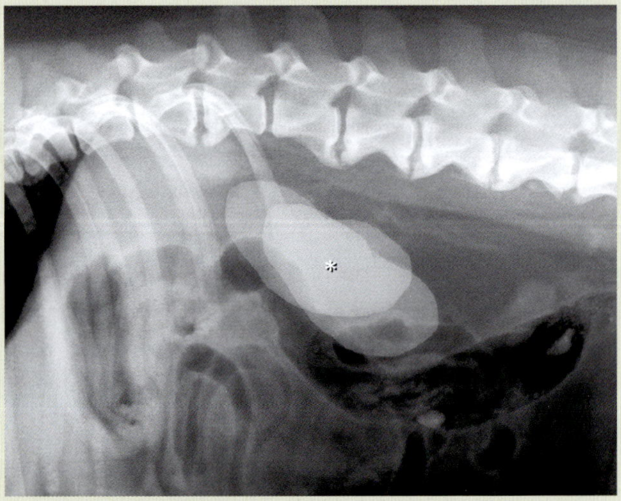

FIGURE 1.18. X-ray of the dorsal and cranial abdomen of a dog showing two semi-transparent silhouettes coinciding with the silhouettes of the kidneys. The overlapping area of both silhouettes (*) appears as a lighter shade of grey due to the "positive" sum of the shades of grey that represent the radiographic densities of both kidneys.

where one structure starts and the other finishes in the contact area. This is known as a **positive silhouette sign**, **silhouette blending** or **edge obliteration sign** (fig. 1.20). Something with a different radiographic density must be placed between adjacent structures with identical radiographic density (e.g. two soft tissues) in order to differentiate between them. Several intra-abdominal structures (liver, spleen, kidneys, bladder, etc.) have a similar soft tissue/water radiographic density. However, radiographers can often partly or fully differentiate between their silhouettes because of the intra-abdominal fat, with its

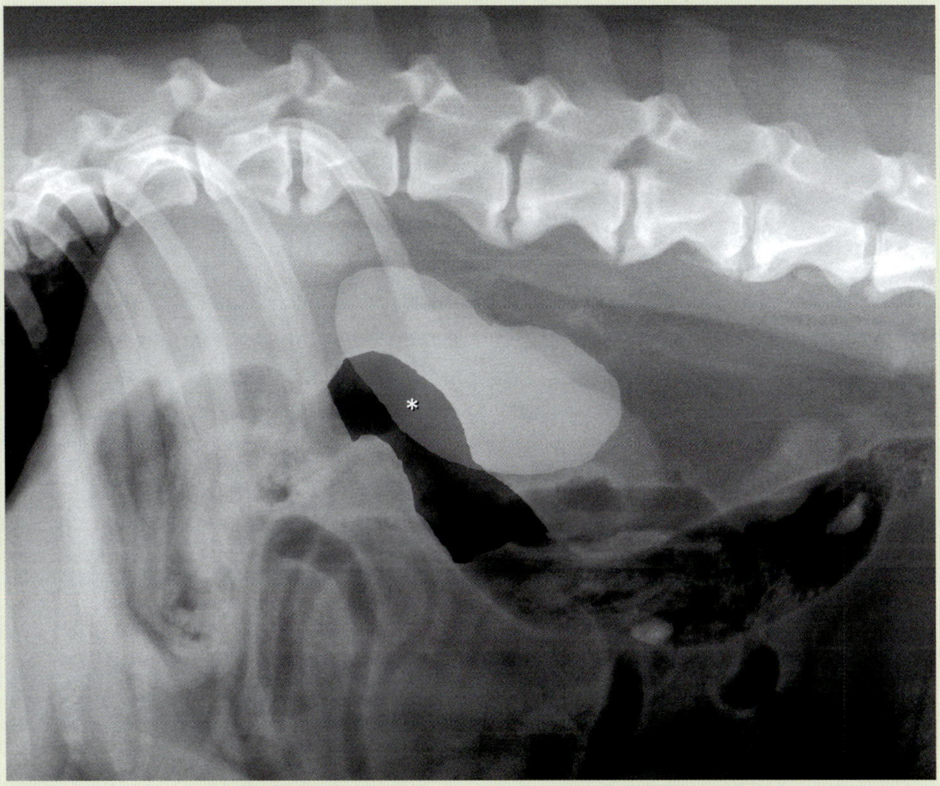

FIGURE 1.19. X-ray of the dorsal and cranial abdomen of a dog showing two semi-transparent silhouettes, one coinciding with the right kidney and the other with a segment of the colon containing gas. The overlapping area of both silhouettes appears as a darker shade of grey than that of the rest of the kidney due to the "negative" sum of the shades of grey representing the radiographic densities of both structures.

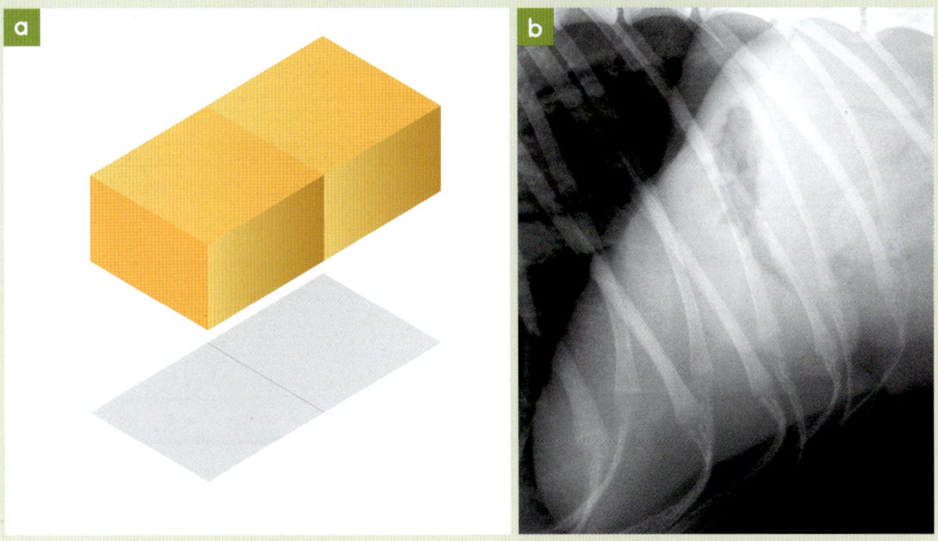

FIGURE 1.20. Schematic diagram of the silhouette sign (also known as silhouette blending or edge obliteration sign) (a): When two adjacent structures have the same radiographic density, distinguishing the contour of one from the other in the area of contact is not possible in an X-ray. X-ray of the cranial abdomen of a dog (b) showing this sign between the silhouettes of the liver and stomach. As the stomach wall and fluid or mucosal contents are of the same radiographic density as the adjacent hepatic parenchyma, it is not possible to distinguish the caudal edge of the liver or cranial edge of the stomach in the image.

lower radiographic density (darker grey) intercalated between them (fig. 1.21).

Similarly, blood vessels in the liver cannot be differentiated from the surrounding parenchyma in X-rays because they share the same radiographic density, whereas pulmonary blood vessels can clearly be distinguished from the adjacent parenchyma which has a very low density because of its high gas content.

The cassette

The radiographic film cassette is a rectangular box designed to hold the X-ray film and protect it from any exposure to light. The front cover of the tube is located in front of the X-ray beam and must be made of a material with a low atomic number, such as aluminium, glass or carbon fibers, to minimise beam attenuation. The cassette's rear cover is lined with lead to absorb as much radiation as possible, and stop X-rays from passing through the cassette and reaching the table, floor, walls, etc., where they could scatter and strike the patient, X-ray film or operator. Cassettes are available in various sizes, the most common are 13 × 18, 18 × 24, 24 × 30, 30 × 40, 35 × 35 and 35 × 43 cm.

Radiographic film

The most used film in non-digital radiography consists of a rigid support, typically of polyester, coated with a photosensitive emulsion, usually on both sides (photographic film is coated on just one side). An adhesive layer is applied between the support and emulsion to prevent the emulsion from peeling. The two emulsion layers are protected from external stresses by a protective coating of pure gelatine. Hence, a double emulsion X-ray film comprises seven layers (fig. 1.22) and its total thickness ranges from 0.2 to 0.3 mm.

As explained in the next section, the X-rays and light emitted from intensifying screens interact directly with the emulsion. It consists of a homogeneous mixture of gelatine and silver halide crystals (generally 98 % silver bromide and 2 % silver iodide). The size and concentration of the silver halide crystals are the main determinants of film speed (or sensitivity) and film contrast.

The silver halide atoms form a crystal lattice. When the radiation reaches the film, it disrupts the crystal lattice and breaks the bonds between the bromine and iodine atoms and the silver atoms. In areas unexposed to the radiation, the crystal lattice remains intact. The silver ions bind with free electrons (released by the interaction with the X-rays) to

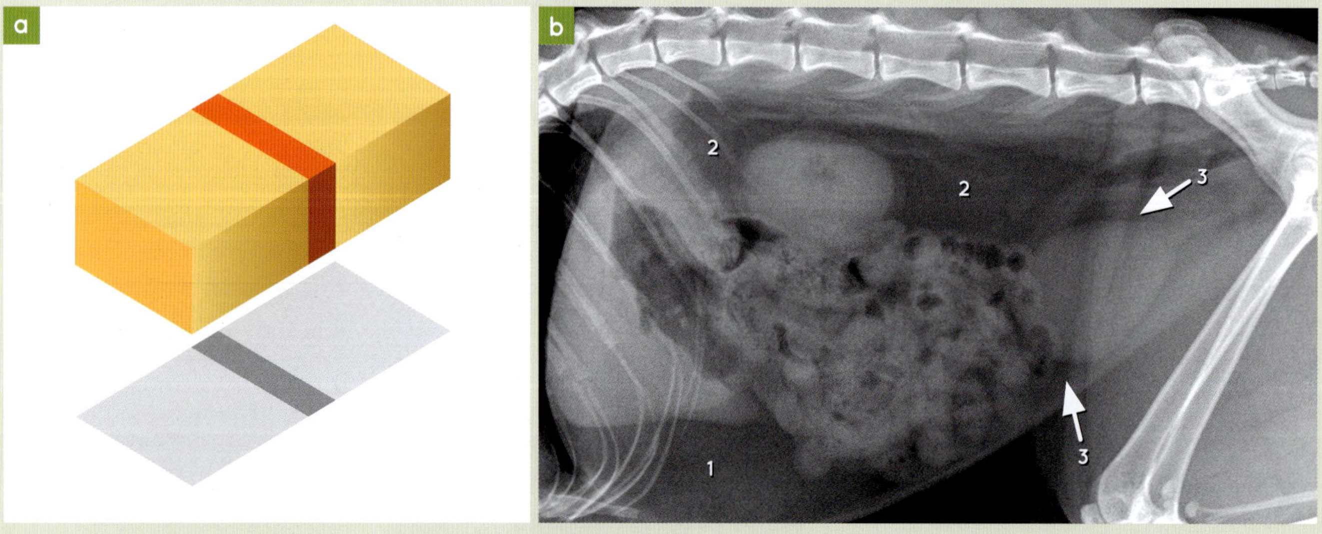

FIGURE 1.21. Schematic diagram of the interposition of an object of lower radiographic density (darker grey) between two objects of equal density, thereby allowing the margins to be differentiated (a). X-ray of the abdomen of a cat (b) with abundant fat ventral to the liver (1), surrounding the kidneys (2) and surrounding the bladder (3), making it easier to identify the margins of these structures, all of which are soft tissue/fluid density.

form silver atoms which are deposited locally. Silver atoms are not visible to the naked eye. Conversely, these silver deposits acquire a black colour during the development process, while the crystals that have not been irradiated retain their crystal lattice structure and remain transparent.

The **contrast** and **sensitivity** of the film depend on the size and distribution of silver halide crystals.

Image intensifying or strengthening screens

Intensifying screens are used in non-digital radiography. They are sheets of luminescent phosphor crystals mounted on a cardboard or plastic base. When the X-rays strike these sheets, the crystals fluoresce, in other words, the crystals convert the X-rays into visible light. For every X-ray photon that strikes a phosphorescent crystal, hundreds of photons of visible light are generated. Radiographic film is more sensitive to light than to X-rays, so the use of intensifying screens greatly reduces the amount of X-rays required to obtain an X-ray image. Approximately 5 % of the density observed in a non-digital radiograph is due to the direct effect of X-rays on film, while 95 % is due to light emitted from the intensifying screen.

Two screens are normally used, attached to the inside of the two cassette covers. When using two screens, each of the emulsions in the film is imprinted by one screen, which produces an image in each emulsion, with the final image being the overlap of both (fig. 1.23).

In general, the larger the phosphorescent crystals, the greater the fluorescent light emission (less X-rays are required), but the radiographic detail of the image is reduced (poorer image quality). With smaller crystals, the image definition is better, but more rays are required. The type of film must be adapted to the type of intensifying screen you are working with.

The drawback of using of intensifying screens is that they provide a lower quality, less sharp radiographic image than if not used. Generally, the reduction in radiation doses compensates for the loss of image quality. However, for special radiological studies in which maximum detail is necessary, radiographs without intensifying screens can be used. This would be the case, for example, of non-digital dental X-rays. These are exposed without screens, with each film wrapped in a paper inside a special plastic cassette with a lead coating on the back. For non-digital mammography, a single high-resolution intensifying screen is used.

FIGURE 1.22. Schematic diagram of an open conventional X-ray cassette, with the X-ray film partially extracted from the inside of the cassette and the different layers into which the film is divided.

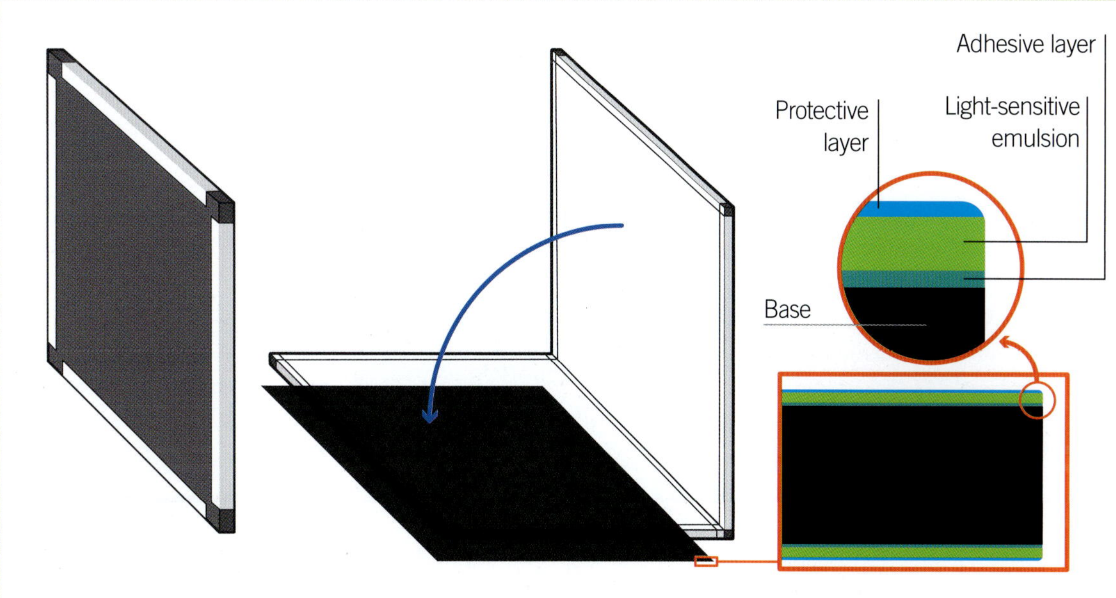

The development process

When X-rays pass through an object or a patient, an emerging beam of rays with different intensities is obtained that create what is called the **X-ray image**. In conventional radiography, when the radiation image interacts with the silver halide crystals in the X-ray film it forms the **latent image**. The development process transforms the latent image into a **visible image**, which can be carried out manually or using an automatic film processor.

The whole development process involves five steps: developing, rinsing, fixing, final washing and drying. Two process uses two different types of chemicals:

- The **developer**, which converts the silver halide crystals exposed to light or X-rays into metallic silver. The metallic silver deposits will appear black on the X-ray. The developer transforms the latent image into a visible image.
- The **fixer**, which converts unexposed silver halide crystals into a soluble compound that can be removed in the subsequent washing step, leaving clear areas on the film.

Film development is time- a temperature-dependent chemical process. The film should remain in contact with the developer for about 5 minutes. The longer the film is in contact with the developer, the darker the image. The film is then rinsed with water to remove any residual developer. The fixing time should be about twice the developing time. Leaving the film in the fixer for longer than necessary does not affect the quality, but the image may look milky if it is removed too soon. The final washing removes any excess chemicals and residual silver halides. If the final washing is not thorough, any residual fixer will react with the silver in the film to form silver sulphide, which causes the film to turn a brownish colour over time. With manual development, the final wash should take about 20 to 30 minutes. Finally, the X-ray can be air dried or placed in a purpose-built dryer.

Vertical trays and tanks are often used for manual development. One tray is needed for the developer, one for the fixer and one or two filled with water for washing. The trays have lids to prevent light (photolysis) and oxygen (oxidation) from deteriorating the developing

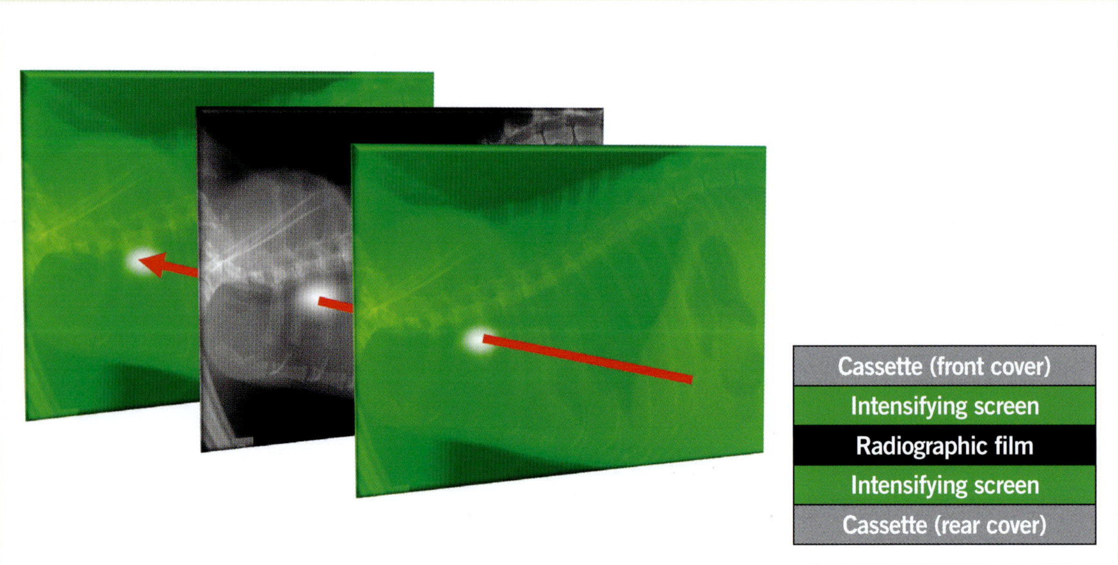

FIGURE 1.23. Schematic diagram of the interposition of the intensifying screens between the X-ray film and the two cassette covers, as well as the phosphorescent light (shown in green) emitted by each of the two screens to imprint the film located between them.

solutions when not in use. Frames or racks are used to hold films while immersing them in the trays.

With automatic processors, the film is developed, fixed, washed and dried inside the machine within an average of approximately 90 seconds. The film travels through the processor via a roller system. When the processor is maintained in perfect working, the development is technically very good.

Since X-ray films are photosensitive, they must be developed in a darkroom (fig. 1.24) and shielded from both light and X-rays from adjacent rooms. The room must be equipped with a darkroom safelight, which can be kept on during development, thanks to a filter system that prevents film fogging.

Negatoscope or X-ray film viewers

This is a box that is illuminated from the aside with one or more fluorescent tubes. The front is covered with an opal glass panel used to illuminate and help examine X-rays. The light should be as homogeneous as possible, although some negatoscopes feature a stronger light source ("warm light") in the centre, with its own switch for a better view of small areas of the image, specially if these have developed darker than expected.

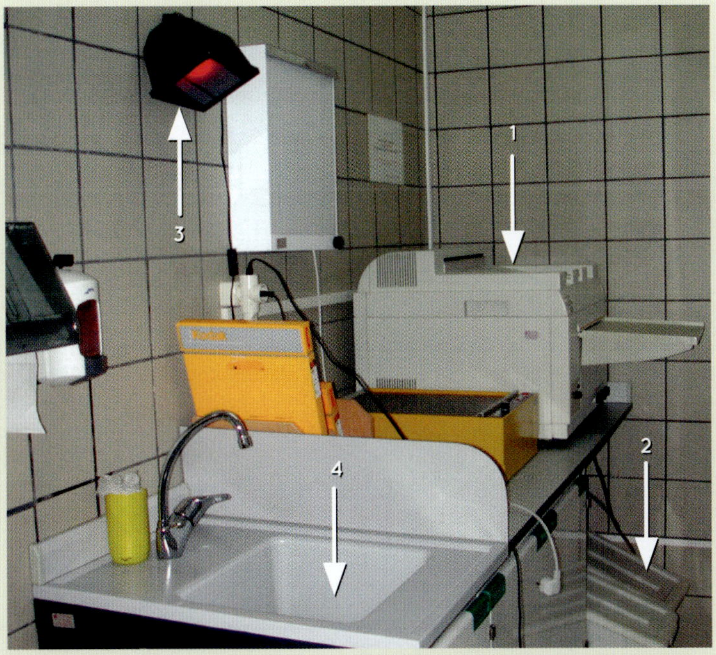

FIGURE 1.24. Darkroom for the developing of conventional radiography. 1: automatic developer; 2: developer solution collection trays; 3: lamp with safety light that can remain on during the developing process; 4: sink.

Digital radiography

Over the past decade, there has been a steady transition from conventional to digital in veterinary medicine. While the acquisition of a digital X-ray system is a relatively expensive investment for a veterinary clinic, the technique offers significant advantages over conventional X-ray systems, including its speed and simplicity in obtaining images of a high diagnostic quality.

Digital X-ray systems

There are two types of digital X-ray systems with very different means of capturing images: computed radiography (CR) and digital radiography (DR). The latter may also be called digital X-rays (DX), although this book uses the term DR. A conventional X-ray tube is still used in both cases, what changes is the way the X-ray image is recorded.

CR systems (fig. 1.25) use **special cassettes** containing a **photostimulable phosphor plates** instead of a conventional radiographic film. When X-ray is taken, the X-rays emerging from the patient print on the phosphor plate creating a latent image. The cassette is then inserted into a **reader**. The reader removes the plate, scans it with a laser beam and sends the information to a **computer**, which displays the X-ray image that has already been converted into a digital file. The average cassette scan time ranges from around 30 to 45 seconds.

DR systems (fig. 1.26) function without neither cassettes nor readers. Instead, DR uses a **detector plate**, which is usually fixed to the X-ray table tray. The plate is connected directly to **a computer**, either by a cable or Wi-Fi. It usually takes just few seconds for the X-ray to be displayed on the screen after it has been taken. Portable detectors, combined with portable X-ray devices, are also available but are mainly reserved for use in equine veterinary medicine.

There are two basic types of detectors in DR systems: the charge-coupled device (**CCD**) and flat-panel detectors (**FPD**).

CCD detectors consist of a scintillation screen that converts X-rays into visible light and a sensor much like those found in modern digital cameras and video recorders. The sensor converts the light into electrical signals and sends them to the computer system. However, the image quality of this technology has been superseded by that of FPD.

There are two classes of FPD, either **direct conversion** or **indirect conversion**. Direct conversion detectors comprise a photoconductor material that converts X-ray photons into electrical signals, and a layer of transistors (thin-film transistors, TFTs) that capture the signals and send them to the computer system. Indirect FPDs contain a layer of scintillator material that converts X-rays into visible light, one of photodiodes that converts light into electrical signals and a layer of TFTs that sends the signals to the computer system.

The photoconductor in direct conversion FPDs is usually made of amorphous selenium. While these detectors offer high-quality images, there can present some disadvantages, such as an image lag due to the persistence of residual electrical charges after reading the image. This issue has largely been resolved in modern machines by incorporating specific charge elimination measures.

Indirect conversion FPDs generally require lower radiation doses while maintaining optimal image quality, which is considered a major advantage in human radiography (the patient's dose may be reduced by as high as much 40 %). This should also considered in veterinary medicine, as besides apart from being beneficial to the animal, in many cases the owner, a technician or the vet must hold the patient. Either caesium iodide (CsI) or gadolinium oxysulfide (oxysulfide) (Gd_2O_2S, also called Gadox or GOS) are generally used as the scintillating material, with the former being more efficient. The photodiode layer is normally amorphous silicon. Most flat-panel systems currently available for use in veterinary medicine are based on indirect conversion with a CsI scintillator.

The consensus is that DR produces higher quality images than CR. However, such a broad statement must be taken with a pinch of salt as it also depends on the technical characteristics of both types of equipment. The latest generation of CR equipment offers extremely high-quality images, equivalent to some DR systems. A good-quality CR system is generally cheaper than an equivalent DR system.

CR and DR systems sold in veterinary medicine must always be adapted and calibrated to optimise

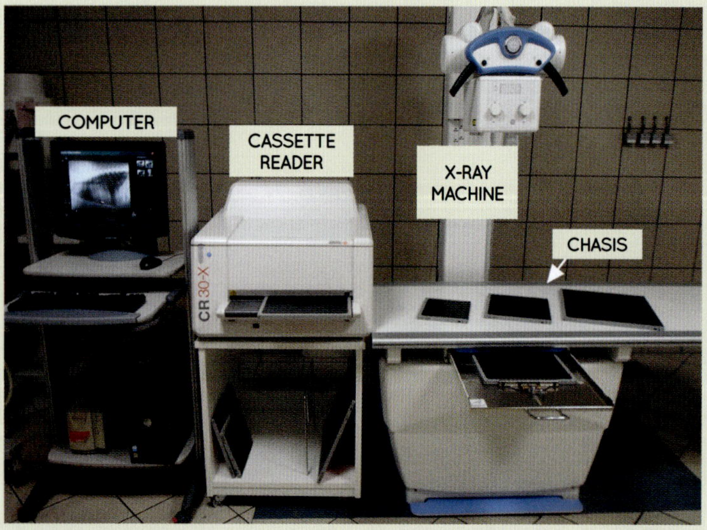

FIGURE 1.25. CR digital radiography system consisting of cassettes containing photostimulable phosphor screens, the cassette reader device and a computer. A standard X-ray machine is used.

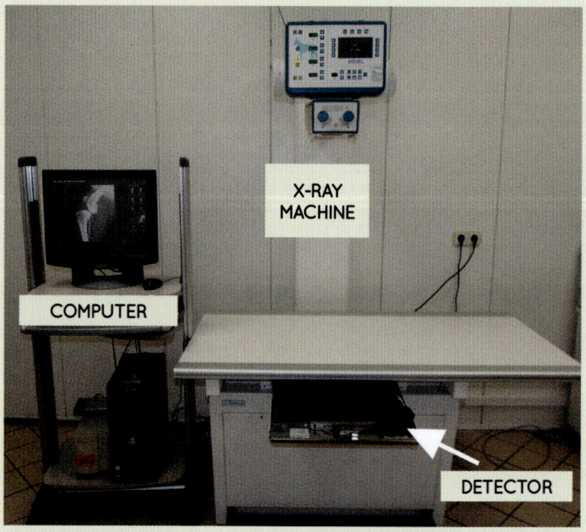

FIGURE 1.26. DR digital radiography system consisting of the detector plate installed on the X-ray system table tray and a computer. A standard X-ray machine is used.

imaging for large and small animals. An X-ray machine intended for use in humans will have different image setting (algorithms), so even if high-performance equipment is used for veterinary purposes but without the relevant modifications, the resulting images may be of unacceptable quality. Calibration for veterinary must be carried out by the manufacturer.

Native data and image algorithms

The data read from the phosphor screens or the electrical signals generated by the detectors are sent to the computer system as raw data which must then be converted into an optimised X-ray image (fig. 1.27). To this end, manufacturers develop algorithms specific to each type of examination, which are classified by anatomical region and projection. These algorithms determine the level of brightness assigned to each pixel in the image based on the radiation received at each point on the phosphor screen or detector, and the contrast ratio between different shades of grey.

Each manufacturer develops specific algorithms specific for their own equipment. The final image quality largely depends on how well these algorithms fit the data for each type of exploration.

DICOM format

The most popular digital image file format used in medical diagnostic imaging is DICOM (Digital Imaging and Communication in Medicine). Files saved in this format retain all the original characteristics of the image at the time it was acquired and include patient demographic information, data of the equipment used, image date and time, etc. (fig. 1.28).

Digital X-ray systems save X-rays in DICOM format but the images can still be exported in more universal formats such as JPEG, TIFF and BMP, although these formats are not recommended for diagnostic purposes because they do not retain the information associated with the imaging study.

Software

Digital X-ray systems include software with basic post-processing tools such as zoom, image displacement, window/level adjustment (equivalent to brightness and contrast), edge enhancement, greyscale inversion, and distance and angle measurements (especially useful for surgical planning in traumatology), among others. Some programs incorporate more specific measurements, such as the Norberg angle, cardiovertebral index or even digital orthopaedic prosthesis templates.

Post-processing tools must be used efficiently, as excessive computer processing can lead to a substantial deterioration in image quality.

Viewing

Monitors used to view digital radiographs must meet some minimal technical specifications in terms of quality. The use of medical diagnostic monitors is mandatory in human radiography. The monitors comply with the DICOM standard, with a minimum resolution of 2 megapixels for general radiography and 5 megapixels for mammography. As they are expensive, the use of cheaper, conventional monitors is common in veterinary medicine, but they must meet the minimum requirements for contrast ratio (at least 1000:1) and luminance (300 cd/m^2) to optimise the X-ray images displayed.

Images can also be printed on film using dry laser imager, but the technique is rarely used in veterinary medicine and on the decline in human radiography its use is in decline. The printed films look very similar to those developed in conventional radiography.

Image archiving and management

The use of digital radiography introduces the need to archive and manage X-rays, once they are converted into computer files. The software on the digital X-ray system's computer can usually store the images on different devices and in different formats, but there is also limited storage capacity and no guarantee of file security.

Specific computer systems, known as picture archiving and communication systems (PACSs,) are used in human radiology to safeguard the security of digital medical images. PACSs are basically medical image archiving and processing systems that enable fast, secure management of each patient's digital images.

PACSs were not widely used in veterinary medicine until a few years ago as they were very expensive when introduced. More affordable systems are now available that can perform the same functions for fewer patients but at a much more affordable price.

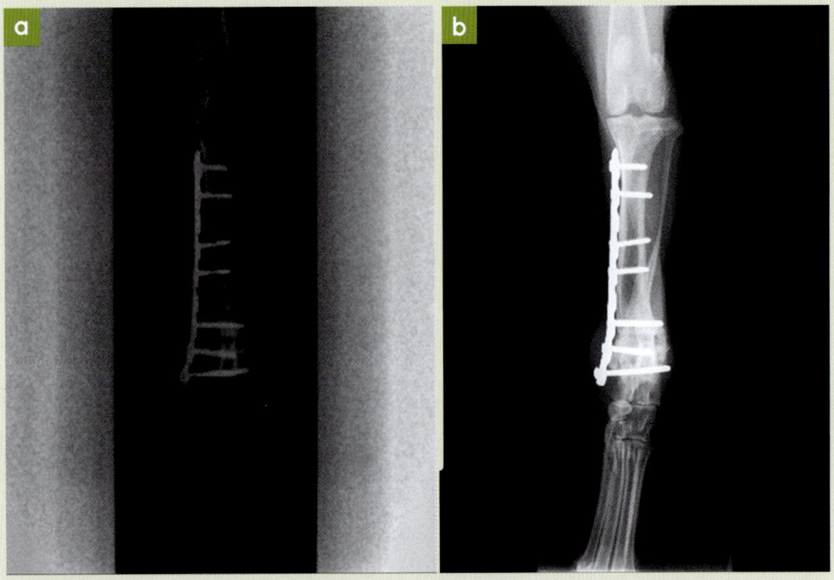

FIGURE 1.27. The raw (native data) image before applying the appropriate image algorithms according to region and projection (a) and final image after applying those algorithms (b).

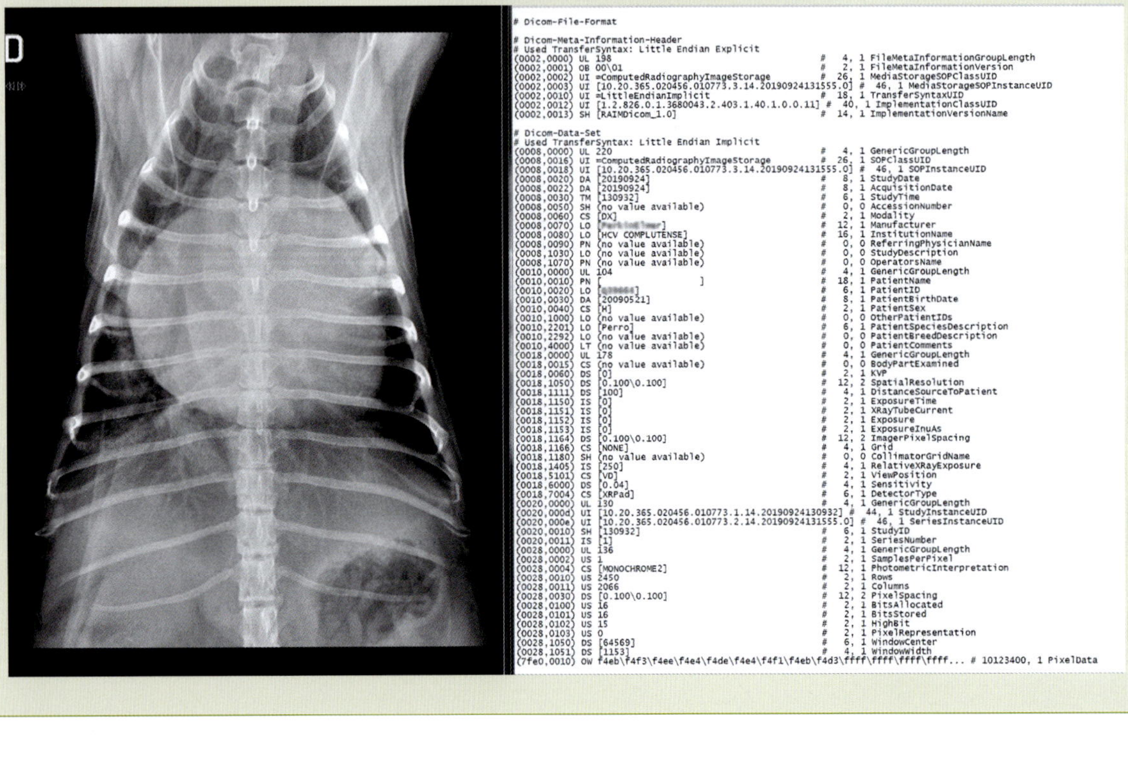

FIGURE 1.28. An X-ray dorsoventral projection of the thorax of a dog with its associated DICOM data.

Technical recommendations in digital radiography

Digital radiography has a much broader dynamic range than that of analogue radiography. In practice, this means that DR produces diagnostic-quality X-rays by working with a much wider range of exposure parameters than in conventional. Consequently, DR greatly reduces the need to repeat X-rays after choosing the incorrect exposure parameters.

Remember that a good X-ray must be centred, collimated and exposed correctly and with the patient positioned correctly. Of all these factors, the shift to digital radiography only improves X-ray exposure.

Proper collimation of the region to be X-rayed has always been an essential technical measure to optimise image quality, while also reducing the patient's exposure to direct radiation and the operator's exposure to scattered radiation. This is particularly important in digital radiography because the algorithms applied to the images are adjusted for each specific anatomical area. For example, when interested in a larger area, the filter enhances the image in the selected region, but it could reduce the image quality for other anatomical areas that are accidently or incorrectly included in the collimation area.

Some early DR systems required higher exposure doses than those used in conventional radiography, although most current DR have now resolved this problem and even operate with lower radiation doses. Some CCDs on the market also require a significant increase in the radiation dose to obtain high-quality images.

Digital radiography image quality

Before delving into digital X-ray image quality, it is important to bear in mind a few concepts regarding spatial resolution and contrast resolution. Spatial resolution is the ability to differentiate small structures in an image (determines the degree of detail), while contrast resolution refers to the ability to distinguish between structures with minimal differences in radiographic density (image intensity).

Two-dimensional digital images are divided into pixels. The set of pixels that make up the image is called a matrix, which is measured by its length and width (in pixels). The smaller the pixel (larger matrix), the higher the spatial resolution of the image. The smaller the pixel (the larger the matrix), the higher the spatial resolution of the image. Spatial resolution is quantified in line pairs per millimetre (lp/mm).

From a theoretical point of view, conventional radiography always achieves better spatial resolution than digital radiography, because at extremely high zooms the pixel margins become visible in digital X-rays, whereas this is impossible with CR. However, as such large magnifications are unnecessary for practical purposes, this defect is imperceptible to the human eye.

DR, on the other hand, offers much better contrast resolution than CR, which means that anatomical structures of very different densities can be viewed properly on the same image. DR's broader dynamic range results in a wider range of greys and therefore both bone and soft tissue can be assessed in a single X-ray. The greater contrast resolution of digital over conventional radiography is particularly evident in chest X-rays.

Lungs are "less black" and healthy large pulmonary vessels and bronchial walls are much clearer in digital X-rays (fig. 1.29). If unaccustomed to assessing digital X-rays, the improved image quality of some structures is sometimes mistaken for certain diseases. Therefore, vets often need to some time to get used to the appearance of healthy animals after acquiring their first digital X-ray system, especially if they previously worked with CR. This is also true when switching from a CR to a DR system given the enhanced spatial and contrast resolution of the latter.

Advantages and disadvantages of digitization

Along with the increased contrast resolution and the ability to enhance images with post-processing, other **important advantages** of digital radiography include:

- Space saving: no longer any need for specially equipped darkrooms nor any need to store patients' X-ray films.
- Cost savings: no X-ray films, automatic developers, trays, developer solutions (which are contaminants and must be collected by specialised companies) are needed.
- Exam speed: in CR systems the cassette scan is usually performed in less than one minute, while with DR, the X-ray image appears on the screen seconds after the X-ray is taken.
- Reduces the need for repeat X-rays due to incorrect choice of exposure values as the range of values at which a quality image is obtained is wider than in conventional radiography. Furthermore, post-processing tools help compensate for incorrect exposures in some cases.
- It is possible to send the X-ray immediately via the Internet to the owner, other veterinarians or remote diagnostic services.
- Many devices allow reduction of exposure doses.

The main **disadvantages** of digital radiography are:

- Initial financial investment: while digital radiography systems can reduce costs (film, solutions, etc.) in the long run, the initial investment is substantial.
- Maintenance costs: this type of equipment requires a specific maintenance service which is provided by the manufacturer. Such contracts can be expensive but are essential after the warranty period has ended.
- Security of the images: digital radiography is converted into a file that is stored on the computer's hard drive. Keeping backups is critical to prevent data loss. However, the most secure system for archiving and managing images is a PACS.
- Improper use of post-processing tools can lead to loss of diagnostic information.

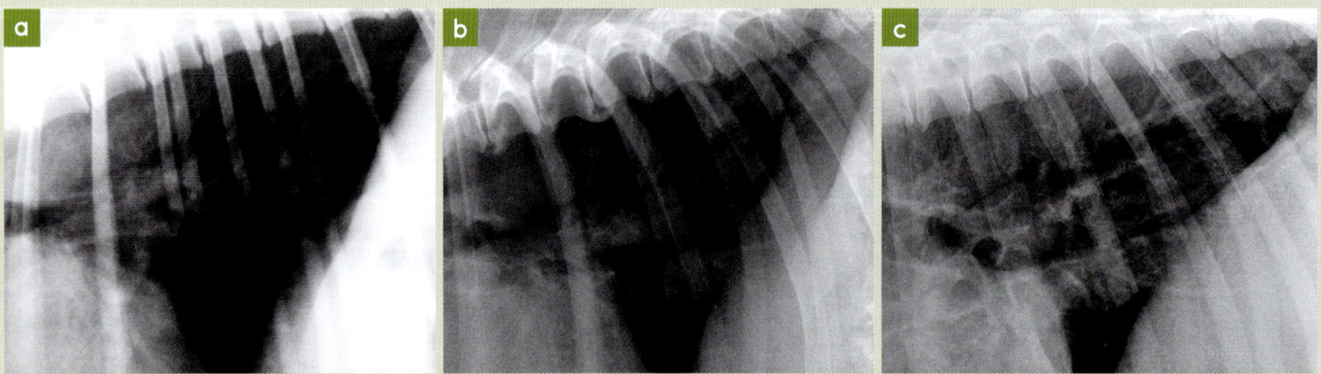

FIGURE 1.29. Radiographs of the dorsocaudal lung obtained with analogue radiology (a), with a CR digital system (b), and with a DR digital system (c) showing substantial improvement in contrast resolution of digital versus analogue radiology, and DR versus CR systems.

Radiation protection

All types of radiation capable of producing ionisation in the matter through which they pass are called **ionising radiations**.

X-rays are a type of ionising radiation.

Ionisation is the process by which an electron is ejected from the atomic or molecular structure to which it belongs. When the electron is "expelled" from the atom, a pair of ions are created: a positive ion from the atom deprived of the electron and a negative ion produced by the expelled electron.

Ionisation is the process that causes biological damage due to radiation. There are two different types of damage:

- Genetic: causing damage to chromosomes or gene mutations in reproductive cells, affecting future generations.
- Somatic: this is evident during the lifetime of the individual (radiation burns, development of tumours, cataracts, etc.).

Radiobiology is the science that studies the phenomena that occur in living organisms after the absorption of energy from ionising radiation.

The biological effects of ionising radiation on living organisms can be classified from various points of view:

1. According to **time of onset**:
   - Early: appearing within minutes to hours of exposure to radiation (e.g. erythema, nausea).
   - Late: appearing months or years after exposure (e.g. radiation-induced cancer, chronic radiation dermatitis, genetic mutations).
2. From **a biological point of view**:
   - Somatic effects: occur only in the person exposed to the ionising radiation.
   - Hereditary effects: these do not manifest in the person exposed to the radiation, but in his or her offspring due to damage to the germ cells of the exposed individual (e.g. genetic mutations).
3. Depending on **the dose:**
   - Stochastic or probabilistic effects: the probability of the effect increasing with the dose received. They are usually late-type effects such as radiation-induced cancer and genetic mutations.
   - Non-stochastic or deterministic effects: these appear almost inevitably when a certain amount of radiation, called threshold doses, is exceeded. These are usually early type effects such as cutaneous erythema.

The characteristics of the biological effects of ionising radiation include:

- Randomness: the interaction of radiation with cells is a probability function and occurs randomly. A photon or particle may reach one cell or another, may or may not damage it and, if so, the damage may be in the nucleus or cytoplasm.
- Fast energy deposition: the energy deposit in the cell occurs extremely rapidly in fractions of a millionth of a second.
- Non-selectivity: radiation shows no predilection for any part or biomolecule, i.e. the interaction is not selective.
- Non-specificity: lesions caused by ionising radiation are always non-specific or, in other words, they could be caused by radiation or some other cause.
- Latency: biological alterations that occur in a cell due to radiation are not immediate but take time to become visible; this is called the "latency period" and it can range from a few minutes to many years, depending on the dose and time of exposure.

Radiation sensitivity or **radiosensitivity** is defined as the sensitivity of cells of different organic tissues to the effects of ionising radiation. Cells undergoing active mitosis (rapidly dividing), that are undifferentiated or have a long future of divisions ahead are more radiosensitive. Based on the radiosensitivity of the cells, the following classification has been established:

- Highly radiosensitive: leukocytes, erythroblasts, spermatogonia.
- Relatively radiosensitive: myelocytes, intestinal crypt cells, basal epidermis cells.
- Intermediate sensitivity: endothelial cells, gastric gland cells, osteoblasts, chondroblasts, spermatocytes, etc.
- Relatively radioresistant: granulocytes, osteocytes, spermatozoa, erythrocytes.
- Very radioresistant: fibrocytes, chondrocytes, muscle and nerve cells.

International Commission on Radiological Protection

The International Commission on Radiological Protection (ICRP) aims to establish a philosophy of radiation protection based on scientific knowledge of the biological effects of ionising radiation. Its findings, which are made known through recommendations, provide advice on the basic principles of radiation protection.

ICRP recommends that all required exposure be kept as low as reasonably achievable (known as the **ALARA Principle**), taking into account both economic and social factors as well as ensuring that the dose received by individuals does not exceed certain established limits.

Legal exposure limits

The **absorbed dose** is the amount of energy deposited by the radiation per unit weight of the biological tissue and is measured in units of gray (Gy). The **equivalent dose** is the radiation dose absorbed by an organ or tissue, weighted according to the type and quality of radiation and measured in sievert units (Sv). The **effective dose** is the weighted sum of the equivalent doses in the various organs and tissues of the body due to internal and external irradiations and is measured in Sv units.

Radiation doses received by persons must not exceed the dose limits established in national regulations, following ICRP recommendations (Table 1.1). In Spain, ICRP recommendations are incorporated into the Regulation on Health Protection against Ionising Radiation (Royal Decree 783/2001 of 6 July 2001). **Occupational exposure** refers to the radiation dose a person may receive for the purpose of his or her professional activity, as opposed to the dose to which the general public is exposed.

Training for exposed workers

Training for staff responsible for running and operating nuclear and radioactive installations is considered an essential element to ensure that these installations are operating under due safety conditions thereby ensuring suitable protection for both workers in the premises and the general public.

Table 1.1. Dose limits for exposed workers and general public recommended by ICRP.

	Occupational exposure	General public
Effective dose	100 mSv/5 years (maximum 50 mSv/year)	1 mSv/year
Equivalent dose, lens of eye	150 mSv/year	15 mSv/year
Equivalent dose, skin and extremities	500 mSv/year	50 mSv/year

In Spain, any person wishing to direct or operate radiation installations for human or animal radiology diagnosis must hold **an accreditation** granted by the Nuclear Safety Council (*Consejo de Seguridad Nuclear* [CSN]). One way to obtain these accreditations to manage or operate an X-ray facility for radiodiagnosis is to take the **training courses** authorised by the CSN. Two types of licenses can be obtained:

- Radiology / diagnostic imaging director.
- Radiology / diagnostic imaging practice operator.

Every X-ray installation must have an accredited director. All personnel working in Radiology Diagnostic Units must participate in ongoing training activities on a regular basis.

Pregnant workers exposed to ionising radiation during the course of their professional activity are a special group, requiring additional radiation protection measures to protect the foetus. In accordance with current legislation, the owner of the radiation installation must ensure, from the moment the worker communicates her pregnancy status, that the dose received by the foetus is no more than 1 mSv. A freely accessible informative leaflet is available on the website of the Nuclear Safety Council: "The radiological protection of pregnant workers exposed to ionizing radiation in the hospital setting".

Classification of work areas

Based on the expected annual doses and the potential exposure risk, the working areas of diagnostic radiology rooms are classified and marked as follows (fig. 1.30):

- Supervised area (indicated with a grey trefoil): there is a possibility of receiving effective doses between 1 and 6 mSv/year or equivalent doses in lens of the eye, skin or extremities between 1/10 and 3/10 of the legally established dose limits.
- Controlled area (indicated with a green trefoil): there is a possibility of receiving effective doses over 6 mSv/year or equivalent doses in lens of the eye, skin or extremities over 3/10 the legally established dose limits.
- Limited stay area (indicated with a yellow trefoil): there is a risk of receiving a dose over long periods of time that exceeds the legally established dose limits.
- Regulated stay area (indicated with an orange trefoil): there is a risk of receiving in short periods of time a dose higher than the legally established dose limits.
- Prohibited access area (indicated with a red trefoil): there is a risk of receiving, in a single exposure, a dose higher than the legally established dose limits.

Staff dosimetric control

Dosimeters are used for the dosimetric control of personnel. They measure the cumulative dose for each individual person. In Spain, dosimeters must be read, calibrated and controlled by a centre duly authorised by the Nuclear Safety Council. Each staff member receives a monthly dosimetric report and must pass an annual medical examination.

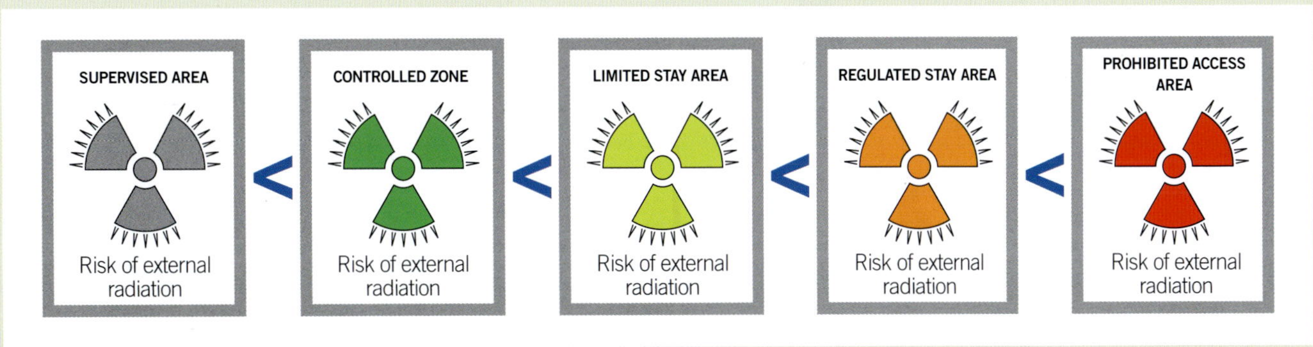

FIGURE 1.30. Marking of work areas according to expected annual doses and potential exposure risk.

General principles to limit radiation exposure

The three general principles to be followed to limit the X-ray exposure are (fig. 1.31):

1. Time: the shorter the exposure time, the lower the dose received.
2. Shielding (lead, concrete): the thicker the shield, the lower the dose received. Depending on the energy and type of radiation, different shielding materials and thicknesses may be desirable.
3. Distance: the greater the distance to the radiation-emitting focus, the lower the dose received. The relationship between distance and exposure is inversely proportional to the square of the distance.

Radiation protection systems

Patient and operator exposure is minimised by applying all available protective measures. The basic protection systems are:

1. **Filtration:** filters (usually aluminium or copper) are fitted to the aperture of the lead housing of the X-ray tube and absorb low-energy X-rays (if they reached the patient they would be absorbed and not reach the film, so they have no diagnostic value).
2. **Collimation:** by reducing the beam size to the absolute minimum needed, we minimise both main radiation and scatter radiation (radiation that is deflected upon reaching the patient).
3. **Image intensification:** in conventional film-screen systems, the intensifying screen allows greatly reduced exposure doses.
4. **Protective clothing:** apron, thyroid collar, gloves and goggles made of lead impregnated materials (fig. 1.32).
5. **Protective barriers:** the X-ray control panel must be located behind a protective barrier, which can be either a lead wall with a lead glass window (fig. 1.33), or a specially designed lead partition (fig. 1.34).

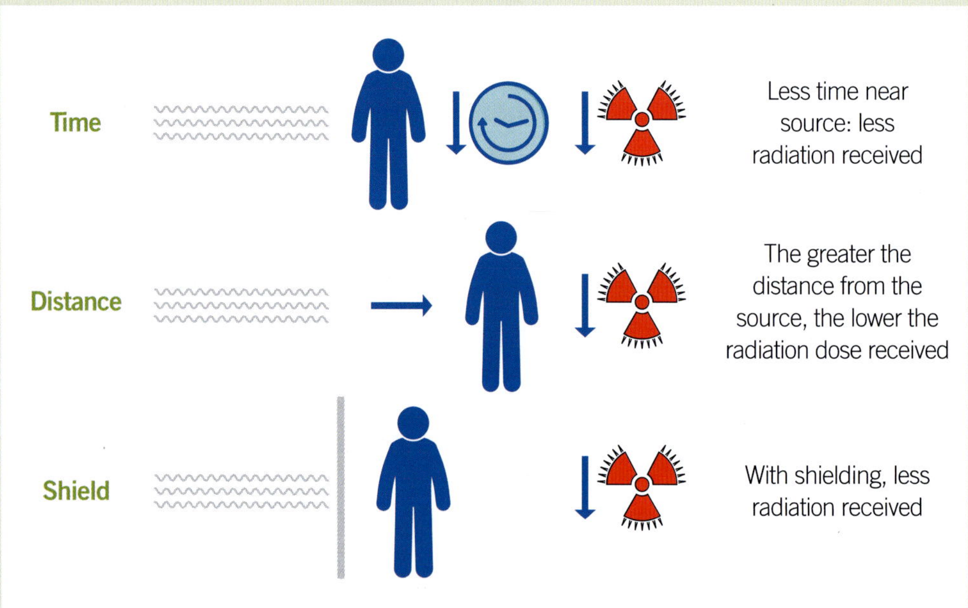

FIGURE 1.31. Schematic diagram of the three basic principles to be followed to limit X-ray exposure: time, distance and shielding.

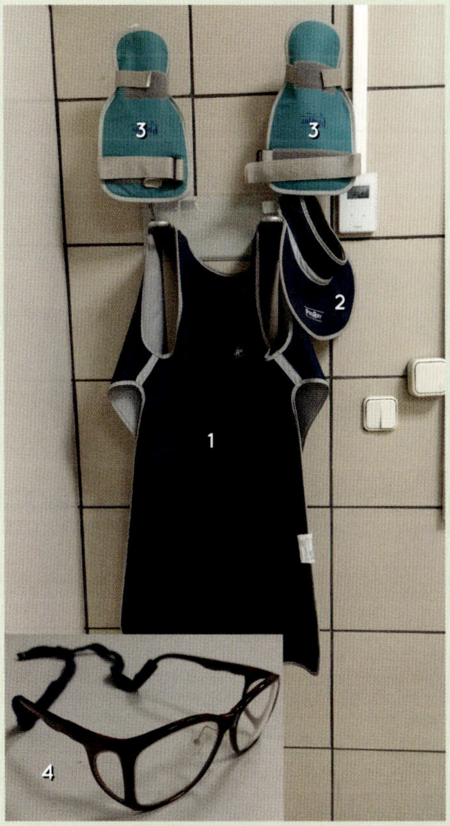

FIGURE 1.32. Radiation protective equipment made from lead impregnated materials.
1: apron; 2: protective thyroid collar;
3: gloves; 4: glasses.

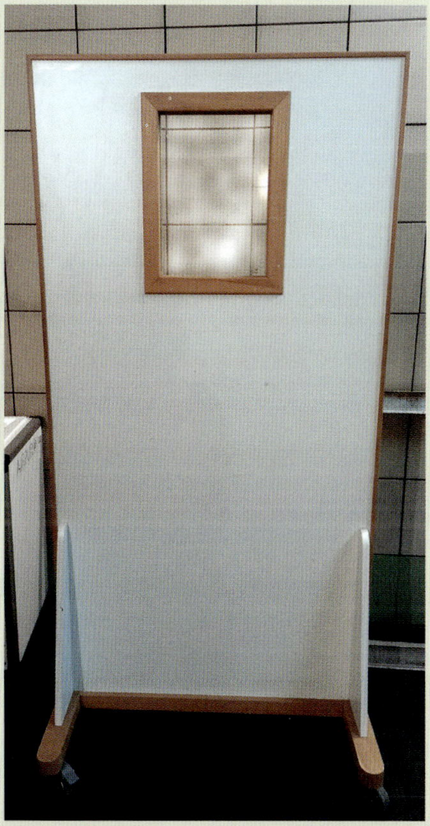

FIGURE 1.34. Radiation shielding partition with small leaded glass window.

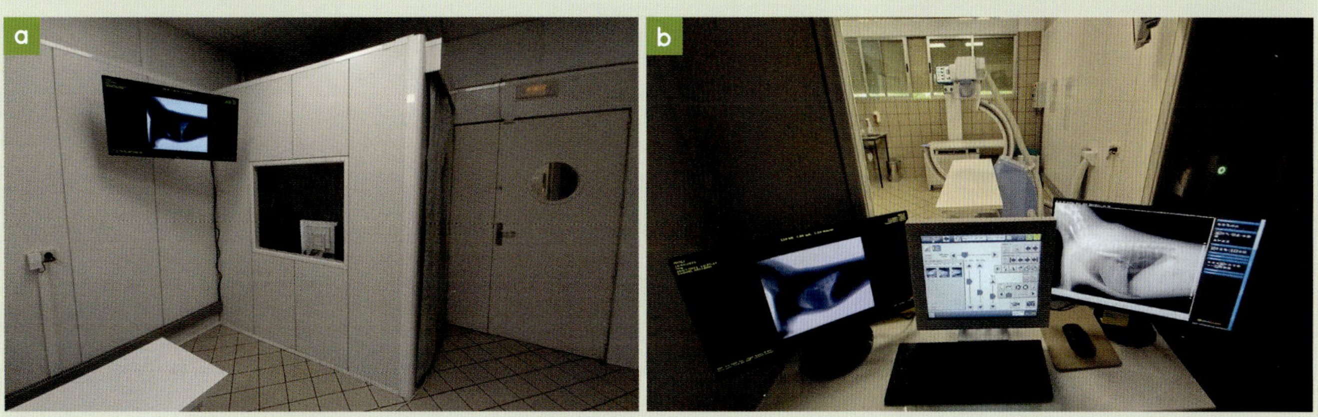

FIGURE 1.33. Enclosure with lead-lined walls, ceiling and glass window (a) and control panel with computer screens inside the cabinet (b) where the operator can operate them avoiding exposure to X-rays.

Critical recommendations for radiology diagnostic facilities

1. Understand and apply the three basic principles of radiation monitoring: Time (minimise), distance (maximise) and shielding.
2. Avoid all exposure to the primary beam.
3. Always wear lead protection equipment (apron, collar, glasses and gloves) if not behind a protective barrier (leaded glass, partition or wall).
4. Always wear a dosimeter and place it **under** the apron.
5. Always collimate to the smallest possible field size.
6. Do not hold the patient personally unless absolutely essential. Use mechanical restraining whenever possible (fig. 1.35). In human radiology, family members are asked to hold patients who are unable to remain still during the radiological examination (young children, the elderly, etc.). The equivalent of this in veterinary medicine would be to ask the owner to hold the animal during examination when it is not feasible to use mechanical restraint.
7. The person holding the patient (including family members or carers) must always wear lead protection equipment as listed in point 3.
8. Pregnant women should never remain in the room during the X-ray examination (except if she is the patient and the examination is considered essential).

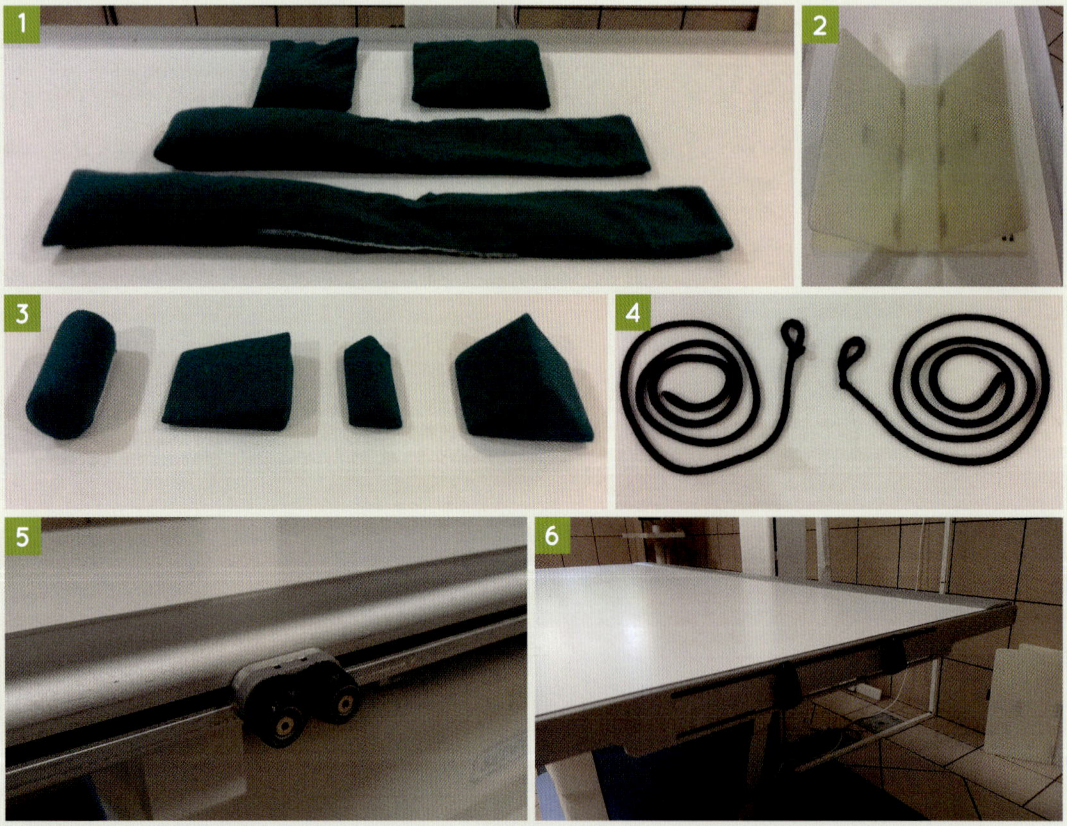

FIGURE 1.35. Mechanical restraint materials. 1: sandbags; 2: rigid positioner; 3: set of radiolucent foam-rubber wedges of various shapes and sizes; 4: straps; 5 and 6: different types of sliding winders attached to the edge of the table.

General principles of X-ray interpretation

The location and **conditions of viewing** X-rays are important to ensure correct evaluation and interpretation. It is, therefore, recommended that X-rays be always examined in a quiet room that is as dark as possible. This is because in dark or dimly lit rooms we can better appreciate the different shades of grey in the image, whether we are viewing the X-ray film on the light box or on our screen in the case of digital radiography. It is also important to examine the image when we have enough time to do so carefully. Haste often leads to misdiagnoses as enough attention is not paid to the finer detail of the image.

We can use a magnifying glass to see finer details in a conventional X-ray. While in the case of digital radiography, post-processing programs include specific tools for general or focal image magnification. However, if we overuse these tools, we may lose some of the overall information provided by a radiographic image.

For conventional X-rays, a strong focal light (e.g. a halogen bulb) could be used to examine areas that appear very dark, bringing the X-ray film close to the bulb but without contact as the heat would damage the film. The region of interest can be more clearly observed with the more intense light focus. This is attained in digital radiography by increasing the brightness of the image with the post-processing program.

Other **computer post-processing tools** that help improve the examination of a digital radiograph are the navigation tool, edge enhancement, measurement tools, etc. Grey inversion can help identify small lung or bone injuries. However, remember that excessive use of post-processing tools can erode the image quality and lead to diagnostic errors.

Standardised criteria are used for the orientation of X-rays when examining them, whether on a view box or computer screen, since consistently viewing them in the same way makes them easier to interpret. These criteria are:

- The right side of the animal is placed to the observer's left.
- The cranial, rostral or proximal part of the animal is placed at the top of the view box or screen, and the caudal or distal part at the bottom.

Incorrect **positioning** of the patient is one of the main sources of diagnostic errors. Patient sedation and the use of mechanical immobilisation devices (sandbags, radiolucent positioners, straps, adhesive tape) facilitate correct positioning which has a major influence on the interpretation of the images.

Other **technical defects** such as overexposure or underexposure also affect X-ray interpretation. We should be familiar with these influences to avoid confusing them with pathologies.

Failure to perform a sufficient number of **radiographic projections** is also another common source of diagnostic error. It is advisable to always obtain at least two orthogonal projections, as this makes it easier to get a three-dimensional idea of the radiographed area and provides additional information. A pleural and mediastinal effusion, for example, may appear as a very similar image in the lateral projection, but they are completely different in a dorsoventral or ventrodorsal view of the thorax.

A clear **understanding of patient anatomy** is essential for correct image interpretation. For this, having reference books on anatomy and radiographic anatomy is often extremely useful. In some cases, the patient itself may serve as a reference for normal anatomy. For example, in patients with an injury on one limb, X-raying both the injured and uninjured limb allows comparisons and aids correct interpretation. It is also important to understand how normal anatomy varies with age, race, etc., so as not to confuse these with pathologies.

The **overlapping of structures** on radiographic images can, on the one hand, lead to the loss of diagnostic information and, on the other, create overlapping silhouettes that can resemble pathological images. This negative effect of overlapping structures may be even more accentuated in digital radiography.

For the correct interpretation of the image, it is essential **to always correlate information with the patient's clinical data**. It is also important **to correlate all findings that appear in the image**. Thus, for example, if we observe signs of megaesophagus and also an alveolar pattern in the cranioventral area of the lung, this latter finding may be due to aspiration pneumonia and not to pulmonary oedema or haemorrhage, which can also cause alveolar patterns.

A systematic viewing order is recommended to fully examine the image. The image should be reviewed from the outside in, from the peripheral to the centre of the image, as we tend to focus our attention on the central area often overlooking details in the peripheral parts. We sometimes sit in front of an image and believe that we see everything in it without paying attention to every detail, less obvious findings can be overlooked.

In radiography, the following principle can be applied: **"to see you have to look, and you have to know"**. In other words, it is not enough just to look closely at the X-ray films. We have to be able to understand what we see and interpret it correctly and this requires a thorough understanding of the radiographic signs specific to each disease.

Radiographic technique

Radiograph identification

The information on each film should include at least the animal's identity (e.g., medical record number) and the date the X-ray was taken. Other information such as the patient's name, the owner's name, the veterinarian's name, the radiographic projection, the age, sex and race of the animal, etc. may be included.

In conventional radiography, a method should be used that allows permanent and unalterable identification of X-ray films, otherwise they cannot be used as legal evidence. Lead markers (letters or templates which can be written on) are often used that are stuck to the cassette prior to exposure. Alternatively, light markers are used post exposure in the darkroom before processing. In digital radiography, the DICOM format includes all patient data that has been entered into the computer system.

X-ray image quality

When performing radiography, the technique needs to be duly adjusted to attain high quality images that can be properly evaluated and interpreted.

The term radiographic quality refers to the ease with which details can be perceived on a radiographic image.

Radiographic quality depends directly on radiographic density, radiographic contrast and a number of geometric factors that affect the image detail. Other factors also affecting image quality include scatter radiation, patient position and the appearance of technical artifacts and errors on the radiograph.

Radiographic density and contrast

Radiographic density refers to the degree of blackness on a film and is directly proportional to the amount of radiation reaching the film.

Radiographic contrast refers to the density difference between two adjacent areas on a radiograph. If the density difference is great, the image is said to have high contrast (exhibits many blacks and white tones with few in between grey tones), while if the density differences are less marked (many shades of grey), the image is said to have low contrast.

Both density and contrast are highly dependent on the selected exposure values (milliamperage, kilovoltage and time), but many other factors may also come into play, such as the type of screen/film system or conventional X-ray development, the type of digital system, the characteristics of the X-ray tube, etc. It is, therefore, not possible to provide universal exposure value tables that are suitable for all X-ray machines and all patients. These tables must be devised by each operator working with a specific machine, with a particular type of film, screen or digital detection system and depending on the type of patients he or she works with. Many modern X-ray machines are already available with these tables adapted for veterinary use. With daily practice on the machine and with real patients, the operator can fine tune the values given by the manufacturer, but as an initial guide they are generally quite useful. Table 1.2 shows the optimised exposure parameters for a given X-ray machine with a 125 kV/400 mA tube and a CR digital system, while Table 1.3 shows the optimised parameters for a specific 150 kV/500 mA tube X-ray equipment and a specific DR system. These tables can serve as a rough reference for the reader, but they are not directly applicable to any X-ray machine or any CR or DR digital radiography system. In general, DR systems require lower mAs and higher kV parameters.

Image geometry

The X-rays making up the beam emitted from the tube are not parallel but form a diverging beam. For this reason, radiographic images always have some degree of **distortion** (deformation) and **magnification** (larger than the real object). The higher the distortion, the lower the sharpness and detail in the image.

Some of the geometric factors that influence image quality are:

- **Focal spot size:** the smaller the focal spot size, the greater the sharpness and detail of the image (fig. 1.36).
- Distance from focal spot to object (**focus-to-object distance**): the greater the distance between the focal spot and the object, the lower the magnification and the greater the sharpness and detail of the image (fig. 1.37). This distance is usually around 90 to 100 cm for most veterinary X-ray machines.
- Distance from the object to the film* (**object-film distance**): the closer the object is to the film, the lower the distortion and magnification of the image and, therefore, the greater the sharpness and detail (fig. 1.38).
- **Alignment:** the sharpest part of an X-ray image will always be the area aligned with the central beam of the X-ray, where the rays are almost perpendicular to the film. In peripheral areas, the rays have some degree of obliquity, causing image distortion or deformation (fig. 1.39).
- Distortion will also occur when:
  - The central ray is not aligned with the object.
  - The central ray does not form a right angle with the object or the cassette/detector.
  - The central ray does not form a right angle with the cassette/detector, even if it does form a right angle with the object.
  - The object is not parallel to the cassette/detector.

Scatter or diffuse radiation

Scatter or diffuse radiation occurs when X-rays that change direction upon interaction with the object or patient. They are detriment to both operators in the room and image quality (fig. 1.40).

Scatter radiation originates initially in the patient but when it comes in contact with other objects such as the table, floor or walls, it can deflect again (fig. 1.41). Aprons, goggles, thyroid protectors and lead gloves protect the operator from this radiation which is unavoidable. It can, however, be minimised by collimation, i.e. adjusting as much as possible the size of the X-ray beam to what is strictly necessary (the smaller the beam, the lower the number of rays deflected).

Lead accessories protect operators from scatter radiation, but operators must also protect themselves from direct radiation (X-rays coming directly from the tube) by never exposing any part of their body to it. In veterinary radiographs, it is common to see the hands of the operator or animal owner holding the animal, even without lead gloves. While gloves can absorb scattered radiation, they do not absorb the most energetic X-rays in the beam. Therefore, with or without gloves, if we place our hands under the beam, we are exposing ourselves directly to the harmful action of X-rays.

* Film in conventional radiography and screen/detector panel in digital radiography.

Table 1.2. Exposure parameters used with a specific X-ray machine, 125 kV and 400 mA, and CR digital radiography system.

Region		Projection	Cat Small dog kV	Cat Small dog mAs	Medium dog kV	Medium dog mAs	Big dog kV	Big dog mAs	Giant breed dog kV	Giant breed dog mAs
Thorax		Lateral	55	10	57	12	58	16	60	20
		VD/DV	55	10	57	16	60	20	65	25
Abdomen		Lateral	55	12	57	16	58	20	60	25
		VD/DV	55	12	57	16-20	60	25	65	32
Spine	Cervical	Lateral	55	10	58	12	60	16	63	20
		VD/DV	55	10	58	12	60	16	63	20
	Chest	Lateral	55	12	58	16	60	20	63	25
		VD/DV	55	12	58	16	62	25	65	32
	Lumbar	Lateral	55	12	58	16	60	20	63	25
		VD/DV	55	12	58	16	62	25	65	32
Head		VD open-mouth	55	8	55	10	58	16	58	16
		Oblique lateral	55	8	57	12	60	16	60	20
		Rostrocaudal tangential	55	10	57	12	62	20	62	20
		DV/VD occlusal*	48	3.2	48	3.2	50	4	52	4
Thoracic limb	Shoulder	Mediolateral	52	8	56	10	58	16	63	20
		Caudocranial	52	8	58	12	60	16	65	25
	Elbow*	Mediolateral	43	3.2	45	3.2	46	4	48	5
		Craniocaudal	43	3.2	45	3.2	48	4	50	5
	Carpus/metacarpus*	Mediolateral	43	3.2	45	3.2	46	4	48	4
		Craniocaudal	43	3.2	45	3.2	46	4	48	4
Pelvic limb	Hip	Lateral	55	10	58	16	60	20	65	25
		VD	55	10	58	16	60	20	65	25
	Knee*	Mediolateral	43	3.2	45	3.2	48	4	50	5
		Craniocaudal	43	3.2	45	3.2	46	4	48	5
	Tarsus/metatarsus*	Mediolateral	43	3.2	45	3.2	46	4	48	4
		Craniocaudal	43	3.2	45	3.2	46	4	48	4

* Values for direct radiographs (placing the CR cassette on the X-ray table).

Table 1.3. Exposure parameters used with a specific X-ray machine, 150 kV and 500 mA, and a DR digital radiography system.

Region		Projection	Cat Dwarf dog kV	Cat Dwarf dog mAs	Small dog kV	Small dog mAs	Medium dog kV	Medium dog mAs	Big dog kV	Big dog mAs
Thorax		Lateral	55	3.2	60	5.0	65	5.0/6.4	80	10/12
		VD/DV	52	3.2	55/60	4.5	60	5.0	75	8.0/10
Abdomen		Lateral	60	5.0	65	6.4	70	8.0	85	16
		VD/DV	55	4.5	60	5.0	65	6.4	80	12
Spine	Cervical	Lateral	58	5.0	60	5.0	70	6.4	75	8.0/10
		VD/DV	55	4.5	60	5.0	65	5.0	70	6.4/8.0
	Chest	Lateral	60	5.0	70	6.4	80	10/12	85	12/16
		VD/DV	60	5.0	65	6.4	75	8.0	80	12/16
	Lumbar	Lateral	60	5.0	70	6.4	80	10/12	85	12/16
		VD/DV	60	5.0	65	6.4	75	8.0	80	12/16
Head		Lateral	55	4.5	60	5.0	65	5.0	70	8.0
		VD/DV	55	4.5	60	5.0	65	5.0	70	8.0
		Oblique	55	4.5	60	5.0	65	5.0	70	8.0
Thoracic limb	Shoulder	Mediolateral	53	3.2	55	4.0	58	5.0	60/65	6.3/8.0
		Caudocranial	55	3.2	57	4.0	60	5.0/6.3	65/70	8/10
	Elbow	Mediolateral	45	2.0	48	2.0	5.0	3.2	53	4.0
		Craniocaudal	45	2.0	48	2.0	5.0	3.2	53	4.0
	Carpus/metacarpus	Mediolateral	45	2.0	48	2.0	5.0	3.2	53	4.0
		Craniocaudal	45	2.0	48	2.0	5.0	3.2	53	4.0
Pelvic limb	Hip	Lateral	60	5.0	70	6.4	75	8.0	80	12/16
		VD	60	5.0	65	6.4	80	10/12	85	12/16
	Knee	Mediolateral	45	2.0	48	2.0	5.0	3.2	53	4.0
		Caudocranial	45	2.0	48	2.0	5.0	3.2	53	4.0
	Tarsus/metatarsus	Mediolateral	45	2.0	48	2.0	5.0	3.2	53	4.0
		Craniocaudal	45	2.0	48	2.0	5.0	3.2	53	4.0

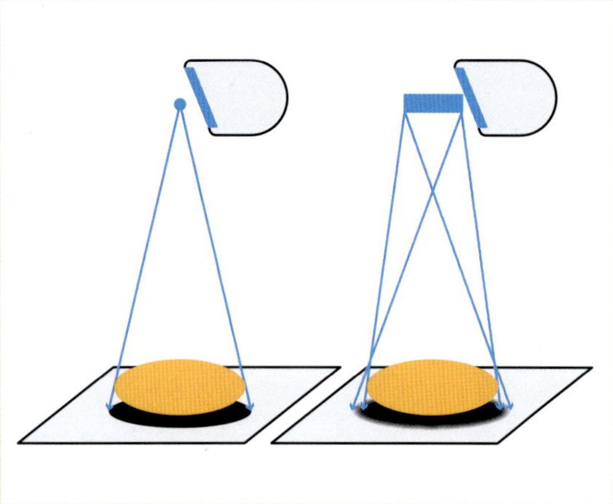

FIGURE 1.36. Schematic diagram of the effect of the focal spot size on image sharpness.

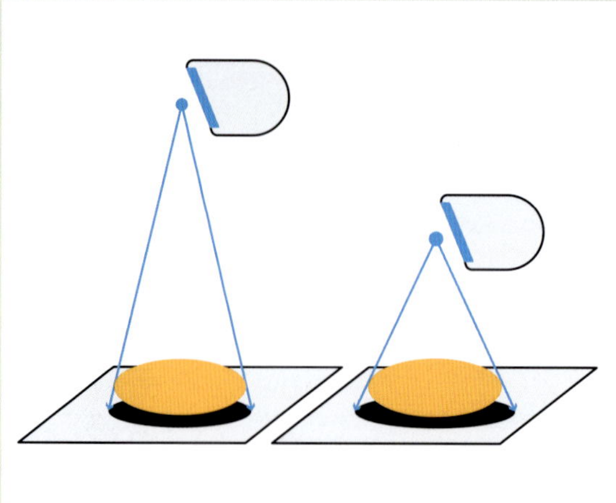

FIGURE 1.37. Schematic diagram of the effect of the focus-object distance on the degree of image magnification.

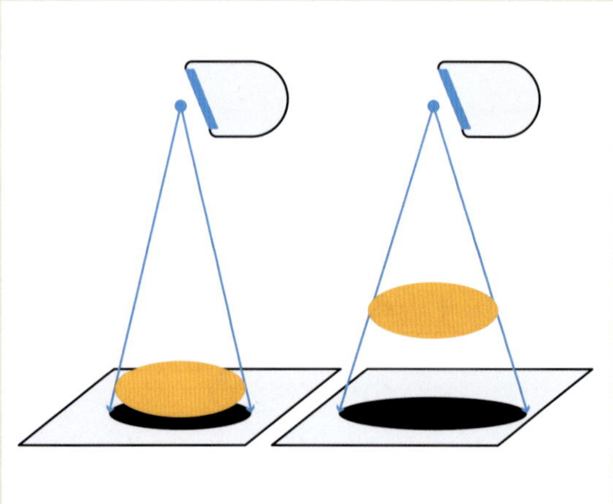

FIGURE 1.38. Schematic diagram of the effect of the object-to-film distance on the degree of image magnification.

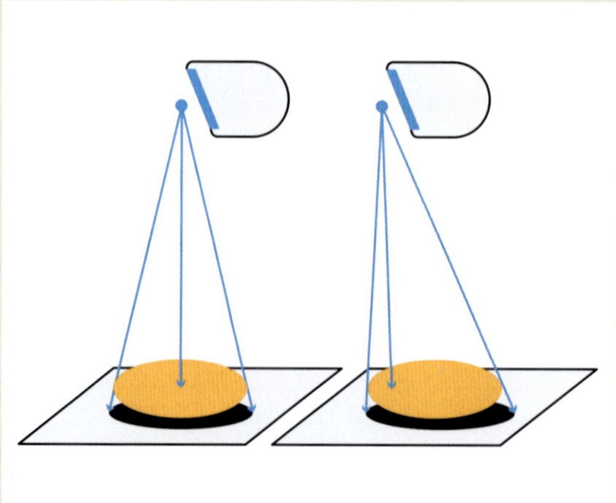

FIGURE 1.39. Schematic diagram of the effect of the alignment of the beam centre with the object on the degree of distortion or deformation in the image.

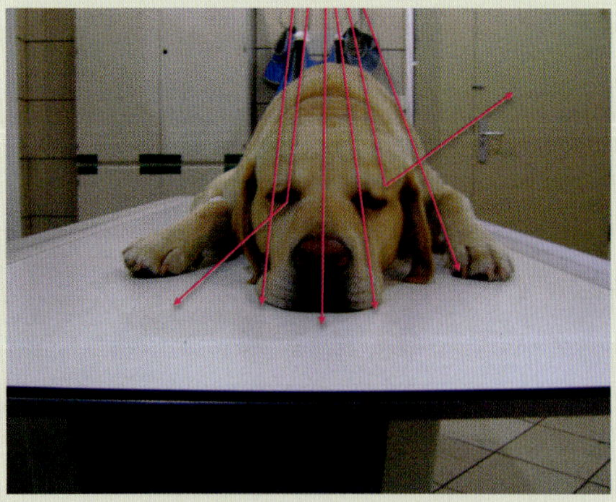

FIGURE 1.40. Scatter radiation represented by arrows that deflect from their original path as they pass through the patient.

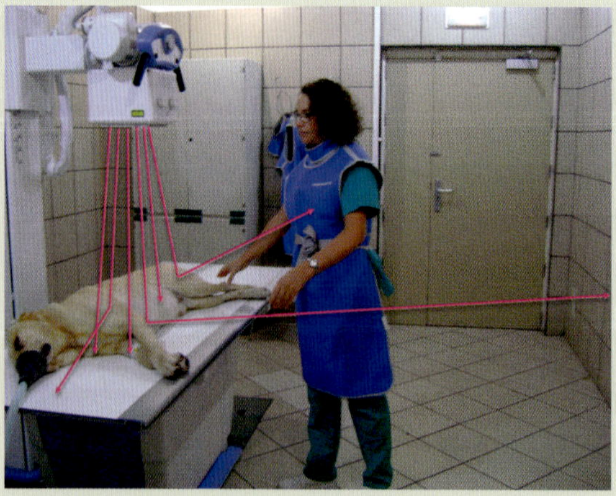

FIGURE 1.41. Scatter radiation (arrows) deflected from their original path as they pass through the patient impacting the X-ray table, operator, walls, etc.

Scatter radiation is also detrimental to image quality as these deflected rays can reach the X-ray film in inappropriate areas resulting in the blurring of the image. The amount of scatter radiation reaching the film can be reduced by using what are called **anti-scatter grids** (fig. 1.42). These are inserted between the patient and the cassette/detector and are intended to absorb a large portion of the scatter radiation heading toward the film. They consist of a large number of lead strips (500 to 1,500) of approximately 0.5 mm thickness arranged next to each other in the same direction, completely parallel (parallel grids) or at different angles of obliquity (focused grids). A radiolucent material is interlaid between these strips. Lead sheets absorb much of the scatter radiation, that is, the radiation deflected from its initial path, while the radiolucent material allows most useful rays to pass through. The strips and radiolucent material are protected by a cover of radiolucent material, usually aluminium.

Using anti-scatter grids helps diminish the influence of scatter radiation on the image by up to 80–90 %. However, the drawback is that they also absorb some of the useful radiation. So when using a grid, the number of rays to be emitted has to be increased, i.e. the mAs value. They are not always used for this reason. In small anatomical regions, the amount of scatter radiation generated is relatively small, so it is not worth using the grid and having to increase the dose.

Use of an anti-scatter grid is recommended when the thickness of the region to be radiographed is over 10 cm.

Grids with parallel strips are only useful when the distance between the tube and the cassette is very large (over 150 cm) or when the radiographed region is very small, because at a distance of 100 cm the strips would absorb not only the scatter radiation but also a substantial part of the useful radiation. Therefore, the most commonly used grids are focused grids in which the strips converge toward the focus, adapting to the shape of the primary X-ray beam (fig. 1.43a). When using focused grids it is important to always check that they are correctly positioned. If placed upside down, the strips would absorb most of the useful radiation (fig. 1.43b). They also absorb more useful radiation than needed when placed right-side up but are off-centre with the X-ray beam (fig. 1.43c). Grids, therefore, are often marked with a central reference line that should be aligned with the beam centre (indicated by the shadows emitted by the collimator on the table). Cross-hatched grids are also manufactured in which the lead strips are arranged in two perpendicular directions.

The taller the lead strips, the greater the amount of scatter radiation they absorb. The grid ratio is the ratio of the height of the lead strips to the distance between two strips. For example, a grid with a ratio of 12:1 will absorb more diffuse radiation than a grid with a ratio of 5:1. This is normally indicated on the top of the grid together with the number of strips per inch or centimetre and the focusing distance (e.g. 100 cm, 88105 cm, etc.). The grid exposure factor is also usually displayed, indicating the number by which to multiply the mAs value.

Radiographic patient positioning and projections

Correct patient positioning is absolutely ESSENTIAL for proper interpretation of the X-ray image. Poor animal positioning, especially when evaluating certain anatomic regions (e.g. head, spine, hip) can lead to significant diagnostic errors.

The terms "position" and "projection" should not be confused. The term **radiographic projection** refers to the path of the X-ray beam as it passes through the anatomical region of the patient, always indicating the entry area first and then the exit area. The projection, therefore, depends on the position of the patient, but these are not equivalent terms. Thus, for a ventrodorsal projection of the chest, the animal is placed in the dorsal decubitus position so that the beam enters the ventral area of the chest and exits through the dorsal part of the chest. Likewise, for a dorsoventral projection, the animal is placed in ventral decubitus so that the beam enters the dorsal part of the chest first and then exits through the ventral part. If the X-ray is performed with the animal in lateral decubitus, the terms right lateral - left lateral should be used if the animal is lying on the left side (left lateral decubitus) and left lateral - right lateral if the animal is lying on the right side (right lateral decubitus). In practice, however, these terms are shortened to left lateral or left latero-lateral in the former, and right lateral or right latero-lateral in the latter, in other words, the side on which the X-ray beam comes out is named at the end.

The compound name given to the X-ray projections is based on the anatomical terminology used depending on the area being examined. We must also remember that there are some differences between the anatomical terminology used for human and veterinary medicine. For example, the term anteroposterior is incorrect in veterinary medicine as anterior and posterior refer to human anatomy.

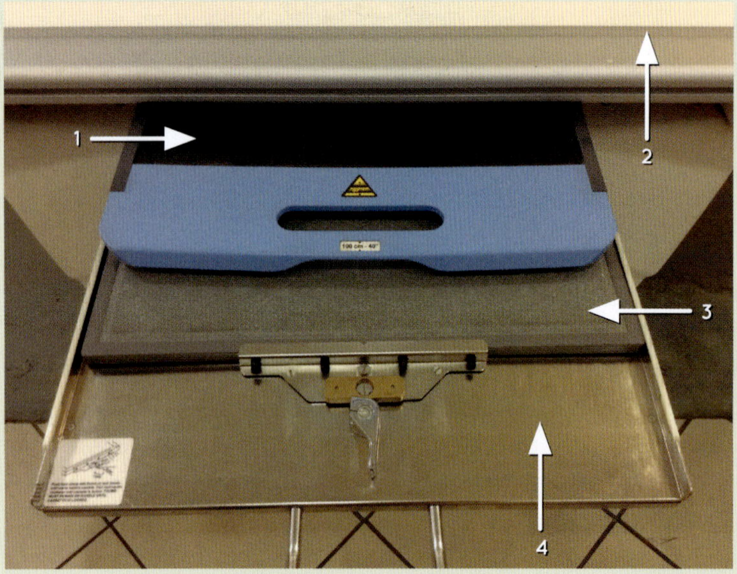

FIGURE 1.42. The anti-scatter grid (1) is placed between the X-ray table (2) and the cassette (3) located in the X-ray machine tray (4).

▼ FIGURE 1.43. Schematic diagram of the correctly positioned anti-scatter grid (a), placed upside down (b) and positioned off-centre to the X-ray beam (c).

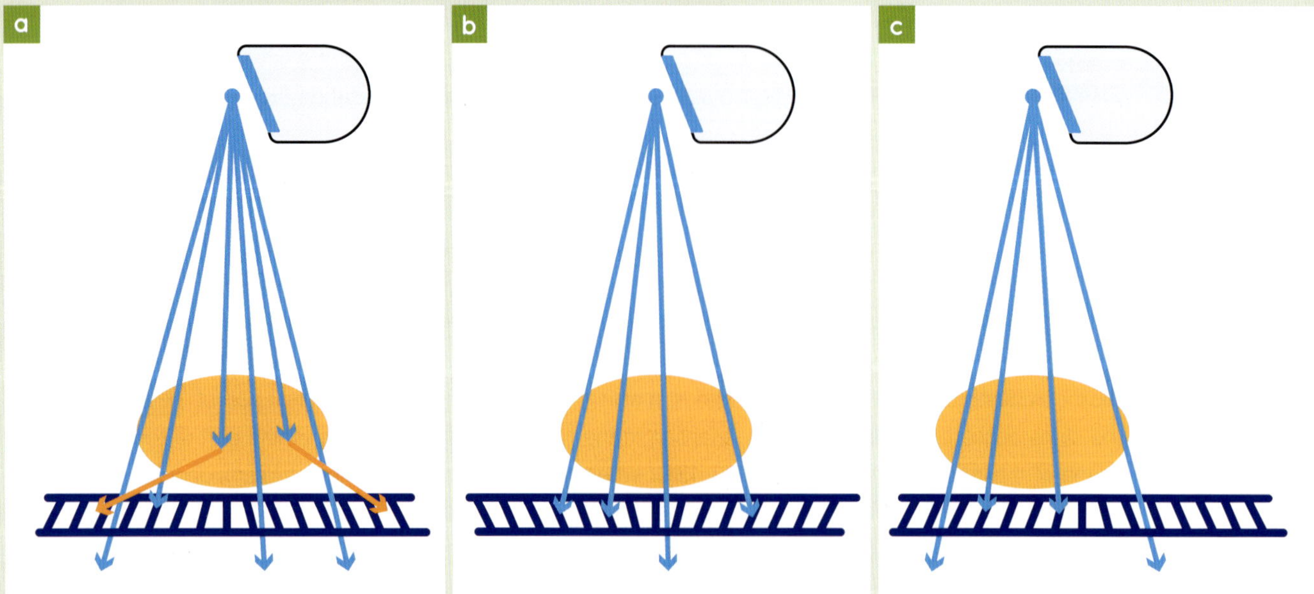

Figure 1.44 shows the terminology used to describe the radiographic projections for each anatomical region.

In the head, the term rostral is used instead of cranial.

In the ribs and extremities, the terms proximal and distal are used instead of the dorsal and ventral.

For the extremities, as with the trunk and tail, the terms cranial and caudal are used up to the carpus and tarsus. Then the terminology changes to dorsal and palmar for the carpus, metacarpals and phalanges of the forelimb and dorsal and plantar for the tarsus, metatarsals and phalanges of the hind limbs.

Technical artifacts and errors

An **artifact** is defined as any factor that decreases the quality of the radiograph making evaluation and interpretation difficult.

The most common artifact seen on veterinary radiographs is blurring of the image caused by patient movement during exposure (fig. 1.45). Proper restraint, either manually or using specific accessories when patient is sedated or anaesthetised, greatly eliminates this artifact. The use of sedation or anaesthesia is highly recommended, especially when examining certain anatomical regions. However, respiratory motion cannot be avoided so the greatest impact of this artifact is seen in chest radiographs. Here we can try to minimise it by reducing the exposure time to the absolute minimum.

The main technical errors that can appear in conventional (non-digital) radiographs are:

- Very dark image: usually due to overexposure (fig. 1.46A). This can be caused by excessively high kilovoltage (kV) or milliamperes-second (mAs), incorrect film development (too long in developer or using it at very high temperature) or incorrect selection of focus-to-film distance.
- Very light image: usually due to underexposure (fig. 1.46B). This can be due to use of excessively low kV or mAs, incorrect film development (not long enough in developer, deterioration or dilution of the developer, or too low developer temperature), incorrect choice of film-screen combination or a voltage input failure.
- Low contrast image (too grey): this is usually caused by the use of a kV that is too high but can also be caused by many other factors such as incorrect development (too high temperature, too long development time, deterioration of chemical solutions), double exposure (repeated X-ray) or the use of expired film.
- Blurring: This is usually due to patient movement, but there are other reasons for this: selecting an object-to-film distance that is too long, inadequate contact between film and intensifying screen, double exposure or poor centring of the object relative to the beam.
- Appearance of marked lines on the image: this is usually associated with incorrect grid position, damage to grid lead strips or faults in rollers in automatic film processors.
- Yellowing of the X-ray: this may be due to inadequate fixing, incomplete washing or when two films come into contact during the fixing process.

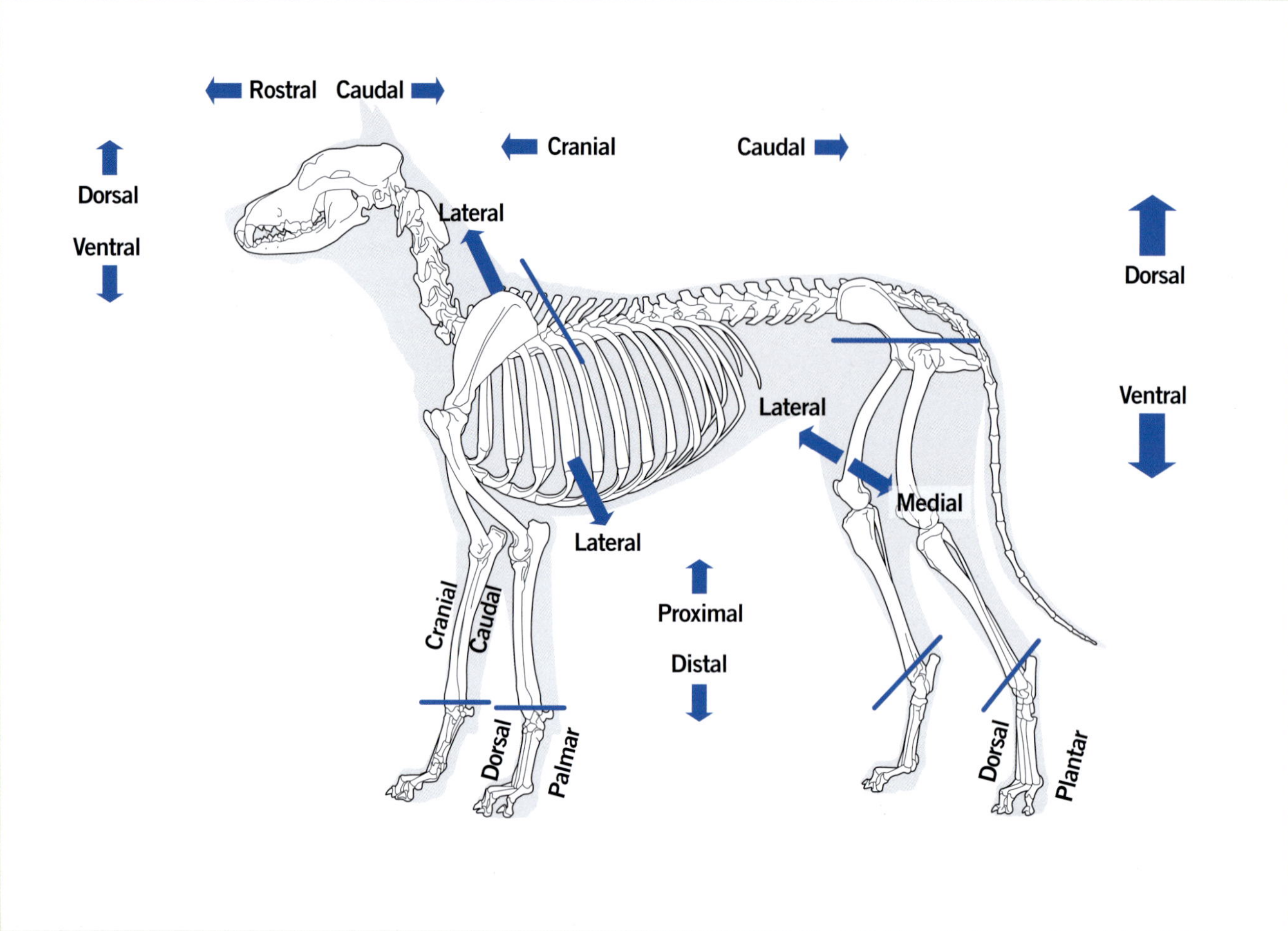

▲ FIGURE 1.44. Schematic diagram of the anatomical nomenclature on which the naming of the X-ray projections is based.

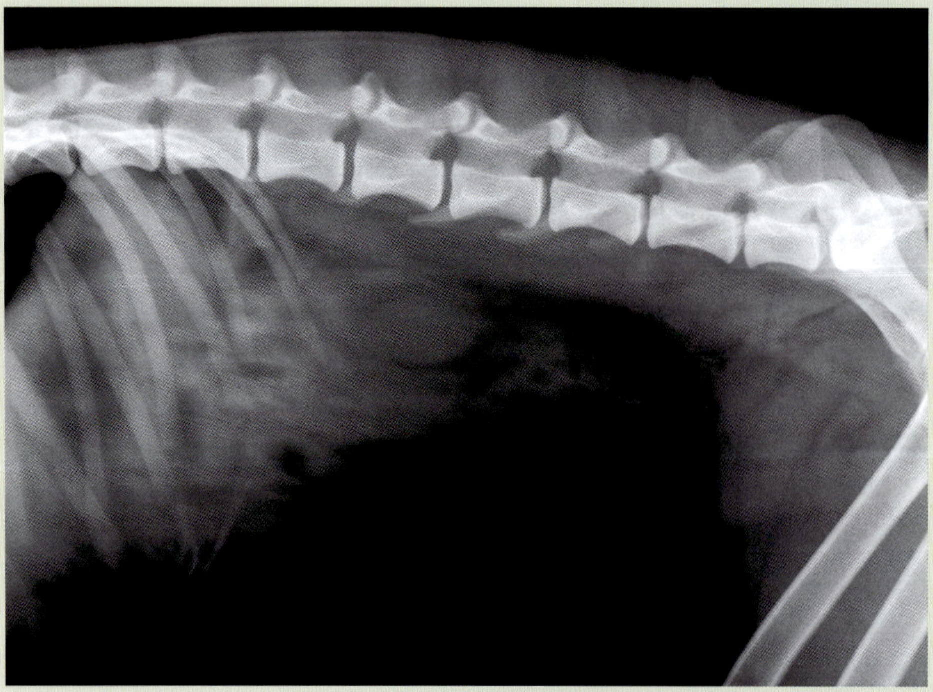

◄ FIGURE 1.45. Lateral projection radiograph of the abdomen of a dog with motion blur.

Some technical artifacts and error characteristic of digital radiography:

- When a digital radiograph is overexposed, it will not appear as generalised darkening of the image as occurs in analogue radiographs, but there will be black focal areas that cannot be clarified with computer post-processing tools (fig. 1.47). This artifact can be corrected by lowering the exposure values.
- When a digital radiograph is underexposed, there will be no lightening of the entire image as occurs in analogue radiographs, but tiny black spots with appear throughout the image and this is what is known as "noise" (fig. 1.48). Increasing exposure values will correct this artifact.
- The appearance of a radiolucent halo between structures of very different radiographic densities, e.g. between bone and soft tissues (fig. 1.49) or between metal and bone. Observing this halo around osteosynthesis material such as bone implants (plates, pins or screws) could be mistaken for a sign of material mobility or rejection. This artifact has generally been corrected by many manufacturers, but it may appear or be accentuated when the edge enhancement computer post-processing tool is overused.
- Use of anti-scatter grids can produce an artifact in which alternating light and dark bands appear on the X-ray, which has been termed a moiré pattern artifact (fig. 1.50). This occurs when the spaces between grid strips coincide with the direction and frequency of the laser beam reading lines in CR systems. Rotating the grid 90° or using a grid that does not match the reading lines resolves this problem. Potter-Bucky grids, which move rapidly when the X-ray is being taken, do not cause this problem.
- When the data from the phosphor screen in CR systems or the electrical signals in DR are sent to the computer, these data are erased. If this erasure is incomplete, part of the silhouette from the previous exposure may be superimposed on the current image. This is called a ghosting artifact. It usually occurs when very high exposure values have been used in a previous X-ray.
- In CR images, the appearance of a white line along the laser beam reading direction indicates a lack of reading of that line (fig. 1.51). This is usually caused by dirt accumulation in the CR laser device.

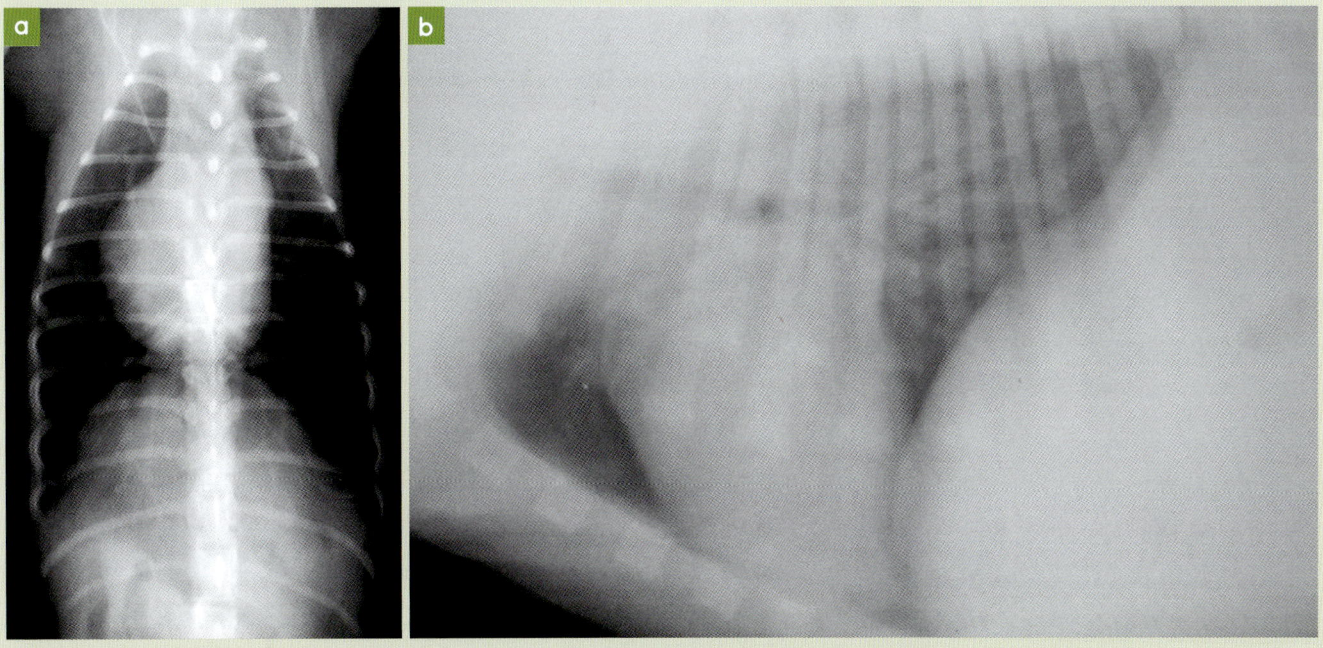

FIGURE 1.46. Conventional (non-digital) lateral projection chest radiographs of two dogs with incorrect exposure parameters: overexposed (a) and underexposed (b). In image (a) a large section of the lung appears uniformly black so unable to visualise the pulmonary vessels. In image (b), the normal lung is a very pale grey, which could be confused with increased opacity of pathological origin.

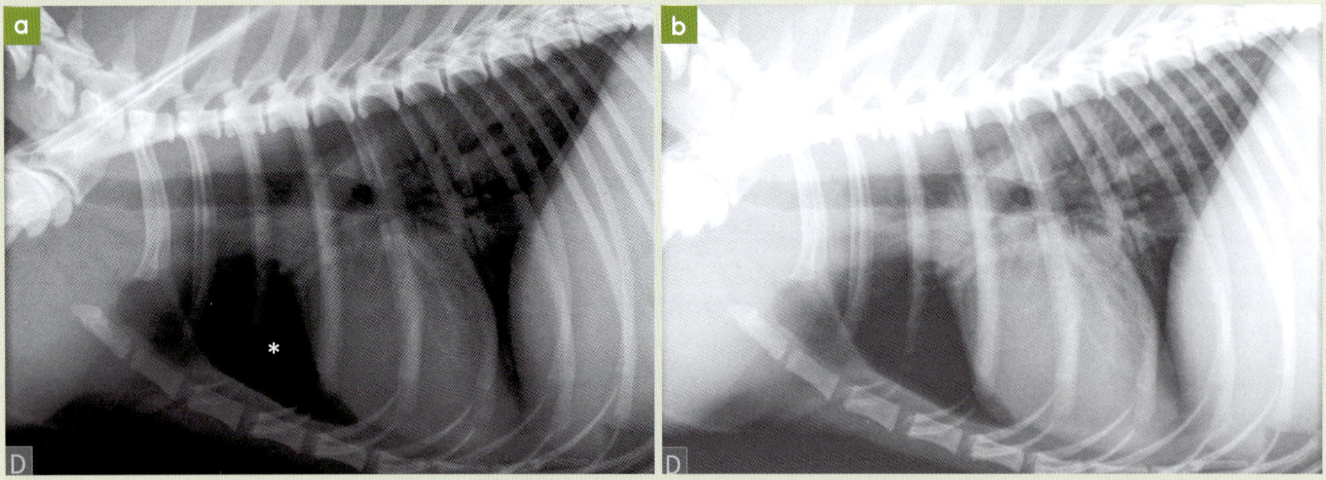

FIGURE 1.47. Digital chest radiograph of a dog which was overexposed before (a) and after (b) computer post-processing. In the cranioventral area of the lung, a black area (*) appears in the lung with no visualisation of a part of the distal third of the third costal pair. This is not corrected by increasing the overall brightness of the image (b) which confirms overexposure. The test must be repeated lowering the exposure parameters.

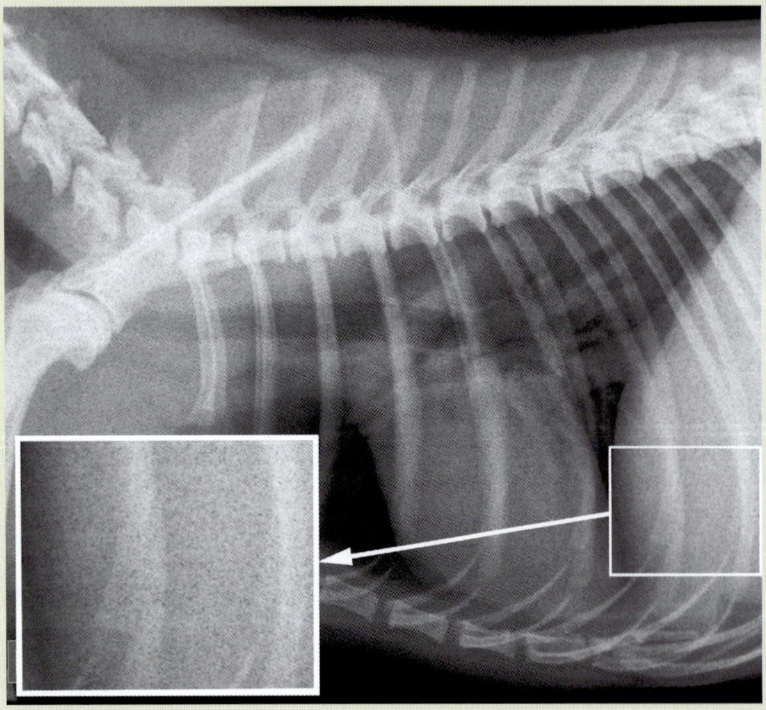

FIGURE 1.48. A digital chest radiograph in a dog which is underexposed, causing tiny dark dots to appear in the image which are termed noise. This error is corrected by raising the exposure parameters, preferably the mAs.

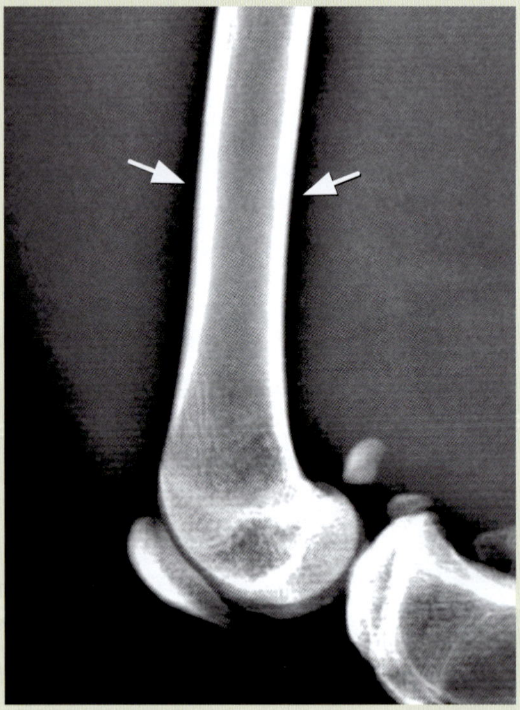

FIGURE 1.49. Digital radiograph of the distal half of the femur in a cat showing a technical error–a radiolucent halo–at the adjacent bone and soft tissue contact areas. This artifact is corrected by varying the image algorithms for which the manufacturer of the digital X-ray system is responsible.

Radiology reports

The following data must be included in a radiology report: patient details, date of X-ray, anatomical region examined and the radiographic projections. It is also useful to explain the reason the X-ray was carried out.

All abnormalities observed in the image (i.e. radiographic signs) should be described in the report using the correct anatomical and radiological terminology. These abnormal findings may include:

- Abnormal radiographic density.
- Abnormal position.
- Abnormal size.
- Abnormal contour or shape.
- Abnormal numbers.

Regarding the degree of detail to include in the description, consider the following as a reference point: A radiographic description will be adequate if a professional who does not see the X-ray can quite accurately imagine it after reading or hearing the description.

After correlating the radiographic findings with the patient's clinical data, the report should establish either a final radiological diagnosis or a list of possible differential diagnoses in the order of likelihood from highest to lowest (the most likely presumptive diagnosis will be placed first on the list).

The report may also include recommendations for further diagnostic tests that we believe could complement the findings of the X-rays.

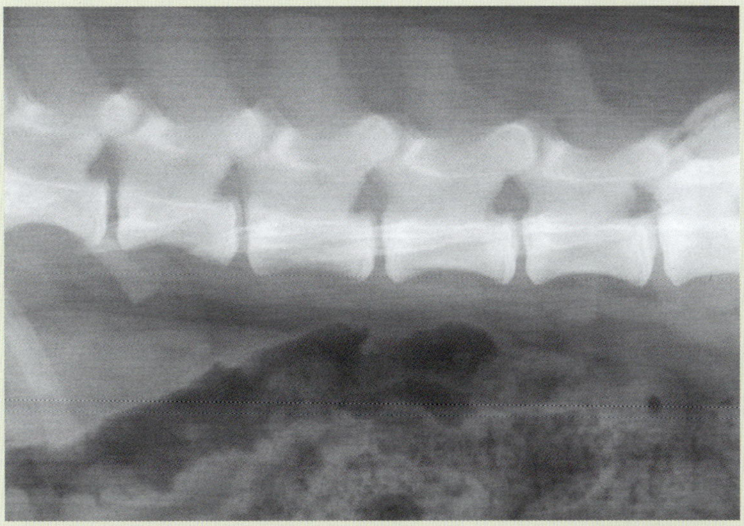

FIGURE 1.50. Digital radiograph showing part of the lumbar spine and dorsal area of the abdomen in a dog. It illustrates alternating light and dark bands as a technical error caused by the incorrect fitting of the anti-scatter grid on the CR cassette. This artifact is called moiré pattern artifact as it is very similar to the fabric pattern known as moiré.

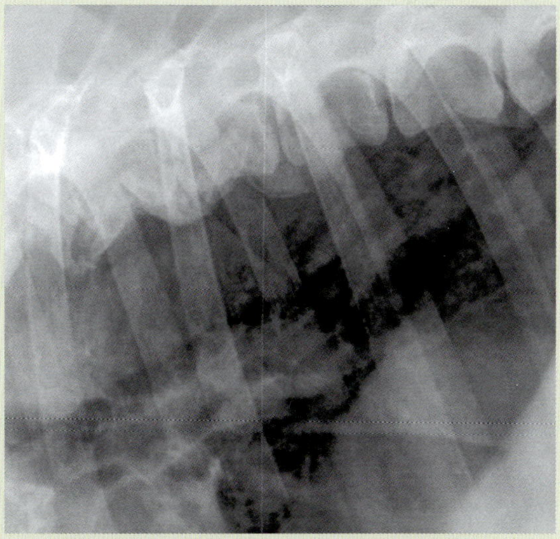

FIGURE 1.51. A digital radiograph obtained with a CR of the dorsocaudal zone of the thorax of a dog. This shows, as a technical error, a white line caused by a defect in the laser light beam reading in that location. This is usually corrected by cleaning the CR laser device.

Atlas of radiographic positioning and anatomy

ABDOMEN

Atlas of normal radiographic anatomy

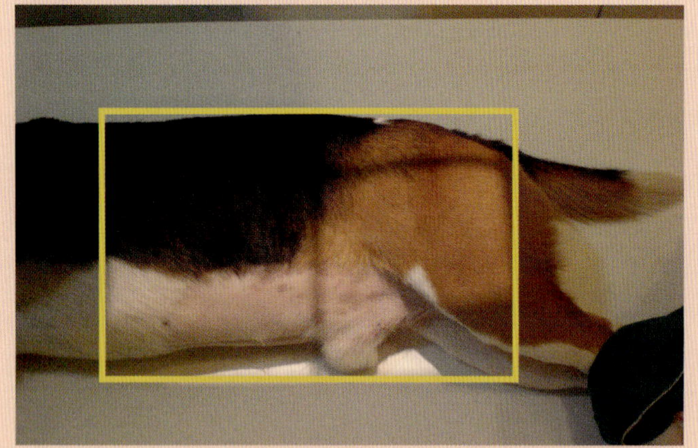

FIGURE P1. Right lateral decubitus position to obtain the right lateral projection of the abdomen.

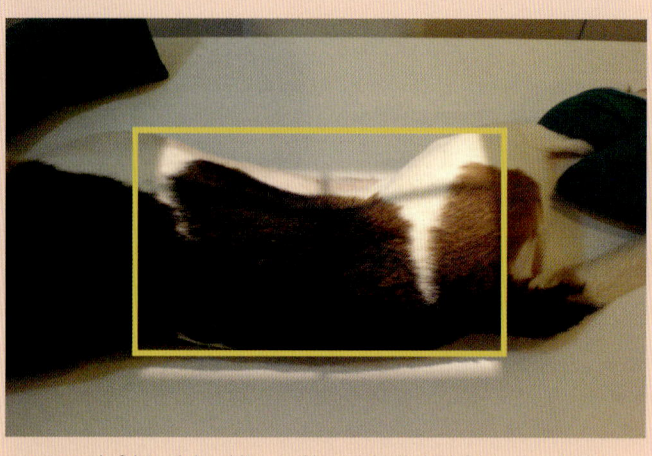

FIGURE P2. Left lateral decubitus position to obtain the left lateral projection of the abdomen.

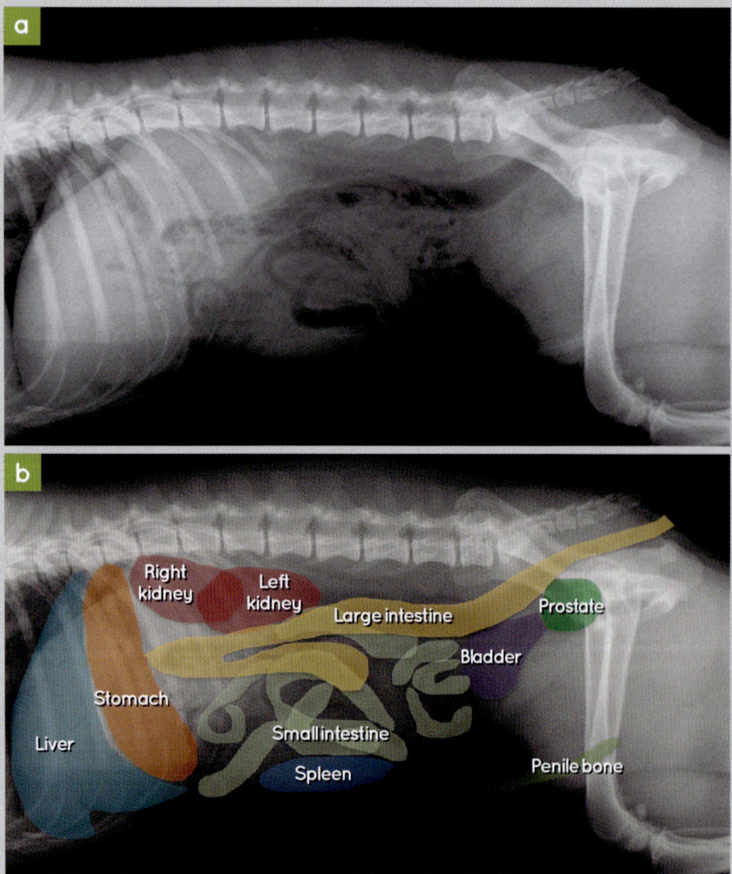

FIGURE A1. Image of the right lateral projection of the abdomen of a male dog. Without (a) and with (b) coloured silhouettes representing the main abdominal structures identifiable in the image.

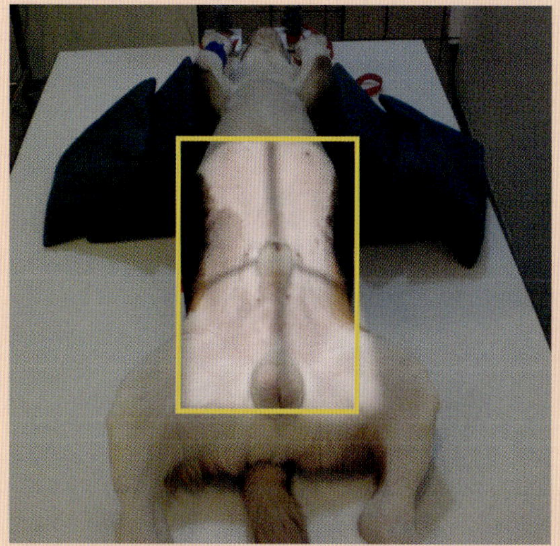

FIGURE P.3. Dorsal decubitus position to obtain the ventrodorsal projection of the abdomen.

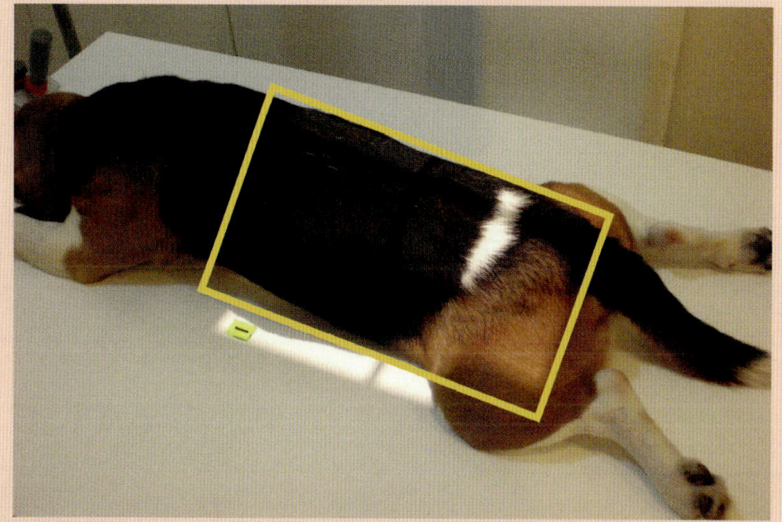

FIGURE P.4. Ventral decubitus position to obtain the dorsoventral projection of the abdomen.

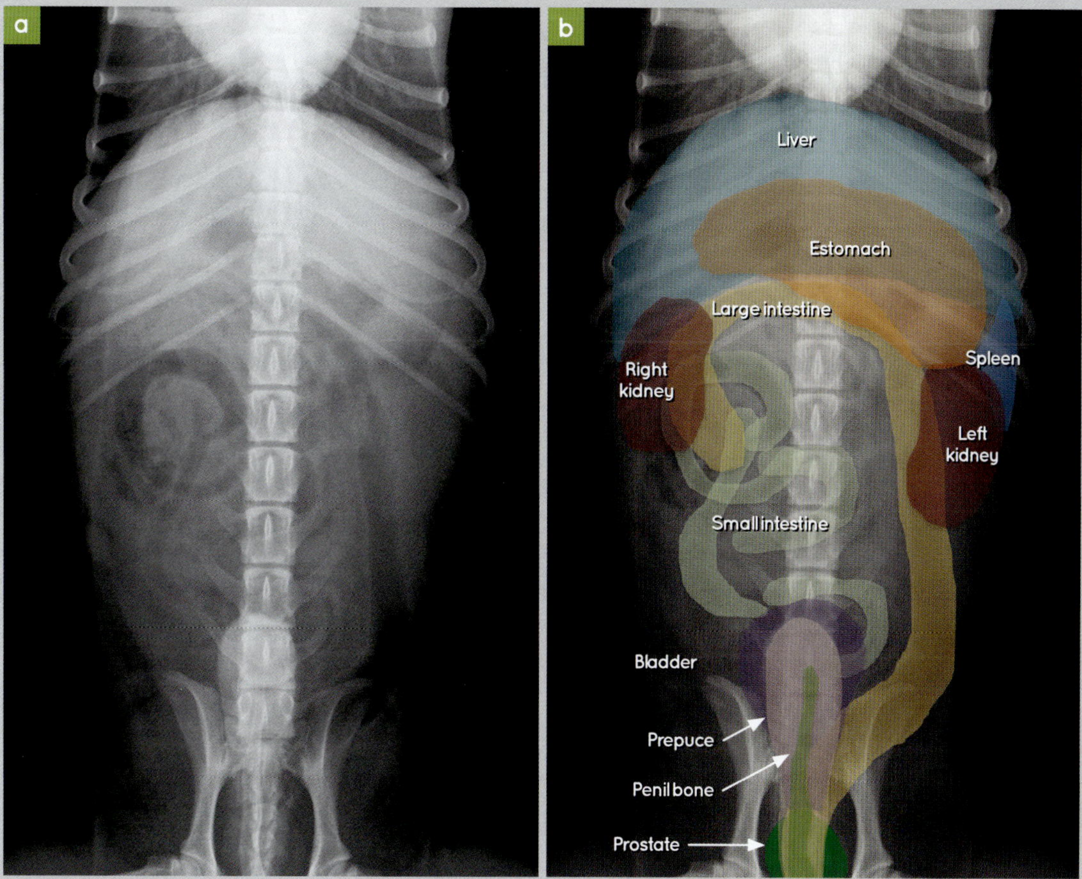

FIGURE A.2. Image of the ventrodorsal projection of the abdomen of a male dog. Without (a) and with (b) coloured silhouettes representing the main abdominal structures identifiable in the image.

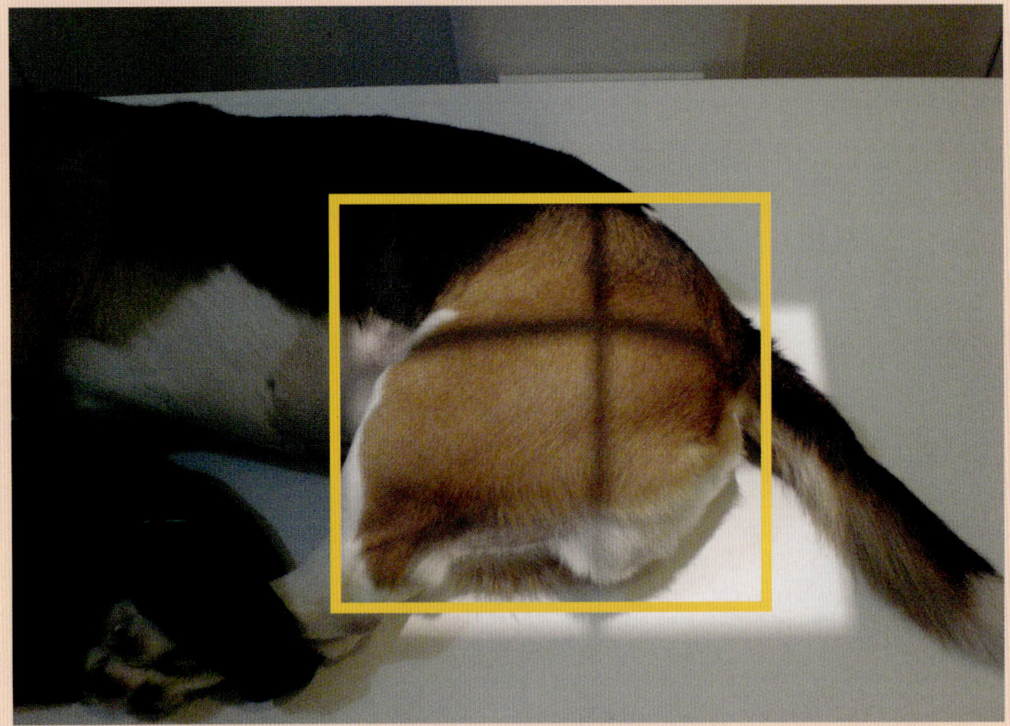

FIGURE P5. Right lateral decubitus position to obtain the lateral projection of caudal abdomen and pelvic region with cranial extension of hind limbs (avoiding overlapping of femurs with penile urethra).

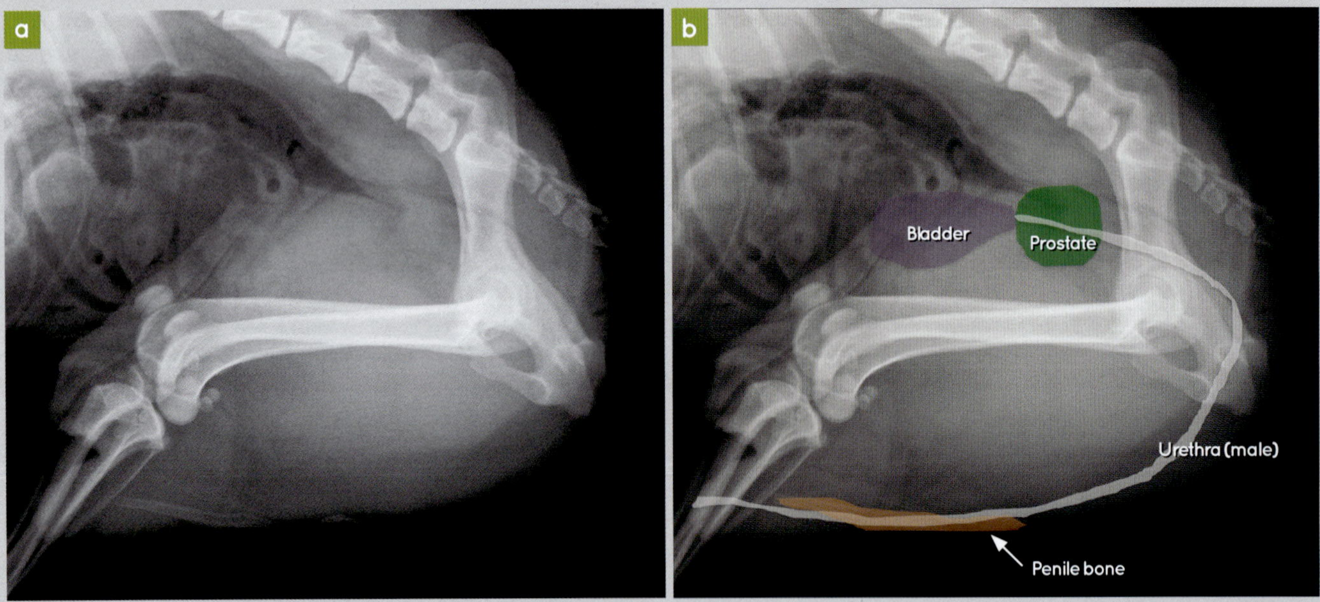

FIGURE A3. Image of the lateral projection of the caudal abdomen and pelvic region with cranial extension of the hind limbs of a male dog. Without (a) and with (b) coloured silhouettes representing the position of the bladder, prostate, urethra and penile bone.

NECK

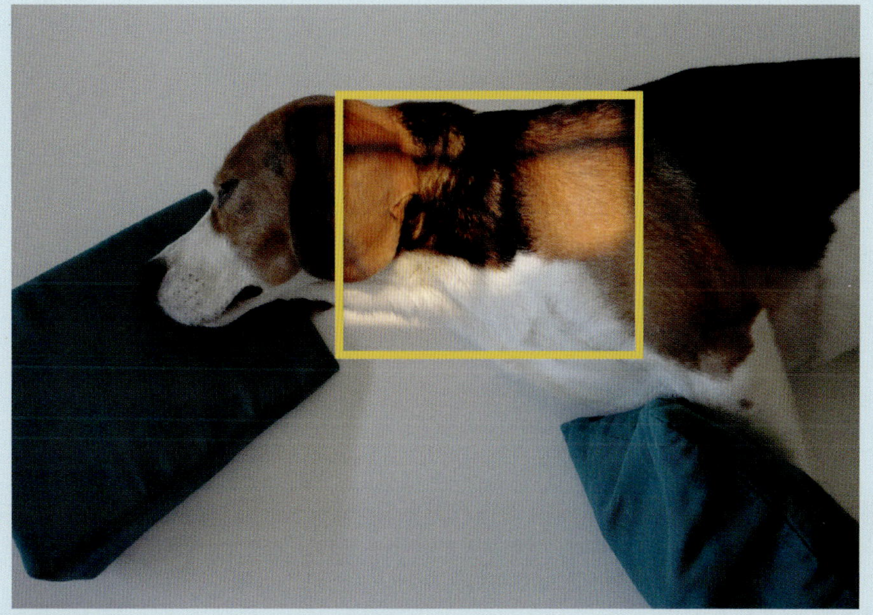

FIGURE P.6. Right lateral decubitus position to obtain the right lateral projection of the neck (for soft tissue assessment) of a dog.

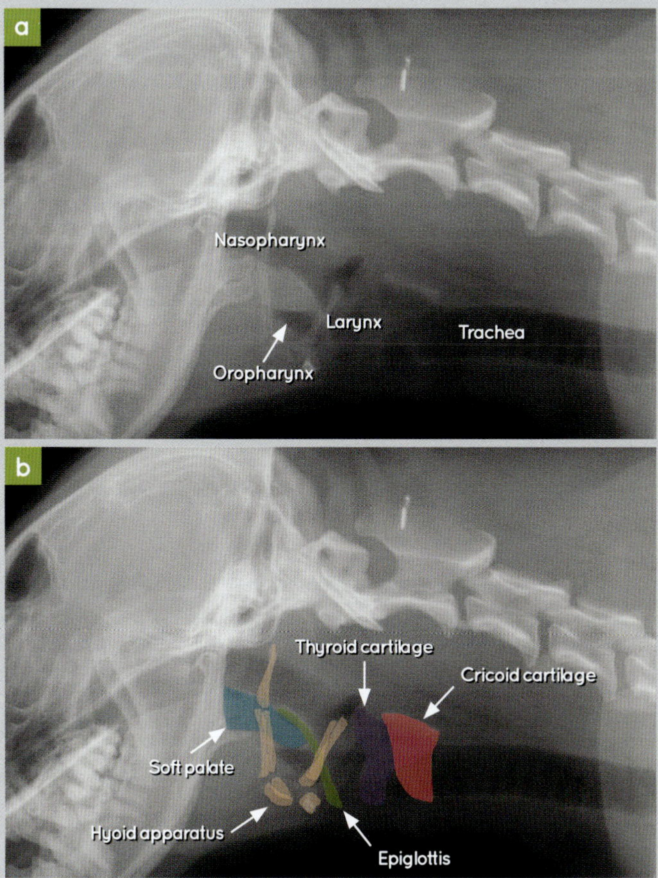

FIGURE A.4. Image of the lateral projection of the neck of a dog. Without coloured silhouettes, with pharynx, larynx and trachea identified (a); with coloured silhouettes showing the soft palate, epiglottis, hyoid apparatus and thyroid/cricoid cartilages (b).

THORAX

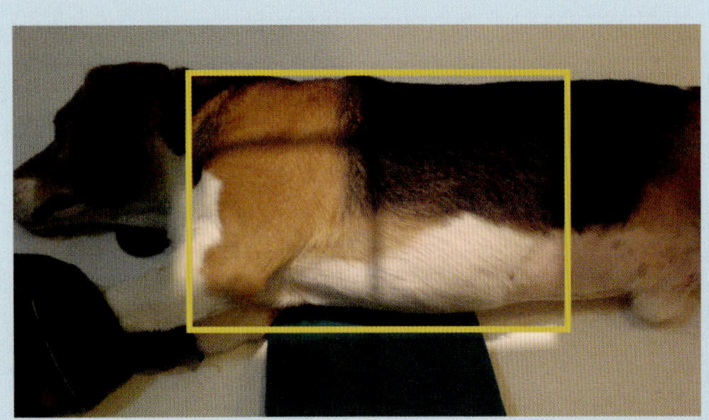

FIGURE P.7. Right lateral decubitus position to obtain the right lateral projection of the thorax.

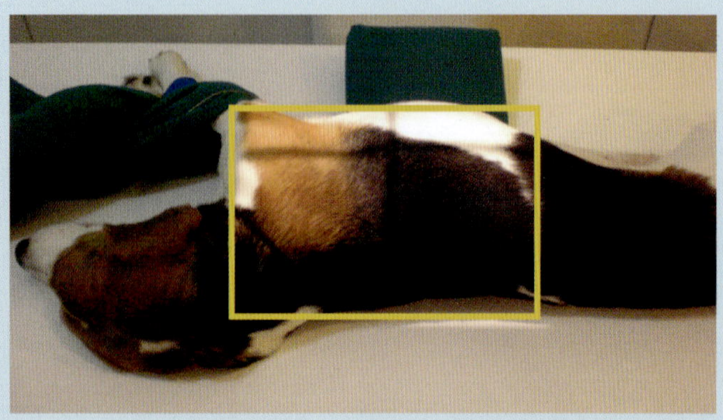

FIGURE P.8. Left lateral decubitus position to obtain the left lateral projection of the thorax.

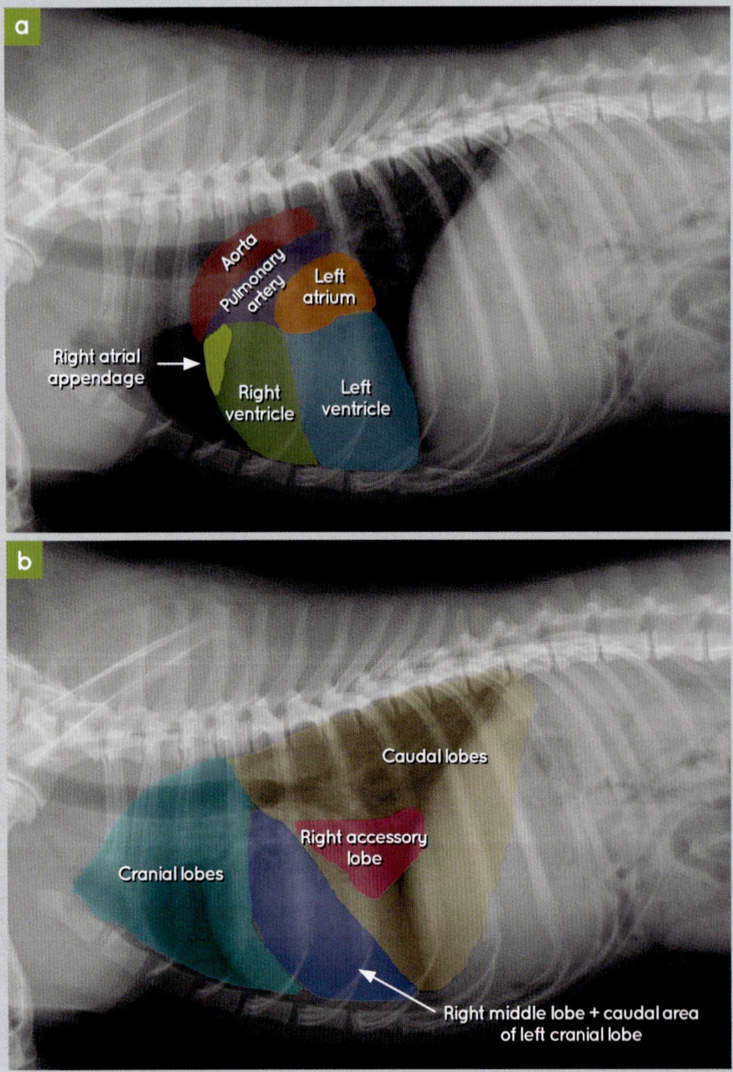

FIGURE A.5. Image of the right lateral projection of the chest of a dog with coloured silhouettes representing heart chambers and large vessels (a), as well as the identifying the lung lobes (b).

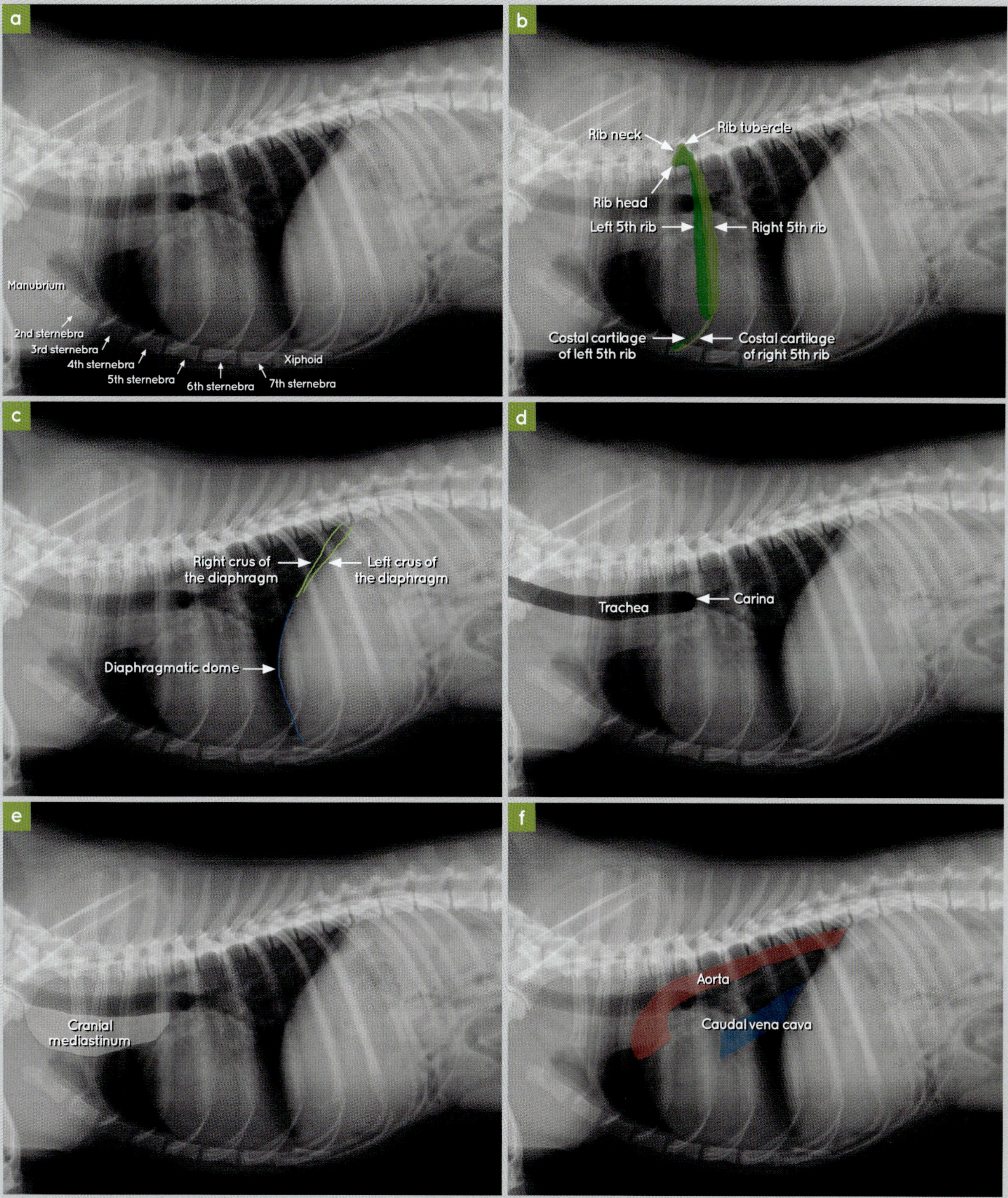

FIGURE A.6. Image of the right lateral projection of the chest of a dog with labelling of the sternebrae (a), ribs (b), diaphragmatic structures (c), trachea and carina (d), soft tissues of the cranial mediastinum (e) and thoracic aorta and caudal vena cava (f).

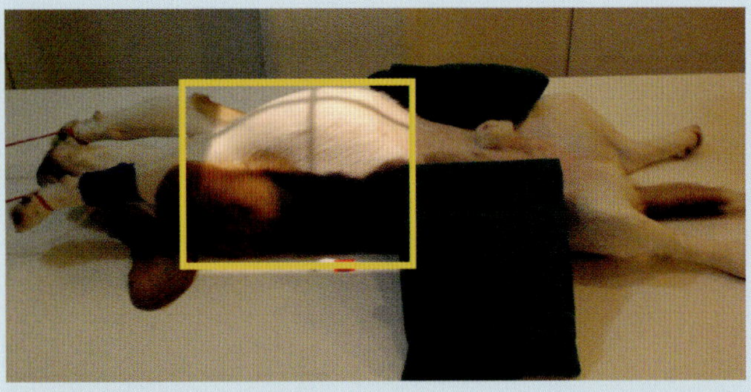

FIGURE P.9. Dorsal decubitus position to obtain the ventrodorsal projection of the thorax.

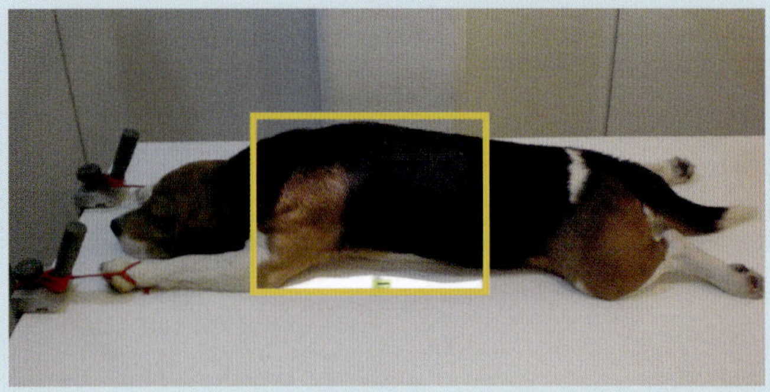

FIGURE P.10. Ventral decubitus position to obtain the dorsoventral projection of the thorax.

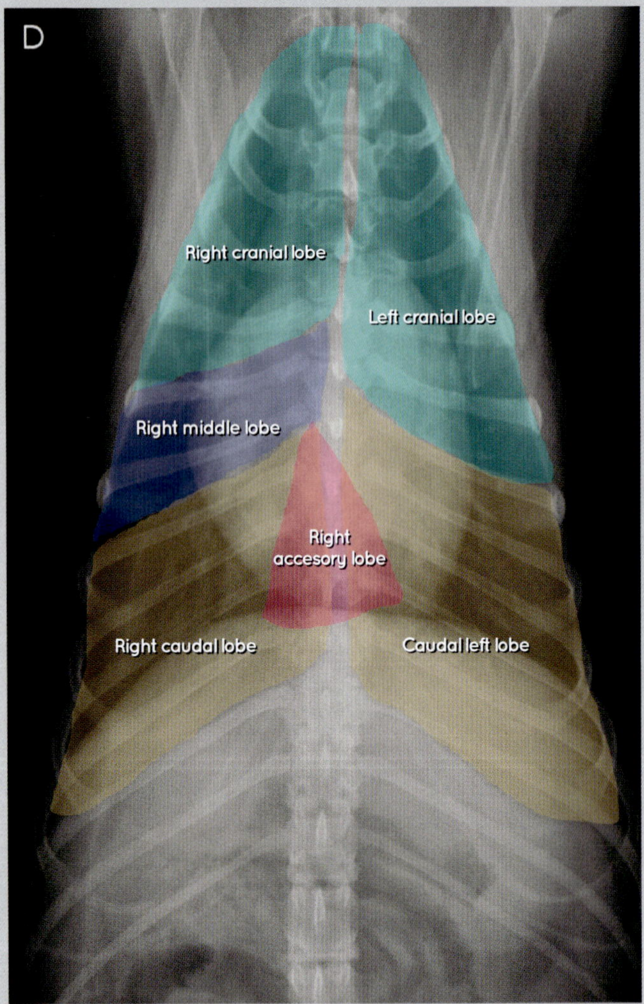

FIGURE A.7. Image of a ventrodorsal projection of the chest of a dog identifying the different lobes of the lung in different colours.

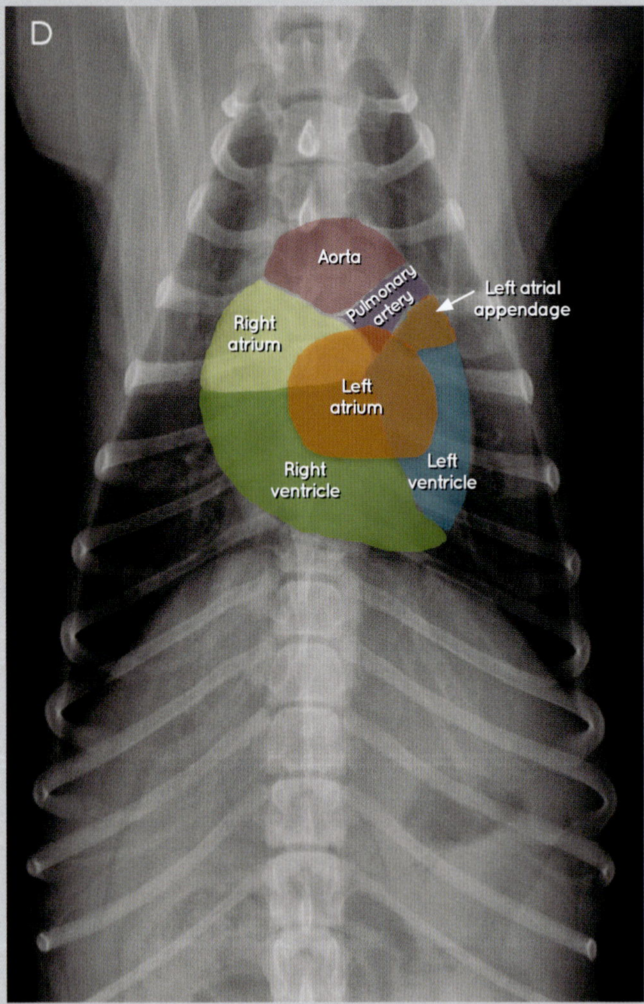

FIGURE A.8. Image of a dorsoventral projection of the chest of a dog highlighting the chambers of the heart and large vessels in colour.

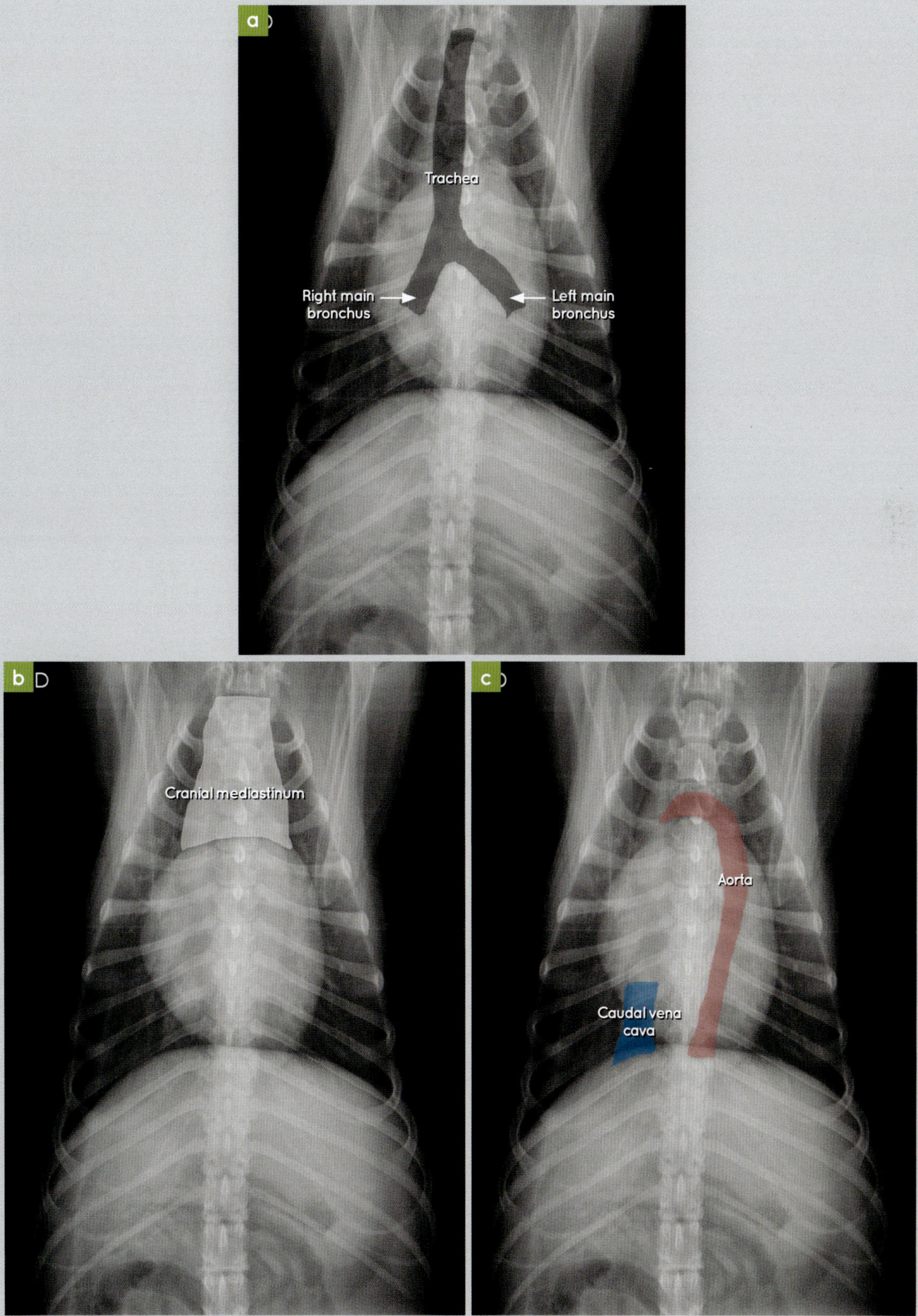

FIGURE A.9. Image of a dorsoventral projection of the chest of a dog showing the trachea and bifurcation of the main bronchi (a), the soft tissues of the cranial mediastinum (b) and the thoracic aorta and caudal vena cava (c).

APPENDICULAR SKELETON

THORACIC LIMB

Scapula

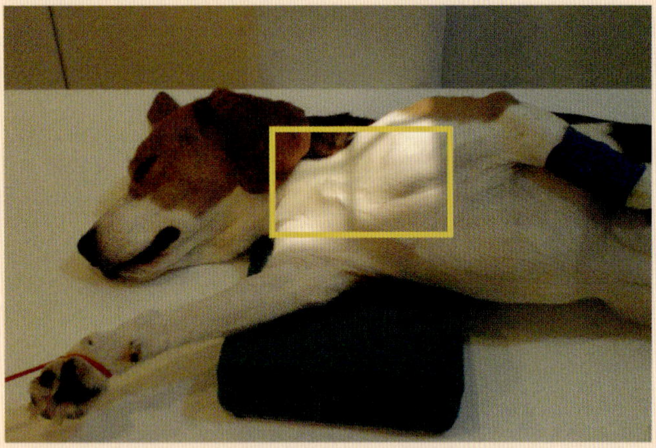

FIGURE P.11. Right lateral decubitus position to obtain the mediolateral projection of the right scapula of a dog.

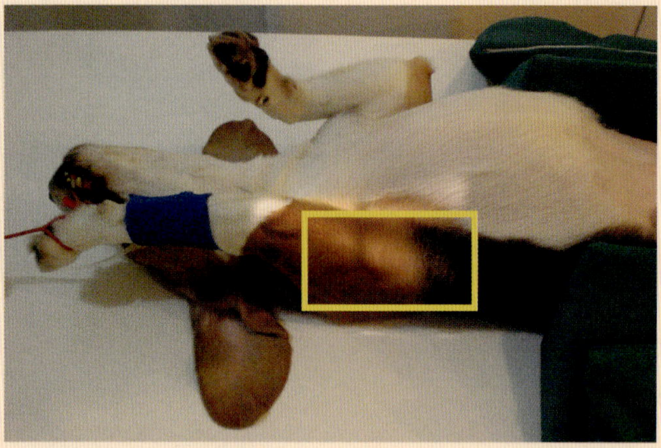

FIGURE P.12. Dorsal decubitus position to obtain the caudocranial projection of the right scapula of a dog.

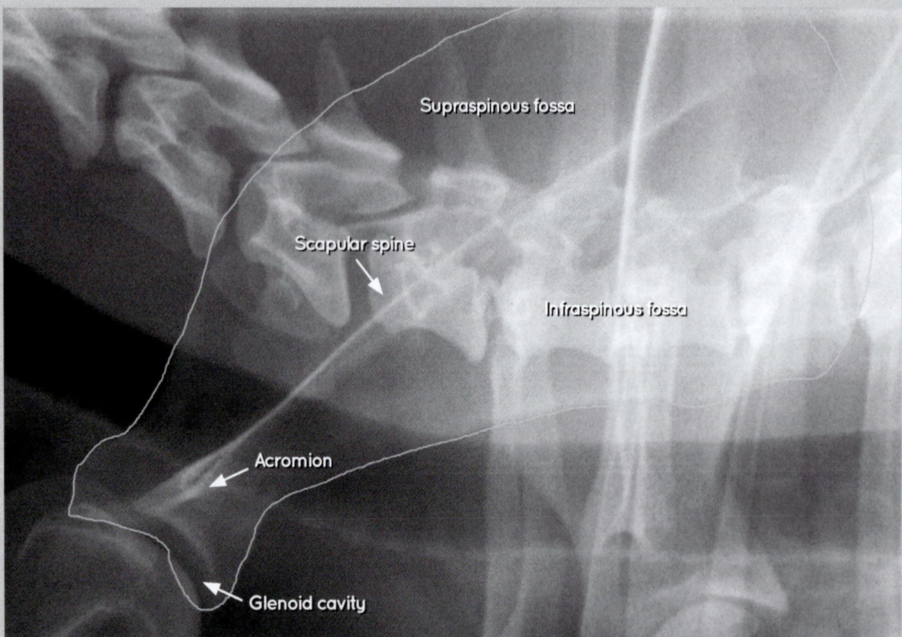

▲ FIGURE A.10. Image of the mediolateral projection of the scapula of a dog.

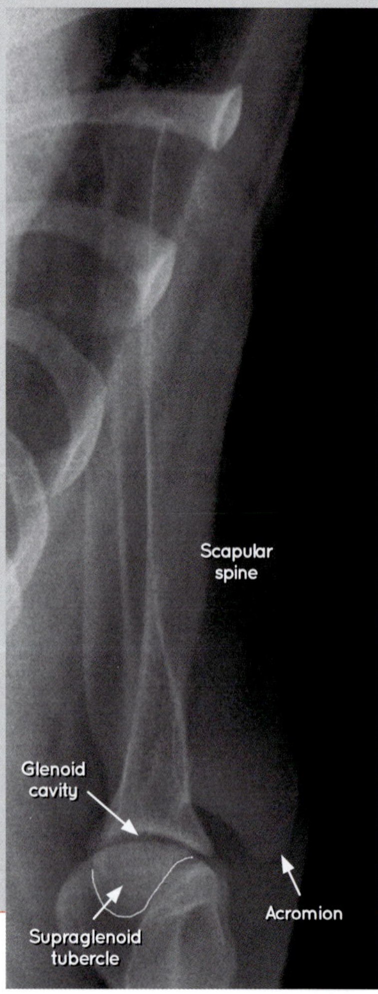

FIGURE A.11. Image of the caudocranial projection of the scapula of a dog. ▶

Shoulder

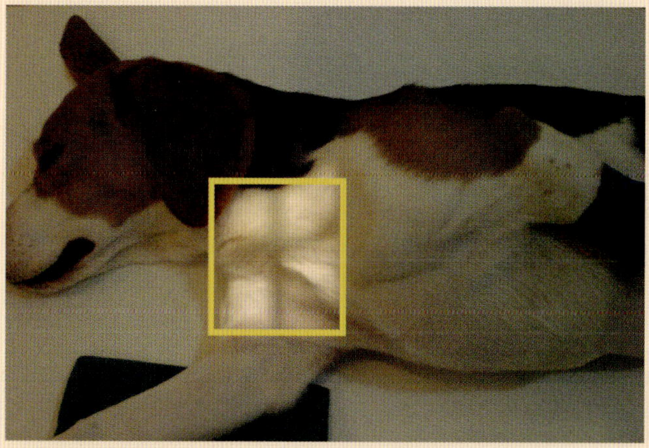

FIGURE P.13. Right lateral decubitus position to obtain the mediolateral projection of the right scapulohumeral joint of a dog.

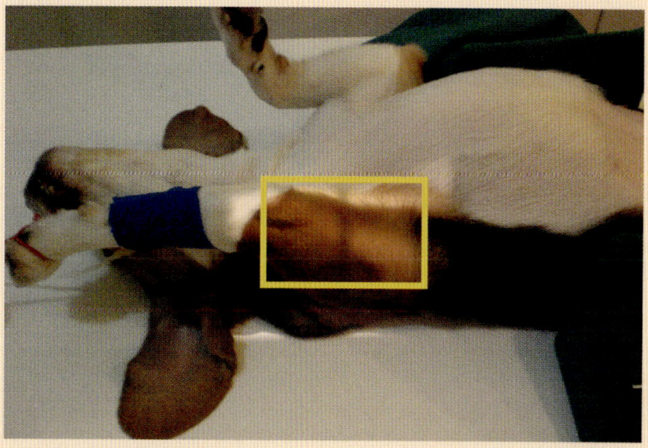

FIGURE P.14. Dorsal decubitus position to obtain the caudocranial projection of the right scapulohumeral joint of a dog.

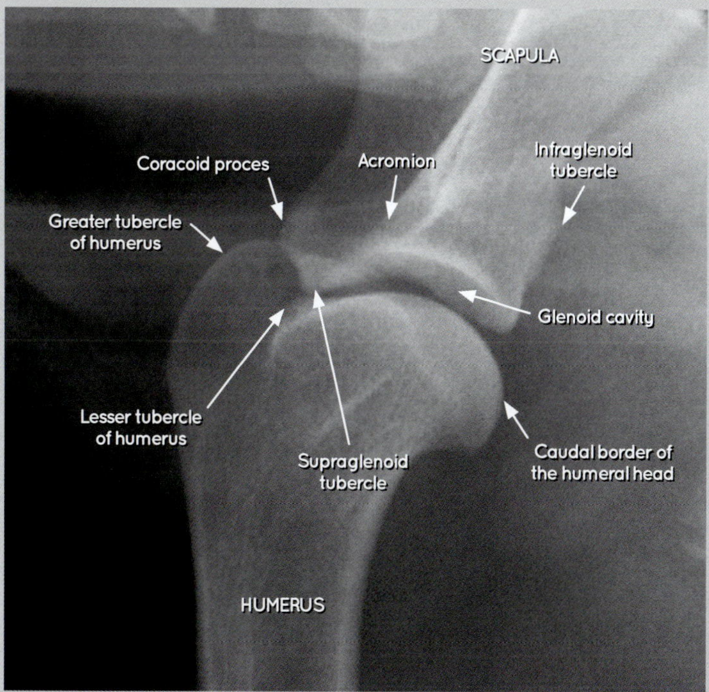

FIGURE A.12. Image of the mediolateral projection of the scapulohumeral joint of a dog.

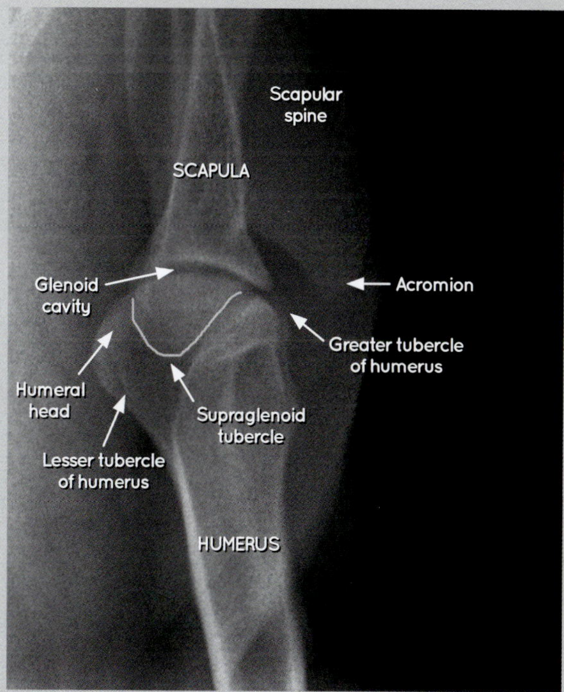

FIGURE A.13. Image of the caudocranial projection of the scapulohumeral joint of a dog.

Humerus

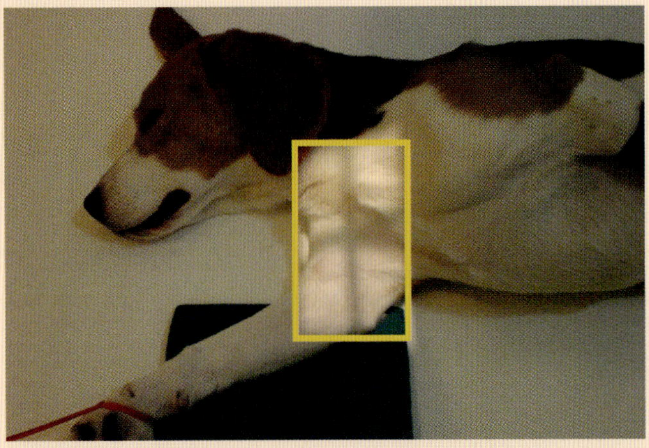

FIGURE P.15. Right lateral decubitus position to obtain the mediolateral projection of the right humerus of a dog.

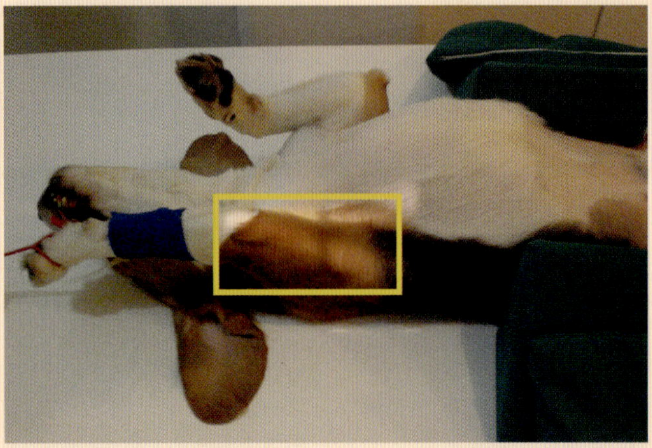

FIGURE P.16. Dorsal decubitus position to obtain the caudocranial projection of the right humerus of a dog.

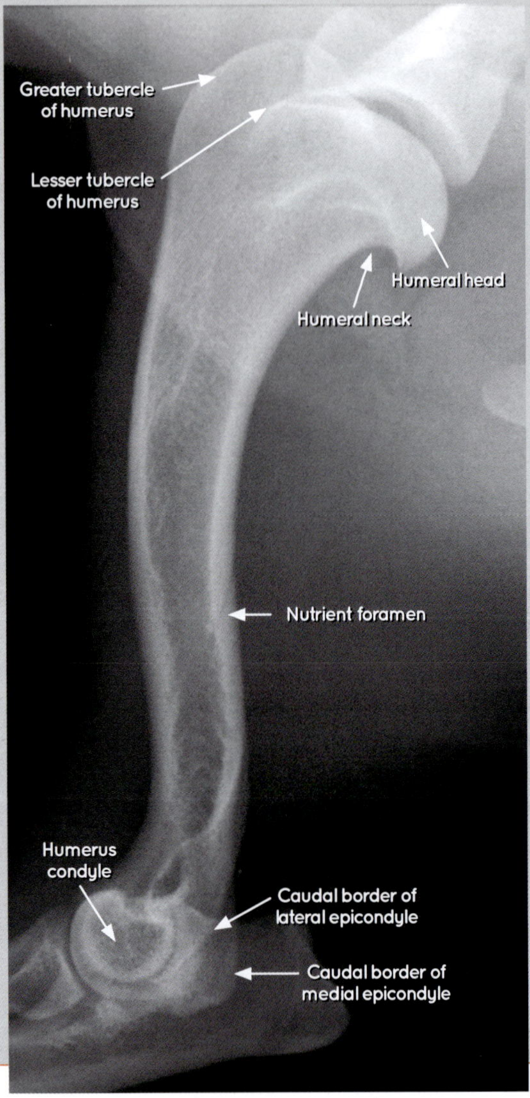

FIGURE A.14. Image of the mediolateral projection of the humerus of a dog.

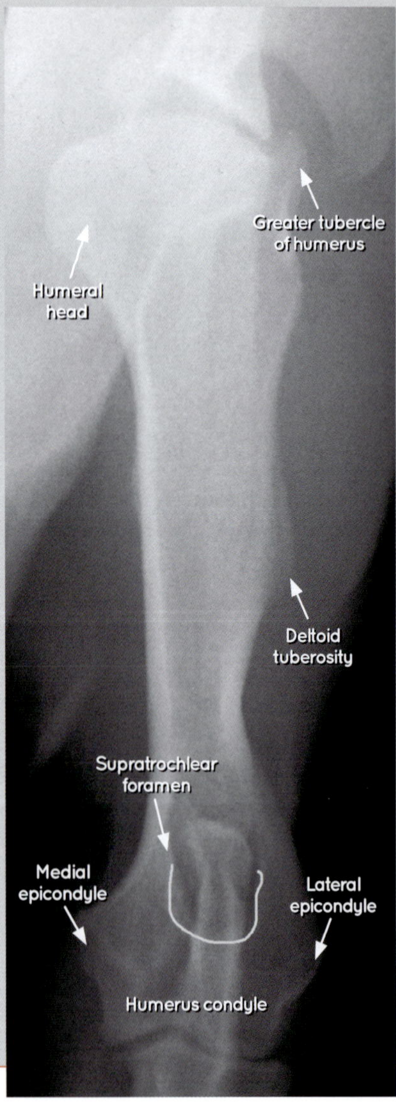

FIGURE A.15. Image of the caudocranial projection of the humerus of a dog.

Elbow

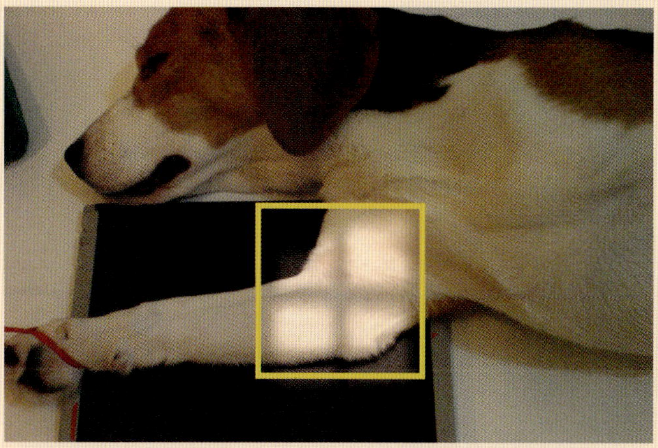

FIGURE P.17. Right lateral decubitus position to obtain the mediolateral projection of the right elbow of a dog.

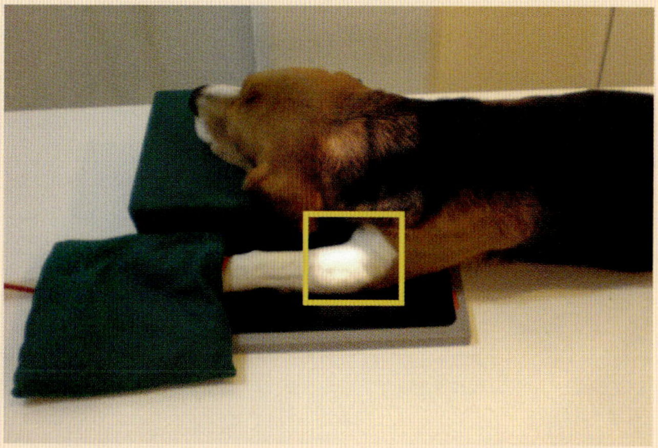

FIGURE P.18. Ventral decubitus position to obtain the craniocaudal projection of the left elbow of a dog.

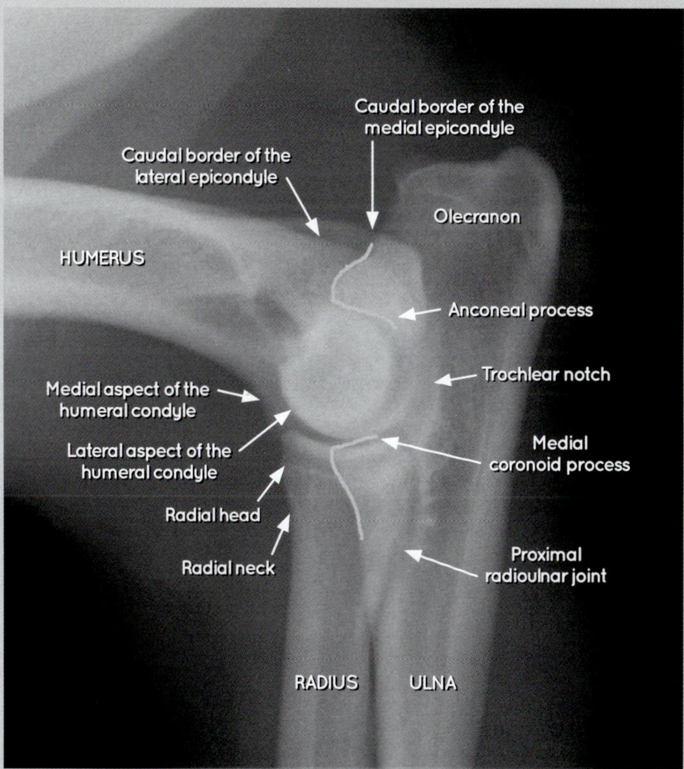

FIGURE A.16. Image of the mediolateral projection of the elbow of a dog.

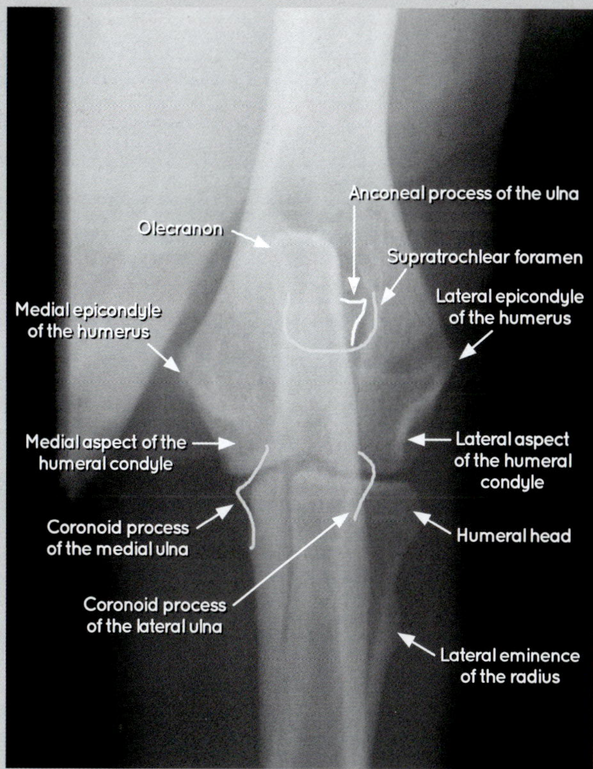

FIGURE A.17. Image of the craniocaudal projection of the elbow of a dog.

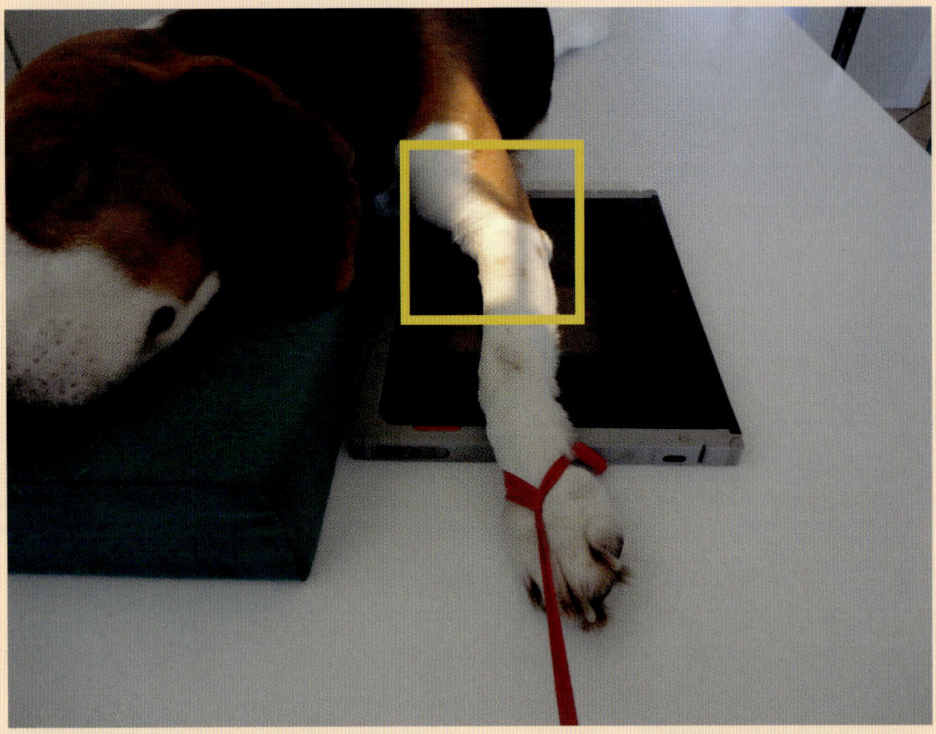

FIGURE P.19. Ventral decubitus position to obtain the craniolateral-caudoventral oblique projection of the left elbow of a dog.

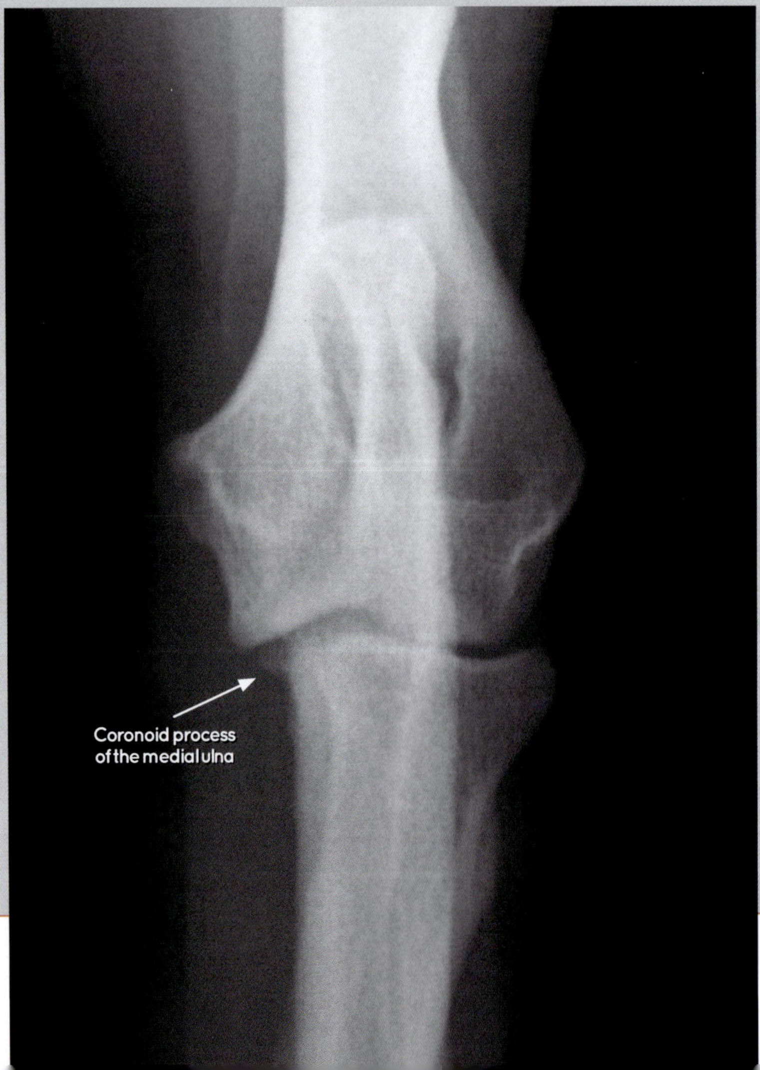

FIGURE A.18. Image of the craniolateral-caudoventral oblique projection of the elbow of a dog (performed to optimise visualisation of the medial coronoid process of the ulna).

Radius-ulna

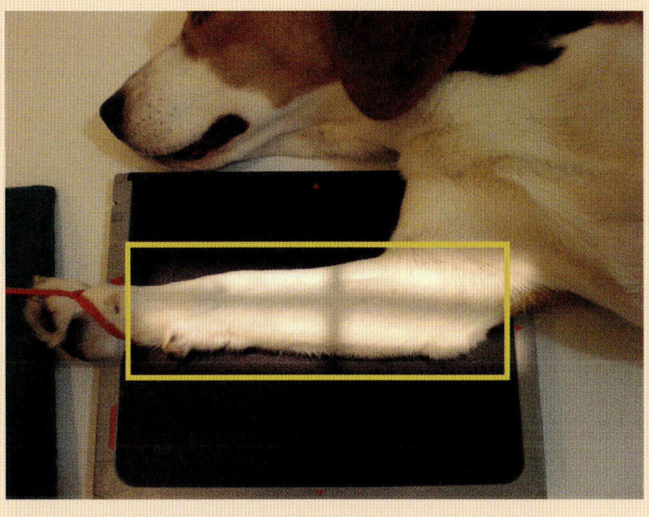

FIGURE P.20. Right lateral decubitus position to obtain the mediolateral projection of the right radius and ulna of a dog.

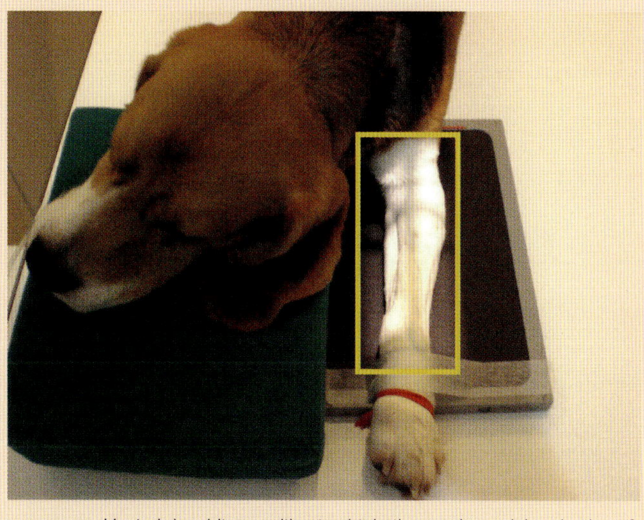

FIGURE P.21. Ventral decubitus position to obtain the craniocaudal projection of the left radius and ulna of a dog.

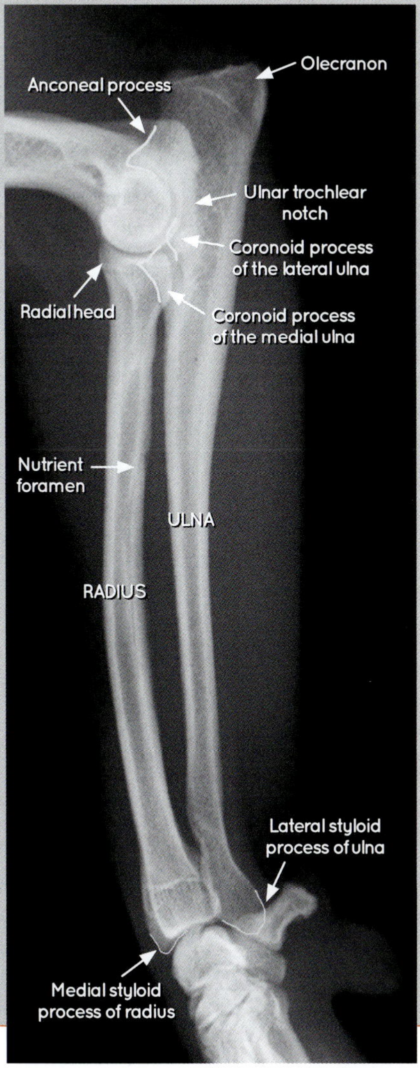

FIGURE A.19. Image of the mediolateral projection of the radius and ulna of a dog.

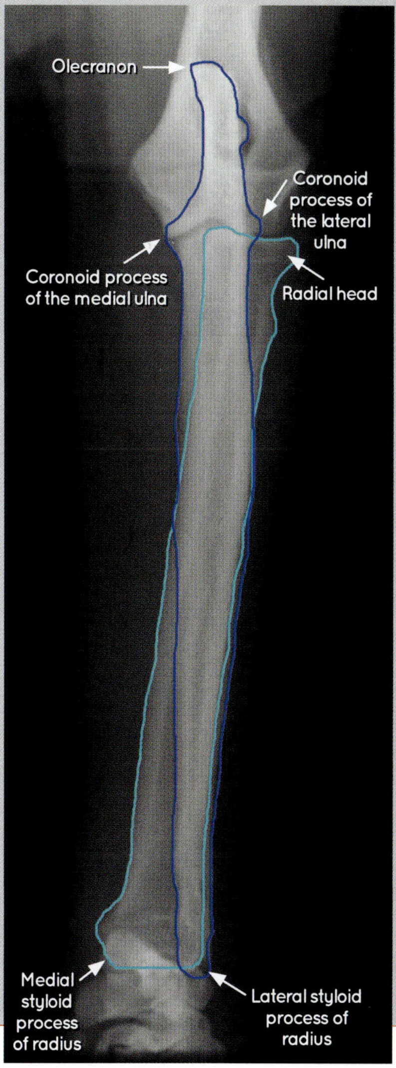

FIGURE A.20. Image of the craniocaudal projection of the radius and ulna of a dog.

Carpus

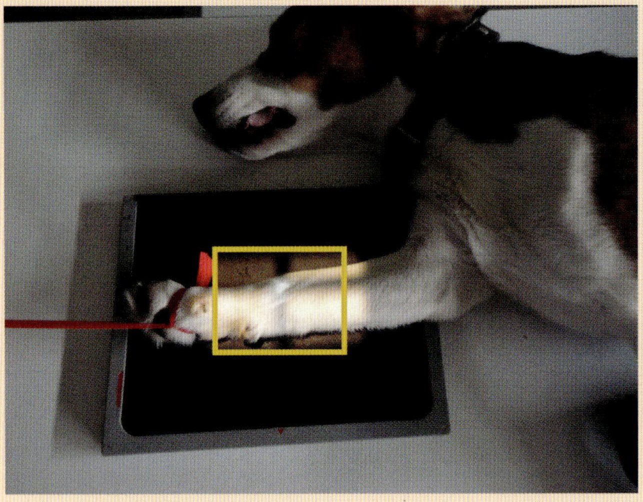

FIGURE P.22. Right lateral decubitus position to obtain the mediolateral projection of the right carpus of a dog.

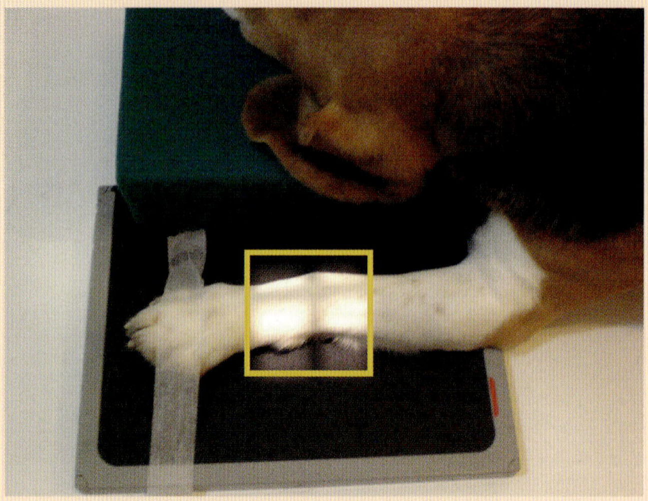

FIGURE P.23. Ventral decubitus position to obtain the dorsopalmar projection of the left carpus of a dog.

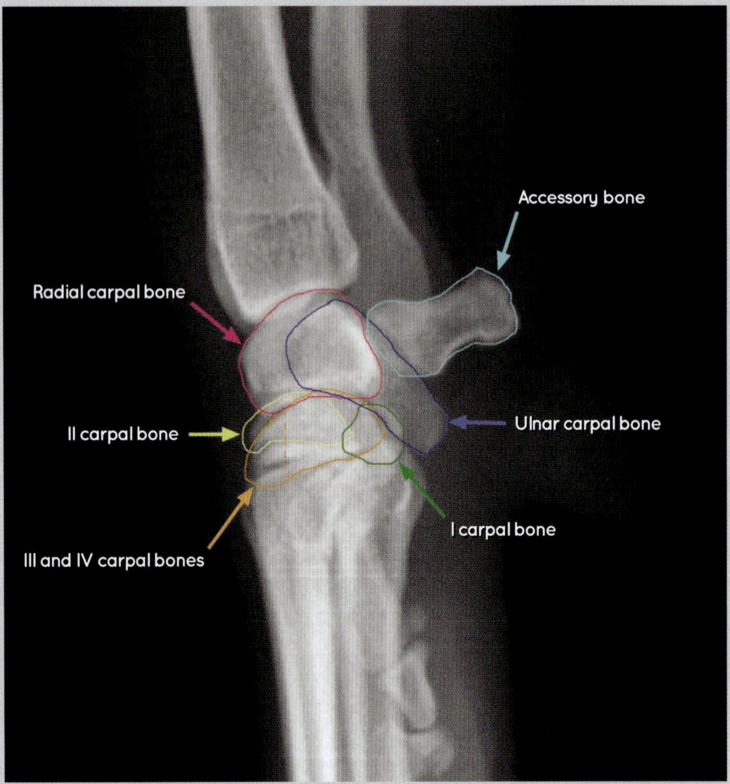

FIGURE A.21. Image of the mediolateral projection of the carpus of a dog.

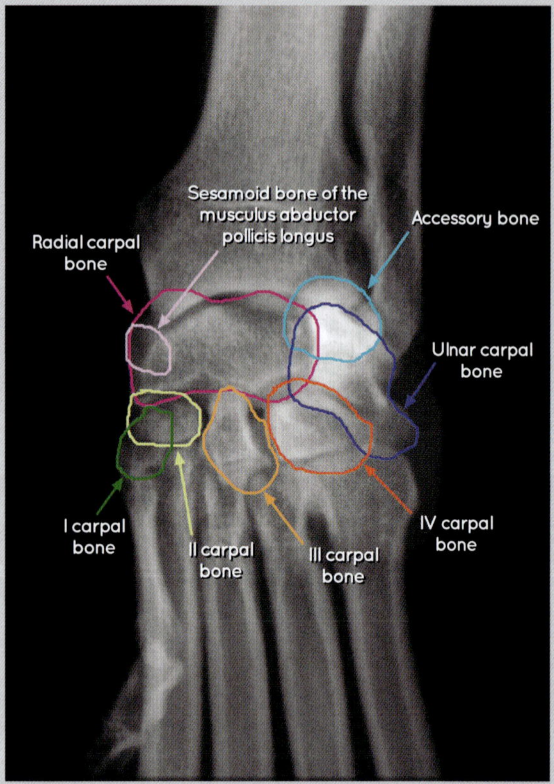

FIGURE A.22. Image of the dorsopalmar projection of the carpus of a dog.

Metacarpus-phalanges

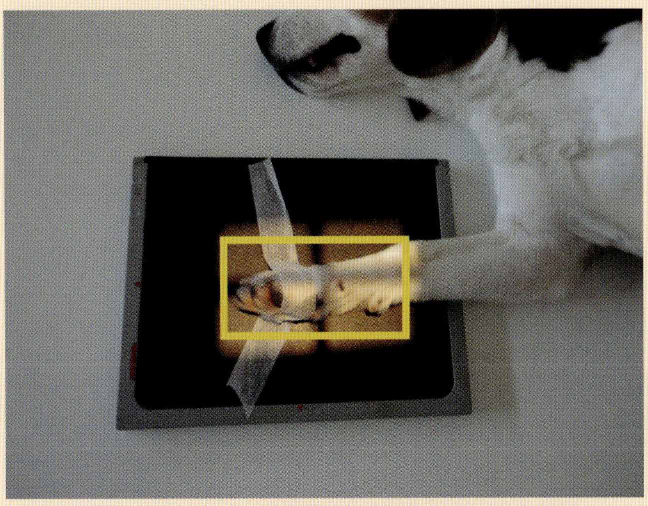

FIGURE P.24. Right lateral decubitus position to obtain the mediolateral projection of the right metacarpals and phalanges of a dog.

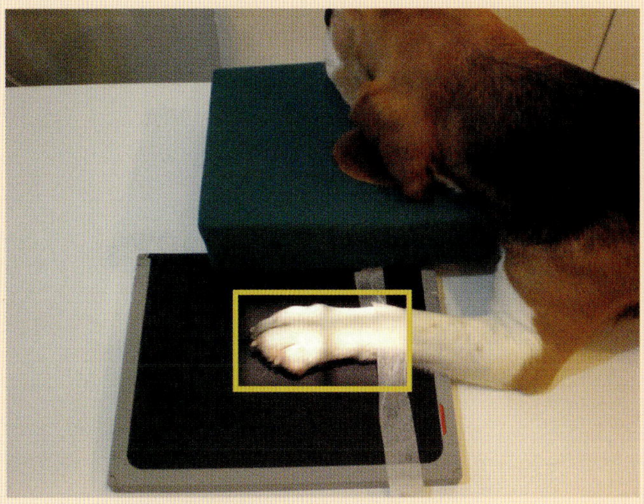

FIGURE P.25. Ventral decubitus position to obtain dorsopalmar projection of the left metacarpals and phalanges of a dog.

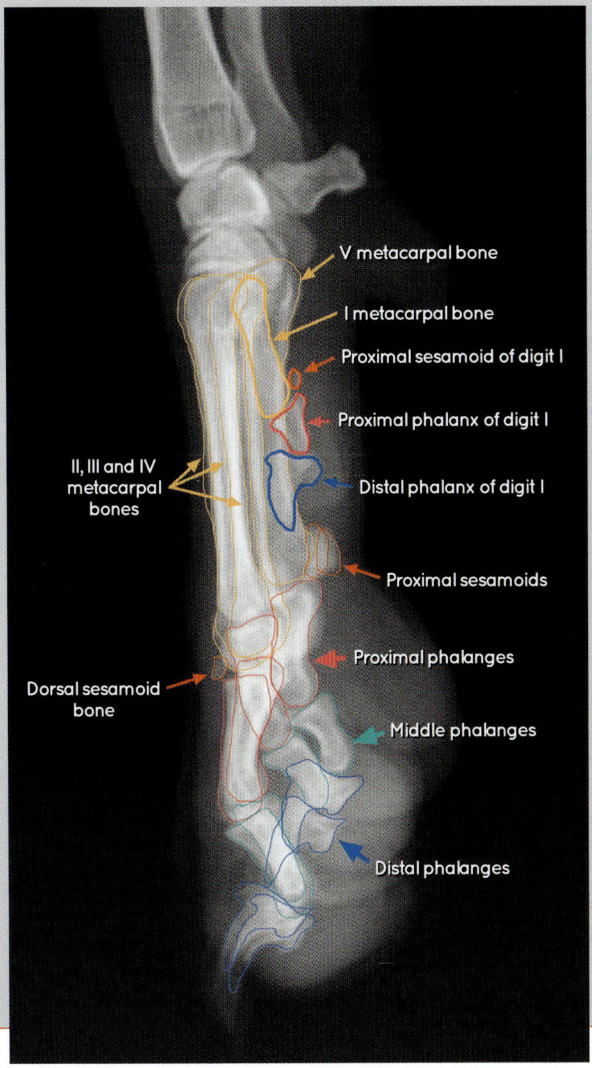

FIGURE A.23. Image of the mediolateral projection of the metacarpals and phalanges of a dog.

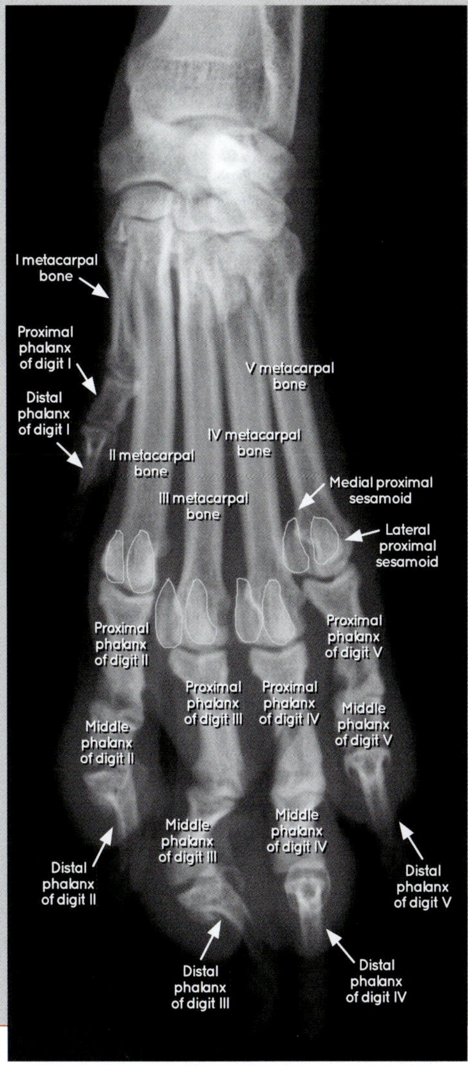

FIGURE A.24. Image of the dorsopalmar projection of the metacarpals and phalanges of a dog.

APPENDICULAR SKELETON

PELVIC LIMB

Hip

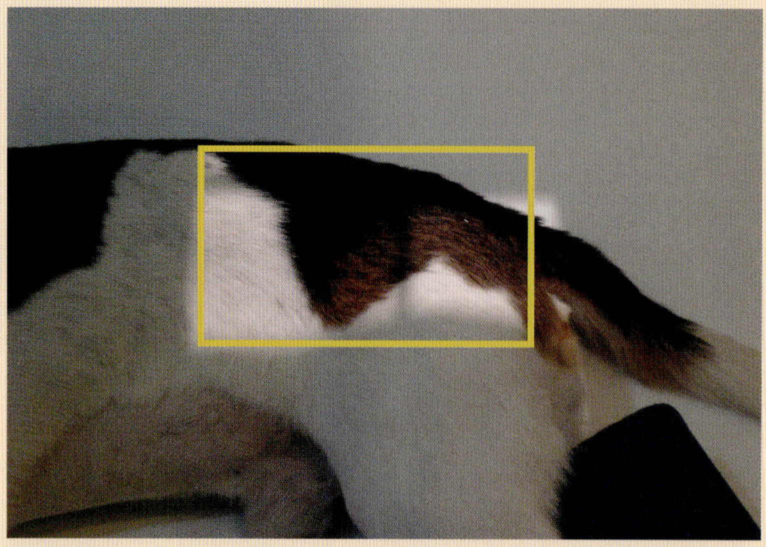

FIGURE P.26. Right lateral decubitus position to obtain the lateral projection of the hip of a dog.

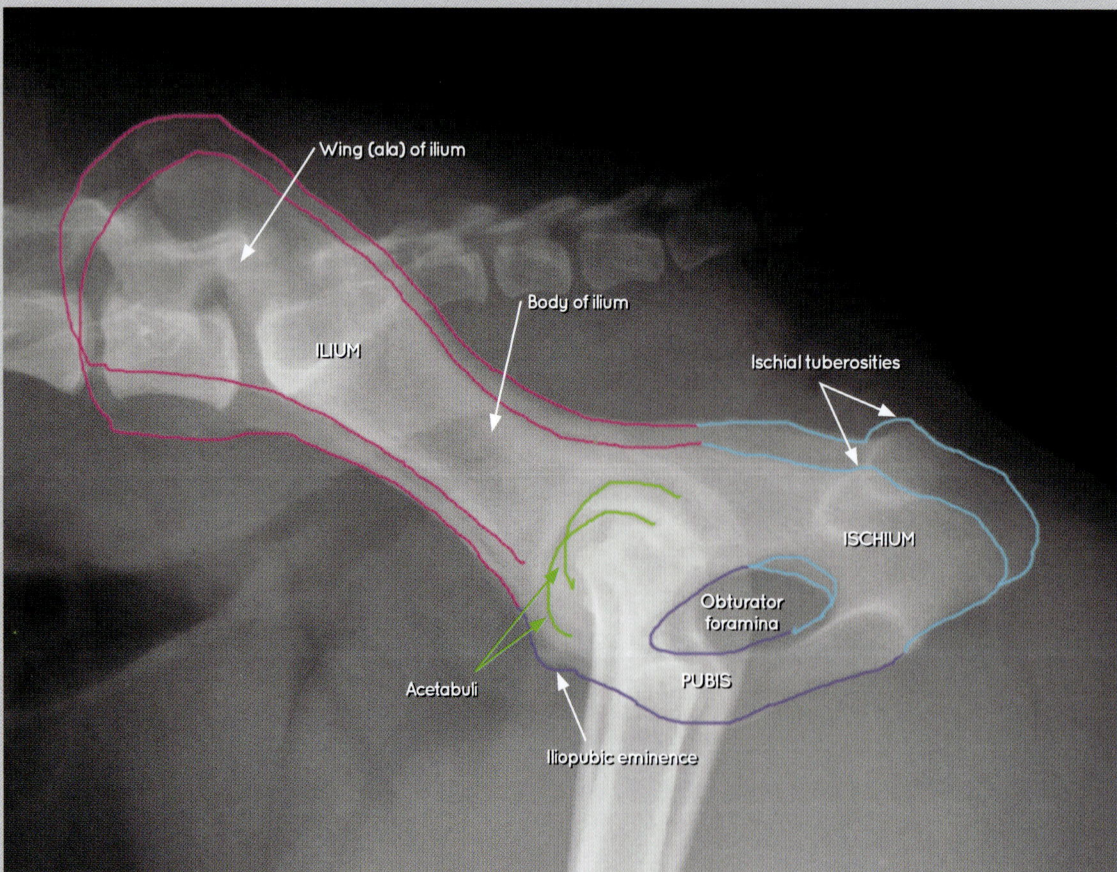

FIGURE A.25. Image of the lateral projection of the hip of a dog.

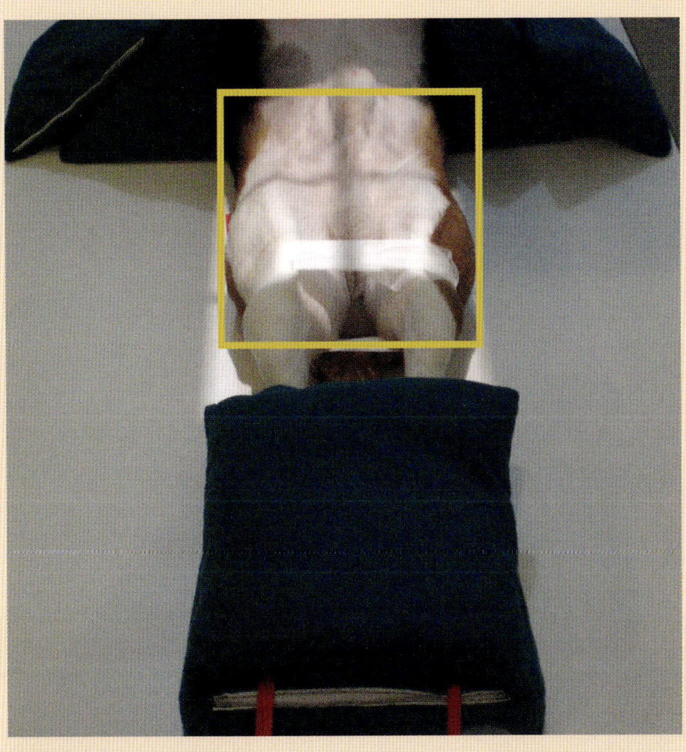

FIGURE P.27. Dorsal decubitus position to obtain the standard ventrodorsal projection of the hip of a dog.

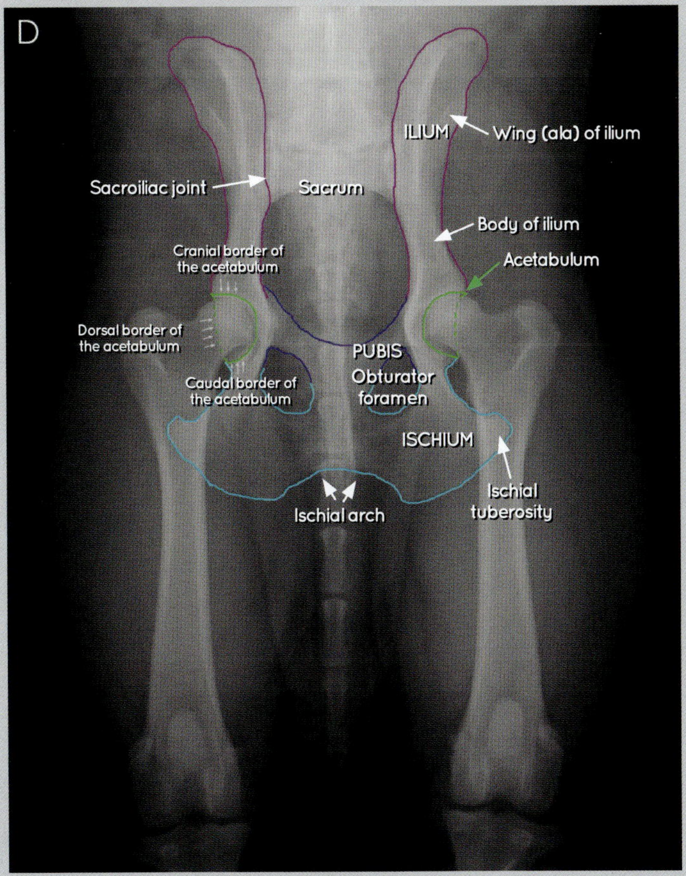

FIGURE A.26. Image of the standard ventrodorsal projection of the hip of a dog.

Femur

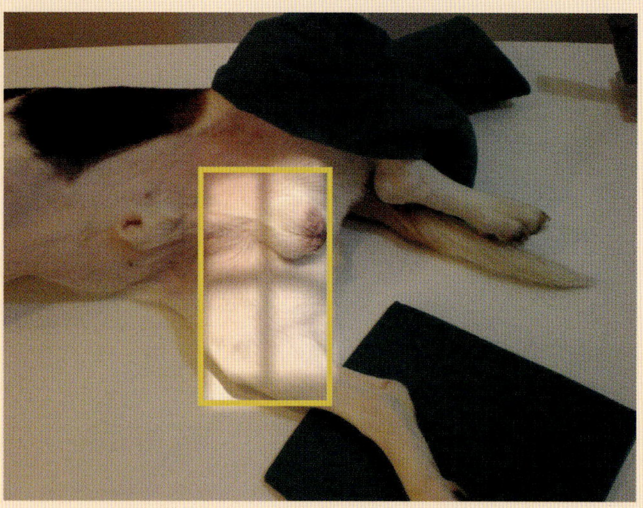

FIGURE P.28. Right lateral decubitus position to obtain the mediolateral projection of the right femur of a dog.

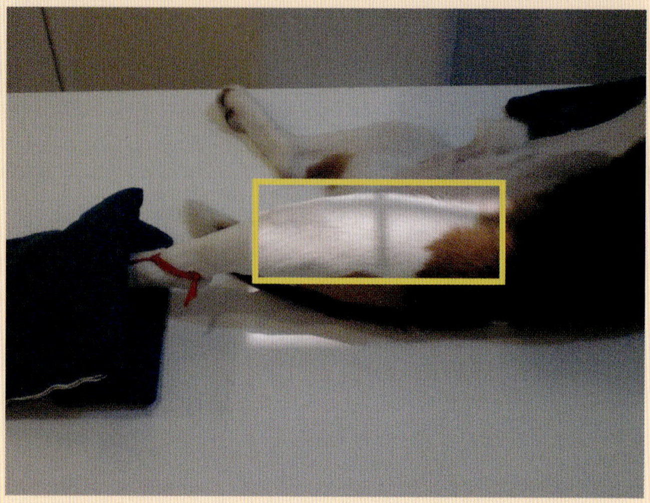

FIGURE P.29. Dorsal position to obtain the craniocaudal projection of the left femur of a dog.

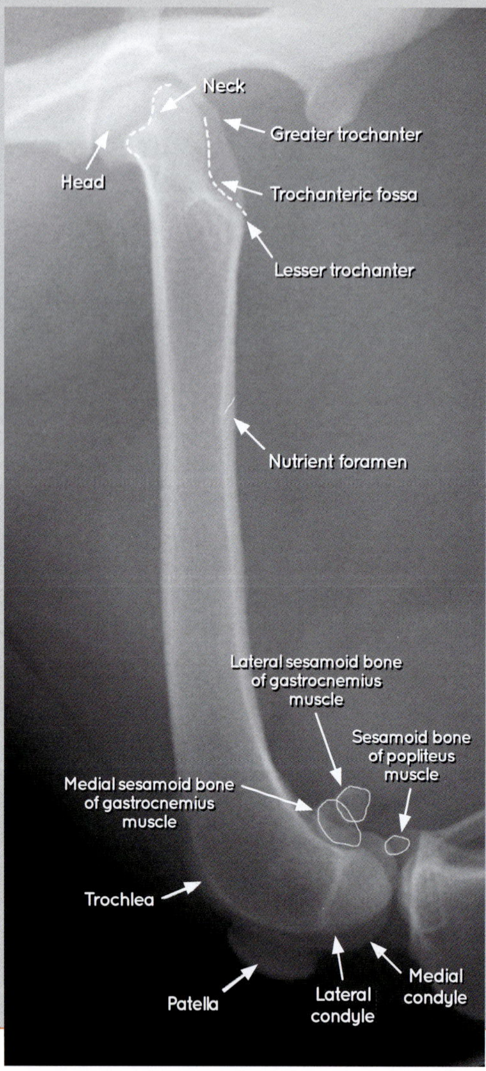

FIGURE A.27. Image of the mediolateral projection of the femur of a dog.

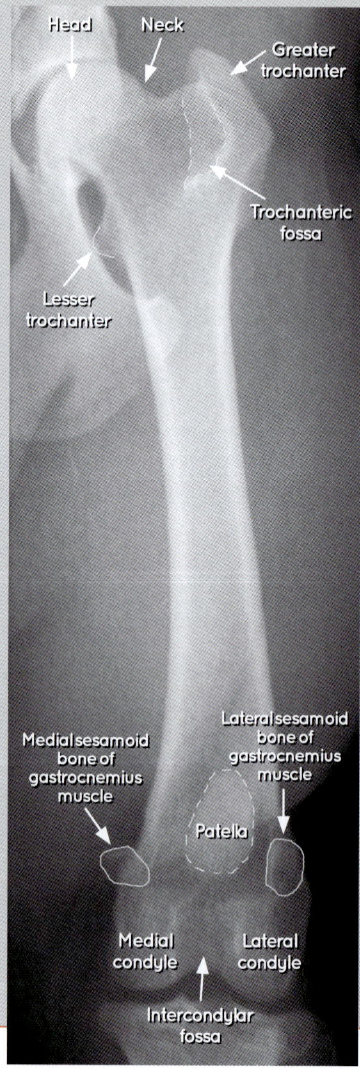

FIGURE A.28. Image of the craniocaudal projection of the femur of a dog.

Knee

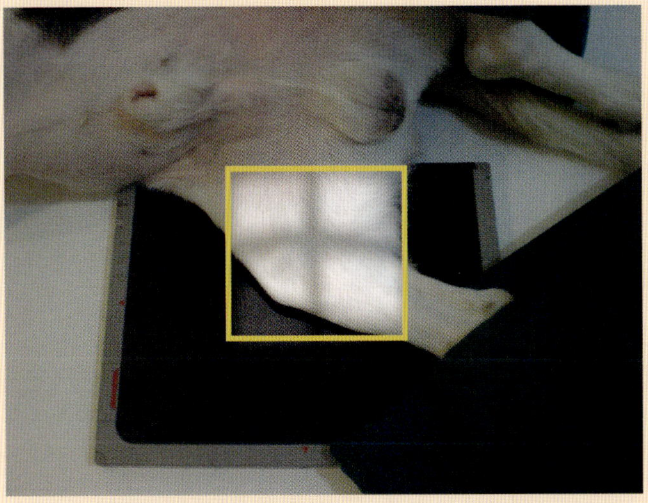

FIGURE P.30. Right lateral decubitus position to obtain the mediolateral projection of the right knee of a dog.

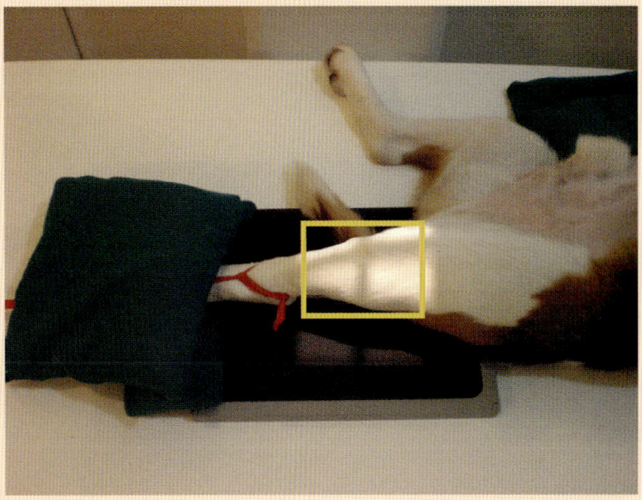

FIGURE P.31. Dorsal decubitus position to obtain the craniocaudal projection of the left knee of a dog.

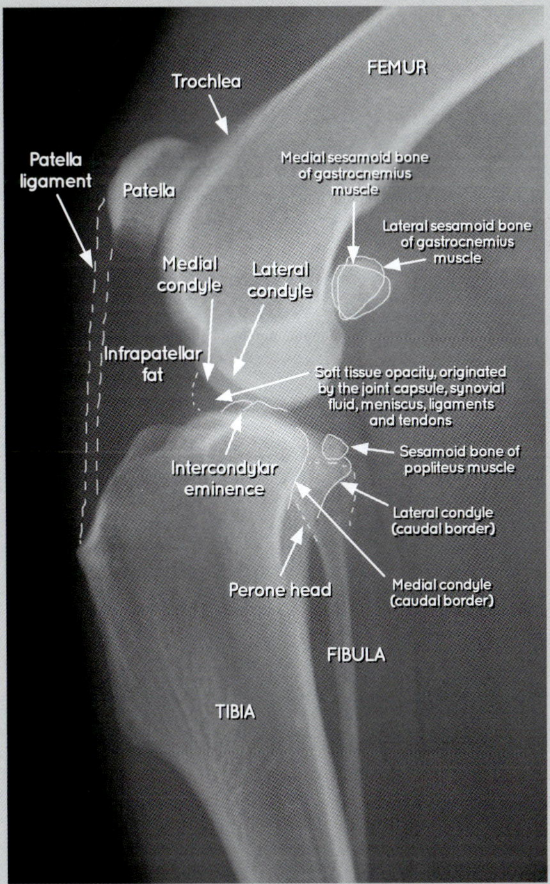

FIGURE A.29. Image of the mediolateral projection of the knee of a dog.

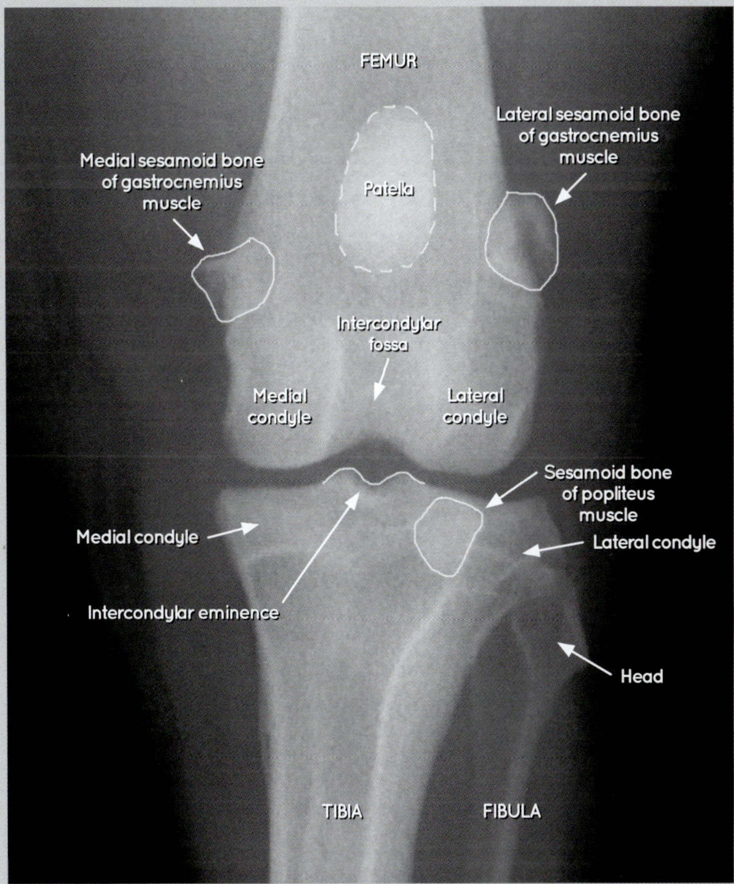

FIGURE A.30. Image of the craniocaudal projection of the knee of a dog.

Tibia-fibula

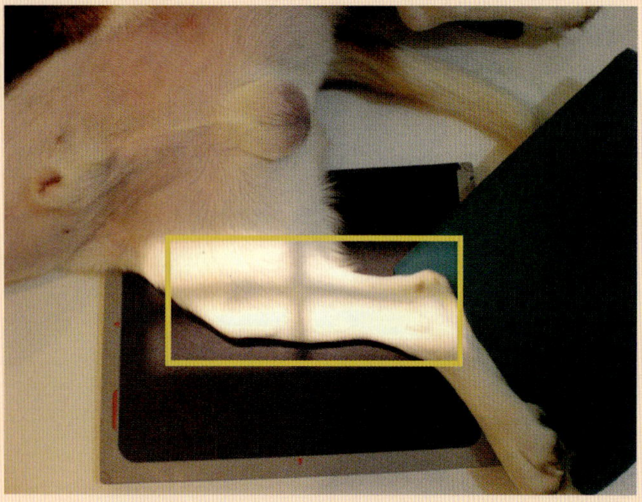

FIGURE P.32. Right lateral decubitus position to obtain the mediolateral projection of the right tibia and fibula of a dog.

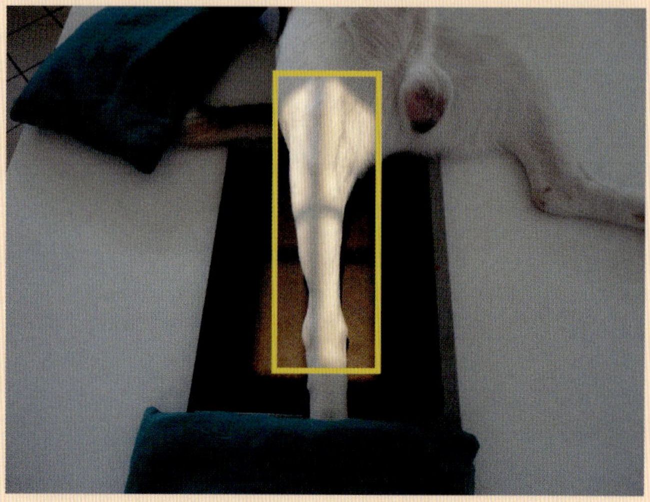

FIGURE P.33. Dorsal decubitus position to obtain the craniocaudal projection of the right tibia and fibula of a dog.

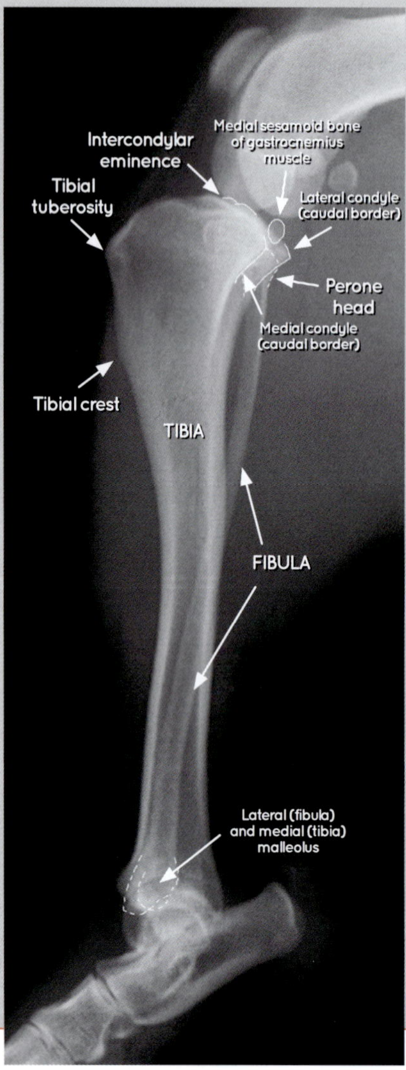

FIGURE A.31. Image of the mediolateral projection of the tibia and fibula of a dog.

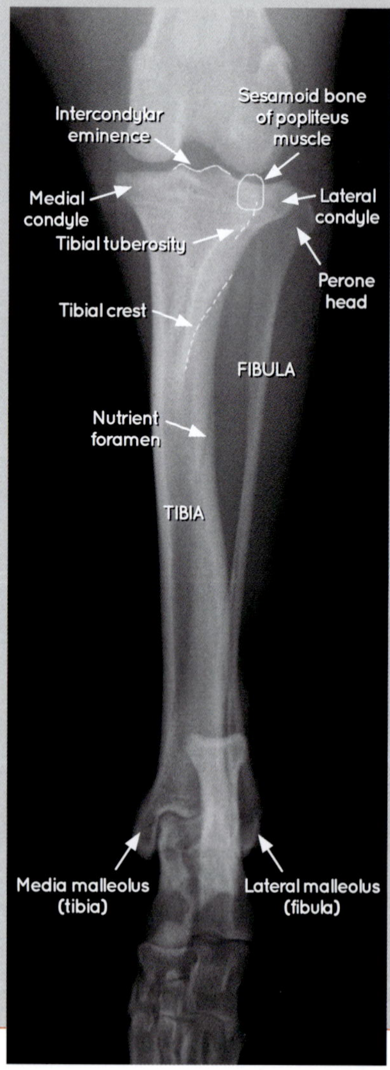

FIGURE A.32. Image of the craniocaudal projection of the tibia and fibula of a dog.

Tarsus

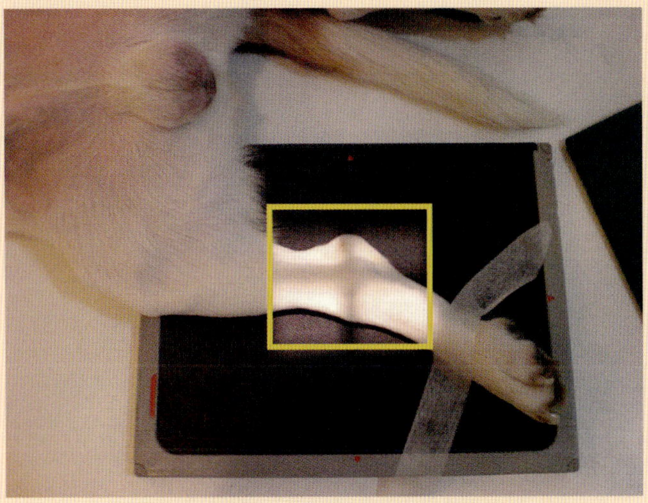

FIGURE P.34. Right lateral decubitus position to obtain the mediolateral projection of the right tarsus of a dog.

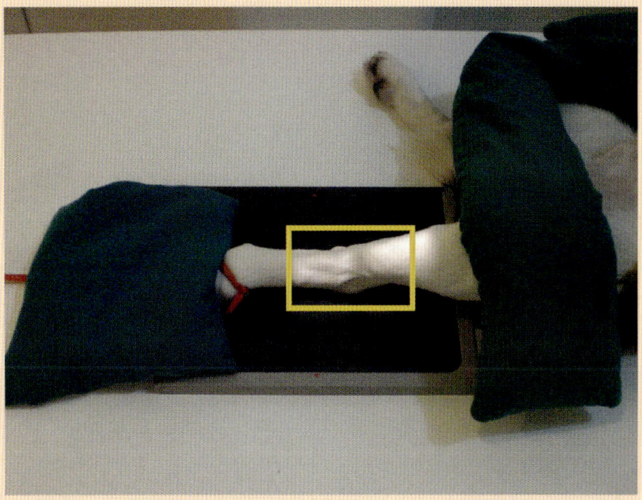

FIGURE P.35. Dorsal decubitus position to obtain the dorsoplantar projection of the left tarsus of a dog.

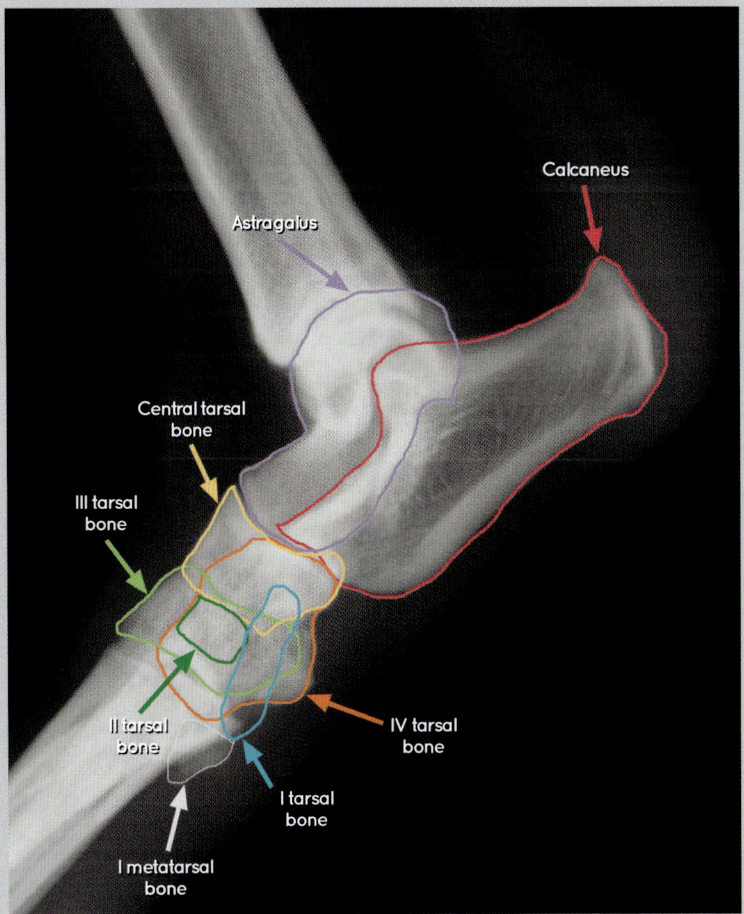

FIGURE A.33. Image of the mediolateral projection of the tarsus of a dog.

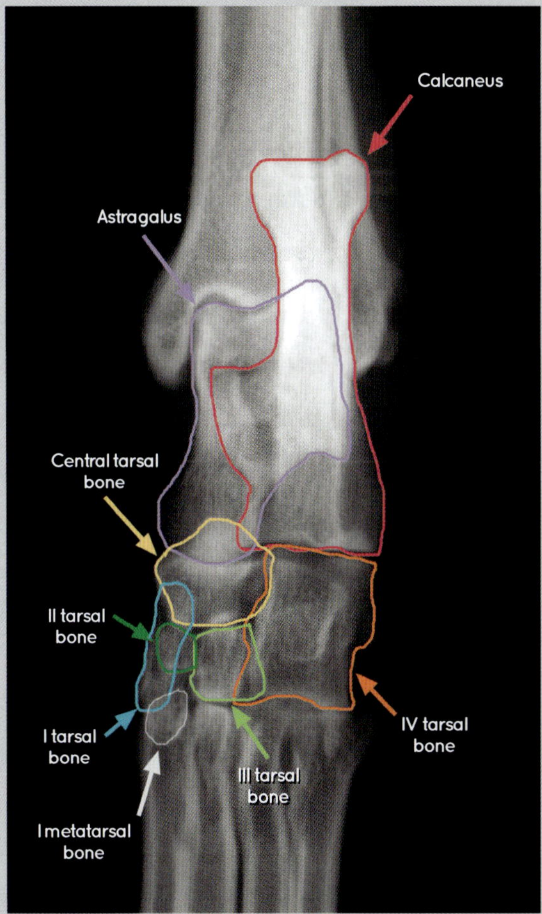

FIGURE A.34. Image of the dorsoplantar projection of the tarsus of a dog.

Metatarsus-phalanges

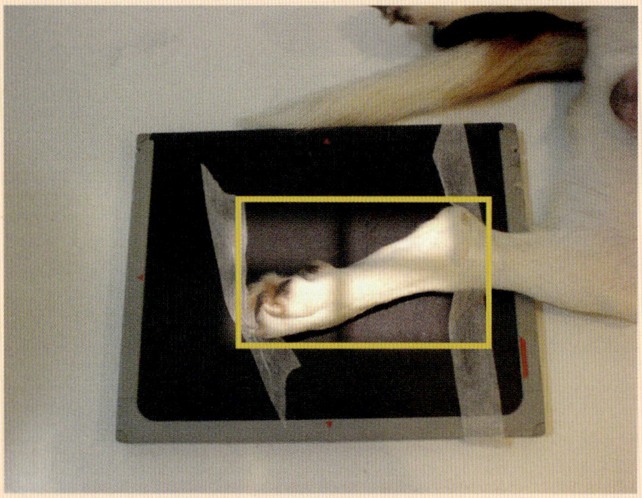

FIGURE P.36. Left lateral decubitus position to obtain the mediolateral projection of the left metatarsal bones and phalanges of a dog.

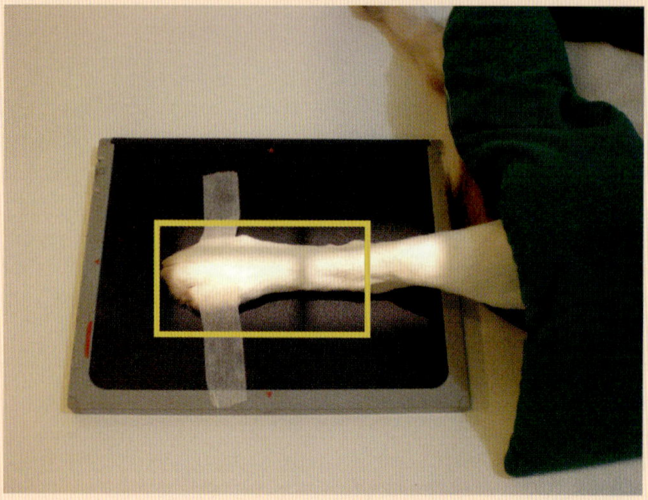

FIGURE P.37. Dorsal decubitus position to obtain dorsoplantar projection of the left metatarsal bones and phalanges of a dog.

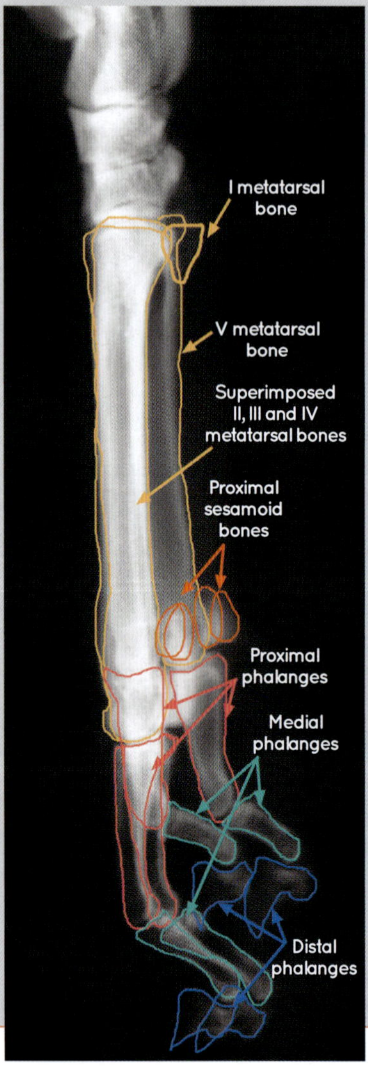

FIGURE A.35. Image of the mediolateral projection of the metatarsal bones and phalanges of a dog.

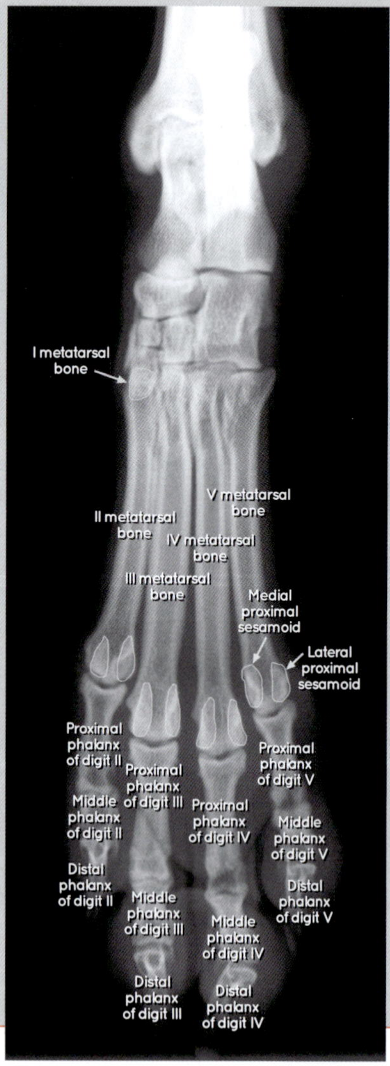

FIGURE A.36. Image of the dorsoplantar projection of the metatarsal bones and phalanges of a dog.

SPINE

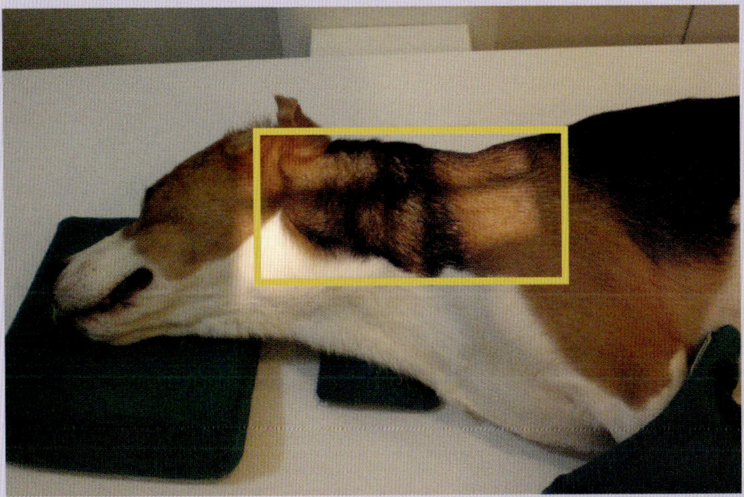

FIGURE P.38. Right lateral decubitus position to obtain the lateral projection of the cervical spine of a dog.

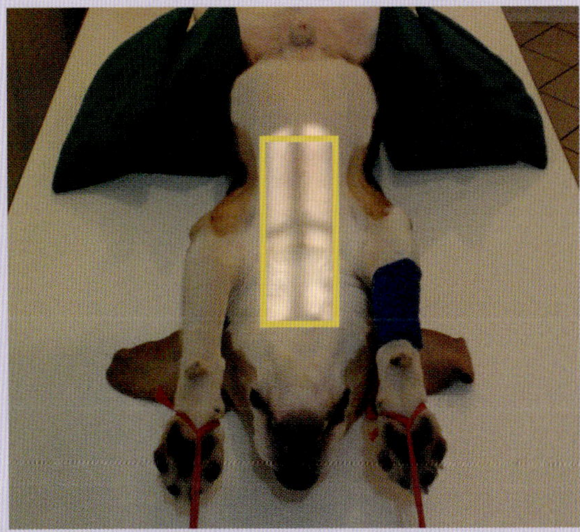

FIGURE P.39. Dorsal decubitus position to obtain the ventrodorsal projection of the cervical spine of a dog.

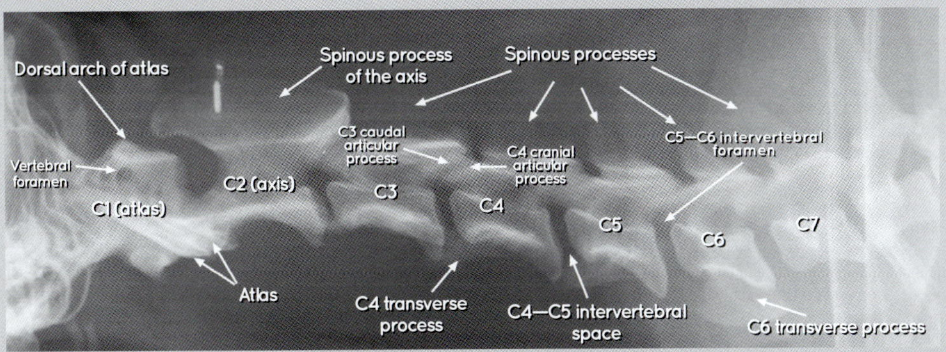

FIGURE A.37. Image of the lateral projection of the cervical spine of a dog.

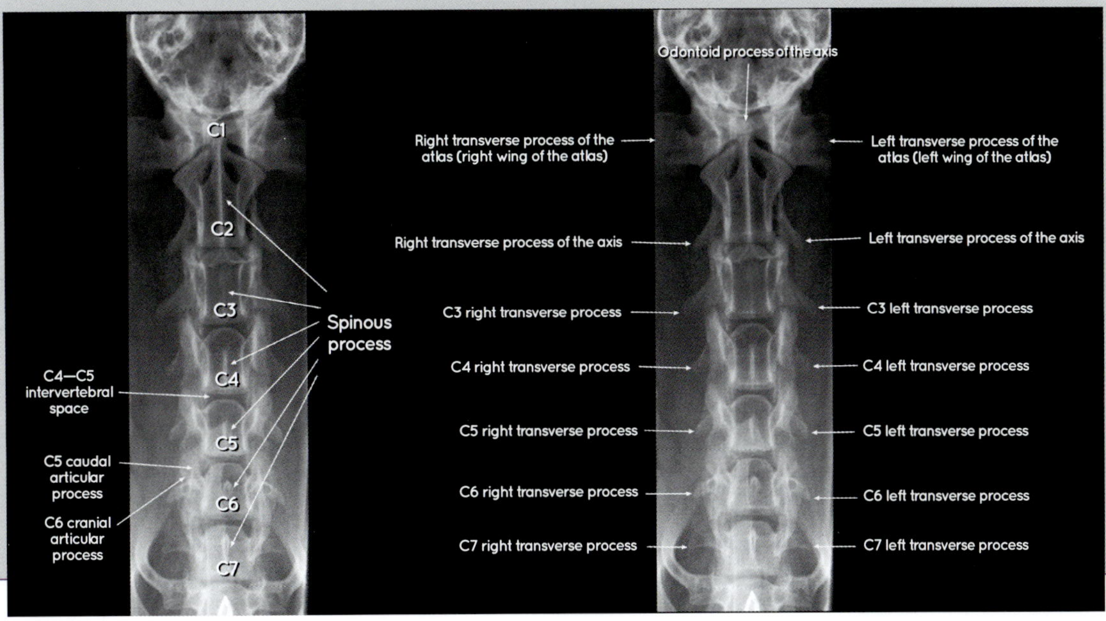

FIGURE A.38. Image of the ventrodorsal projection of the cervical spine in a dog.

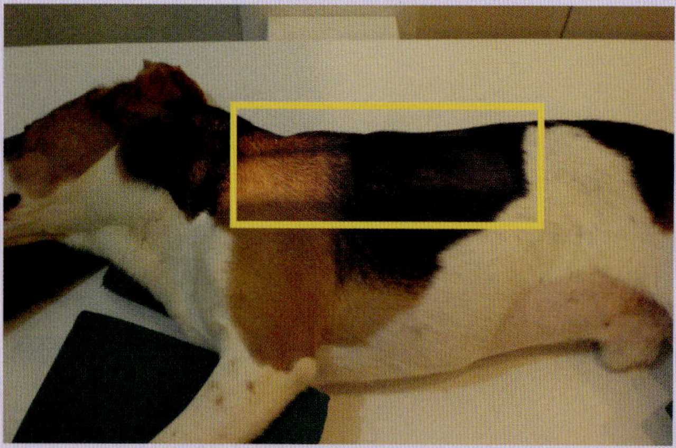

FIGURE P.40. Right lateral decubitus position to obtain the right lateral projection of the thoracic spine of a dog.

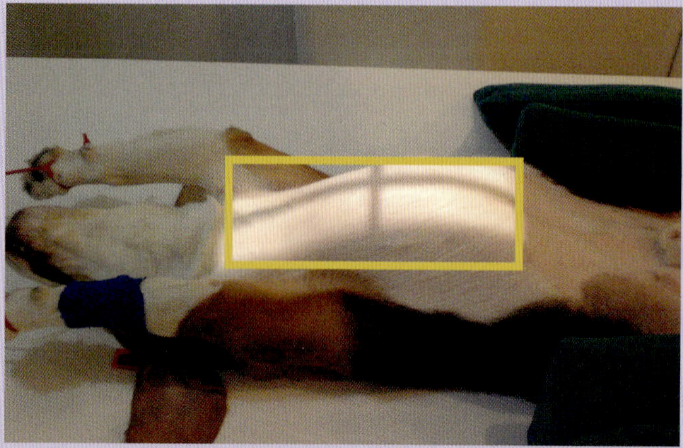

FIGURE P.41. Dorsal decubitus position to obtain the ventrodorsal projection of the thoracic spine of a dog.

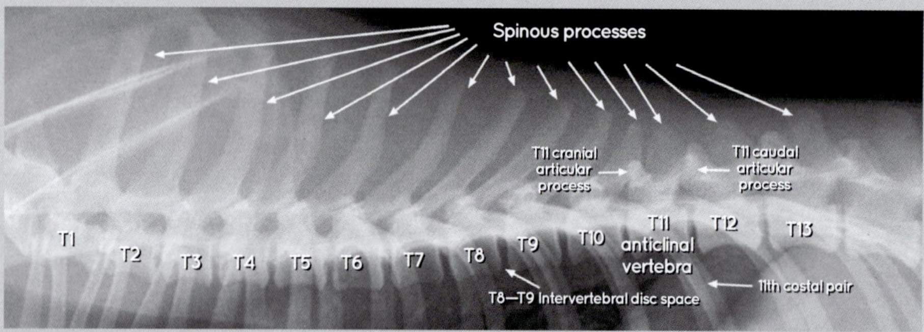

FIGURE A.39. Image of the lateral projection of the thoracic spine of a dog.

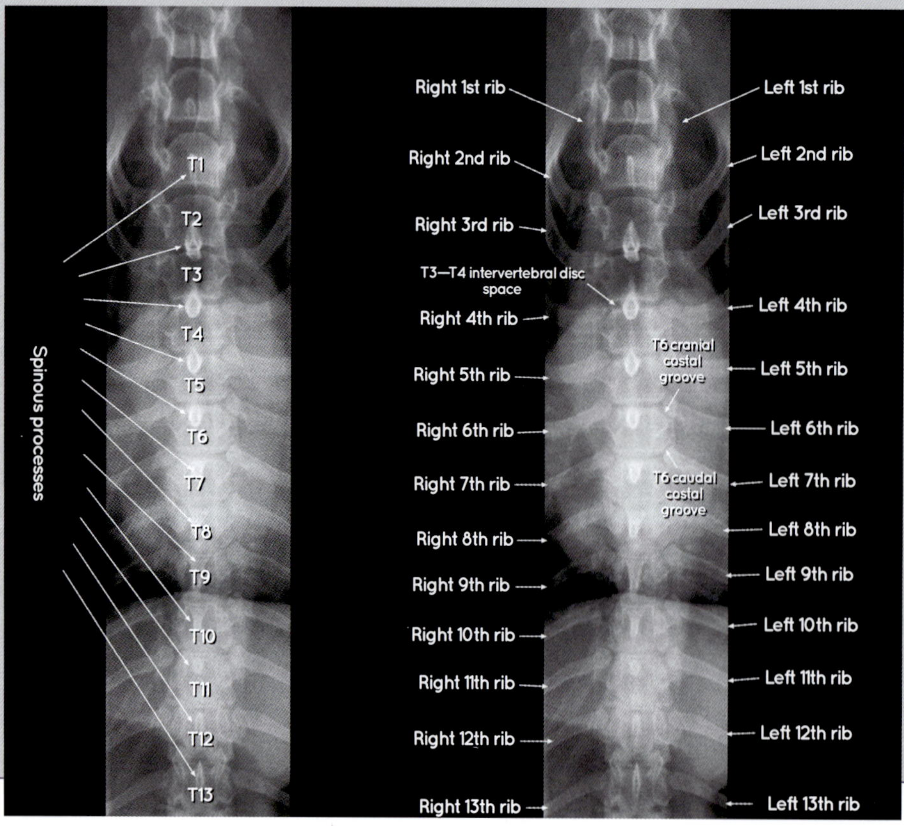

FIGURE A.40. Images of the ventrodorsal projection of the thoracic spine of a dog.

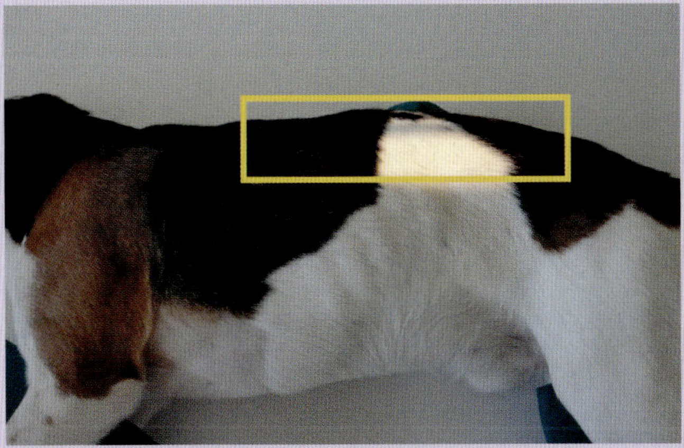

FIGURE P.42. Right lateral decubitus position to obtain the right lateral projection of the thoracolumbar region of a dog.

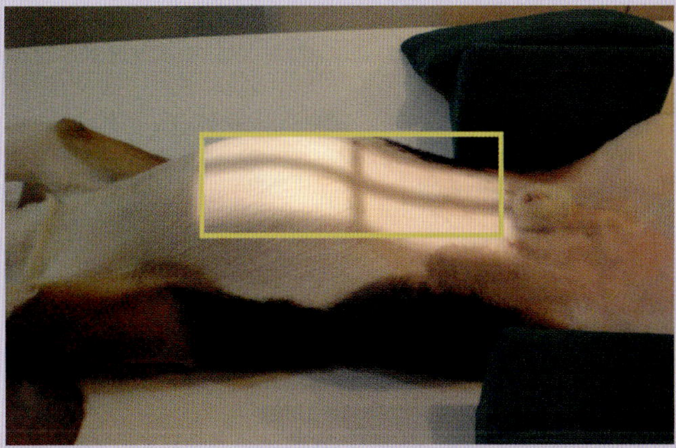

FIGURE P.43. Dorsal decubitus position to obtain the ventrodorsal projection of the thoracolumbar region of a dog.

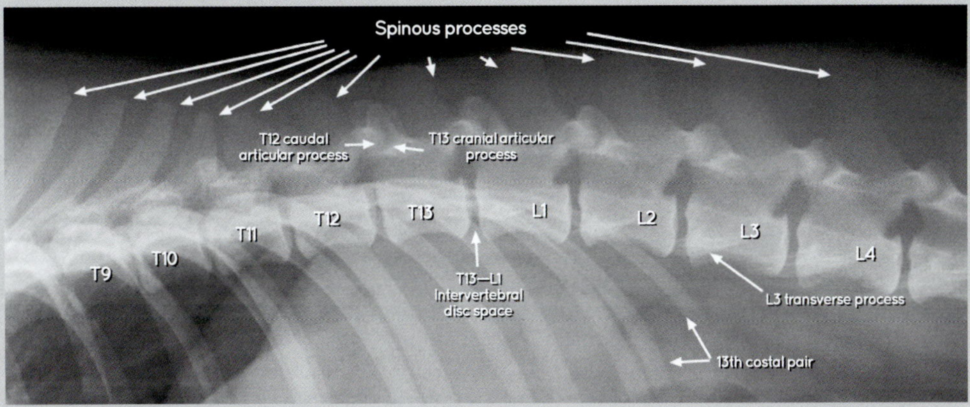

FIGURE A.41. Image of the lateral projection of the thoracolumbar region of a dog.

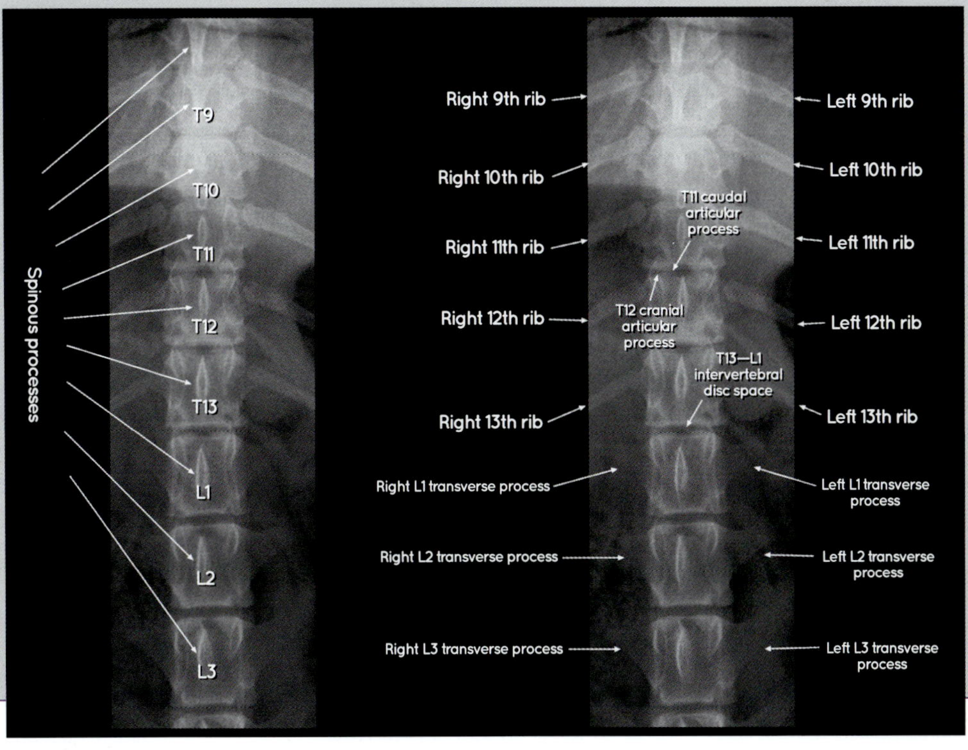

FIGURE A.42. Images of the ventrodorsal projection of the thoracolumbar of a dog.

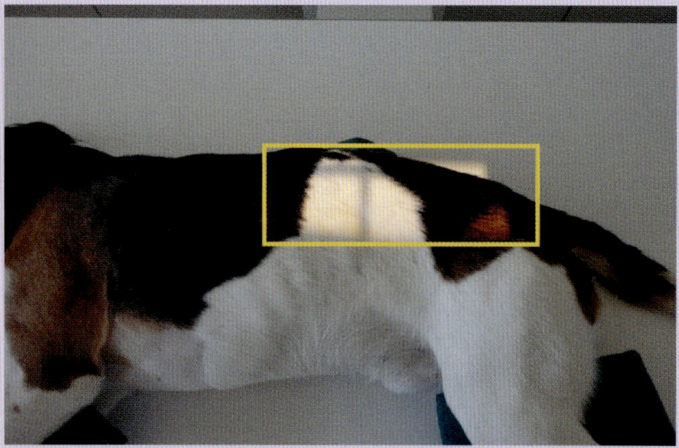

FIGURE P.44. Right lateral decubitus position to obtain the right lateral projection of the lumbar spine of a dog.

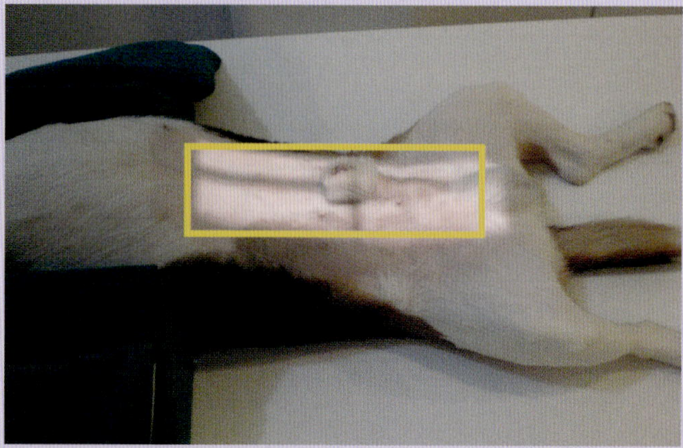

FIGURE P.45. Dorsal decubitus position to obtain the ventrodorsal projection of the lumbar spine of a dog.

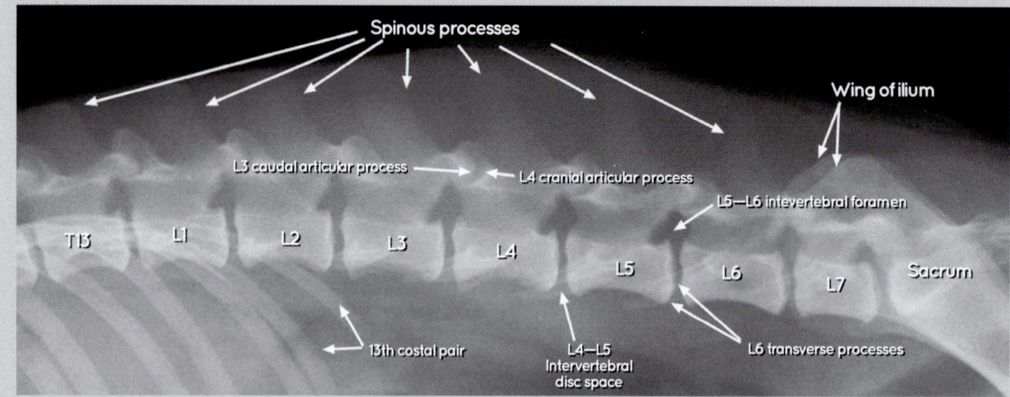

FIGURE A.43. Image of the lateral projection of the lumbar spine of a dog.

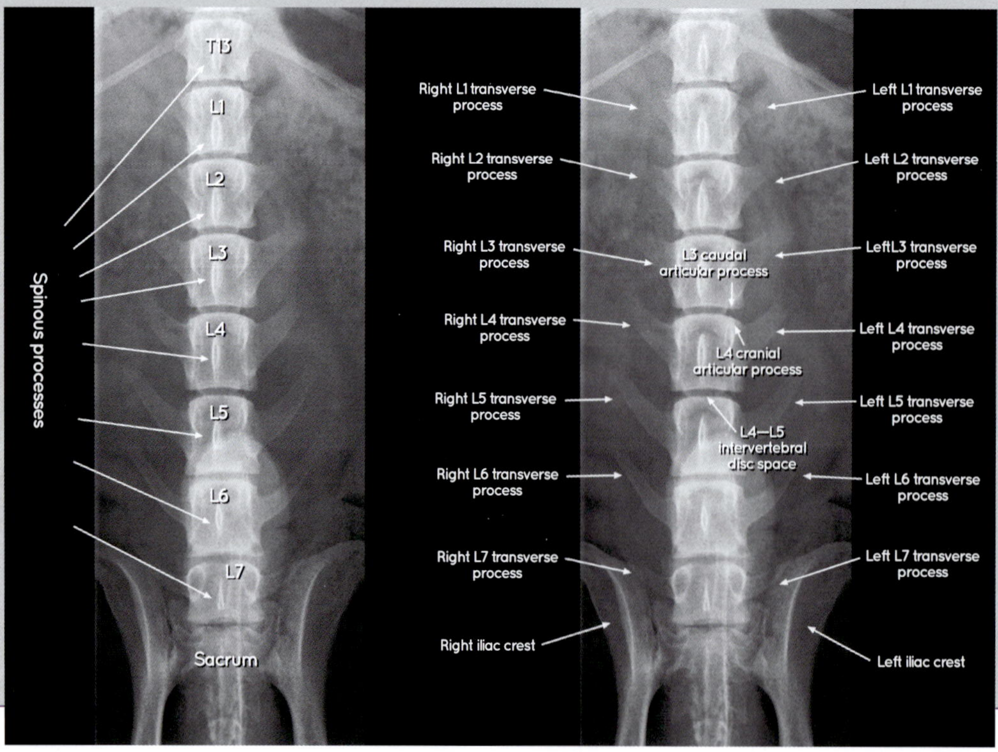

FIGURE A.44. Image of the ventrodorsal projection of the lumbar spine in a dog.

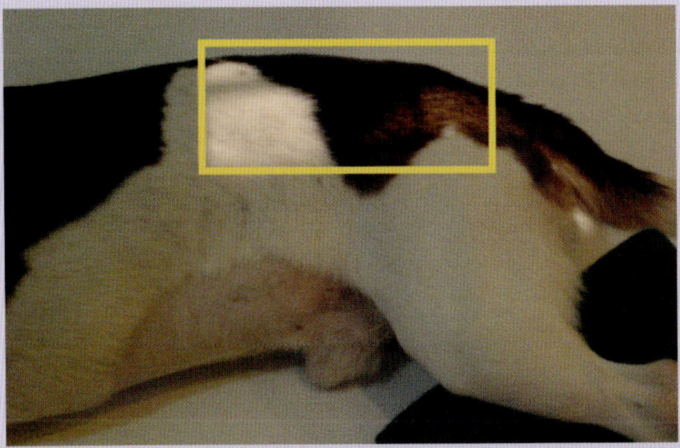

FIGURE P.46. Right lateral decubitus position to obtain the right lateral projection of the lumbosacral region of a dog.

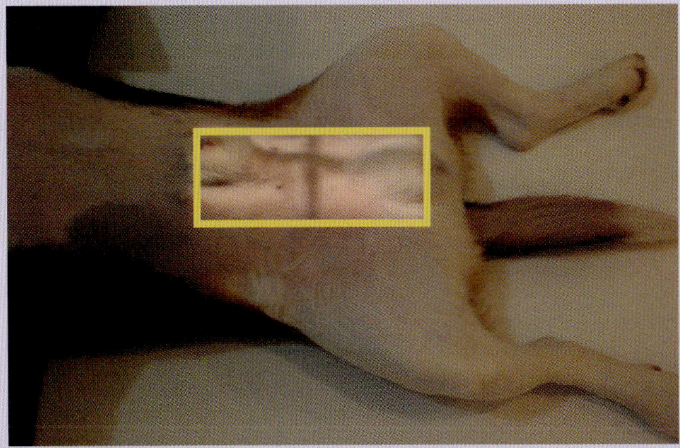

FIGURE P.47. Dorsal decubitus position to obtain the ventrodorsal projection of the lumbosacral region of a dog.

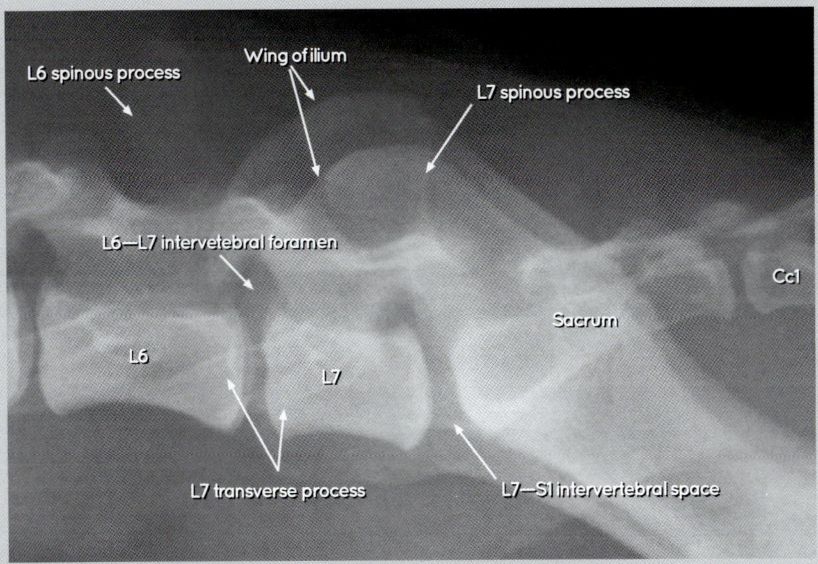

FIGURE A.45. Image of the lateral projection of the lumbosacral region of a dog.

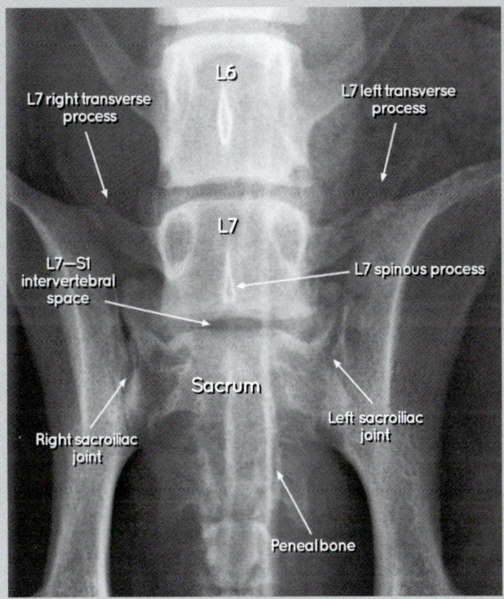

FIGURE A.46. Image of the ventrodorsal projection of the lumbosacral region of a dog.

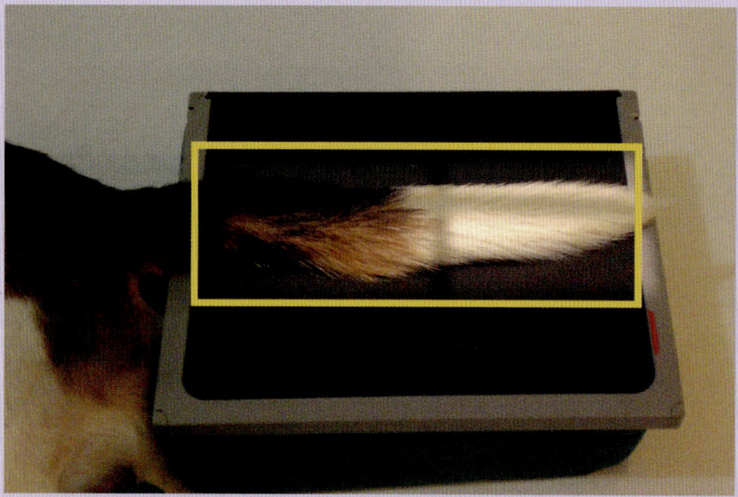

FIGURE P.48. Right lateral decubitus position to obtain the right lateral projection of the coccygeal vertebrae of a dog.

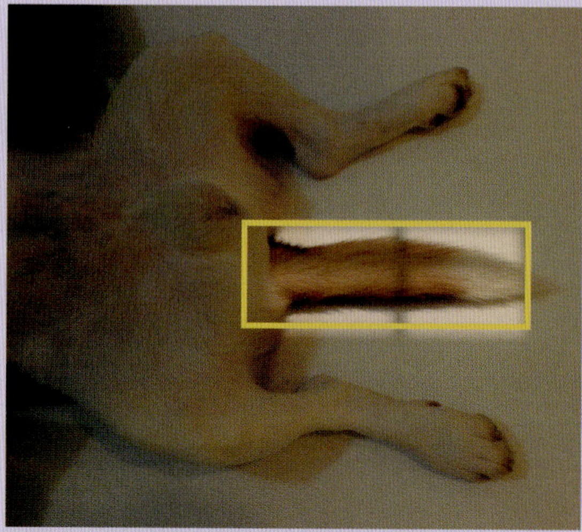

FIGURE P.49. Dorsal decubitus position to obtain the ventrodorsal projection of the coccygeal vertebrae of a dog.

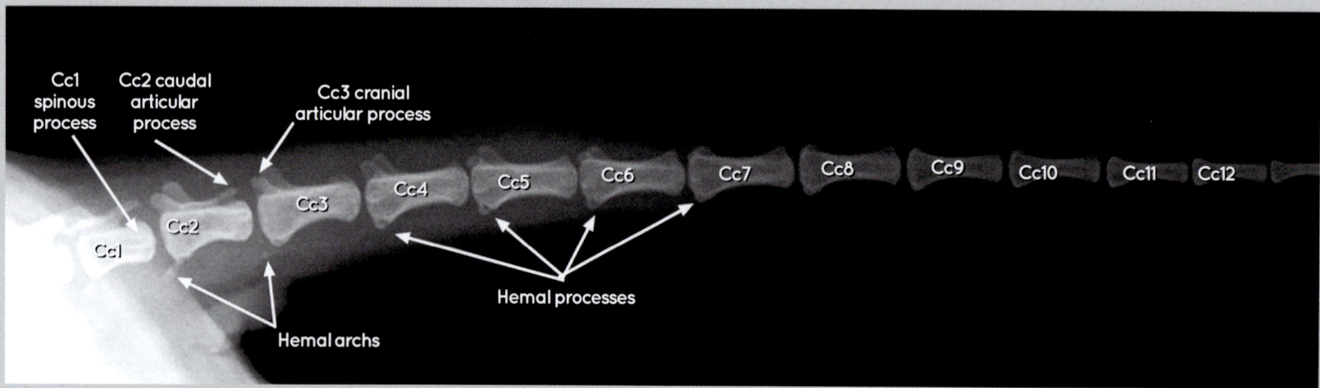

▲ FIGURE A.47. Image of the lateral projection of the coccygeal vertebrae of a dog.

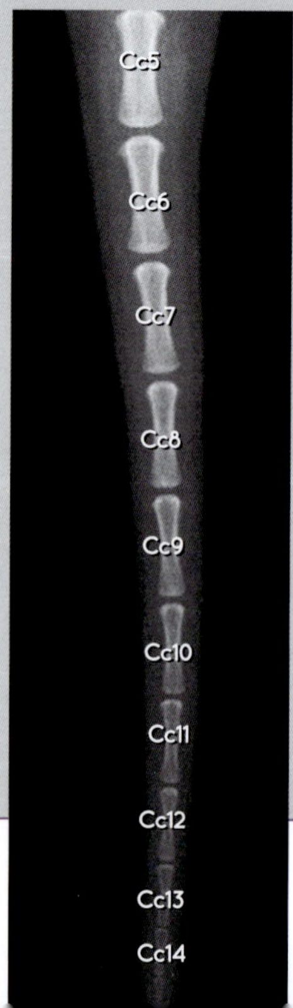

FIGURE A.48. Image of the ventrodorsal projection of the coccygeal vertebrae of a dog. ▶

HEAD

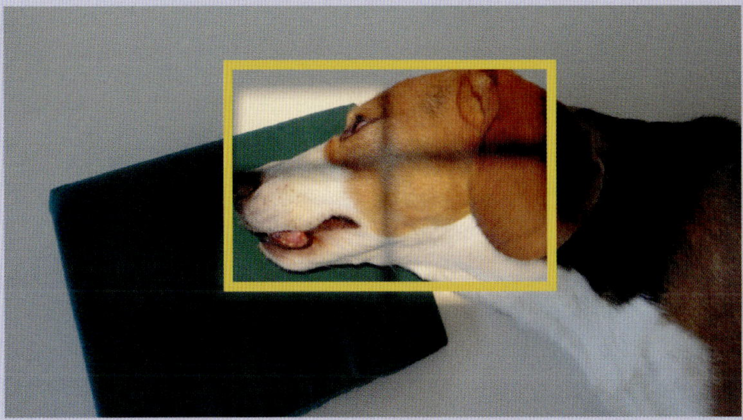

FIGURE P.50. Right lateral decubitus position to obtain the right lateral projection of the head of a dog. Using a 15° radiolucent wedge, the rostral part of the head should be raised to ensure that the sagittal plane of the head is parallel to the X-ray table.

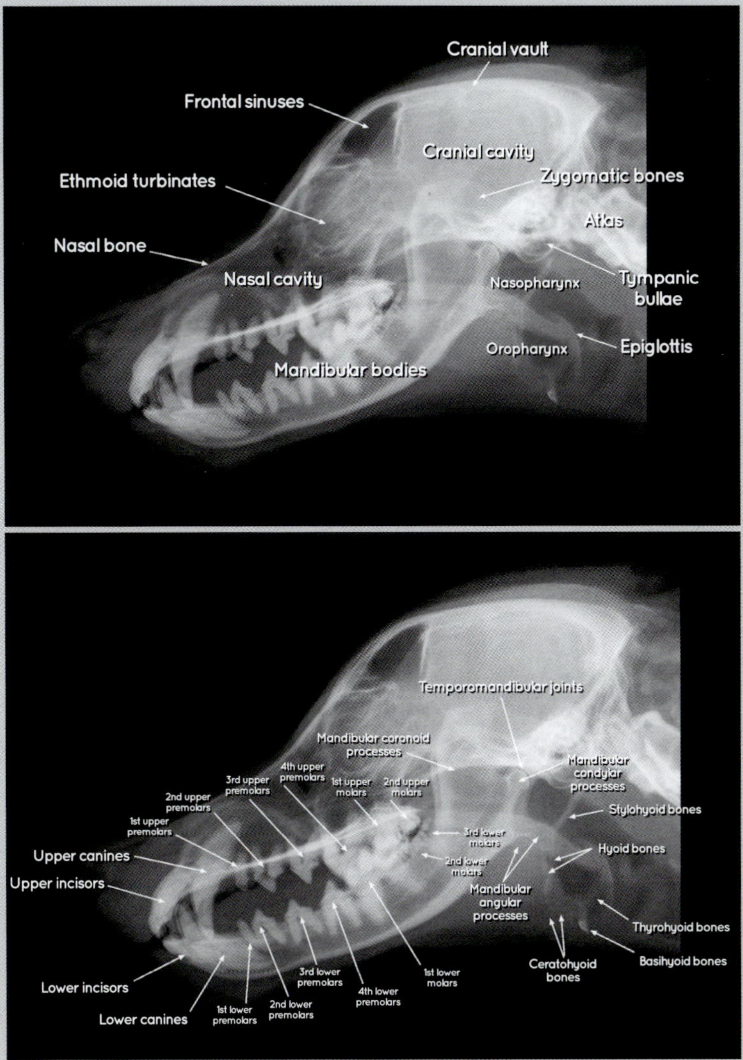

FIGURE A.49. Images of the lateral projection of the head of a dog.

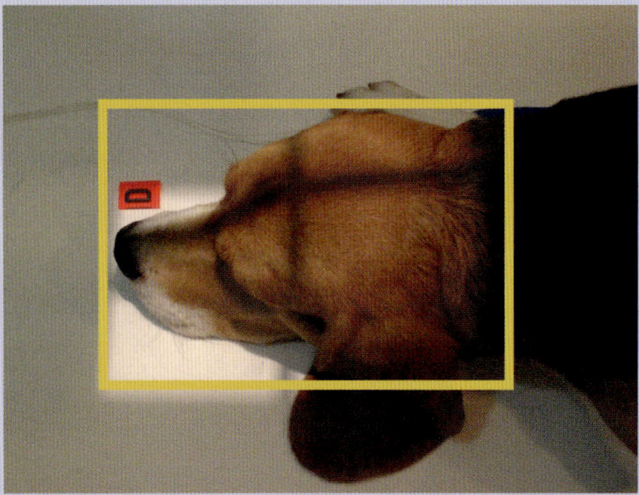

FIGURE P.51. Ventral decubitus position to obtain the dorsoventral projection of the head of a dog.

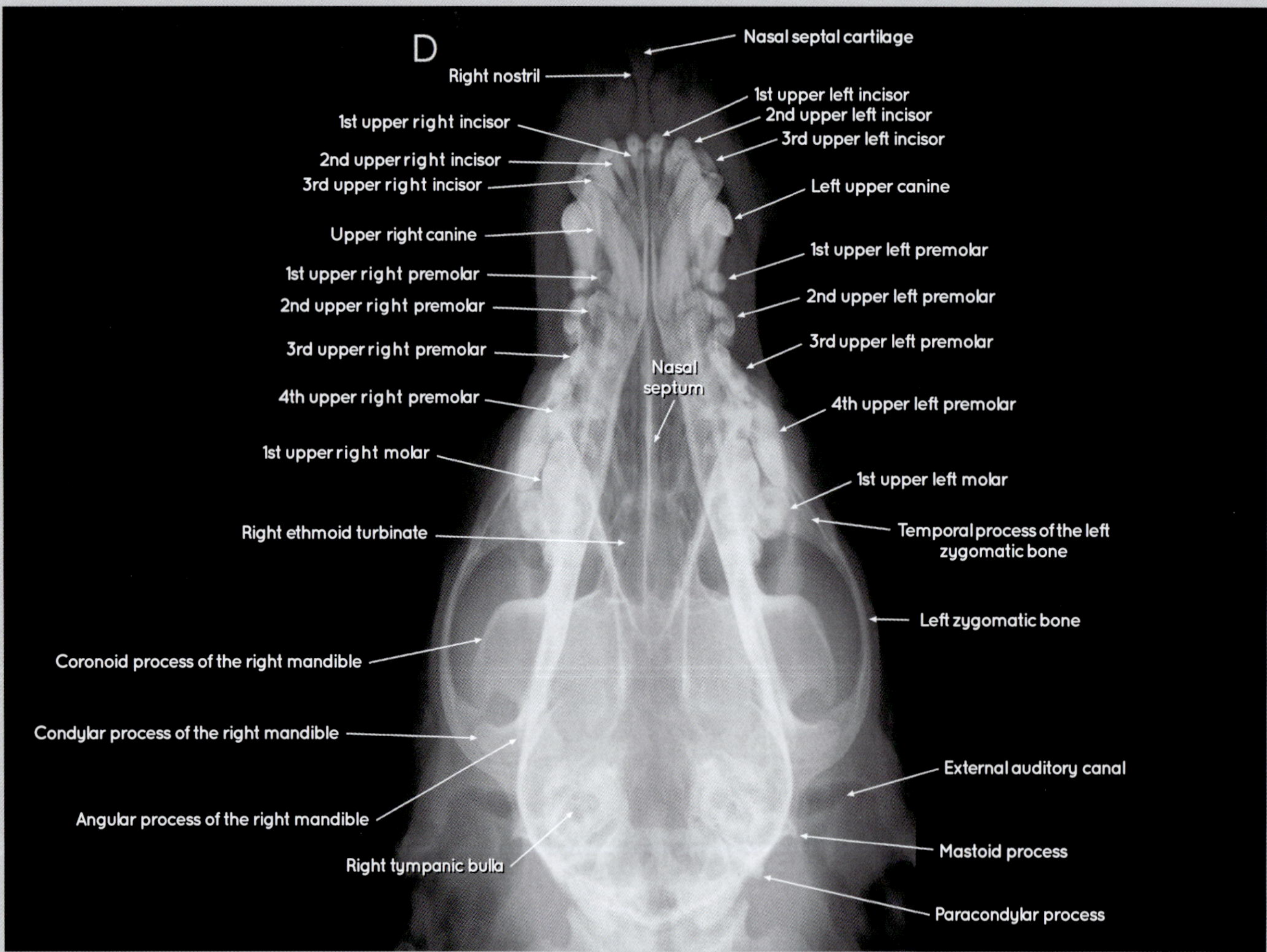

FIGURE A.50. Image of the dorsoventral projection of the head of a dog.

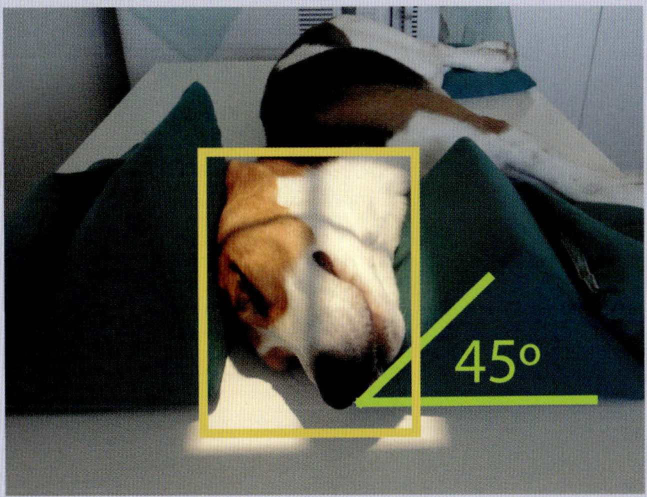

FIGURE P.52. Right lateral decubitus position at a 45° angle of the ventral part of the head to obtain an oblique projection optimising visualisation of the right tympanic bulla in a dog.

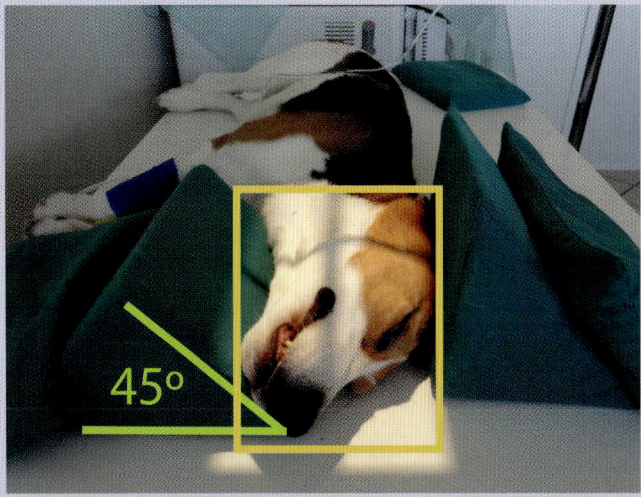

FIGURE P.53. Left lateral decubitus position at a 45° angle of the ventral part of the head to obtain an oblique projection optimising visualisation of the left tympanic bulla in a dog.

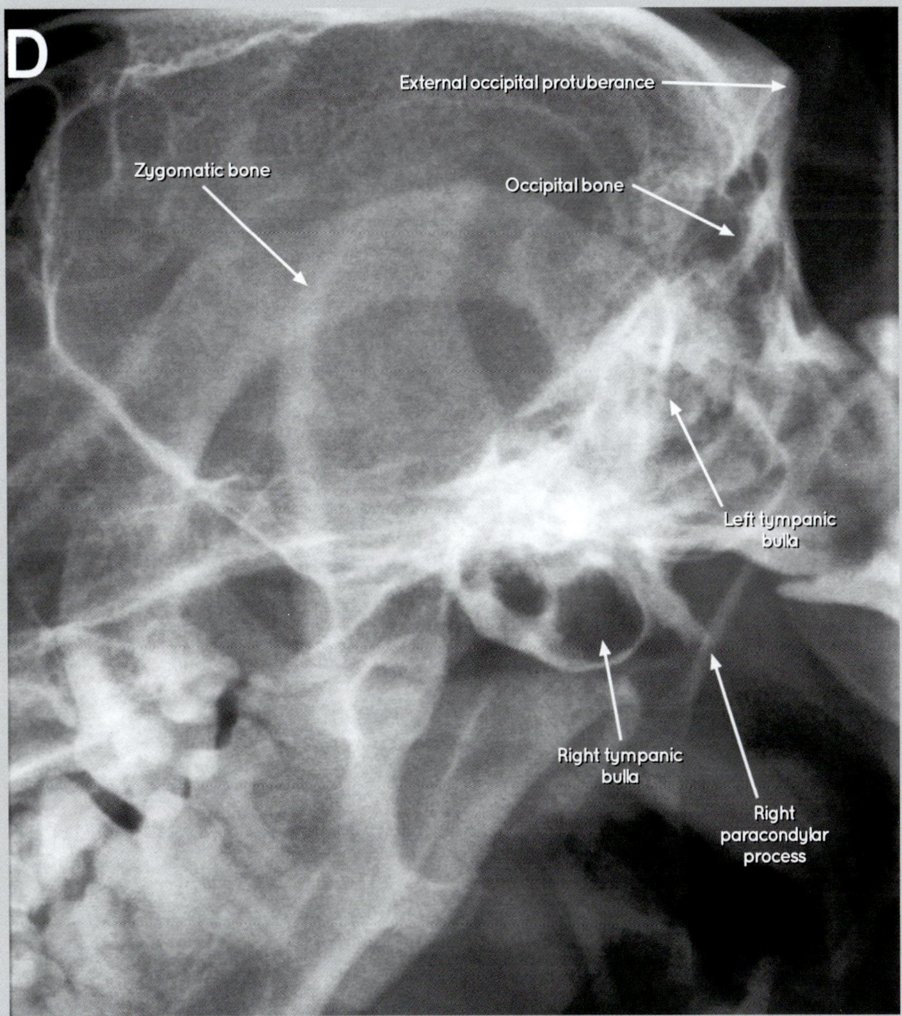

FIGURE A.51. Image of oblique right lateral projection, at a 45° angle, of the ventral part of the head of a dog taken to optimise visualisation of the right tympanic bulla.

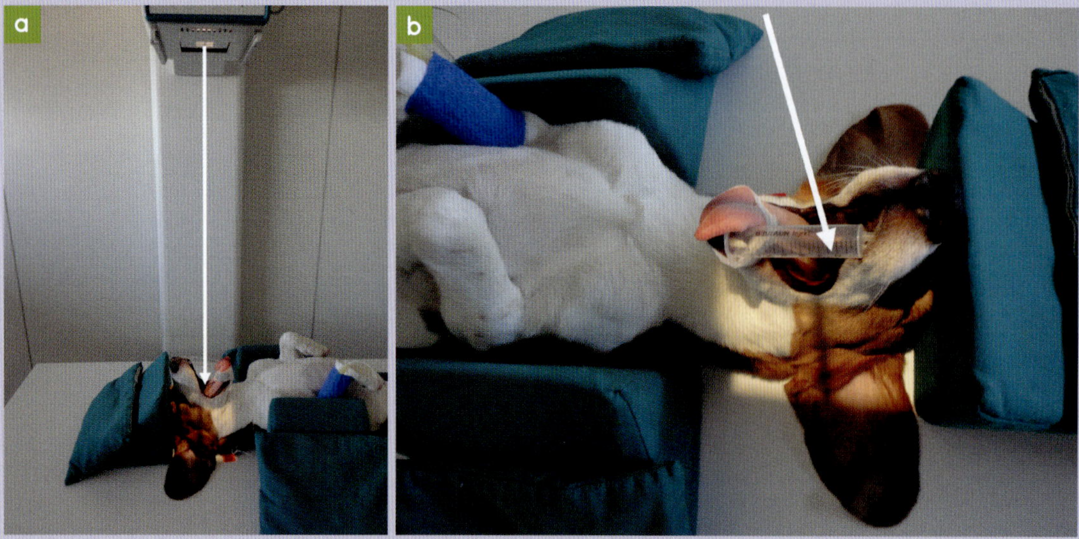

FIGURE P.54. Dorsal decubitus position to obtain the open-mouth rostrocaudal projection to optimise the visualisation of the two tympanic bullae of a dog. The arrow indicates the direction of entry of the X-ray beam. Lateral view (a) and front view (b).

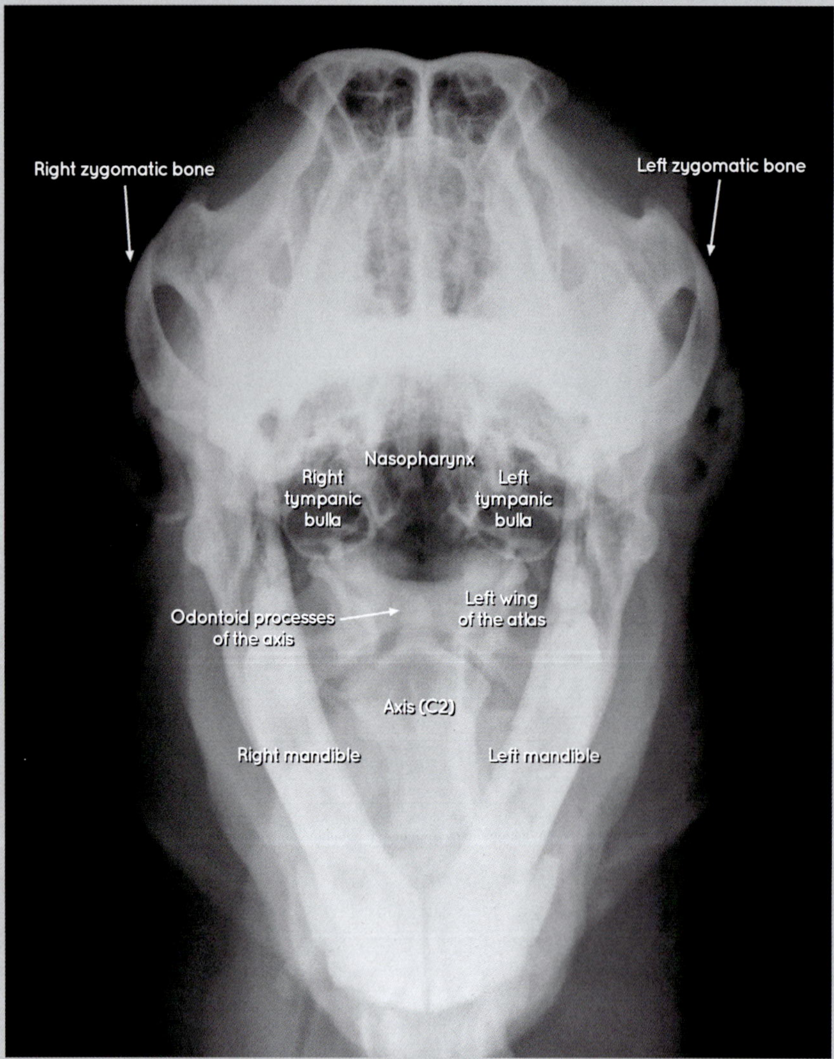

FIGURE A.52. Image of an open-mouth rostrocaudal projection of the head of a dog taken to optimise the visualisation of the two tympanic bullae.

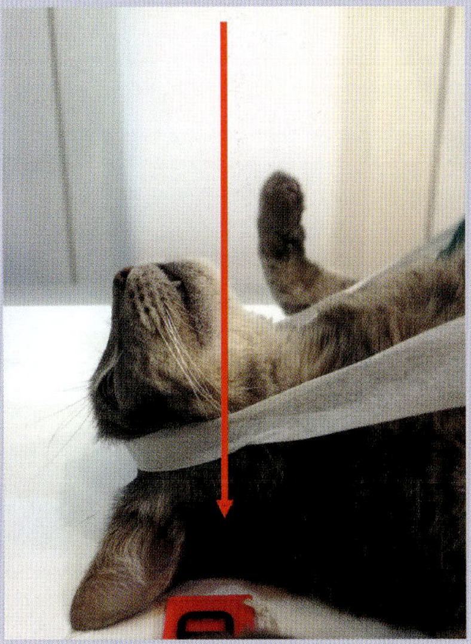

FIGURE P55. Dorsal decubitus position to obtain the 10° angle oblique rostroventral-caudodorsal projection of the rostral part of the head allowing optimal visualisation of the two tympanic bullae of a cat. The arrow indicates the direction of entry of the X-ray beam.

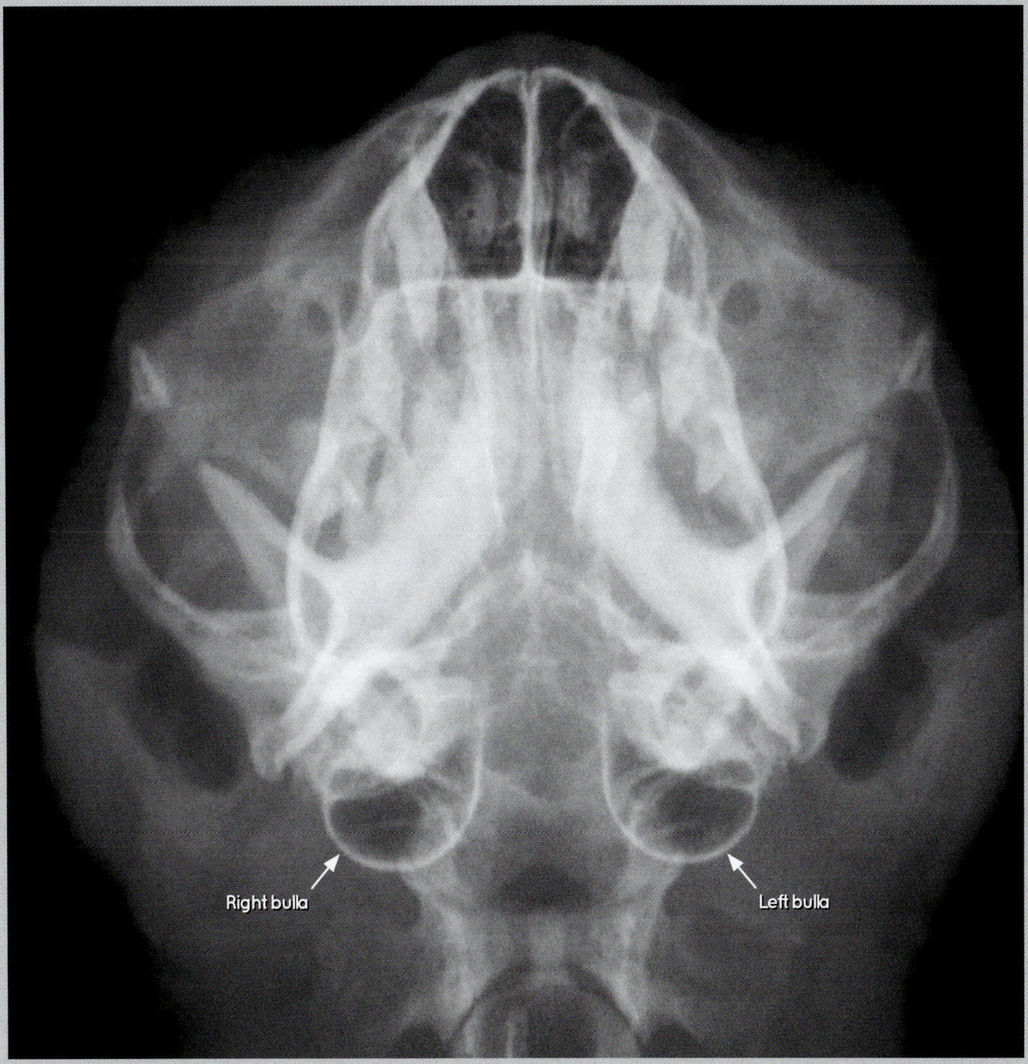

FIGURE A53. Image of an oblique rostroventral-caudodorsal projection with a 10° angle of the head of a cat, allowing optimal visualisation of the two tympanic bullae in this species.

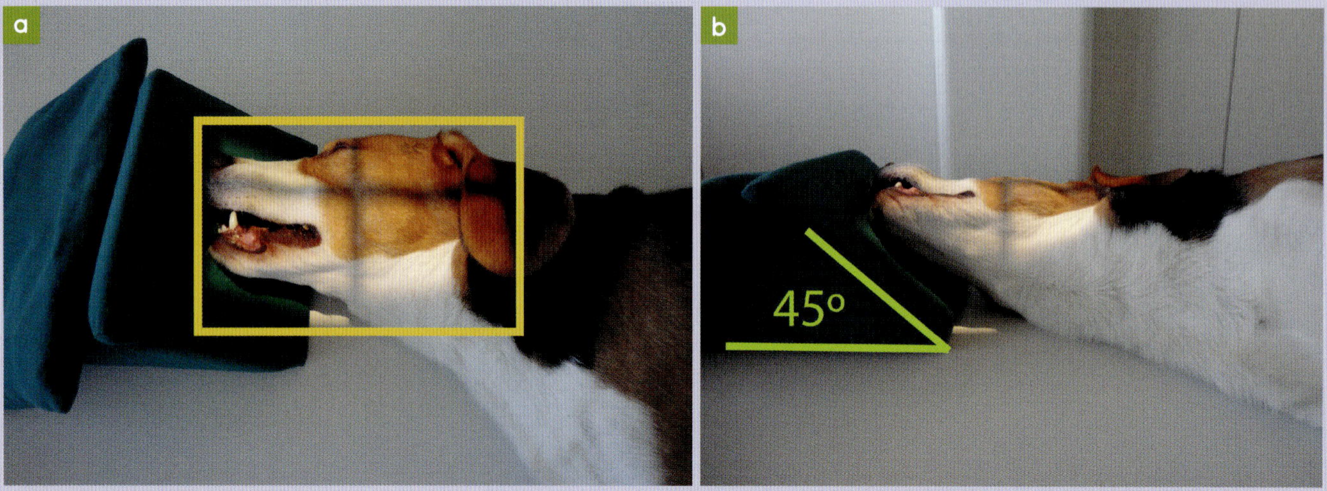

FIGURE P.56. Right lateral decubitus position, at a 45° angle, of rostral part of the head to obtain a right lateral oblique projection optimising visualisation of the right temporomandibular joint in a dog. The tilt angle may vary from 20° to 45° depending on the cranial conformation. Lateral view (a) and ventral view (b).

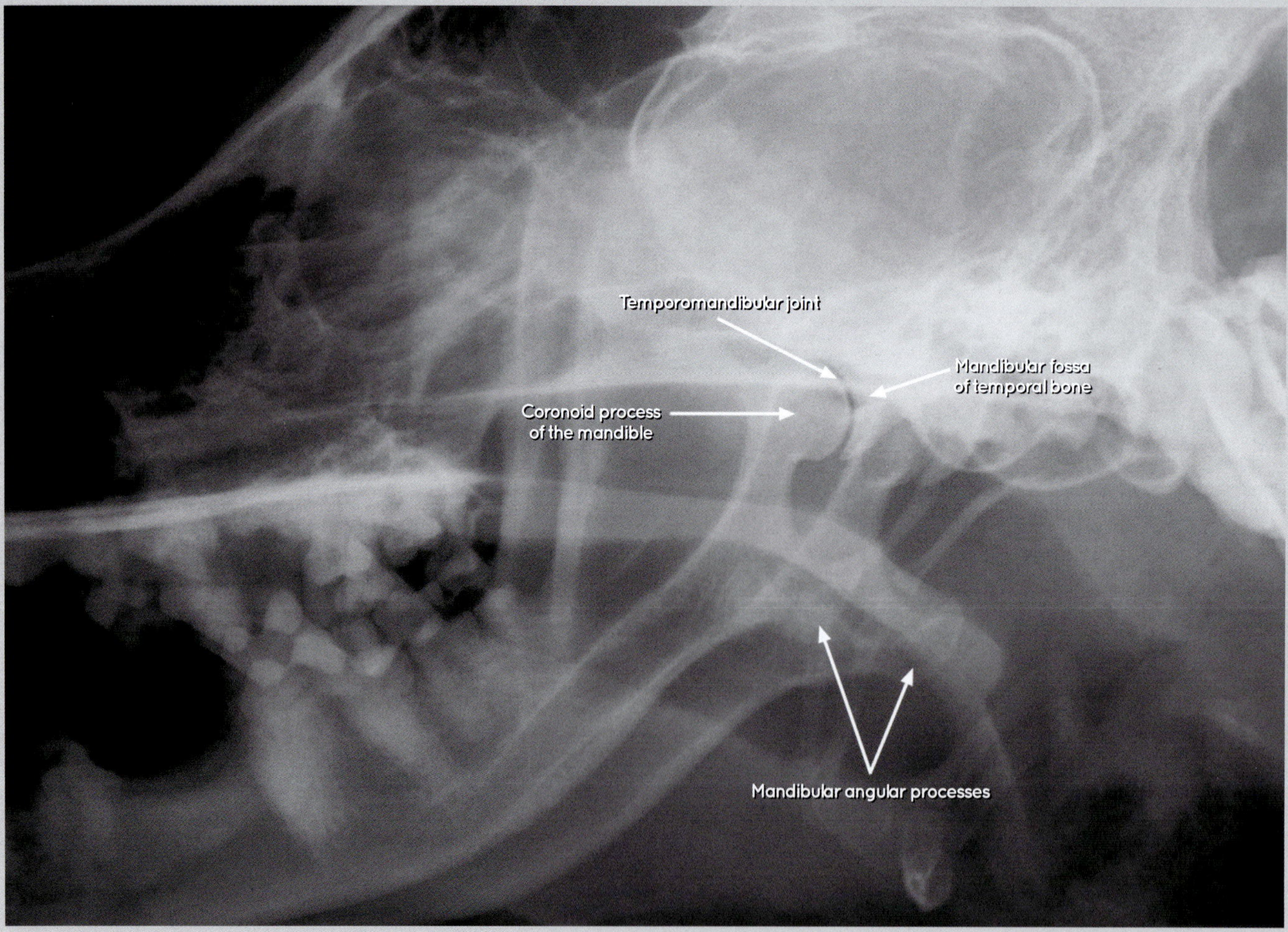

FIGURE A.54. Image of the oblique lateral projection, at 45° angle, of the rostral part of the head of a dog, taken to optimise the visualisation of the temporomandibular joint that appears most rostral in the image, which corresponds to the joint closest to the X-ray table.

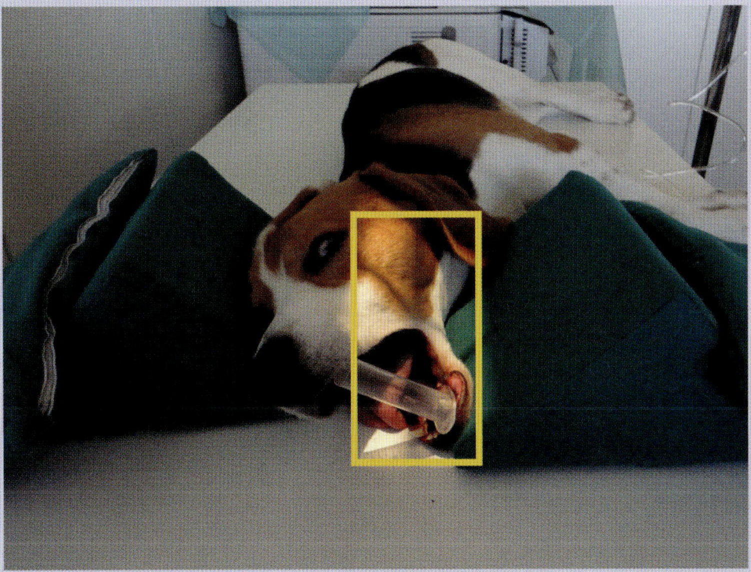

FIGURE P.57. Right lateral decubitus position with a 45° dorsal head angle and mouth open to obtain a right lateral oblique projection optimising visualisation of the right mandibular region of a dog.

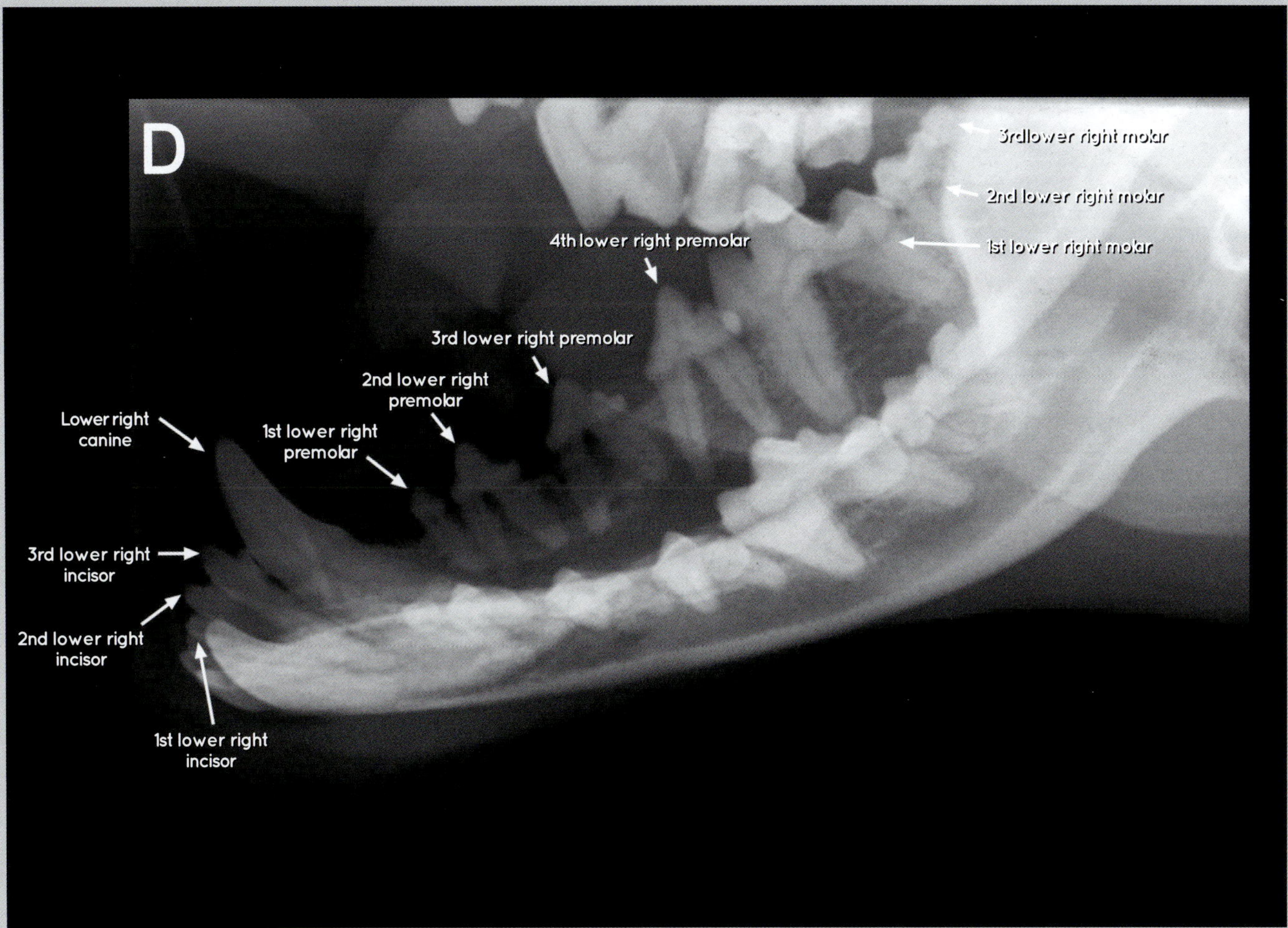

FIGURE A.55. Image of the oblique lateral projection, at a 45° angle, of the dorsal part of the head of a dog with mouth open, taken to optimise the visualisation of the mandibular region located closest to the X-ray table.

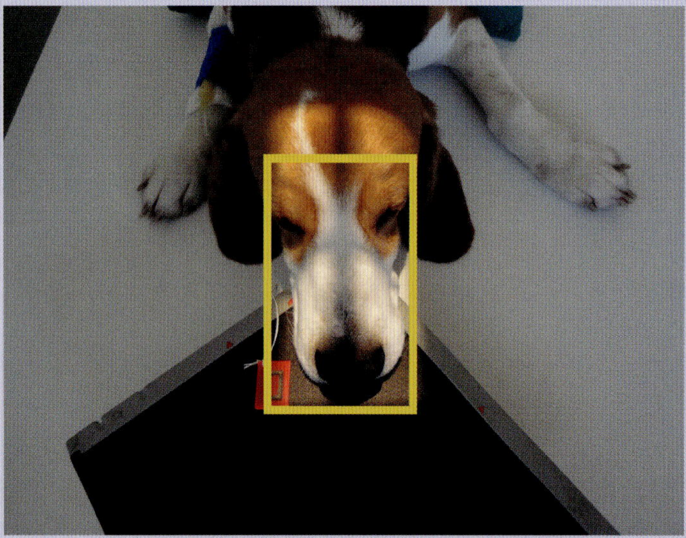

FIGURE P.58. Ventral decubitus position to obtain an intraoral (occlusal) dorsoventral projection allowing visualisation of the rostral part of an upper jaw of a dog.

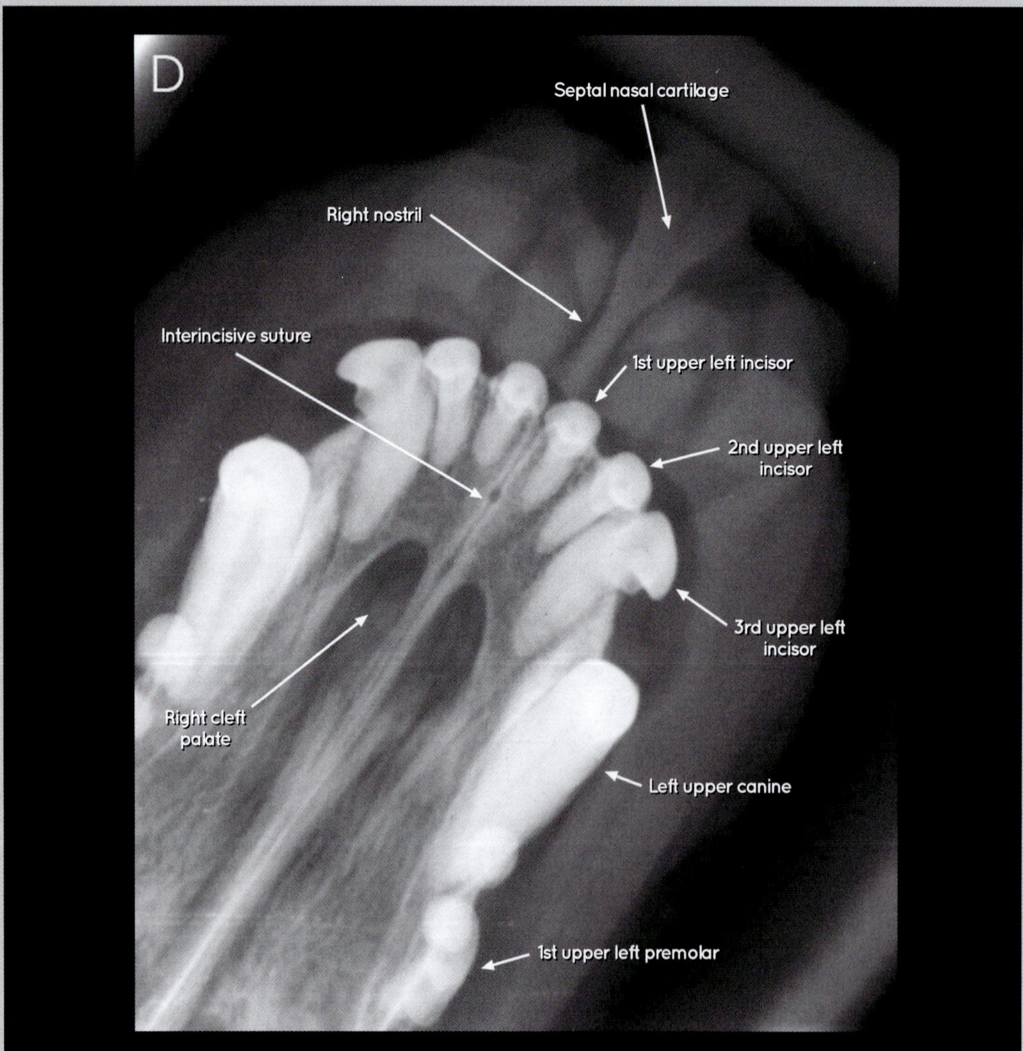

FIGURE A.56. Image of intraoral (occlusal) dorsoventral projection of the upper jaw of a dog, made by inserting the corner of a cassette into the oral cavity.

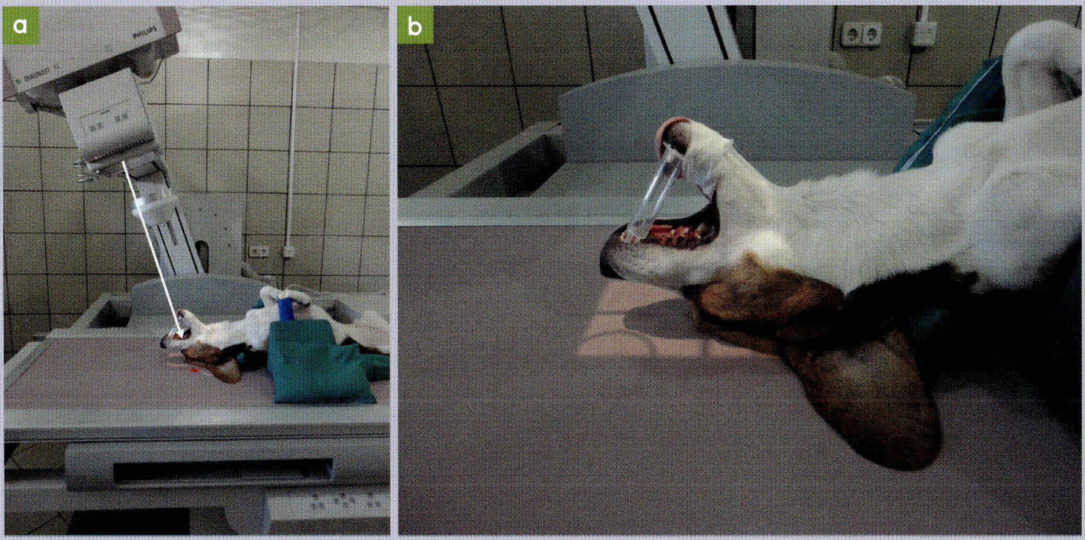

FIGURE P59. Dorsal decubitus position to obtain an open-mouth ventrodorsal projection, with an X-ray beam entry angle of 20°, maximising visualisation of the upper jaw and nasal cavity of a dog. General view (a) and enlarged view of head position (b).

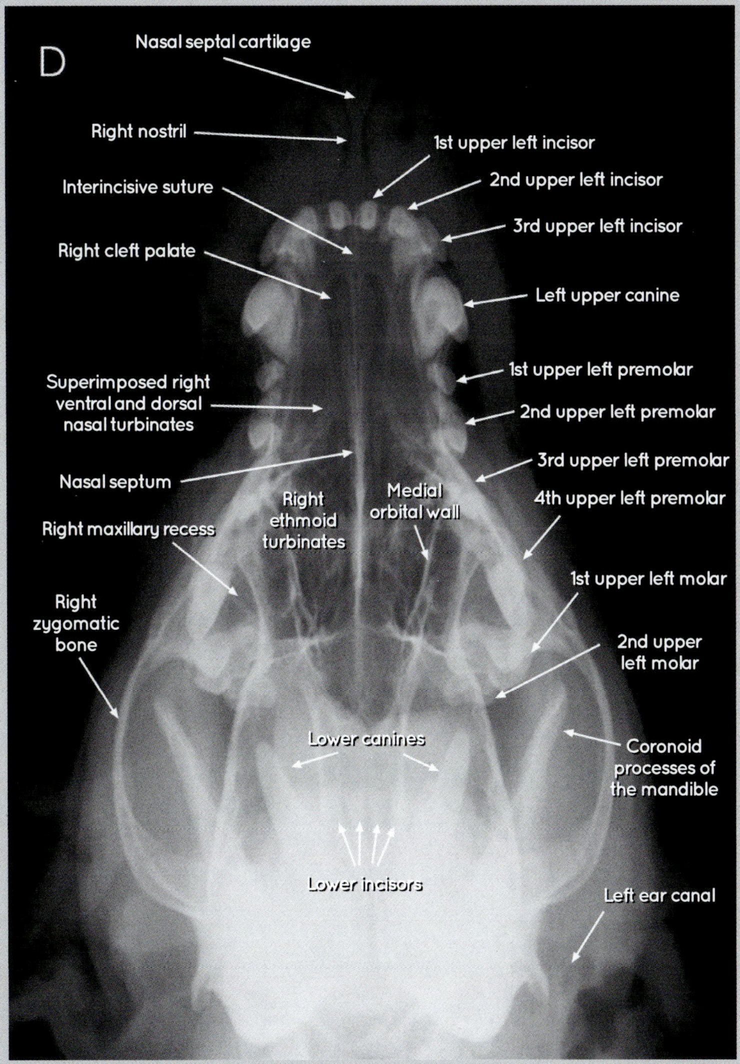

FIGURE A57. Image of open-mouth ventrodorsal projection, with X-ray beam at angel of 20°, showing the entire nasal cavity (overlapping of the jaw is avoided with beam angle).

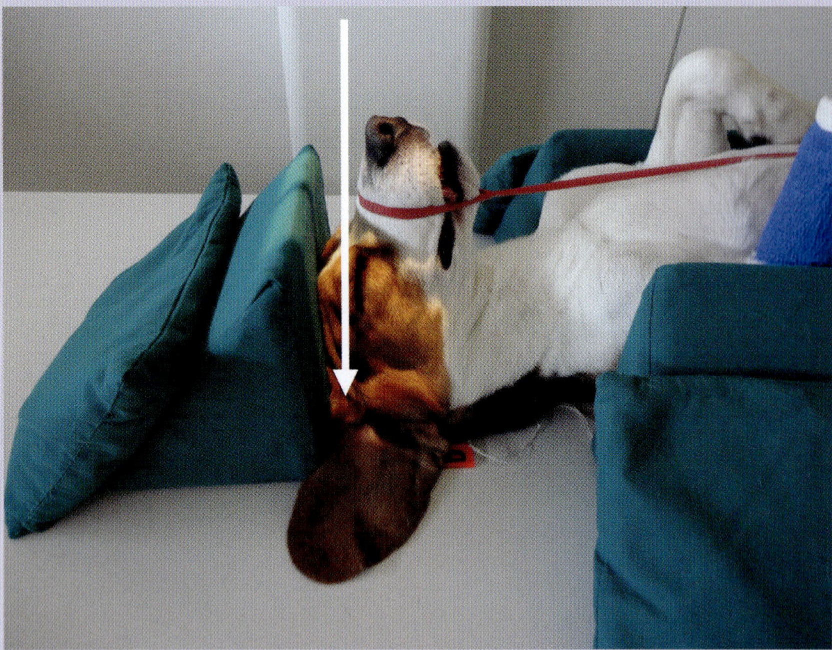

FIGURE P.60. Dorsal decubitus position to obtain the rostrocaudal tangential projection of the frontal sinuses of a dog.

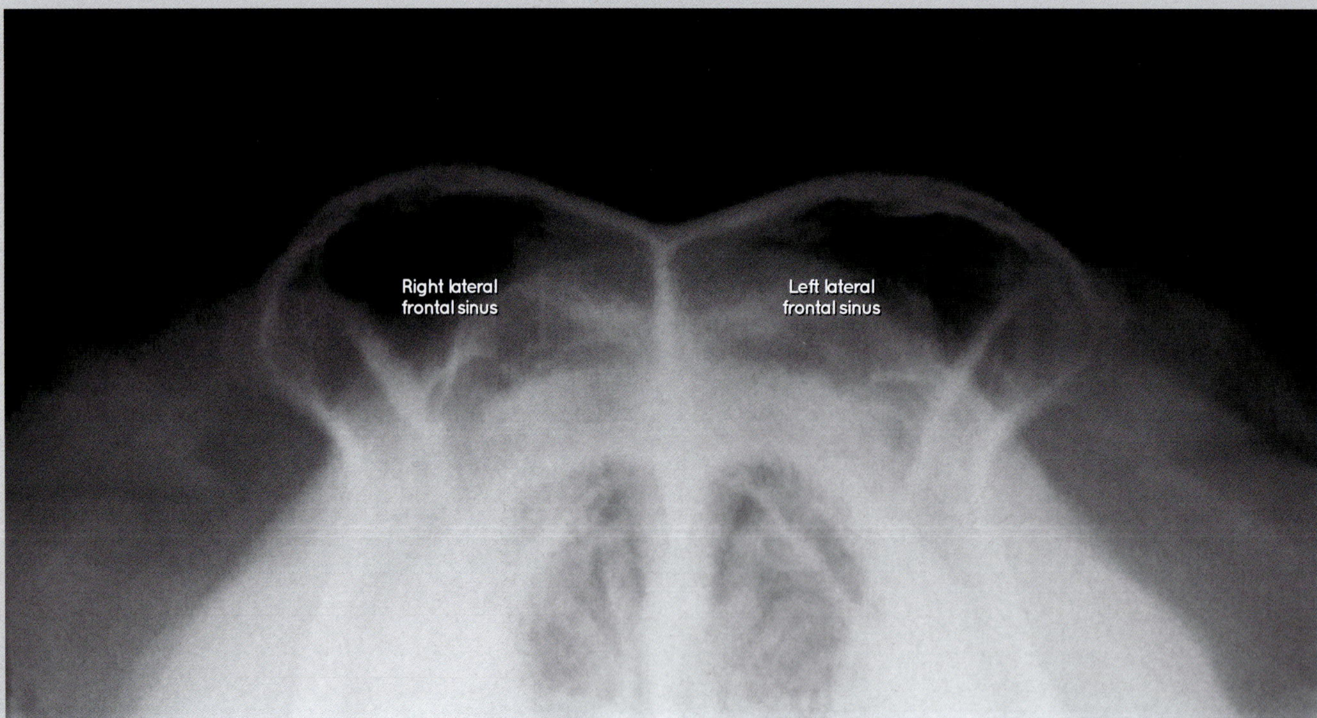

FIGURE A.58. Image of rostrocaudal tangential projection of the frontal sinuses of a dog. This allows viewing and comparison of both sinuses in the same X-ray.

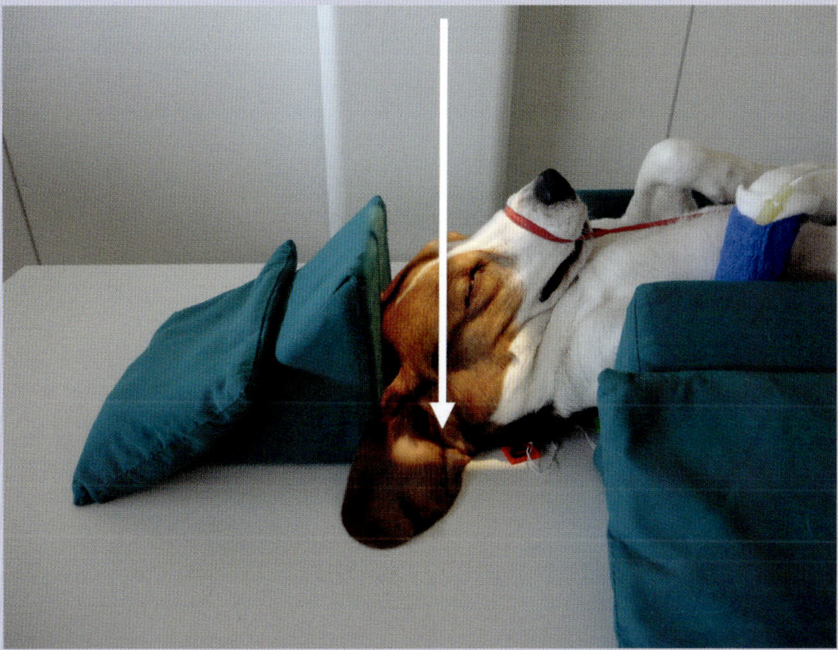

FIGURE P.61. Dorsal decubitus position to obtain the rostrodorsal to caudoventral projection to optimise visualisation of the foramen magnum of a dog.

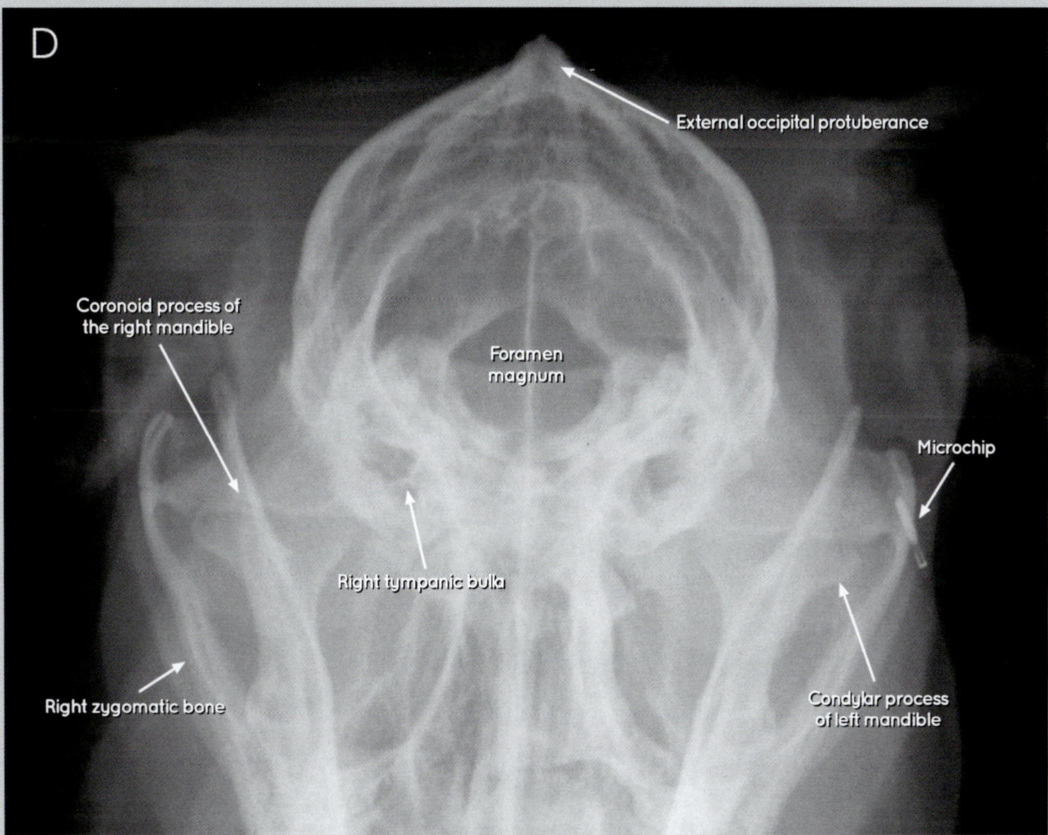

FIGURE A.59. Image of rostrodorsal-caudoventral projection of a dog, optimising visualisation of the foramen magnum

Abdomen 2

Normal radiographic anatomy of the abdomen
https://goo.by/yQEIH

Principles of interpretation

Radiography of the abdomen is one of the most commonly performed diagnostic tests in small animal veterinary practice. Nowadays, the routine use of ultrasonography has reduced the need for radiographs of the abdomen in many cases. However, it is important to highlight that the diagnostic information provided by both techniques remains complementary. For instance, an ultrasound scan is always performed if there is a clinical suspicion of liver disease, but radiography is more accurate when a possible reduction in liver size needs to be confirmed. Another example of the valuable combination of both techniques can be found in the assessment of the gastrointestinal tract, where ultrasonography has acquired great relevance over the past few years, without minimising the importance of the diagnostic information offered by radiography in this aspect.

When taking a radiograph of the abdomen, we should include:

- The diaphragm.
- The lumbar spine.
- The abdominal wall.
- The pelvic inlet.

In large breed dogs, the length of the abdomen may exceed the length of the cassette. This therefore requires taking two radiographs to examine the whole abdomen: one centred on its cranial part and the other centred on its caudal part. It is necessary to use an anti-scatter grid (either stationary or Potter-Bucky) when the height of the abdomen exceeds 10 cm once the patient has been placed on the cassette or table. This measure will improve the sharpness of the image by reducing the influence of scattered radiation on the radiograph.

The radiographic projections that are usually used are the lateral and ventrodorsal projections. On occasions, comparing the images of right lateral and left lateral projections may provide additional information, especially in the case of the gastrointestinal tract. Ventrodorsal radiographs are preferred over dorsoventral ones, since the latter are taken in sternal recumbency and the shadows of the organs therefore appear slightly distorted due to compression. If we want to examine the urethra of a male dog, its course will be better viewed by extending the hind limbs in cranial direction.

It is usually possible to identify the liver, spleen, kidneys, bladder, stomach, small intestine, large intestine, abdominal wall and shadow of the diaphragm on a normal radiograph of the abdomen. In male dogs, it is also possible to observe the os penis, the shadow of the prepuce and part of the prostate (fig. 2.1). In normal conditions, it is not possible to identify the pancreas, adrenal glands, gallbladder, ureters, urethra, lymph nodes, blood vessels, ovaries or a non-pregnant uterus.

The main differences between the radiographic image of the abdomen in cats and dogs (fig. 2.2) are summarised in table 2.1.

The main limiting factors in the interpretation of radiographs of the abdomen are the superimposition of the numerous anatomical structures contained within the peritoneal cavity and the lack of differentiation between many of them, as most of them exhibit similar radiopacity (soft tissue-fluid). The liver, spleen, kidneys, bladder, etc., all have the same radiographic density, the same tone of grey in the image. The walls of the stomach and intestine also have the same radiopacity as the fluid or mucous content that may be present in the lumen of these organs, hindering differentiation on a simple radiograph. The food or gas content of the stomach and gas or faeces in the intestine are more easily identified, precisely because the radiographic density of gas, non-digested or partially digested food and faeces is different from that of the walls and fluid or mucous content

TABLE 2.1. Summary of the main differences in the radiographic appearance of the abdomen between the dog and the cat.

	Dog	Cat
Stomach	Pyloric antrum to the right of the median line.	Pyloric antrum on the median line. A layer of fat is sometimes observed on the wall.
Caecum	Generally visible in the right mid-abdomen.	Not identified.
Spleen	Visible on lateral and ventrodorsal radiographs.	Only visible on ventrodorsal radiographs.
Pancreas	Not identified.	The left lobe is sometimes observed on ventrodorsal radiographs.
Adrenal glands	Not identified.	Calcified adrenal glands with a normal size are sometimes observed as an incidental finding.
Os penis	Visible.	It is not identified as it is minute in size.
Abdominal fat	More or less homogeneous distribution.	Tendency to a greater accumulation of fat in the area of the falcifom ligament (ventral to the liver), surrounding the intestinal mass (which is centred in the mid-abdomen) and in the retroperitoneal space (facilitates the observation of the kidneys).

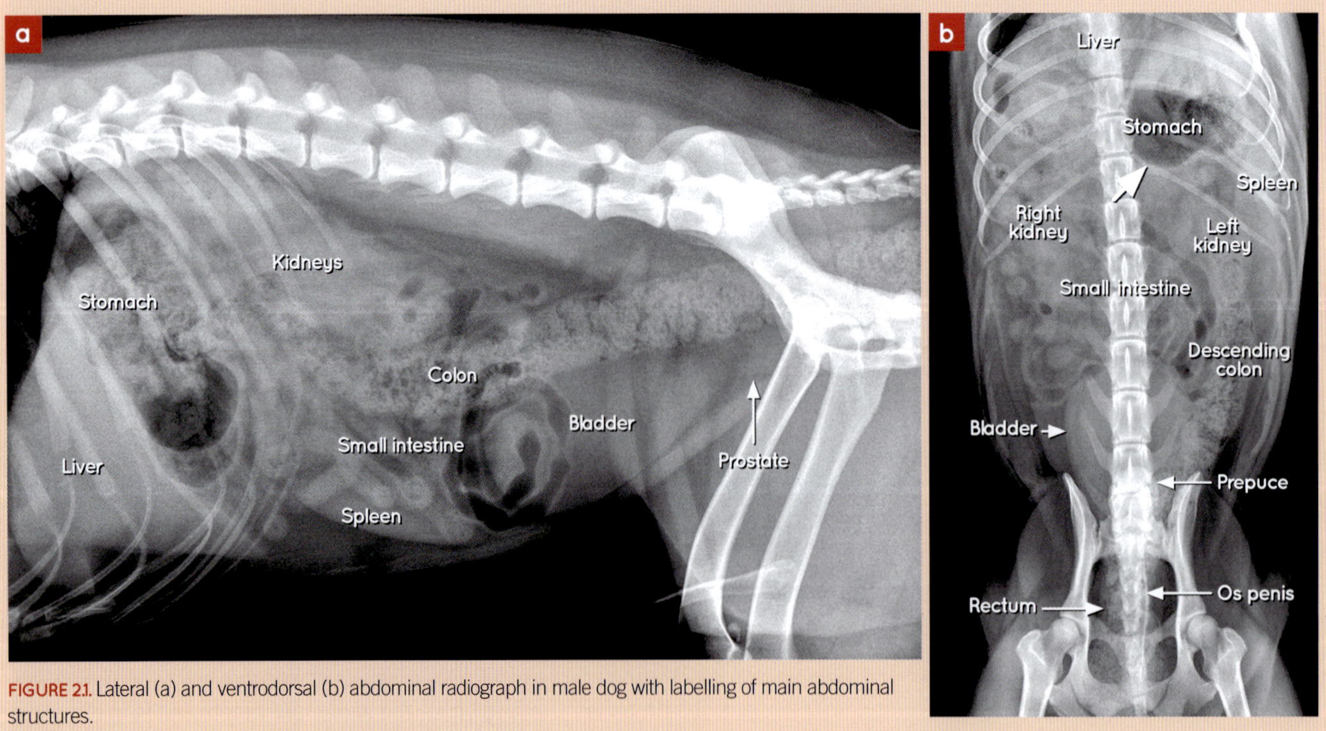

FIGURE 2.1. Lateral (a) and ventrodorsal (b) abdominal radiograph in male dog with labelling of main abdominal structures.

of the gastrointestinal tract, as well as from that of most of the surrounding anatomical structures.

The fat that accumulates in the peritoneum interposes between the abdominal organs, facilitating the differentiation of their contours on the radiograph. The radiographic images of very young or very thin adult animals, which have very little abdominal fat, will show a lack of differentiation of the structures. This may be confused with the image of free fluid or peritoneal reaction. However, an excessive amount of abdominal fat significantly increases X-ray scattering, which may lead to a blurry appearance of the image, even in spite of the use of an anti-scatter grid.

Advanced diagnostic imaging techniques such as computed tomography or magnetic resonance imaging are not often used for the assessment of the abdomen, since the combination of plain or contrast radiography and ultrasonography allows most diagnostic needs to be covered in this anatomical region. Nevertheless, they may be particularly interesting for the evaluation of alterations of the retroperitoneum or blood vessels (e.g. precise diagnosis of portosystemic communications). Both techniques are excellent to examine the pelvic region, as they offer images with great anatomical details of the muscles and bone structures of this area, the rectum, anal sacs, urethra, vagina and vulval vestibule in females, as well as of the prostate, penis and scrotum in males.

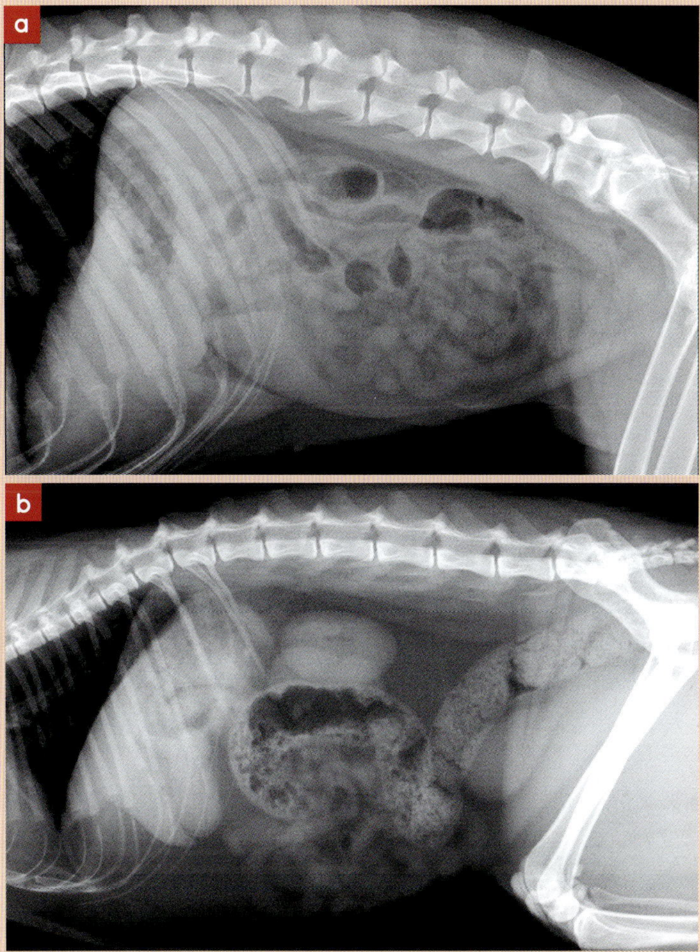

FIGURE 2.2. Lateral radiographs of the normal abdomen of a dog (a) and of a cat (b).

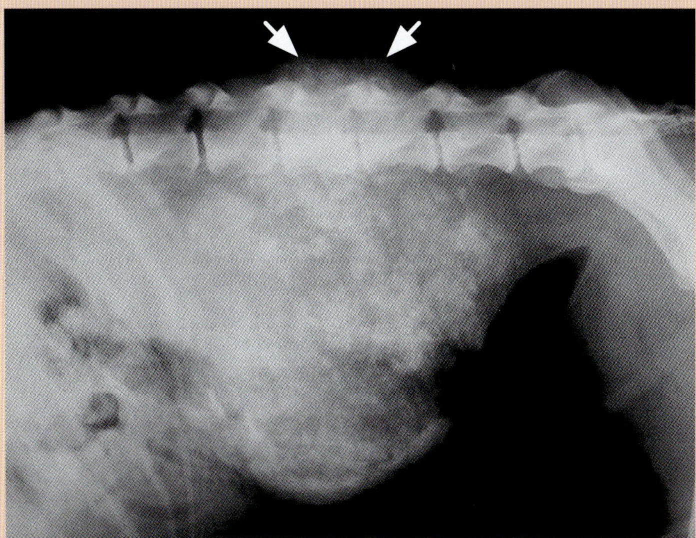

FIGURE 2.3. Lateral radiograph of the abdomen of a dog with a calcified mass located in the abdominal wall. It cannot be confused with an intrabdominal mass, since the dorsal margin of the mass can be seen above the lumbar spine (arrows).

Abdominal wall

The abdominal wall is formed cranially by the diaphragm and costal wall, ventrally and laterally by the abdominal muscles, dorsally by the sublumbar muscles and caudally by the peritoneum.

Radiography allows the detection of alterations in the radiographic density of the wall. The presence of bands of gas lucency is indicative of subcutaneous emphysema, generally associated with penetrating wounds. Lipomas have fat density, while some muscle or skin tumours may appear calcified (fig. 2.3). Areas of calcification that are not associated with masses may also be observed in the wall, for example in patients suffering from Cushing's syndrome with cutaneous calcinosis.

Radiography is also very useful in the diagnosis of **hernias**, which may be congenital or the result of trauma (fig. 2.4). Umbilical or inguinal hernias appear as focal distensions of the ventral abdominal wall. Their radiographic density varies in function of the contents of the hernial sac. It is relatively easy to identify the presence of intestinal loops in a hernia, since they appear as structures with a tubular morphology where gas –or faeces in the case of the colon– generally accumulates to a greater or lesser extent. It is also possible to identify the shadow of the bladder if it is distended (fig. 2.5). When the uterus is displaced into the hernial sac, the uterine horns appear as tubular structures with soft-tissue density. These are difficult to differentiate from intestinal loops with fluid or mucous content, unless the uterus is enlarged due to pregnancy or to a pathological dilatation. It is possible to use contrast techniques to confirm the presence of the intestine or bladder in a hernial sac, but it is usually not necessary as ultrasonography is an excellent complementary technique in those cases and allows a fairly precise examination of the defect in the wall and of the structures contained in the hernia.

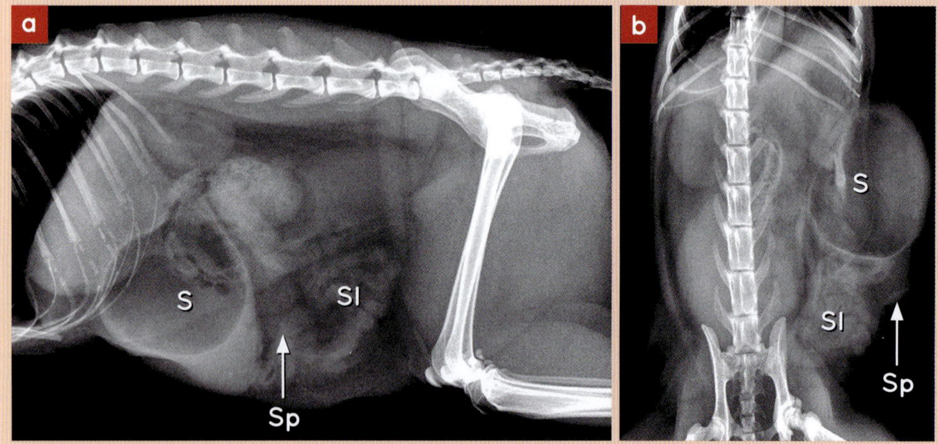

FIGURE 2.4. Lateral (a) and ventrodorsal (b) abdominal radiograph in cat with left lateral abdominal wall hernia due to trauma. The stomach (S), small intestine (SI) and spleen (Sp) appear herniated.

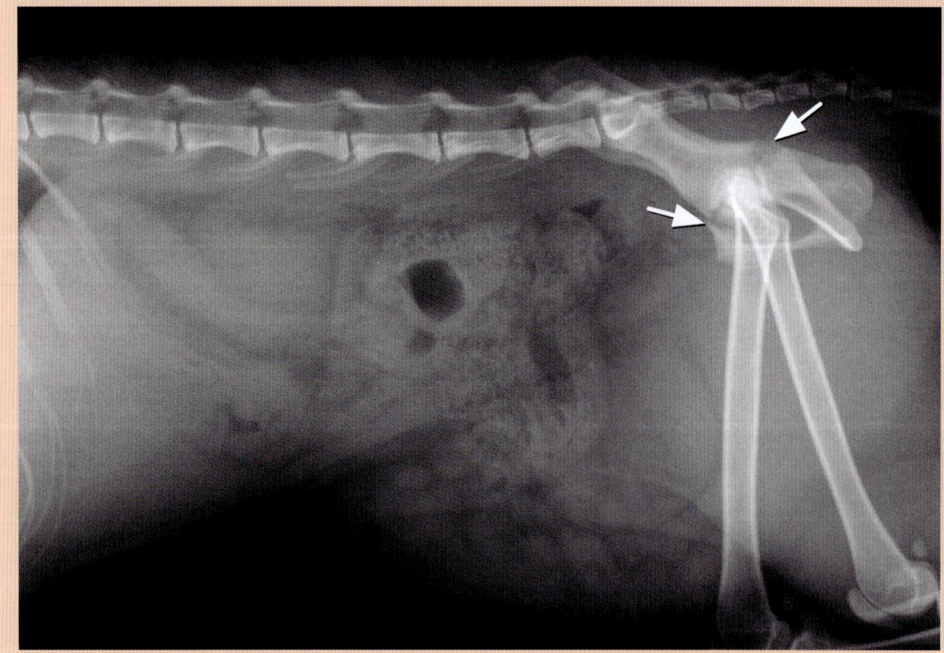

FIGURE 2.5. Lateral radiograph of the abdomen of a cat with an inguinal hernia containing the bladder and segments of the small intestine and colon. Two lines of fracture (arrows) can be observed in the bony pelvis.

The diaphragm is a musculotendinous sheet that separates the thoracic and abdominal cavities. In normal conditions it is not possible to identify the diaphragm on a plain radiograph, since the liver lies adjacent to it and has the same radiographic density. However, the characteristic morphology of the diaphragm, which is divided into two dorsal crura and a ventral dome, allows us to distinguish its shadow on radiograph. The shadow of the diaphragm will vary according to the chosen radiographic projection (fig. 2.6).

The radiographic image of a diaphragmatic hernia varies in function of the size and location of the defect or rupture in the diaphragm. The most characteristic radiographic sign is the identification of abdominal anatomical structures in the thoracic cavity. A stomach or intestine with gas, food or faeces is easier to identify, while organs with soft-tissue density, such as the liver or spleen, may appear less differentiated (fig. 2.7). In some cases, the abdominal cavity may appear partially empty of its contents (fig. 2.8). If an associated pleural effusion appears, this may mask the images of the abdominal organs displaced into the thorax. When the defect in the diaphragm is small, it is more difficult to diagnose as there may be no evident radiological signs, for instance, when only a part of the liver protrudes through the defect. Ultrasonography is sometimes useful to provide complementary information, although small diaphragmatic hernias are also difficult to diagnose with this technique.

Perineal hernias (fig. 2.9) occur more frequently in males and may contain the prostate and bladder. Although a positive-contrast cystogram may be performed to confirm the presence of the bladder in the hernial sac, ultrasonography allows the easy identification of all the structures contained in it.

Peritoneal cavity and retroperitoneal space

The peritoneum is a serous membrane essentially composed of connective tissue, which delimits the peritoneal space. The retroperitoneum is the anatomical space located between the dorsal parietal peritoneum and the vertebrae and paraspinal muscles; the kidneys, adrenal glands, ureters, blood vessels and lymph nodes lie in it.

In dogs, abdominal fat essentially accumulates in the mesentery and greater omentum, which are spaces formed by folds of peritoneum. In cats, on the other hand, more fat is accumulated in the falciform ligament (ventral to the liver) and retroperitoneal space than in the mesentery. In obese cats, the small intestinal loops may appear clumped in the centre of the abdomen due to a more peripheral accumulation of intraperitoneal fat (fig. 2.10).

Pneumoperitoneum

It is defined as the presence of free gas in the peritoneal cavity. The most frequent cause is iatrogenic, due to an accumulation of air after a laparotomy, which may remain up to one month in this anatomical space and is progressively absorbed. The pathological causes of pneumoperitoneum are penetrating wounds and the perforation or rupture of abdominal organs containing gas (stomach and intestine).

The upright lateral view has traditionally been considered the most suitable to demonstrate the presence of free gas in the abdomen, especially when the quantities of gas are low, but recent studies have shown that the left lateral view is equally as sensitive for the detection of mild pneumoperitoneum. The left lateral image is preferred because in the right it is easy to confuse the free gas with gastric fundus gas. The patient should be kept in lateral recumbency for at least 2 minutes before taking the radiograph. This will allow the gas to rise and collect in the upper part of the abdomen and make it easier to identify.

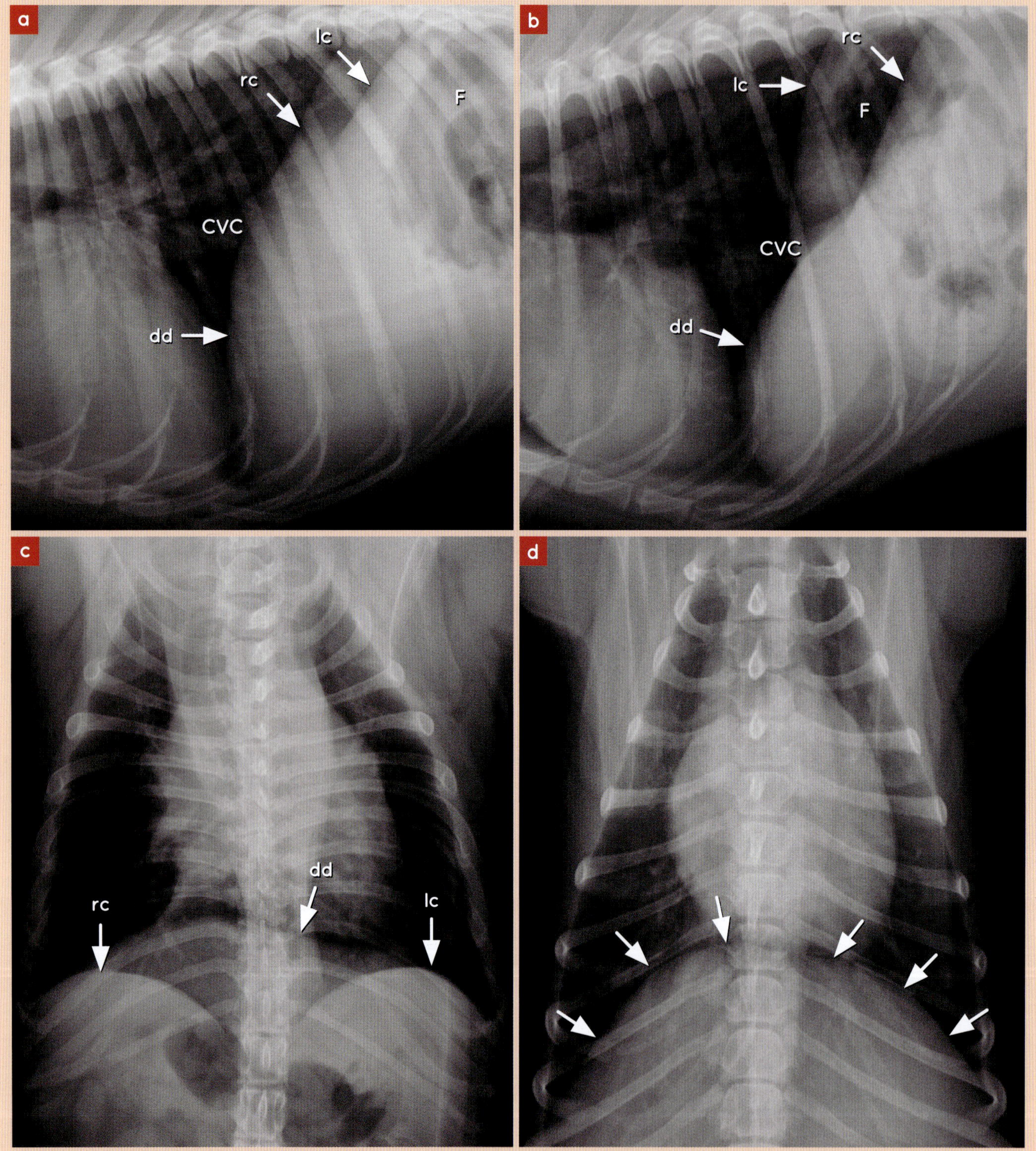

FIGURE 2.6. Right lateral (a), left lateral (b), ventrodorsal (c) and dorsoventral (d) radiographs of the thorax, in which it is possible to see the normal appearance of the diaphragmatic shadow. Right crus of the diaphragm: rc. Left crus of the diaphragm: lc. Diaphragmatic dome: dd. In the right lateral projection, the right crus of the diaphragm is located cranial to the left crus, while in the left lateral projection it is the left crus that has the most cranial position. The two crura of the diaphragm can be differentiated radiographically because the caudal vena cava (CVC) blends with the right crus, while the fundus (F) always appears immediately caudal to the left crus. On the ventrodorsal view, the diaphragmatic shadow may appear as three convex images (the two crura in caudal position and the dome in cranial position), although they are not always easy to identify on radiographs. On the ventrodorsal view, the diaphragmatic shadow always appears as a single convex image (arrows).

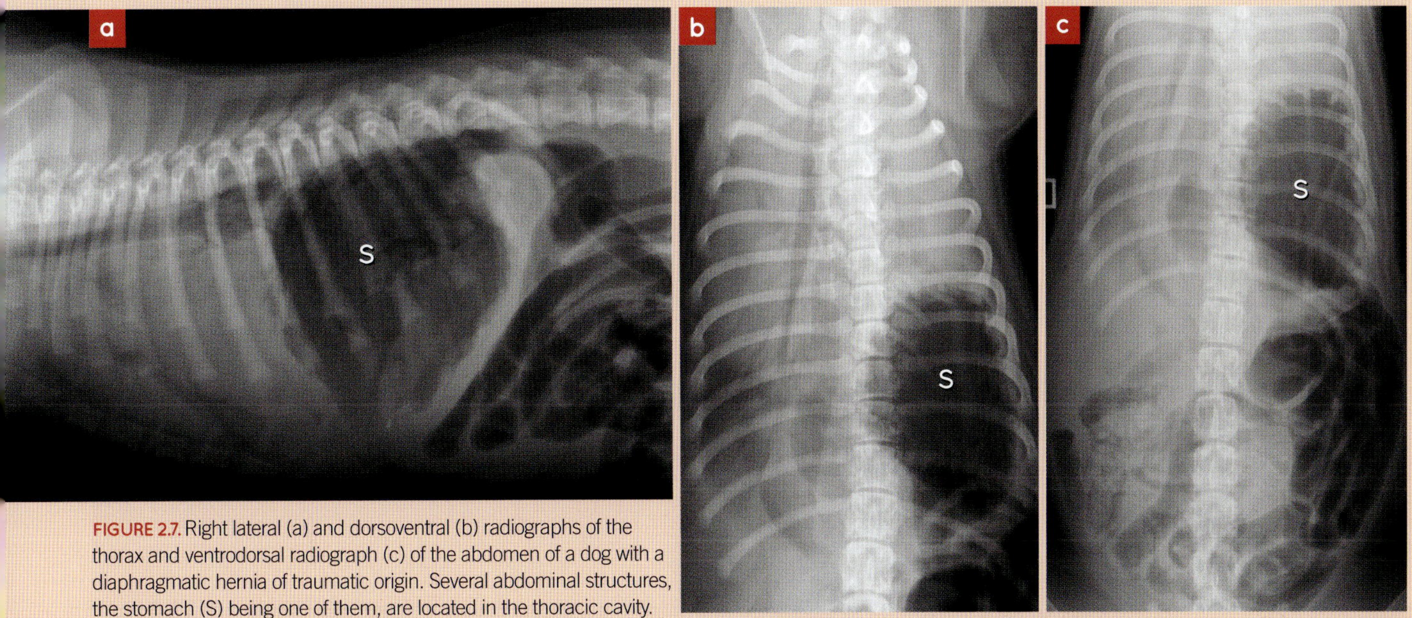

FIGURE 2.7. Right lateral (a) and dorsoventral (b) radiographs of the thorax and ventrodorsal radiograph (c) of the abdomen of a dog with a diaphragmatic hernia of traumatic origin. Several abdominal structures, the stomach (S) being one of them, are located in the thoracic cavity.

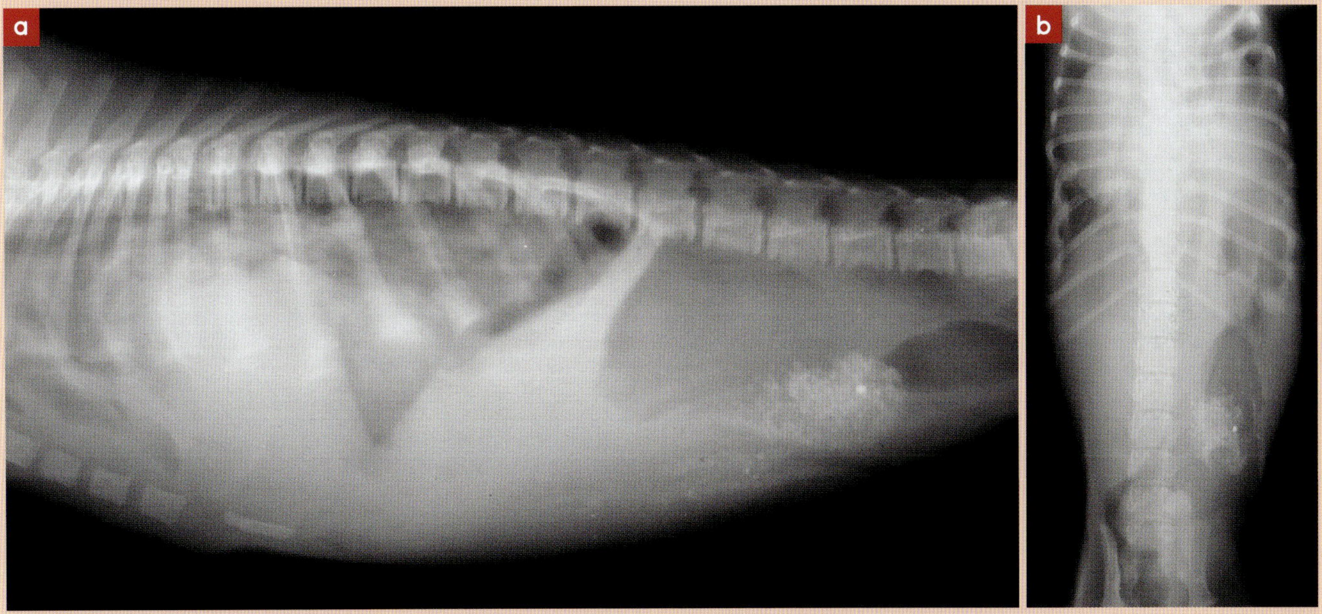

FIGURE 2.8. Right lateral (a) and ventrodorsal (b) radiographs of the abdomen and thorax of a young dog with a diaphragmatic hernia of congenital origin. It is possible to identify intestinal loops with gas content in the thorax, while the abdomen appears partially empty.

The radiographic signs of pneumoperitoneum depend on the amount of accumulated gas in the cavity. When gas accumulates in large amounts, a general reduction of abdominal radiopacity and a greater definition of the contour of the organs due to the accumulation of gas between them are observed (fig. 2.11). On the other hand, it may be difficult to identify small amounts of free gas, since they are usually mistaken for gas contained in the digestive tract. If gas accumulates between the liver and the diaphragm, the latter can be observed as a thin line of soft-tissue opacity limited cranially by the lung and caudally by free peritoneal gas (fig. 2.12). The observation of this radiological finding confirms the diagnosis of pneumoperitoneum.

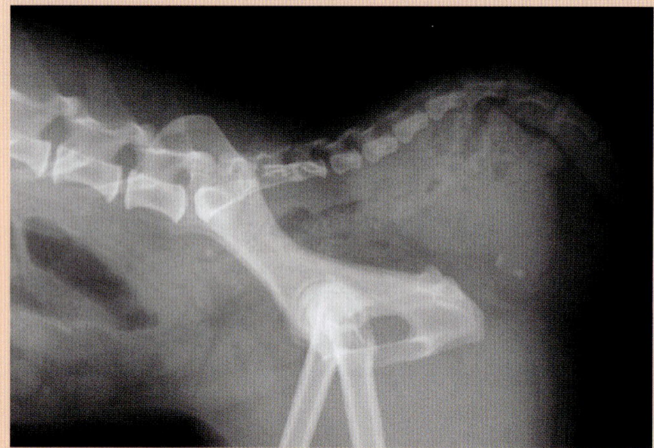

FIGURE 2.9. Lateral radiograph of the caudal abdomen and perineal region of a male dog with a perineal hernia. It is not possible to visualise the shadow of the bladder in the caudal area of the abdomen, as it is located in the hernial sac together with the prostate and part of the rectum.

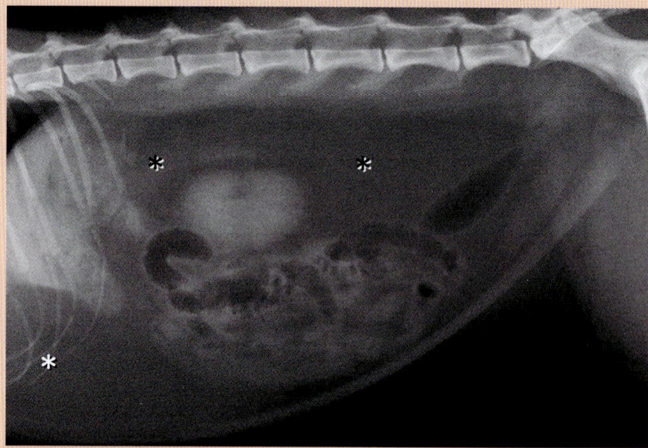

FIGURE 2.10. Lateral radiograph of the abdomen of an obese cat. Cats accumulate more fat in the falciform ligament (ventral to the liver, marked with a white asterisk) and in the retroperitoneal space (marked with black asterisks) than in the mesentery. In obese cats, the intestinal loops appear clumped in the centre of the abdomen due to the greater accumulation of fat in the peripheral areas.

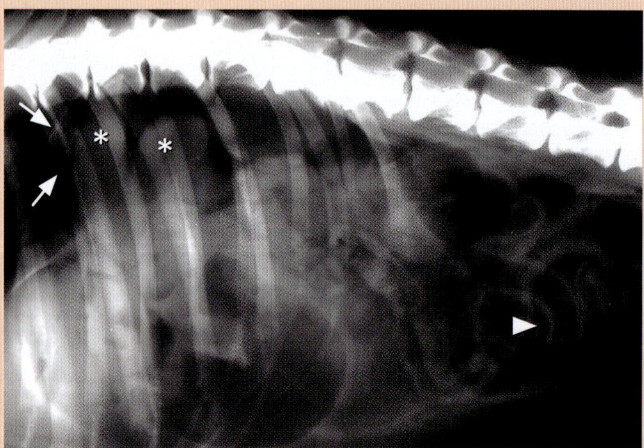

FIGURE 2.11. Lateral radiograph of the abdomen of a dog with a pneumoperitoneum. There is a large amount of intra-abdominal free gas. It is located between the organs, which facilitates the observation of their outline and causes a general reduction of radiopacity of the abdomen. This way, it is possible to identify the liver lobes (asterisks) and the diaphragm (arrows) and to view the external aspect of the gastric and intestinal wall clearly, especially in the segments containing gas, since the soft-tissue opacity of the wall contrasts with the gas lucency on both sides (tip of the arrow).

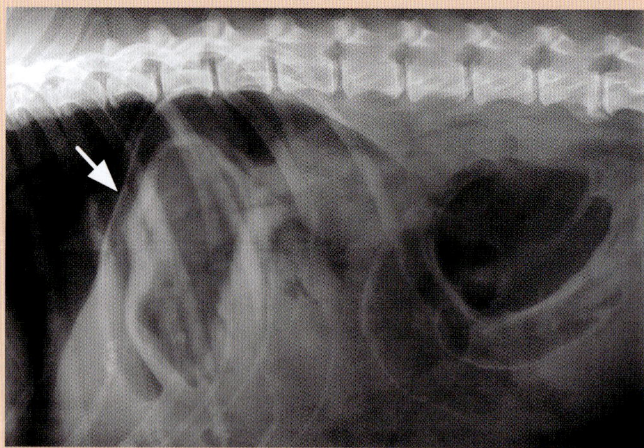

FIGURE 2.12. Lateral radiograph of the abdomen of a dog with a pneumoperitoneum. The amount of intra-abdominal free gas is moderate. When it is located between the diaphragm and the liver, it is possible to identify the diaphragm (arrow), since it contrasts with the gas located cranial and caudal to it, which confirms the pneumoperitoneum.

Free fluid

It may be exudate, transudate, blood, urine, bile or lymph. The most common causes of accumulation of free fluid in the peritoneal cavity are:

- Congestive heart failure.
- Hepatic alterations.
- Trauma.
- Renal disease.
- Hypoproteinaemia.
- Peritonitis.
- Abdominal neoplasia.

The most frequent causes of accumulation of free fluid in the retroperitoneal space are:

- Acute kidney injury (the amount of fluid is usually minimal and accumulates next to the affected kidney or kidneys).
- Extravasation of urine of traumatic origin.
- Haemorrhage associated to trauma.
- Coagulopathies.
- Vessel rupture.
- Rupture of highly vascularised retroperitoneal masses.

The radiographic signs of ascites depend on the amount of accumulated fluid in the peritoneal cavity. In general, increased soft-tissue opacity may be observed in the abdomen due to the accumulation of fluid between the organs. This accumulation of liquid causes a decrease or loss of the differentiation of the contour of the organs. Radiologically, this is termed loss of serous definition or loss of serosal detail. This may be the only evident sign when the amount of liquid is low. If this is very large, the abdomen will have practically homogeneous soft-tissue opacity, and only the gas, food or faeces contained in the stomach and intestine will be discernible (fig. 2.13).

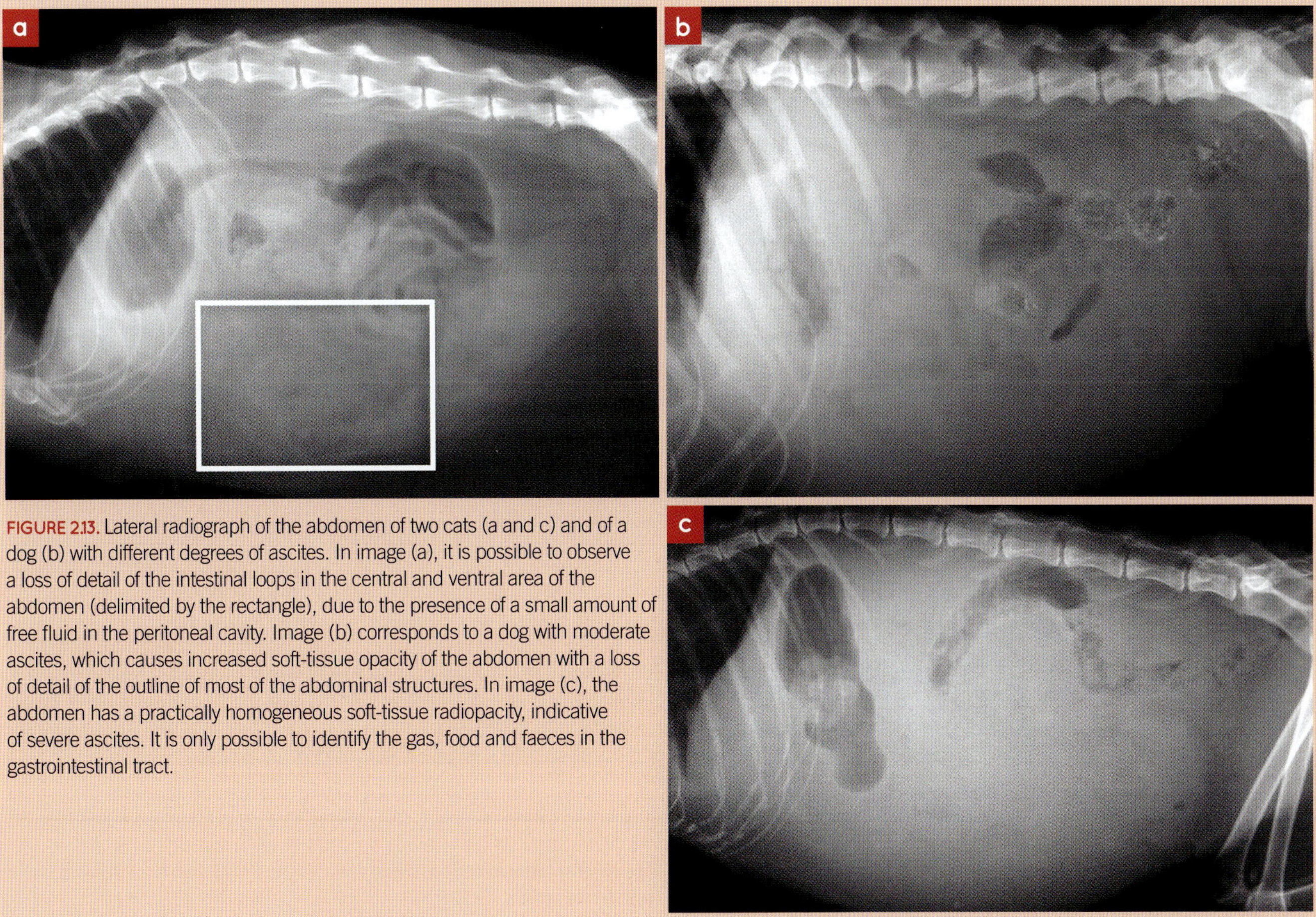

FIGURE 2.13. Lateral radiograph of the abdomen of two cats (a and c) and of a dog (b) with different degrees of ascites. In image (a), it is possible to observe a loss of detail of the intestinal loops in the central and ventral area of the abdomen (delimited by the rectangle), due to the presence of a small amount of free fluid in the peritoneal cavity. Image (b) corresponds to a dog with moderate ascites, which causes increased soft-tissue opacity of the abdomen with a loss of detail of the outline of most of the abdominal structures. In image (c), the abdomen has a practically homogeneous soft-tissue radiopacity, indicative of severe ascites. It is only possible to identify the gas, food and faeces in the gastrointestinal tract.

It may be accompanied by more or less marked abdominal distension, depending on the amount of accumulated fluid.

The presence of free fluid in the retroperitoneal space increases radiopacity in this anatomical cavity, together with a loss of detail of the structures contained in it (fig. 2.14). Ultrasonography is more useful than radiography to detect small amounts of free fluid in the retroperitoneum and also allows the collection of samples under ultrasound guidance.

Peritonitis and retroperitonitis

Inflammation of the peritoneum causes a loss of detail of the outline of the abdominal structures that is similar to that caused by free fluid. In fact, ascites and peritonitis cannot be differentiated on a radiograph. In the case of focal peritonitis, the poorly defined structures (loss of serosal detail) will only be evident in the affected area of the abdomen. The image would therefore be very similar to that caused by the presence of small amounts of free fluid in the peritoneal cavity. If peritonitis is generalised, the image will be very similar to that caused by a large amount of free peritoneal fluid, although it is not usually accompanied by abdominal distension (fig. 2.15). However, it is important to bear in mind that peritonitis is often associated with ascites, in which case there will be two causes leading to the same radiographic image (fig. 2.16).

Ultrasonography allows us to clearly distinguish between free fluid, which appears anechoic and improves the identification of the contour of the structures it surrounds, and peritonitis, which is characterised by increased echogenicity of the mesentery (fig. 2.17).

A common cause of focal peritonitis is pancreatitis. A normal pancreas cannot be identified on radiographs, although in obese cats it may be possible to identify its left lobe as an area of soft-tissue density located between the fundus of the stomach, the spleen and the left kidney (fig. 2.18). When pancreatitis is associated with peritonitis, an irregular increase of soft-tissue opacity in the medial or cranial area of the abdomen may be observed on radiographs (fig. 2.19). The descending duodenum may appear curved and displaced in ventral and lateral direction (fig. 2.20). Pancreatitis is sometimes associated with secondary paralytic ileus, which causes generalised and moderate dilatation of the small intestine.

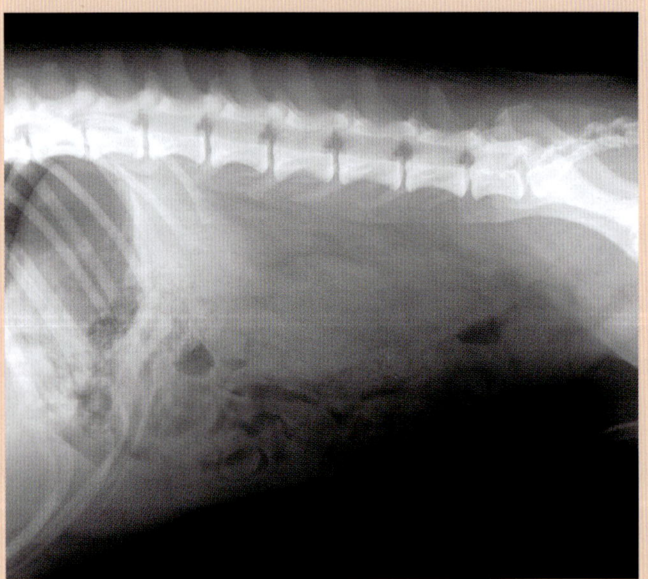

FIGURE 2.14. Lateral radiograph of the abdomen of a dog with free fluid in the retroperitoneal space. An increase in radiopacity in the dorsal area of the abdomen can be observed, with a loss of detail of the renal shadows and ventral displacement of the colon.

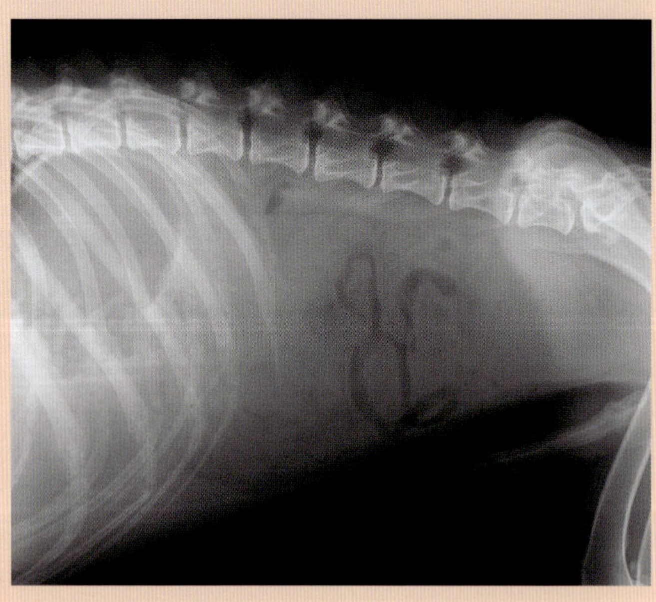

FIGURE 2.15. Lateral radiograph of the abdomen of a dog with peritonitis. Increased soft-tissue opacity may be observed in the abdomen, with a loss of differentiation of the outline of most of the abdominal structures and no abdominal distension. This image cannot be distinguished from that of moderate ascites.

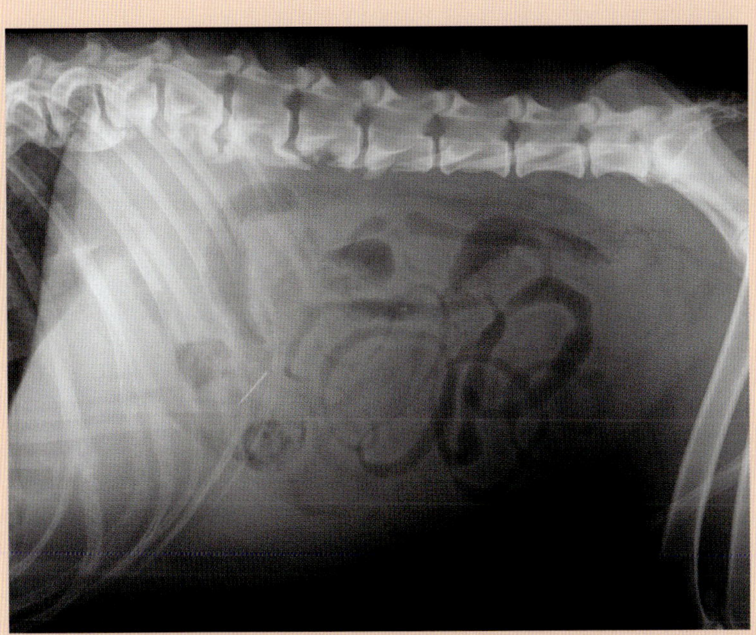

FIGURE 2.16. Lateral radiograph of the abdomen of a dog with peritonitis and ascites due to an intestinal perforation. Increased soft-tissue opacity may be observed in the abdomen, with a loss of differentiation of the outline of most of the abdominal structures and abdominal distension. A sharp metallic foreign body can be seen in the cranial abdomen. Spondylosis deformans of the spine (T11-L4 and L7-S) is worth mentioning as an incidental finding.

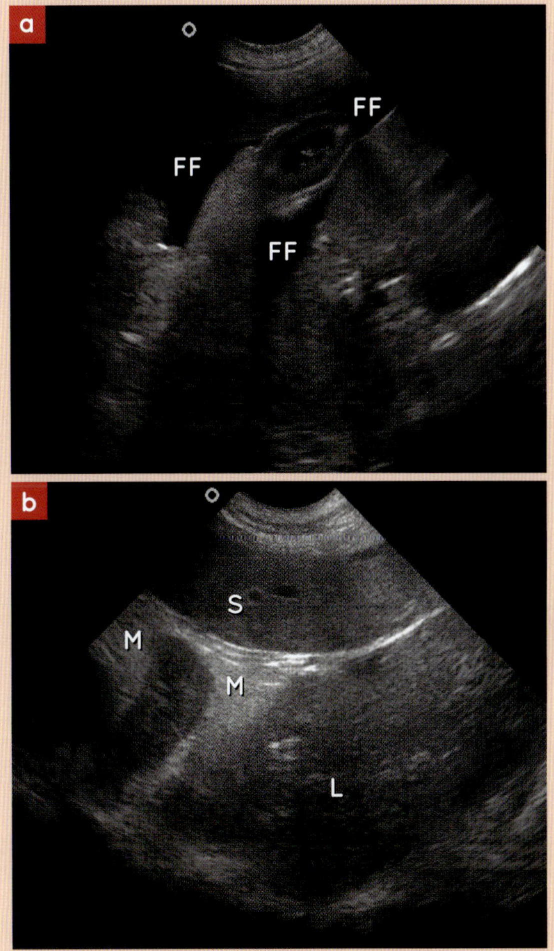

FIGURE 2.17. Ultrasound images of ascites (a) and peritonitis (b). The free fluid (FF) is anechonic and, as opposed to what occurs on a radiograph, it makes the observation of the outline of the organs easier. The inflammation of the peritoneum causes an increase of the echogenicity of the mesentery (M). S: spleen, L: liver.

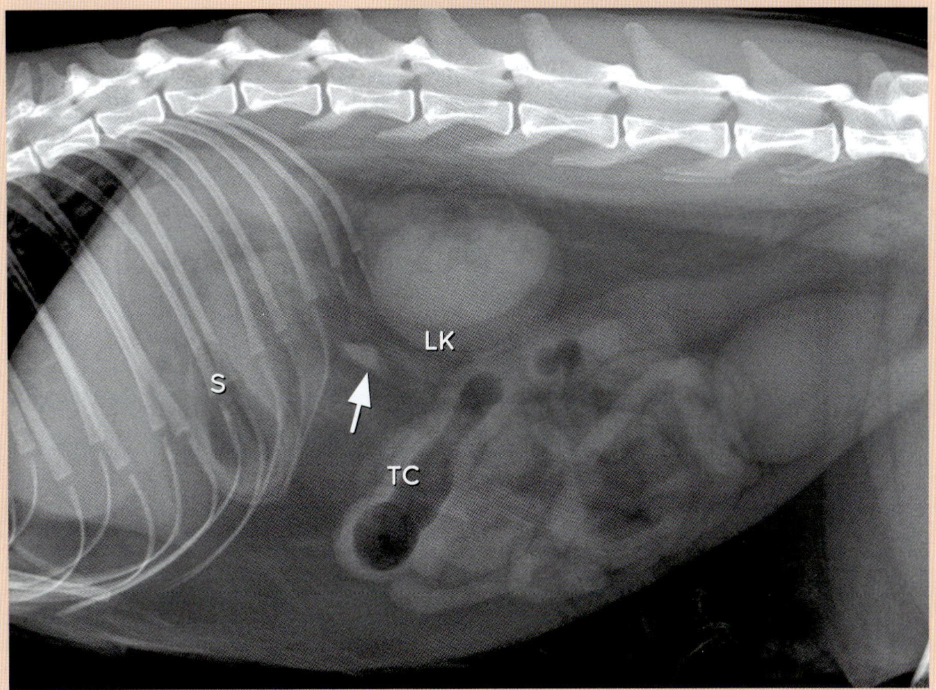

FIGURE 2.18. Lateral abdominal radiograph of a healthy cat. The arrow points to the normal pancreas shadow, surrounded by fat and located between the stomach (S), the left kidney (LK) and the transverse colon (TC).

The most frequent causes of retroperitonitis are the penetration of foreign bodies, penetrating wounds, the extension of local infections (e.g. pyelonephritis) and iatrogenic lesions of the urethra. The most common radiographic finding is increased radiopacity in the retroperitoneal area, with a displacement of the adjacent structures if associated masses appear (e.g. abscess). The appearance of gas in this area may be due to retroperitonitis caused by penetrating wounds or gas-producing anaerobic bacteria (fig. 2.21), but it can also appear in cases of severe pneumomediastinum, due to passage of gas from the mediastinum to the retroperitoneal space (fig. 2.22). In chronic cases, signs of spondylitis may appear in lumbar vertebrae, which are characterised by the appearance of bony overgrowths in the ventral margin of the affected vertebral bodies.

Although ultrasonography is useful to detect accumulated fluid, abscesses, alterations of the renal parenchyma, etc., the information it provides is sometimes limited due to the location and size of the lesions. In these cases, the use of computed tomography or magnetic resonance imaging becomes necessary, as they offer detailed anatomical information of the area and both are very sensitive for the detection of most of the pathological alterations that may be found at this level.

Peritoneal carcinomatosis

The neoplastic infiltration of the peritoneum is termed peritoneal carcinomatosis. This may have a very similar image to that of peritonitis and therefore to that of free intra-abdominal fluid. In addition, carcinomatosis often causes ascites. In the ultrasound examination, it is possible to observe thickening and irregular margins of the mesentery and, on occasions, focal hypo-echoic lesions in it.

Masses

An abdominal mass appears as a consequence of the increase in size of one or various intra-abdominal structures. This increase in size may be due to pathological causes (neoplasia, hyperplasia, haematoma, abscess, granuloma or cyst, essentially), but also occurs in some physiological processes such as pregnancy, or in iatrogenic diseases such as splenomegaly associated with the administration of barbiturates.

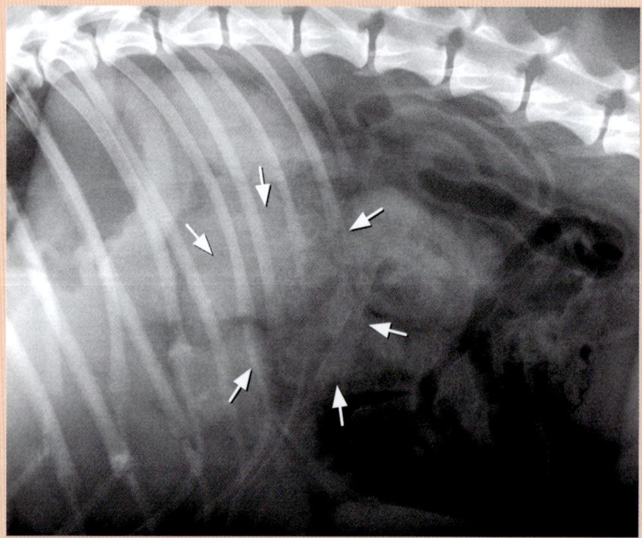

FIGURE 2.19. Enlarged image of the cranial abdomen on a lateral radiograph of a dog with peritonitis secondary to pancreatitis. The area of speckled radiopaque spots indicated by the arrows is due to focal peritonitis. Radiographically, it is not possible to distinguish between peritonitis caused by pancreatitis and other potential causes of inflammation or neoplastic infiltrations (carcinomatosis) of the peritoneum.

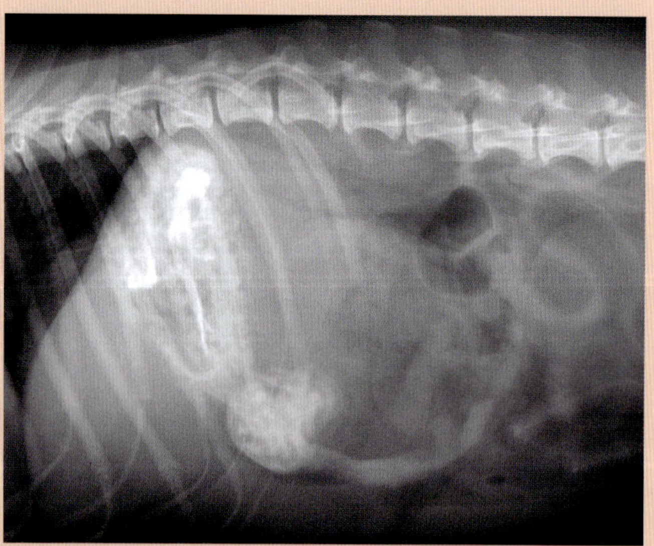

FIGURE 2.20. Lateral contrast radiograph (barium) of the abdomen of a dog with pancreatitis. The presence of the contrast medium in the duodenum shows its displacement and ventral curvature, caused by the inflammatory process of the pancreas. The central area of the abdomen shows a loss of differentiation of the structures due to the peritonitis associated with the process.

Although it is not usually possible to determine with certainty the origin of an abdominal mass based only on plain radiographs, its location in the cavity (table 2.2) and the displacement of other abdominal structures it causes may be of great help when establishing a differential diagnosis. For example, a hepatic mass causes a caudal and dorsal displacement of the stomach (fig. 2.23), while a splenic mass usually appears located in the central and ventral area of the abdomen, generally on the left side, and may displace the caecum and the colon in dorsal direction and the small intestine in dorsal and caudal direction (fig. 2.24). Taking radiographs in the two orthogonal projections, lateral and ventrodorsal, provides more complete information in this aspect.

Abdominal masses usually have soft-tissue opacity, although lipomas appear as fat opacity masses. Exceptionally, gas may be identified in an abdominal mass when there are areas of necrosis or when it is related to the digestive tract.

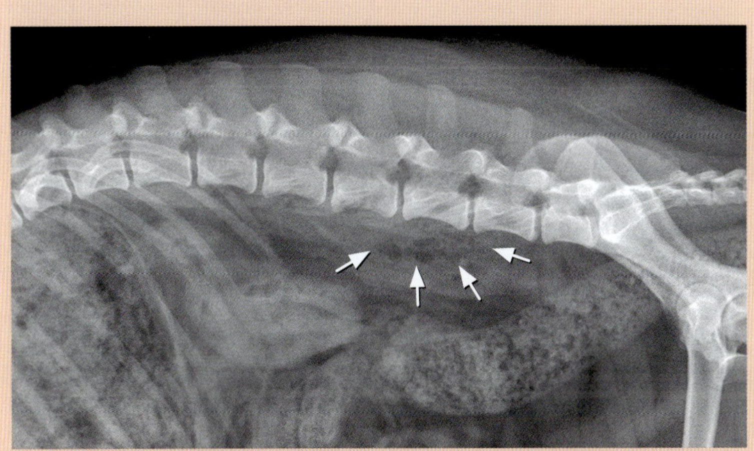

FIGURE 2.21. Enlarged image of dorsal abdomen in lateral radiograph of a dog with retroperitonitis due to *Clostridium* spp. The arrows indicate multiple accumulations of gas in the retroperitoneal area, produced by this pathogen. Image courtesy of María José Ruiz Fernández.

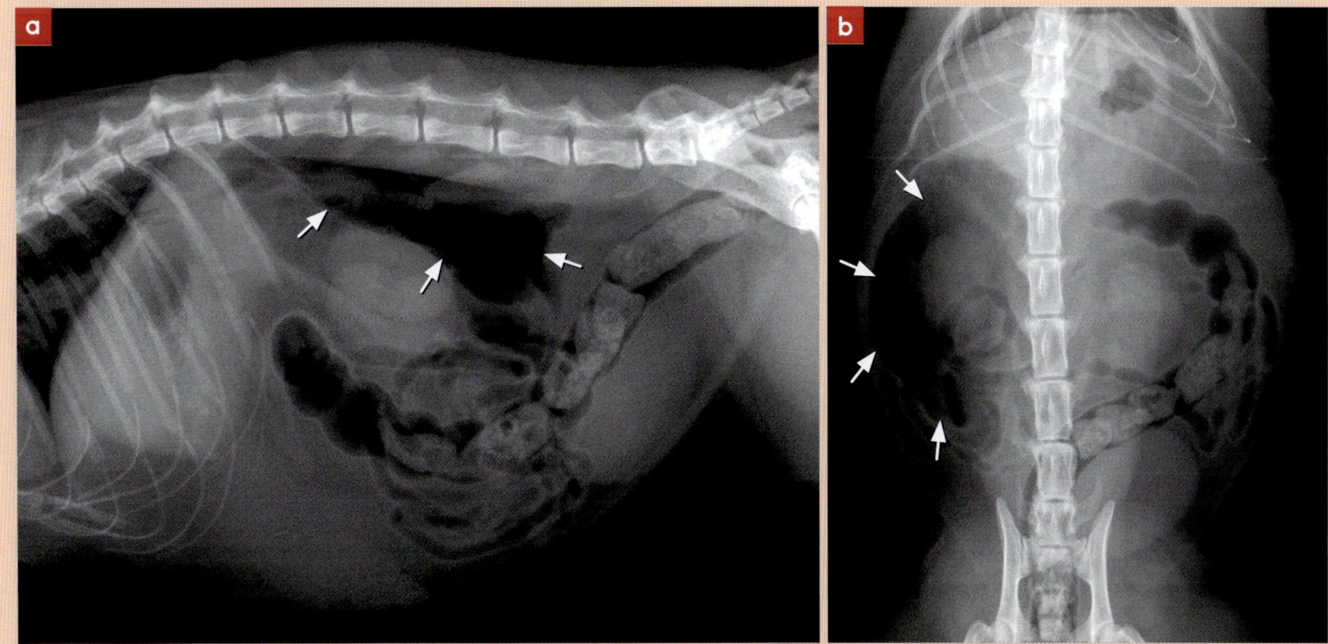

FIGURE 2.22. Lateral (a) and ventrodorsal (b) abdominal radiograph of a cat with pneumoretroperitoneum secondary to tracheal rupture, resulting in secondary pneumomediastinum; gas passed from mediastinal space into the retroperitoneum (arrows).

TABLE 2.2. Most probable organs of origin according to the location of an abdominal mass.

Location		Organ of origin
Cranial abdomen	Dorsal	■ Liver ■ Stomach ■ Pancreas ■ Kidney ■ Adrenal glands
	Ventral	■ Liver ■ Stomach ■ Pancreas ■ Biliary system
Middle abdomen	Dorsal	■ Kidney ■ Adrenal glands ■ Ovary ■ Retroperitoneal lymph nodes ■ Ureter
	Ventral	■ Spleen ■ Intestine ■ Jejunal lymph nodes* ■ Right lobe of the pancreas* ■ Left kidney* ■ Ovary*
Caudal abdomen	Dorsal	■ Medial iliac lymph nodes ■ Large intestine ■ Ureter
	Ventral	■ Bladder ■ Uterus ■ Prostate ■ Abdominal testicle

* The masses originating in these organs may gravitate towards the ventral part of the abdomen if they are very large.

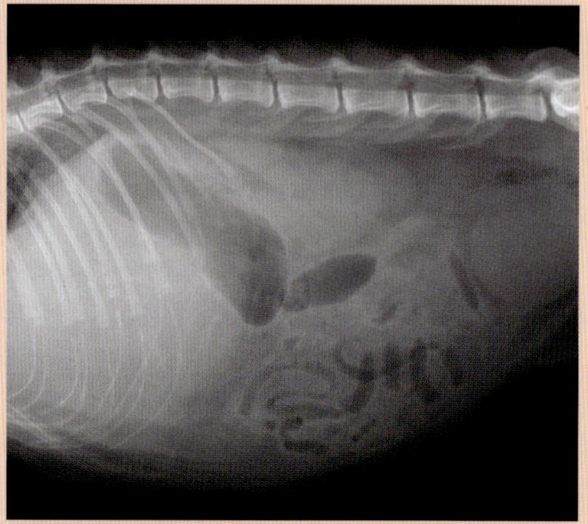

FIGURE 2.23. Lateral radiograph of the abdomen of a cat with a liver mass. The most significant finding is the dorsal and caudal displacement of the stomach. The loss of detail of structures in the central area of the abdomen is due to the presence of free fluid in the peritoneal cavity.

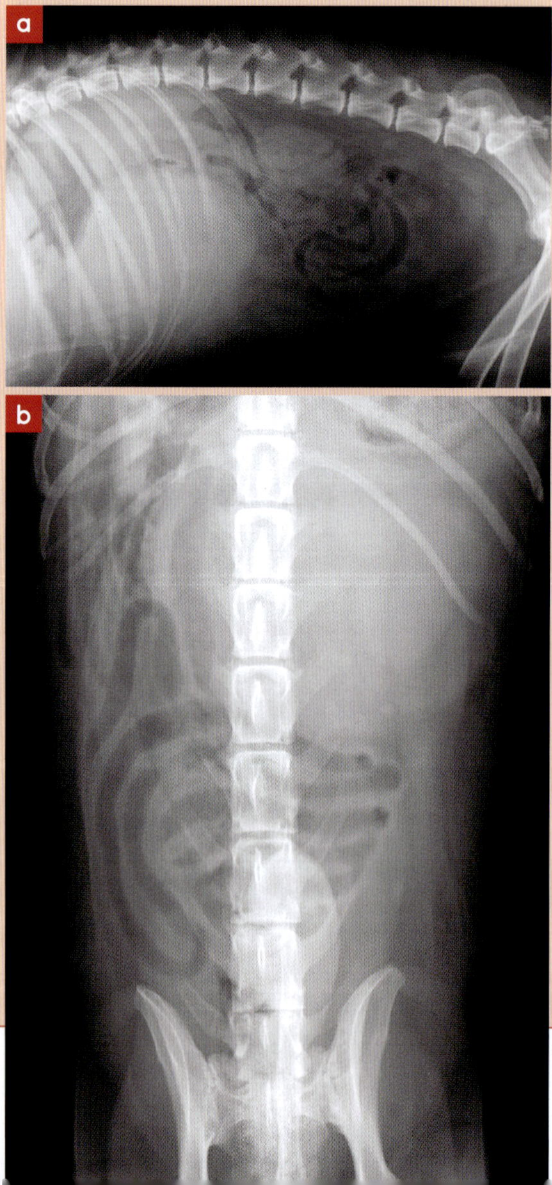

FIGURE 2.24. Lateral (a) and ventrodorsal (b) abdominal radiographs of a dog with a splenic mass, seen in the left cranial area of the abdomen, displacing the colon dorsally and to the right, and the small intestine dorsally, caudally and to the right. In the lateral view, a bladder catheter is visualised.

The visibility of a mass on a radiograph depends on its size and on the degree of definition of its margins, which may be significantly reduced when free fluid is present or if the patient also suffers from peritonitis or carcinomatosis, or is very thin. If the margins of a mass cannot be clearly seen in the image, but there is an evident abnormal displacement of the adjacent anatomical structures, we will use the term "mass effect" (fig. 2.25).

Depending on their size, retroperitoneal masses may displace adjacent abdominal structures in ventral direction (fig. 2.26). They may have a renal, adrenal, muscular, lymphatic or vascular origin, essentially. Computed tomography and magnetic resonance imaging allow us to precisely define the borders of the mass and determine whether the adjacent structures are affected (fig. 2.27).

The adrenal glands can only be identified on a radiograph if they are enlarged or calcified. An adrenal origin should be suspected when a mass (with soft-tissue density or partially calcified) is identified craniomedial to a kidney (fig. 2.28). The radiographic finding of a calcified adrenal mass in patients with Cushing's syndrome is very indicative of a neoplasm. However, it should be borne in mind that in cats, the adrenal glands may be calcified with no pathological significance.

Ultrasonography will allow a more precise assessment of the peritoneal and retroperitoneal masses and in many cases, will enable ultrasound-guided cytology or biopsy.

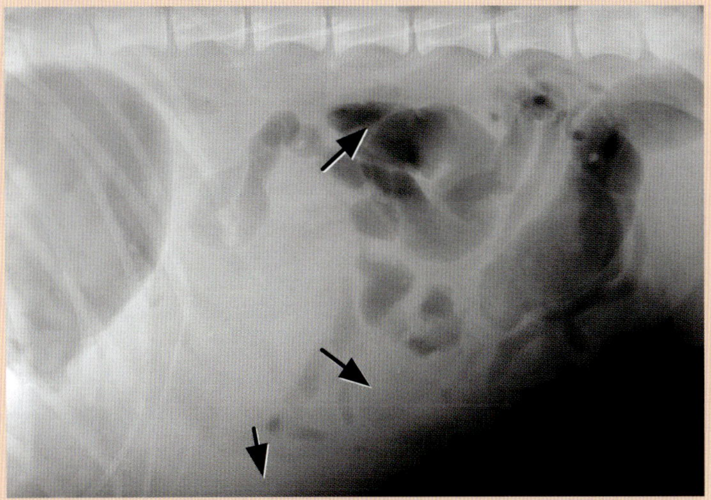

FIGURE 2.25. Lateral radiograph of the abdomen of a dog with a "mass effect" in the cranial area of the abdomen. Immediately caudal to the stomach, it is possible to observe an area of soft-tissue opacity with poorly defined margins, which displaces the adjacent structures dorsally, caudally and ventrally. This finding is due to the presence of a small-sized mass in the central area of the splenic tail.

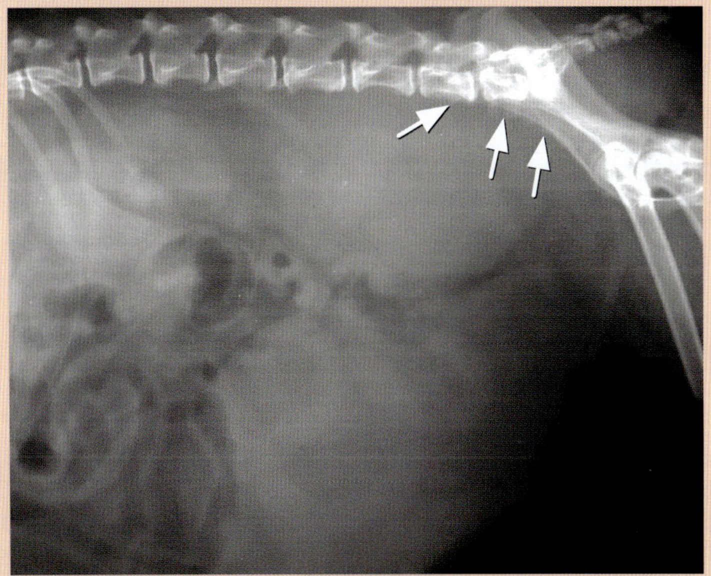

FIGURE 2.26. Lateral radiograph of the abdomen of a dog with a localised tumour in the retroperitoneal space. The mass causes a ventral displacement of the bladder (very distended), descending colon and rectum. In the ventral margin of the last lumbar vertebrae and cranial margin of one of the wings of the ilium, it is possible to identify small bony overgrowths (arrows), compatible with bone metastases. If it were a retroperitoneal abscess instead of a tumour, the bony overgrowths could be due to secondary spondylitis/osteomyelitis.

Liver, spleen and lymph nodes

Liver

On lateral radiographs, the liver occupies a triangular area between the diaphragm and the ventral abdominal wall. Its caudoventral border has an angular shape and does not generally extend beyond the costal arch, or only very slightly. This caudal border is sometimes masked by the splenic shadow. The longitudinal axis of the stomach on this view should be, in normal conditions, perpendicular to the spine or parallel to the ribs. On ventrodorsal radiographs, the liver occupies almost the whole concavity of the diaphragm. Its caudal border appears delimited by the cranial duodenal flexure, the cranial pole of the right kidney and the lesser curvature of the stomach. The left lobes appear superimposed on the fundus on this view (fig. 2.29).

Radiographically, we can detect changes in the size, outline, location and radiographic density of the liver.

A recent publication described a radiographic liver size evaluation method, measuring the area occupied by the liver shadow in digital images (RLA: radiographic liver area) and how this correlates with the patient's T11 body area (fig. 2.30) and body weight. The normal reference values for these ratios are: RLA to T11=32.7±6.2 and RLA to body weight=7.0±1.4.

When the liver increases in size in a generalised manner, the stomach is displaced caudally. The caudoventral border may appear round and is located

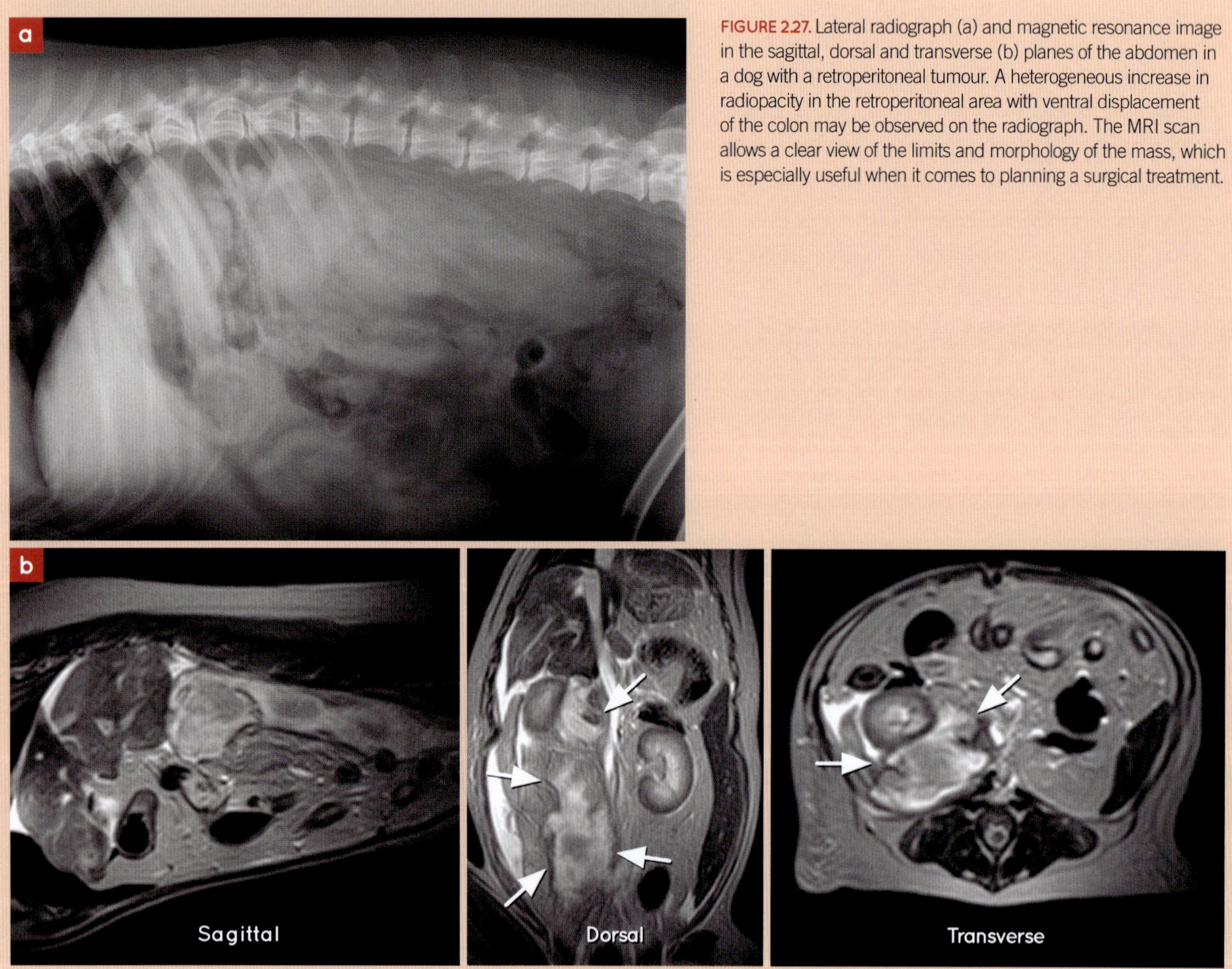

FIGURE 2.27. Lateral radiograph (a) and magnetic resonance image in the sagittal, dorsal and transverse (b) planes of the abdomen in a dog with a retroperitoneal tumour. A heterogeneous increase in radiopacity in the retroperitoneal area with ventral displacement of the colon may be observed on the radiograph. The MRI scan allows a clear view of the limits and morphology of the mass, which is especially useful when it comes to planning a surgical treatment.

farther away from the costal arch (fig. 2.31). If the increase in size is localised, these signs may not be as obvious on the radiograph. The radiographic image of liver masses depend on their size and location in the organ, but if they are large, they occupy the most cranial part of the abdominal cavity and significantly displace the stomach caudally and dorsally (fig. 2.32).

Radiography is a fairly precise tool to detect a reduction of the size of the liver (microhepatia). The axis of the stomach appears displaced cranially and the distance between the margin of the diaphragmatic dome

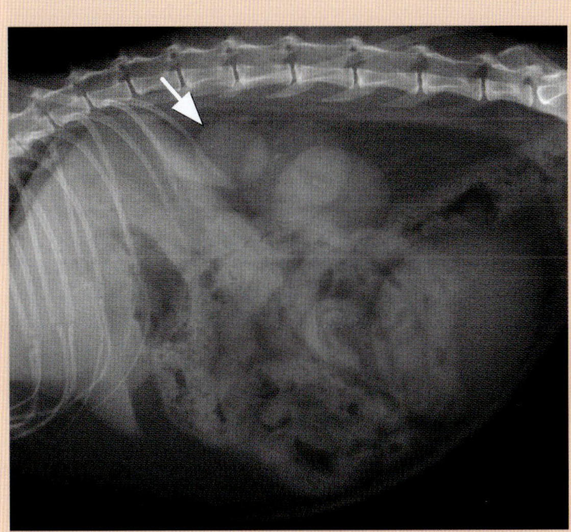

FIGURE 2.28. Lateral radiograph of a cat with an adrenal mass (arrow). Although its size is small, the large amount of retroperitoneal fat allows it to be clearly identified in the image. The fact that it is located cranial to the renal shadows indicates that it is of adrenal origin, although masses of other origins (e.g. glandular) may also appear in this location.

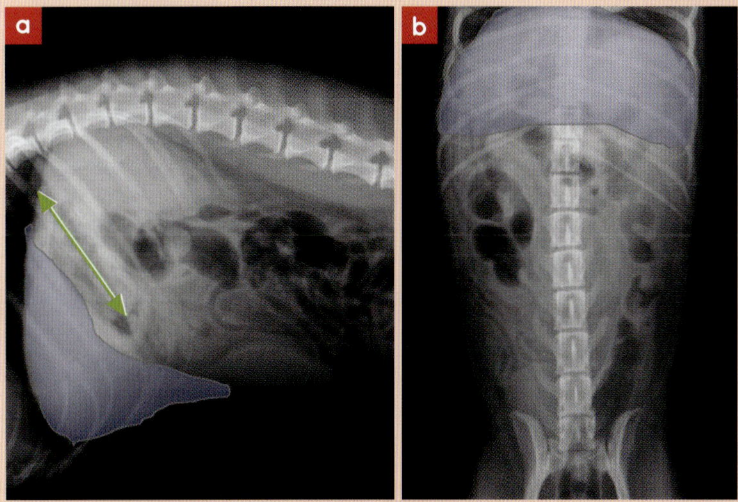

FIGURE 2.29. Lateral (a) and (b) ventrodorsal radiographs of the abdomen of a healthy dog, in which the shadows of the liver are highlighted with blue areas. The green line represents the longitudinal axis of the stomach, drawn from the centre of the fundus to the centre of the pyloric area.

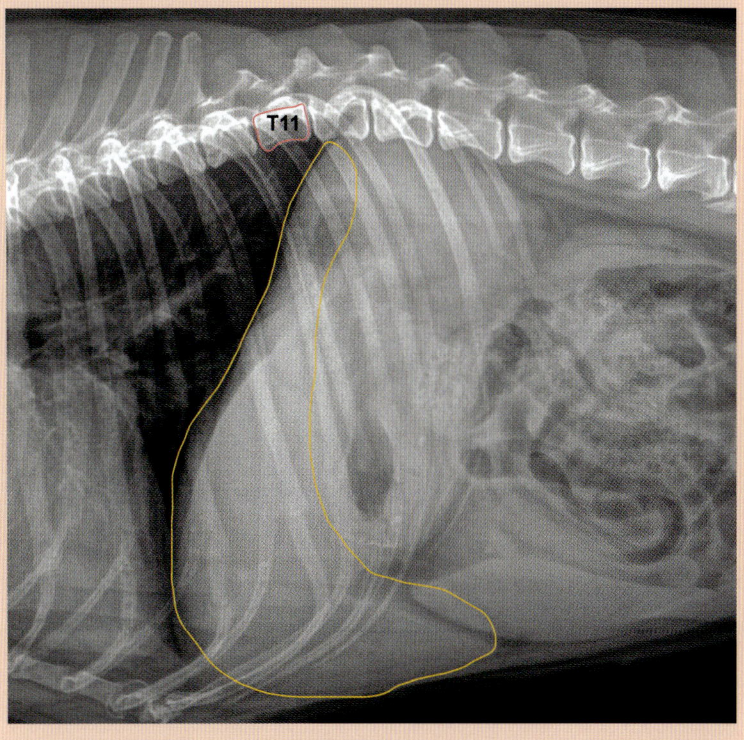

FIGURE 2.30. Enlarged image of the cranial abdomen in lateral view of a healthy dog to illustrate the liver size measurement method based on the ratio between liver area and T11 thoracic vertebra area. The normal reference value of the liver area:T11 area ratio=32.7±6.2.

and caudal hepatic border (fig. 2.33). Doubts about the size of the liver may sometimes arise with ultrasonography, but this technique provides much more information about alterations of the liver parenchyma and margins, which is why both methods are used in a complementary manner to diagnose a reduction of the size of this organ.

It is not uncommon to observe areas of mineral opacity in the liver. Gallbladder sludge or calcified gallbladder stones are often identified on plain radiographs

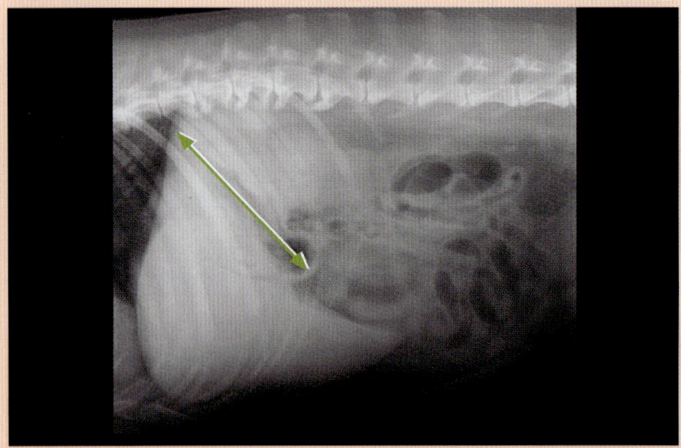

FIGURE 2.31. Lateral radiograph of the cranial abdomen of a dog suffering from hepatomegaly. The axis of the stomach appears displaced caudally and a great part of the caudoventral border extends beyond the costal arch. As an incidental finding, it is possible to observe spondylosis deformans in the T11-L2 segment.

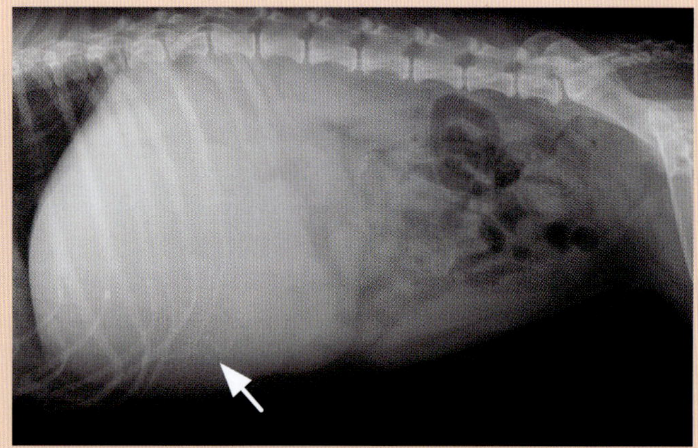

FIGURE 2.32. Lateral radiograph of the abdomen of a dog with a liver mass, which occupies a great part of the cranial abdomen and displaces the stomach, intestine and spleen caudally. The mass shows a region with small areas of calcifications (arrow).

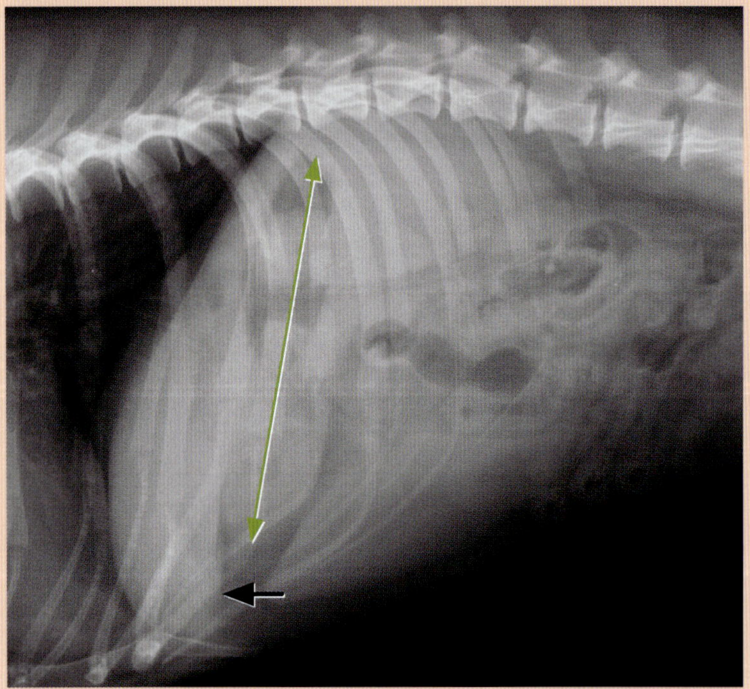

FIGURE 2.33. Lateral radiograph of the abdomen of a dog with an abnormally small liver (microhepatia). The axis of the stomach is displaced in cranial direction and the distance between the dome of the diaphragm and the caudoventral border of the liver appears reduced (indicated by the black arrow).

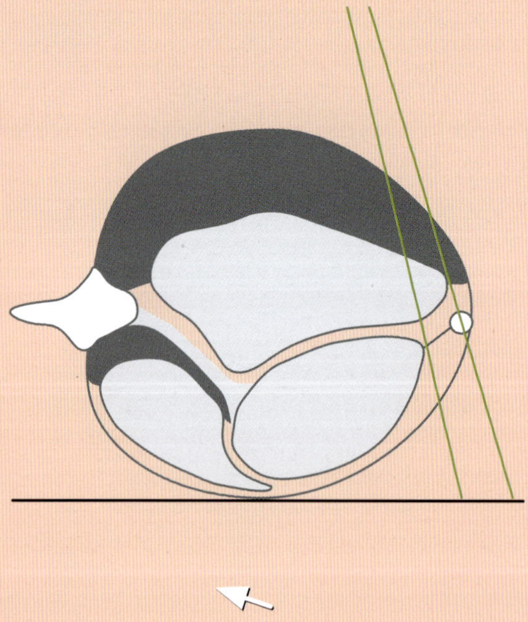

FIGURE 2.34. Enlarged image of the cranial abdomen on a lateral radiograph of a dog with calcified sludge in the gallbladder (arrow).

and are in many cases a casual finding (fig. 2.34). If the calcified areas have a linear pattern, the most probable diagnosis is that of calcification of the biliary tract (fig. 2.35), which is sometimes an incidental finding in small breed dogs. Abscesses, haematomas, cysts and tumours may also appear partially calcified in this organ. In addition, the presence of gas may be detected in the liver parenchyma or in the gallbladder and biliary tract. This may be due to an infection caused by anaerobes or, in diabetic patients, by microorganisms that ferment glucose, giving rise to the formation of carbon dioxide. If the morphology of the gas opacity areas is linear, this suggests involvement of the biliary tract (neumobilia), if it is oval, of the gallbladder, and if it is irregular, this is more suggestive of the presence of an abscess or of a tumour with a necrotic centre in the parenchyma. In any case, both calcifications and the presence of gas in this organ can be assessed and confirmed by means of ultrasonography.

Spleen

The spleen is an organ with a relatively variable size and location, especially in dogs. The head of the spleen has a more stable position in the left craniodorsal area of the abdomen, thanks to the gastrosplenic ligament. On ventrodorsal radiographs, it appears as a shadow with a triangular morphology superimposed on the last ribs of the left side (fig. 2.36), and it is visible both in dogs and cats. The position of the tail of the spleen, by contrast, may considerably vary. On lateral radiographs, the canine spleen usually appears as a triangular or oval shadow in the mid to ventral abdomen.

The feline spleen is proportionally smaller than the canine spleen. Its distal end is generally not identified in the lateral view while its proximal end may be visualised in some cases dorsally and caudally to the fundus of the stomach. In the ventrodorsal projection, the head of the feline spleen appears similar to the canine spleen, i.e. a triangular shadow superimposed on the

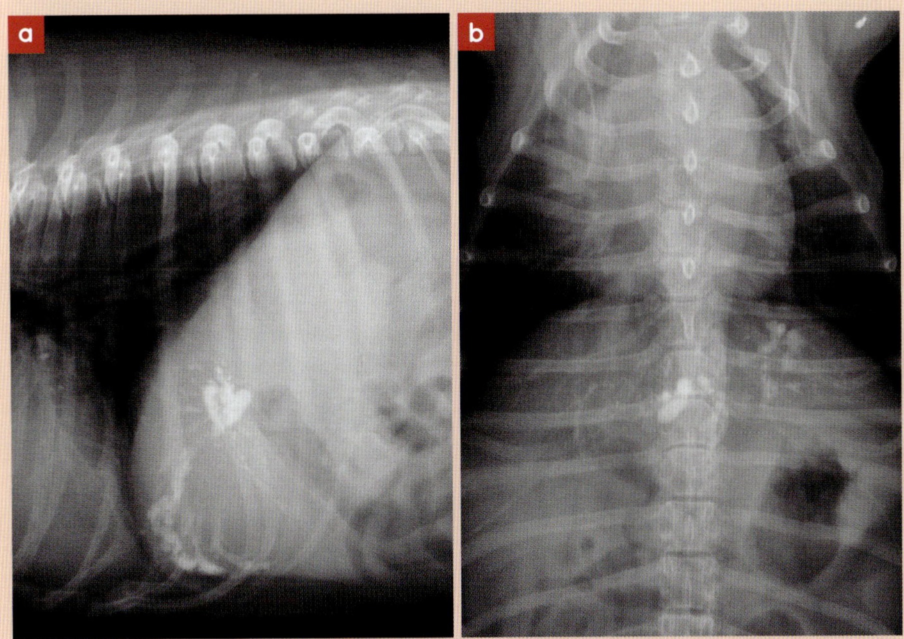

FIGURE 2.35. Enlarged images of two lateral (a) and ventrodorsal (b) radiographs of the cranial abdomen of a dog with calcification of the bile ducts. This finding may be incidental in small breeds.

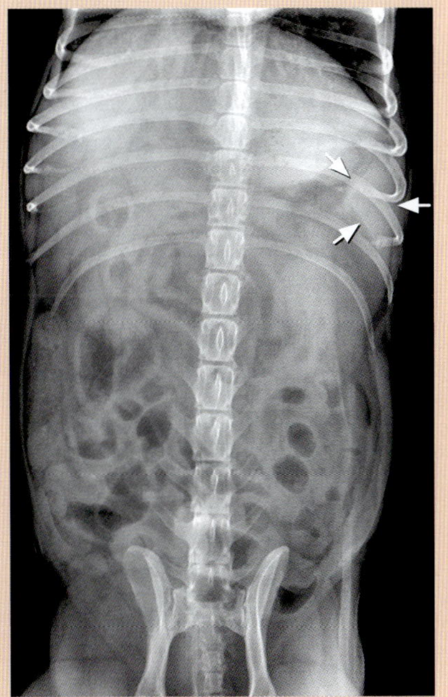

FIGURE 2.36. Ventrodorsal radiograph of the abdomen of a healthy dog. The shadow of the head of the spleen (arrows) has a triangular morphology on this view and is located in the left cranial abdomen, superimposed on the most caudal ribs of the same side.

most caudal ribs in the left hemithorax. Sometimes in ventrodorsal views, a normal splenic tail can be seen adjacent to the left abdominal wall (fig. 2.37).

The length of the splenic shadow in dogs will vary on lateral radiographs depending on the position of the tail of the spleen. If the latter is almost completely located in the cranial part of the mid-abdomen, the shadow will be relatively short; if it is in an oblique position in the mid-abdomen, the shadow will be longer; and if it is located along the left side of the animal, the shadow will then be very long on the radiograph (fig. 2.38).

We should not confuse a longer shadow of the spleen with splenomegaly. Splenomegaly is assessed in a subjective manner but is always accompanied by an enlargement (fig. 2.39) and in many cases rounded borders of the organ. It should be borne in mind that healthy German Shepherd dogs have a larger spleen than other breeds of a similar size. With lateral views, a clear visualisation of the distal extremity of the spleen is considered indicative of splenomegaly in cats (fig. 2.40). In the case of a splenic torsion, the organ usually appears very enlarged, with rounded margins and an abnormal position in the abdomen.

The image of splenic masses varies in function of their size and location (fig. 2.41). If there is a haemorrhage, the tumour margins may appear totally or

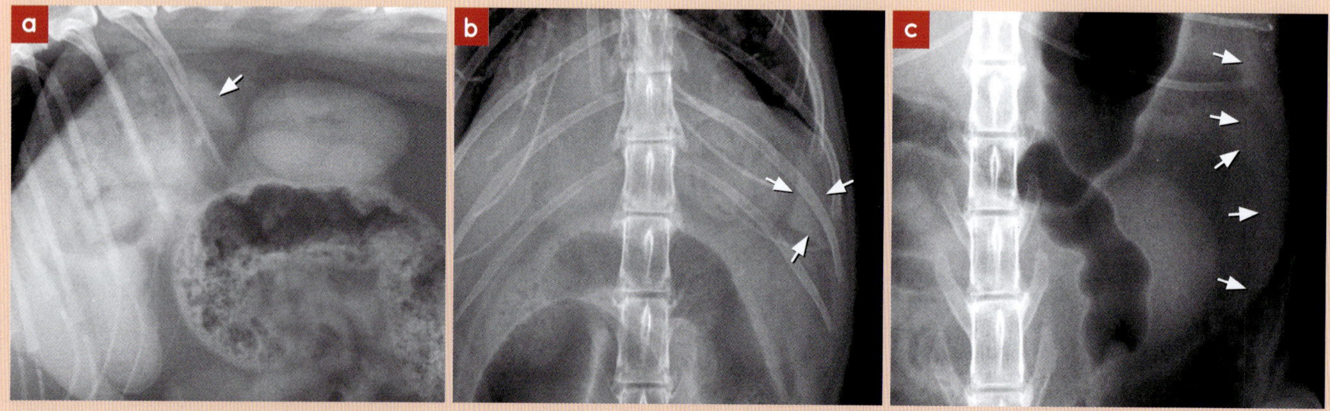

FIGURE 2.37. Enlarged images of the cranial abdomen in lateral (a) and ventrodorsal (b and c) radiograph of healthy cats. The silhouette of the proximal aspect of the spleen (arrow) can be seen between the gastric fundus, the colon and the left kidney (a). The triangular shadow of the splenic head (arrows) superimposed with the caudal left ribs (b) is identified, as is the shadow of the spleen adjacent to the left abdominal wall (c) (arrows).

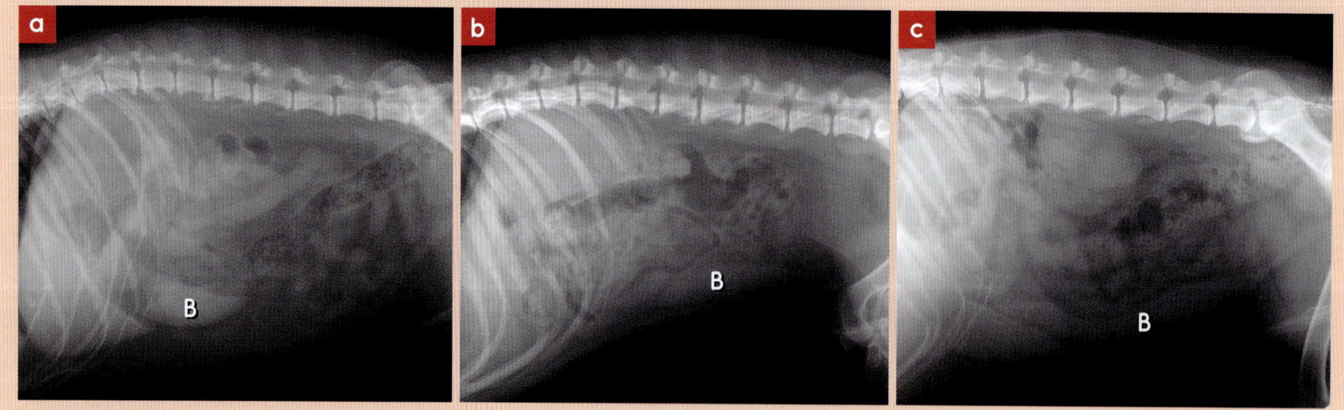

FIGURE 2.38. Lateral radiographs of the abdomens of three healthy dogs showing different positions of the tail of the spleen. In image (a), the shadow is short because the tail of the spleen (S) is located in the cranial abdomen. In image (b), the shadow is slightly longer because the tail of the spleen is located obliquely in the mid-abdomen. In image (c), the tail of the spleen is located along the left side of the animal, thus creating a longer shadow on the lateral view. In the three cases, the spleen has a normal size.

partially masked, although the displacement of the adjacent viscera will be an evident sign of its presence in the abdominal cavity.

Changes in the radiographic density of the spleen are rare. The organ may show areas of calcification associated with dystrophic calcification of neoplasms, abscesses, granulomas or haematomas.

A recently published report described 3 cases of emphysematous splenitis secondary to *Clostridium* spp. infection, all in Golden Retrievers. With such a small number of patients, no conclusions can be drawn as to whether or not there is a predisposition in this breed. This is a rare pathology in human medicine, only described in severe forms of sepsis produced by anaerobic pathogens. In dogs, radiography shows a focal or multifocal coalescing gas pattern in the splenic region, which may be accompanied by signs of loss of serosal detail and pneumoperitoneum. Other causes of

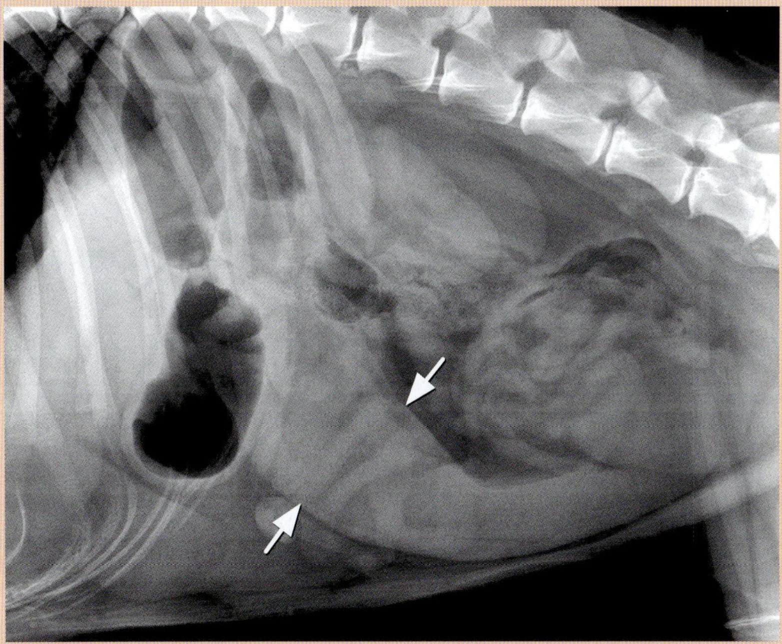

FIGURE 2.39. Lateral radiograph of the abdomen of a dog with splenomegaly. The spleen appears enlarged (arrow), which indicates an increase in the size of the organ.

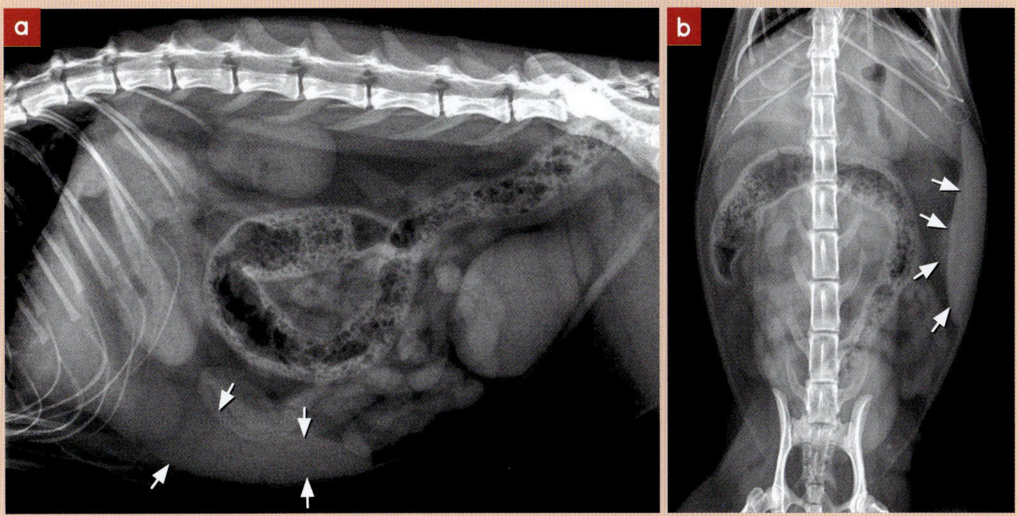

FIGURE 2.40. Lateral (a) and (b) ventrodorsal abdominal radiographs of a cat with splenomegaly. Visualisation of the distal part of the spleen (arrows) on the lateral view is considered indicative of splenomegaly. In the ventrodorsal projection, the spleen appears enlarged.

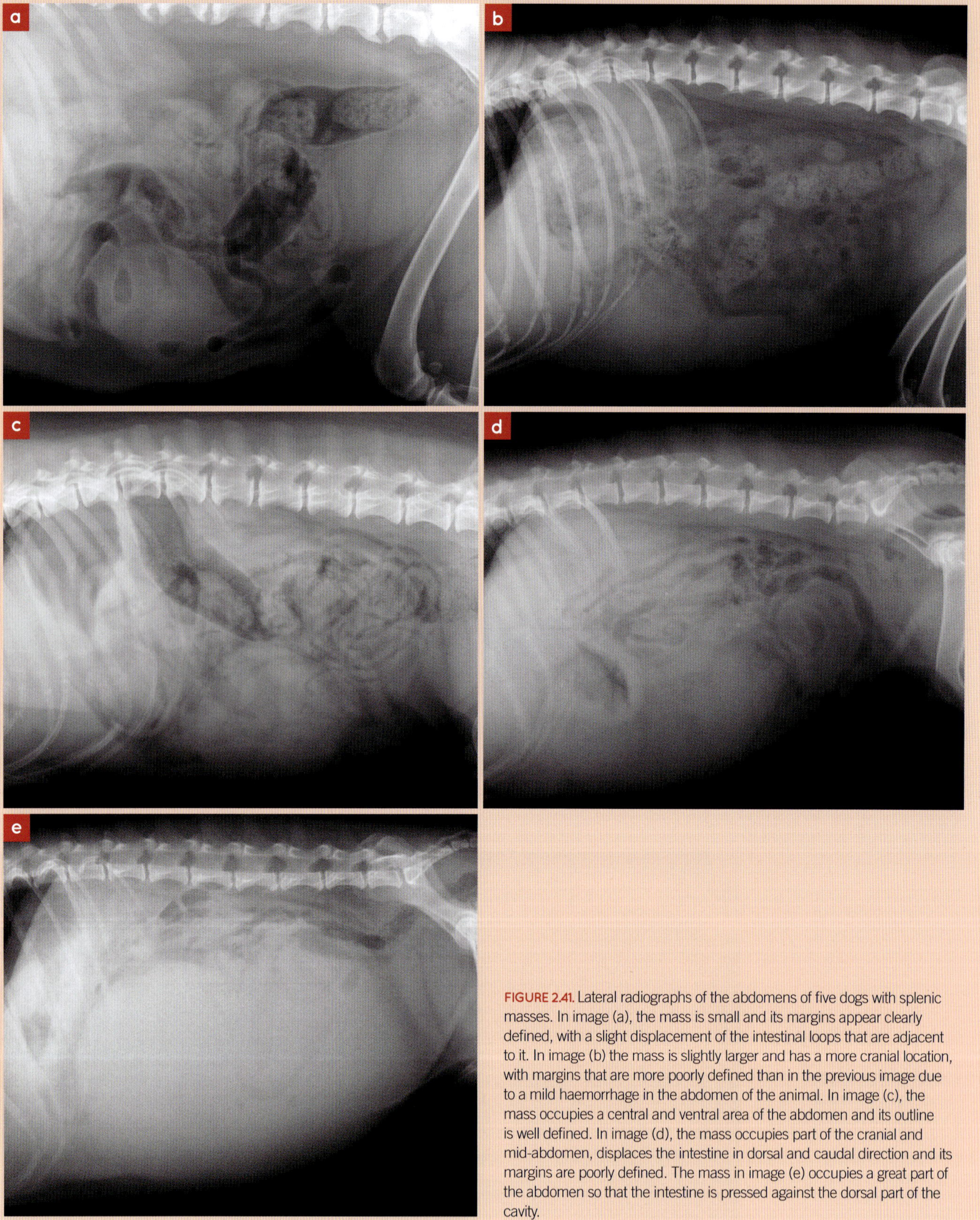

FIGURE 2.41. Lateral radiographs of the abdomens of five dogs with splenic masses. In image (a), the mass is small and its margins appear clearly defined, with a slight displacement of the intestinal loops that are adjacent to it. In image (b) the mass is slightly larger and has a more cranial location, with margins that are more poorly defined than in the previous image due to a mild haemorrhage in the abdomen of the animal. In image (c), the mass occupies a central and ventral area of the abdomen and its outline is well defined. In image (d), the mass occupies part of the cranial and mid-abdomen, displaces the intestine in dorsal and caudal direction and its margins are poorly defined. The mass in image (e) occupies a great part of the abdomen so that the intestine is pressed against the dorsal part of the cavity.

gas accumulation in the splenic parenchyma include abscesses or neoplasms infected by gas-producing bacteria and gas embolism secondary to splenic torsion or infarction. These are also uncommon.

Lymph nodes

Abdominal lymph nodes are only identified on radiographs when they are enlarged or calcified. The more retroperitoneal fat a patient has, the easier it will be to observe them.

The medial iliac (sublumbar) lymph nodes are the easiest to identify on radiographs of the abdomen when they are enlarged. They are located ventral to the lumbar vertebrae L6 and L7. If the enlargement is very pronounced, their silhouette can extend more cranially (fig. 2.42) and produce conspicuous displacement of the descending colon and rectum ventrally (fig. 2.43). The enlargement may be due to lymphadenitis, hyperplasia or neoplasia. A tumoral infiltration of these lymph nodes may be primary (e.g. lymphoma) or metastatic (e.g. in the case of localised tumours in the caudal area of the abdomen or in the pelvis).

Urinary system

Conventional radiography is a very important diagnostic technique in the study of diseases of the urinary system, although it has now been replaced to a great extent by ultrasonography, since this latter allows a direct assessment of the internal architecture of the kidneys and bladder. However, contrast radiographic techniques still are the standard method of choice to examine the ureters and urethra.

Kidneys

A plain radiograph allows the observation of alterations in the number, size, outline, position and radiographic density of the kidneys, but it does not offer any information about their internal architecture. That is why the diagnostic imaging technique of choice to assess the kidneys is ultrasonography, since this technique does offer detailed information about the normal internal structure and its possible alterations.

The contrast technique used to examine the kidneys and ureters is excretory urography. It involves

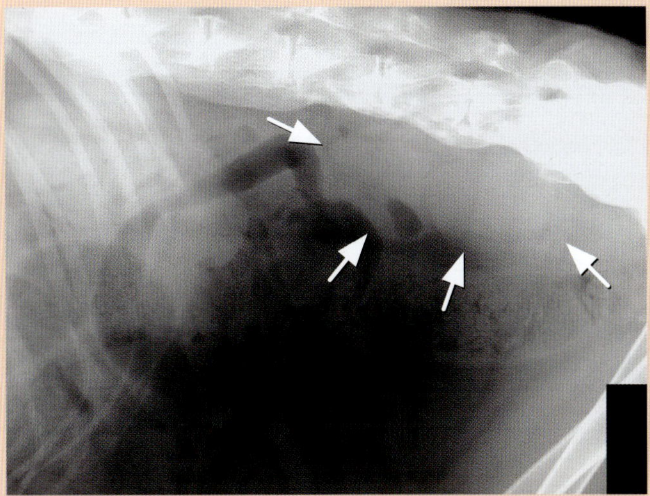

FIGURE 2.42. Enlarged image of the caudal abdomen on a lateral radiograph of a dog with sublumbar lymphadenopathies. Its outline cannot be seen properly due to the presence of surrounding retroperitoneal fat.

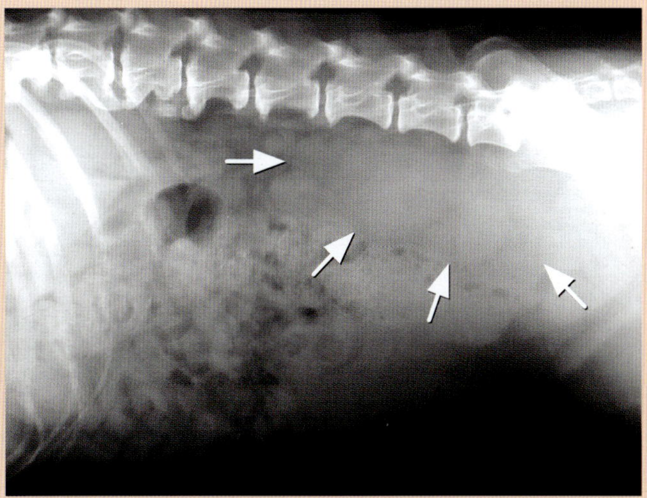

FIGURE 2.43. Lateral radiograph of the abdomen of a dog with very large sublumbar lymphadenopathies due to a lymphoma. The "mass effect" is located ventral to L5-L7 and causes the ventral displacement of the descending colon.

the intravenous administration of a positive contrast medium that is selectively excreted by the kidneys. With this technique it is possible to obtain a certain amount of information about the internal structure of the kidney (although not as complete as that offered by ultrasonography), and functional information based on the qualitative assessment of the degree of filtration of the contrast agent through the renal parenchyma.

The kidneys are located in the retroperitoneal space. On lateral radiographs, they appear located in the craniodorsal area of the abdomen and partially superimposed, while on ventrodorsal radiographs they are not superimposed on one another but on other structures, which masks the shadow of one or the two kidneys, particularly in dogs. The greater the amount of retroperitoneal fat an animal has, the more defined the renal shadows will be in the image. Cats accumulate more fat in this anatomical location, which significantly improves the visualisation of the kidneys. The anatomical location of the right kidney is more cranial than that of the left one, which allows their differentiation on lateral radiographs.

The evaluation of the size of the renal shadows is based on the comparison of their length with that of the vertebral body of the L2 vertebra. In healthy animals, the maximum length of the renal shadows should be comprised between 2.5 and 3.5 times the length of L2 in dogs (fig. 2.44), and between 2.4 and 3 times its length in cats (fig. 2.45), although lower ranges have been published in older cats with no clinical symptoms of kidney disease (2.1 to 3.2 in non-neutered cats and 1.9 to 2.6 in neutered cats.)

An increase in the size of the renal shadows may be due to very different diseases. A decrease in the size of the kidneys in young animals is usually caused by congenital diseases such as renal dysplasia or hypoplasia, while in adult animals it is usually attributed to chronic renal diseases at an advanced or terminal stage.

The relative assessment of the kidneys, that is to say, comparing the size, shape and outline of a kidney with those of the other, may be more useful in practice than evaluating the actual size of each kidney. If the two renal shadows appear enlarged, the differential diagnosis will include renal lymphoma (fig. 2.46), bilateral hydronephrosis, polycystic kidney disease, bilateral perinephric cyst (fig. 2.47) and bilateral neoplasia. If the two kidneys appear decreased in size, the most probable cause is chronic interstitial nephritis (fig. 2.48). When one of the shadows maintains a normal size and the other one is enlarged, this suggests

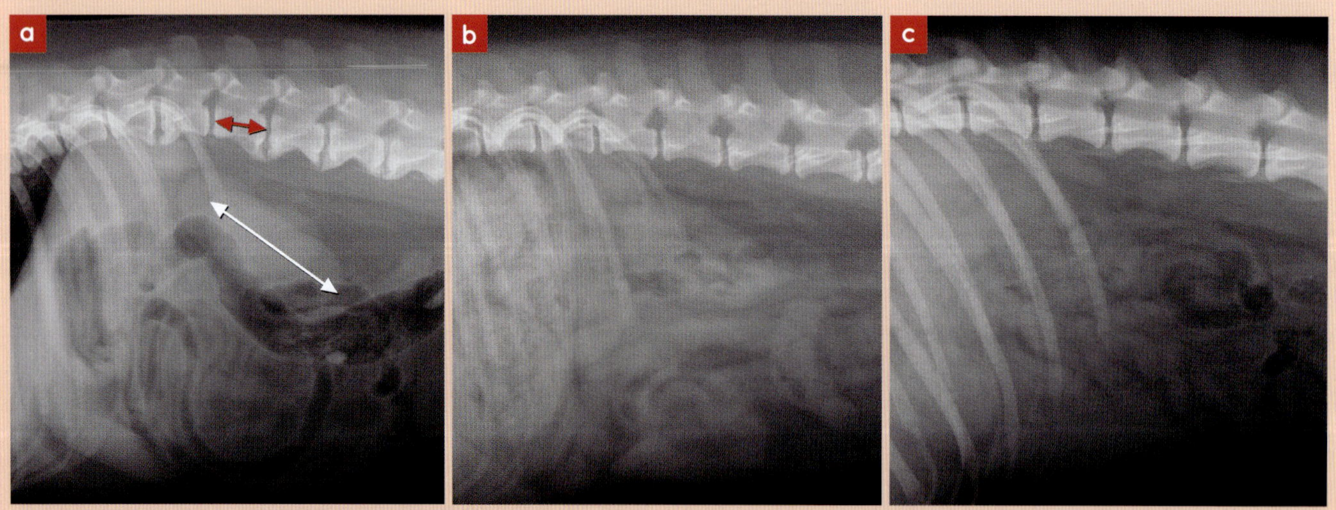

FIGURE 2.44. Enlarged images of the cranial abdomens on lateral radiographs of three dogs with normal kidneys. In image (a), the two renal shadows are perfectly differentiated due to the large amount of retroperitoneal fat of the animal. In normal conditions, the length of the renal shadows (shown in the left kidney with a white arrow), should be comprised between 2.5 and 3.5 times the length of the L2 vertebra (shown with a red arrow). In image (b), only the shadow of the left kidney, which is anatomically located in a more caudal position, is well defined, while the right renal shadow is masked by other structures. In image (c), none of the renal shadows can be clearly distinguished because of the lack of retroperitoneal fat and other superimposed structures.

neoplasia, renal trauma, unilateral perinephric cyst or unilateral hydornephrosis. Finally, if the shadow of a kidney is enlarged and the other one is reduced, the most probable cause is chronic interstitial nephritis in a kidney with compensatory hypertrophy of the other one (fig. 2.49).

Plain radiography also allows the visualisation of alterations in the outline of the kidneys, although

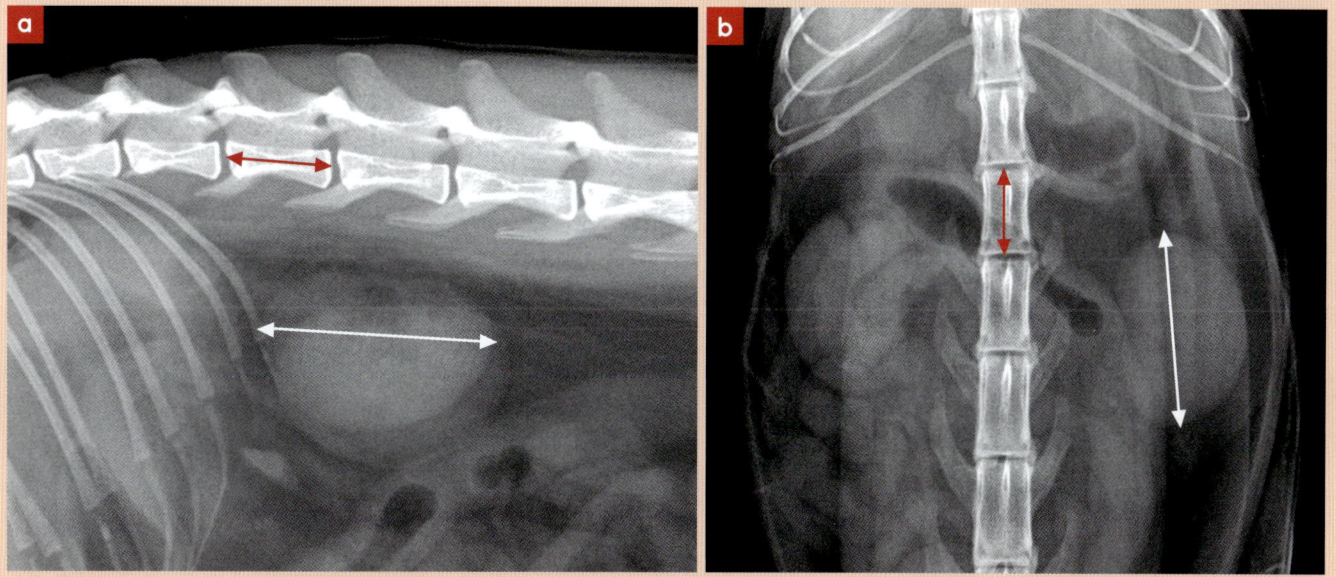

FIGURE 2.45. Enlarged images of lateral (a) and ventrodorsal (b) abdominal radiographs of a healthy cat showing renal length measurement references. As a general reference for normality, the length of the renal shadows in cats should be between 2.4 and 3 times the L2 length, although lower ranges have been published in older cats (2.1 to 3.2 in non-neutered cats and 1.9 to 2.6 in neutered cats). Measuring the length of the renal shadow in the ventrodorsal view is considered more accurate as in lateral decubitus the kidneys may acquire a certain degree of obliquity.

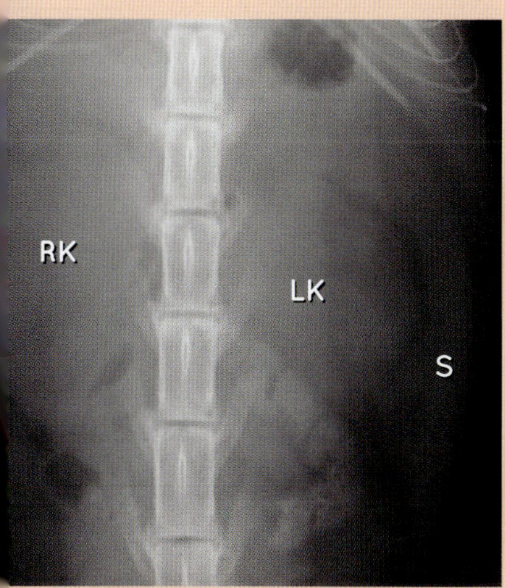

FIGURE 2.46. Enlarged image of the abdomen on a ventral radiograph of a cat with renal lymphoma. The two renal shadows (RK, LK) appear enlarged in size with an irregular contour. The spleen (S) also appears enlarged.

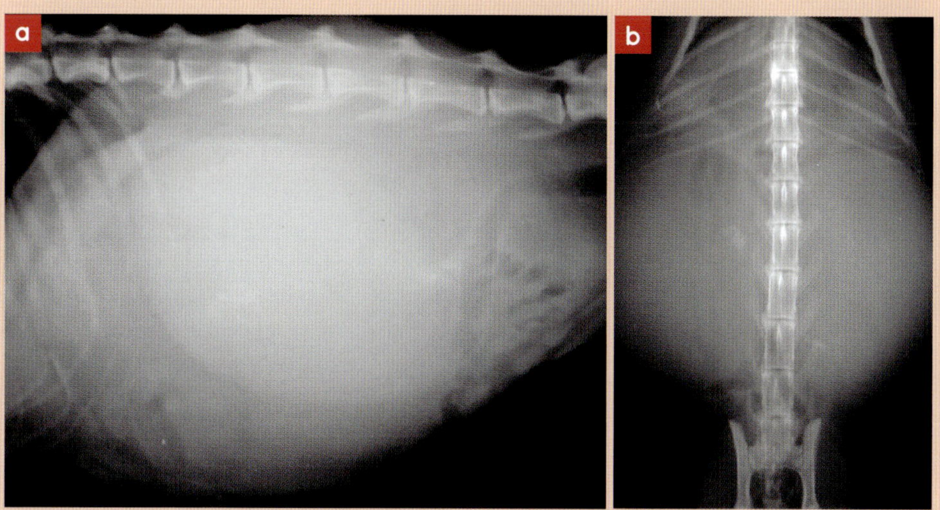

FIGURE 2.47. Lateral (a) and (b) ventrodorsal radiographs of the abdomen of a cat with bilateral perinephric cysts (perinephric pseudocysts). This disease is very uncommon and mainly affects older cats. It is characterised by an accumulation of a large amount of fluid (urine, transudate, lymph, or blood) that totally or partially surrounds one or the two kidneys. In this case, it gives rise to the appearance of large masses in the region of the kidneys.

ultrasonography is more precise in this aspect. The most common causes of changes in the contour of the kidneys are: polycystic renal disease, neoplasia, abscess, simple cysts, haematoma, cortical infarction or chronic renal disease at an advanced stage (fig. 2.50).

It is uncommon to detect significant anomalies in the position of the kidneys. When they appear displaced from their normal position, this is generally due to an increase in the size or displacement of the structures that are adjacent to the kidneys, although they may also have an abnormal location due to congenital alterations (renal ectopy) or to trauma causing their avulsion.

Calcification of the renal parenchyma due to the presence of calculi (fig. 2.51) or to dystrophic calcification is frequent, especially in older animals. Not all calculi are observed as mineral opacities. Those composed of ammonium urate and cystin have a similar radiopacity to that of soft tissues and fluids, which is why they are usually qualified as radiolucent in plain radiography. Ultrasonography allows the detection of all types of calculi, although if they are small it will be difficult or impossible to distinguish them from calcifications in the renal parenchyma. Excretory urography may offer more precise information in this sense, especially if it is evaluated by means of computed

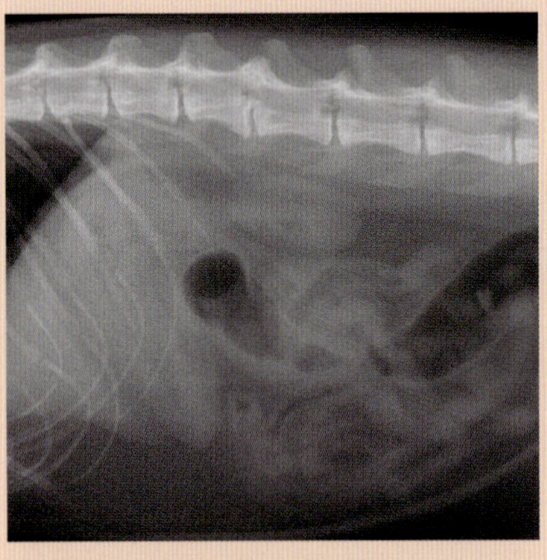

FIGURE 2.48. Lateral radiograph of the abdomen of a cat with abnormally small kidneys.

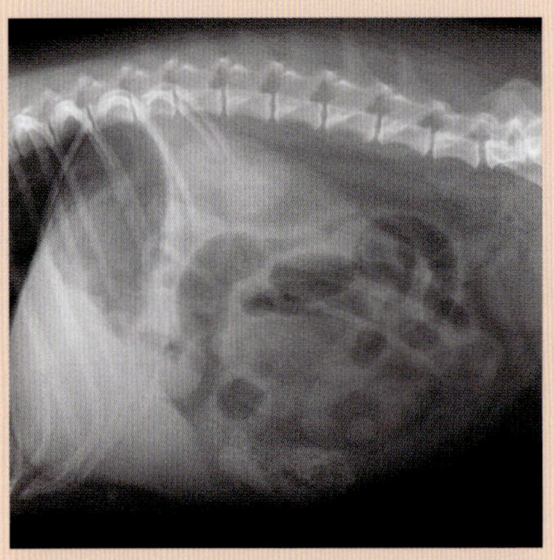

FIGURE 2.49. Lateral radiograph of the abdomen of a dog with an abnormally small right kidney. The left kidney is slightly enlarged, which could be due to compensatory hypertrophy.

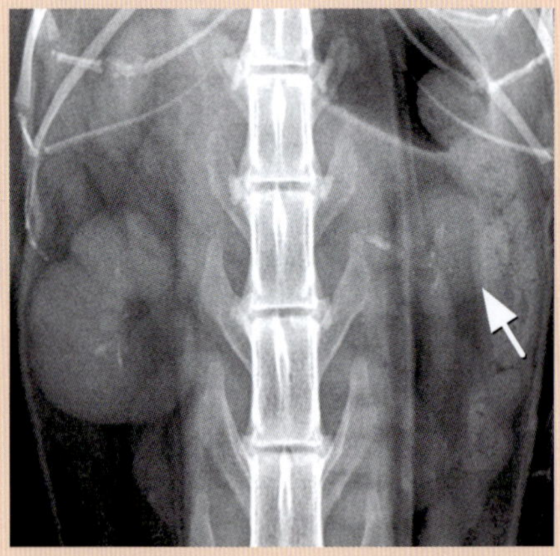

FIGURE 2.50. Ventrodorsal abdominal radiograph of cat with altered contour of both kidneys and decreased left kidney size (arrow). Both renal silhouettes also present small parenchymal mineralisations.

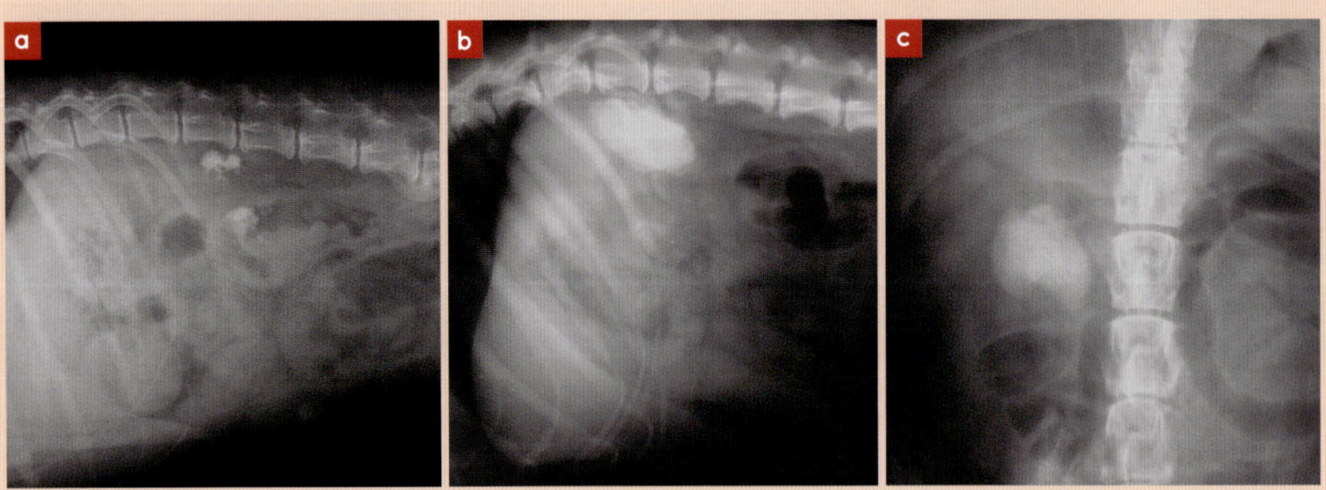

FIGURE 2.51. Enlarged images of the cranial abdomen on lateral (a and b) and ventrodorsal (c) radiographs of three dogs with radiopaque renal calculi.

tomography. Dystrophic calcification alone does not usually have any pathological significance, although it sometimes coincides with the appearance of other signs of chronic kidney disease in the patient.

In some healthy cats, it is possible to identify the normal renal pelvis due to the presence of fat in this area, which contrasts with the soft-tissue opacity of the surrounding parenchyma. Negative-contrast or double-constrat cystography also allows the identification of the presence of gas in the kidneys as a consequence of vesicoureteral reflux. The non-iatrogenic presence of gas in the kidney may suggest the presence of anaerobic bacteria that produce gas.

Patients with chronic renal failure may show secondary signs on plain radiographs, such as dystrophic calcification of the folds of the gastric wall or osteopaenia caused by secondary renal hyperparathyroidism, which essentially affects the maxilla and mandible (see chapter 6).

Excretory urography

Compared with plain radiography, excretory urography provides additional morphological information as well as qualitative information about renal function. Taking into account the information that other imaging techniques can provide, it would currently be recommended to perform excretory urography in cases of urinary incontinence, uroabdomen (suspicion of rupture of the kidney, bladder or ureter), or to investigate haematuria or locate the kidneys in the presence of a retroperitoneal mass. It would be contraindicated in patients suffering from anuria, dehydration and allergy to iodine. Excretory urography is not an appropriate technique to specifically examine the bladder, since the contrast medium mixes with urine in this organ and, in addition, an adequate degree of bladder distension is not usually achieved. However, it may be used as an alternative technique to conventional cystography when it is impossible to catheterise the patient.

The intravenous administration of hyperosmotic iodinated contrast media (e.g. diatrizoate or meglumine amidotrizoate) may cause adverse reactions in some patients, although the incidence is low. Nausea and vomiting are the most frequent adverse effects, while systemic hypotension and acute kidney injury induced by the contrast agent are possible, although less probable, complications. There is a risk of anaphylaxis but it is very uncommon. However, the necessary medication to treat it should always be available before starting the procedure and the intravenous catheter should be maintained until the end in case administration of emergency medication is required.

It is recommended to obtain a signed informed consent from the pet's owner every time a contrast technique is performed.

The risk of adverse effects is reduced with the use of low osmolarity, non-ionic iodinated contrast media, such as iohexol or iopamidol, although their much higher cost limits their indication to those patients that have previously been diagnosed with renal disease.

The preparation of the patient prior to an intravenous urogram is very important. The animal should be kept on an empty stomach for 12–24 hours, a mild laxative should be administered and an enema should be performed 2 hours before starting the procedure. This will avoid the loss of information due to superimposition of food or faeces on the renal shadows. If a urinalysis or urine culture is necessary, the sample should be collected before administering the contrast agent, since this may affect the results and inhibit the growth of some bacteria.

It is very convenient to perform urography with the animal under sedation or anaesthesia. This a procedure requires obtaining numerous radiographs in a short time, and the intervals given in the protocol have to be respected, which will be easier if we do not have to restrain the patient manually. Anaesthesia also somewhat reduces the incidence of vomiting and nausea associated with the administration of contrast media.

Before administering the contrast medium, lateral and ventrodorsal radiographs should be taken to evaluate the appropriate preparation of the patient (absence of food in the stomach and of faeces in the colon), adjust the exposure values and rule out any evident alterations that would exclude the need to perform a contrast technique. It should be borne in mind that small renal calculi can be detected on a plain radiograph and, in contrast, can be masked by the contrast media.

If the objective is to assess the entry of the ureters into the bladder with precision, it is highly recommended to perform a pneumocystogram before the intravenous administration of the iodinated contrast medium. In order to do so, the bladder should previously be emptied from urine and, next, gas should be introduced (air, carbon dioxide or nitrous oxide) until it is adequately distended. This way, the gas contained in the bladder will clearly contrast with the distal end of the ureters when these are filled the with positive contrast agent during the urography procedure. Oblique lateral radiographs will help to differentiate a ureter from the other.

Although two methods for intravenous administration of the iodinated contrast agent are usually described, slow infusion and bolus administration, it is more common to use the latter, with a dose of 600 to 800 mg of iodine per kg of live weight (mg I/kg). Box 2.1 summarises the protocol to take radiographs.

The phases into which a urography procedure is divided (fig. 2.52) are:

1. Vascular phase: the renal arteries become radiopaque 5–7 seconds after the start of contrast medium injection, which is why it will only be observed on a radiograph if this is taken at the same time as the contrast medium bolus is injected.
2. Nephrogram: the renal parenchyma becomes opaque 10–20 seconds after the start of contrast medium injection, which is when maximum opacification is reached. Opacity will then progressively decline in healthy animals.
3. Pyelogram: the renal pelvis and ureters become radiopaque. Their visualisation starts 1–2 minutes after the start of contrast medium injection. In normal conditions, the pelvis has a curvilinear shape and is less than 2 mm long. In some dogs and in the majority of cats, normal pelvic diverticuli, measuring less than 1 mm, can be identified. Given the ureteral peristalsis, which pumps the urine forward, often only an opacified part of the ureter appears in each radiograph.
4. Cystogram: opacification of the bladder. If air has previously been injected in the bladder to improve the visualisation of the openings of the ureters, the iodinated contrast material will progressively mix with the negative contrast material. If this does not allow an appropriate evaluation of the ureters, it will be useful to empty the bladder and introduce additional negative contrast medium during the course of the study.

The excretion of the contrast medium depends on the degree of glomerular filtration. A delay in the excretion of the contrast medium may be indicative of renal failure, but it is not a precise method for its evaluation. The nephrographic phase should gradually disappear throughout the procedure, although up to 25 % of dogs with no kidney disease may still have a detectable nephrogram up to 2 hours after the contrast medium injection.

Some of the abnormal patterns (fig. 2.53) that may be observed on excretory urograms are:

- Lack of renal opacification: insufficient dose of contrast medium, severe renal disease, renal aplasia or atrophy, avulsion or obstruction of the renal artery, extreme hydronephrosis, severe neoplasia.
- Heterogeneous renal opacification: cysts, abscesses, haematomas, neoplasia, infactus, nephritis, pyelonephritis.
- Normal initial opacification, which then persists or increases: severe renal disease, acute renal obstruction, systemic hypotension or acute renal injury caused by the contrast.
- Dilatation of the pelvis and/or ureters.
- Abnormal location of the end of the ureters.
- Filling defects: calculi or blood clots.

Computed tomography optimises the information that can be obtained from excretory urography, since it prevents the loss of information due to superimposition of structures. The dose of contrast medium may be reduced to 400 mg I/kg (important for patients with kidney disease) and allows a more precise calculation of the degree of glomerular filtration.

Percutaneous pyelography

Percutaneous pyelography may be used as an alternative to excretory urography. This technique involves the direct administration of a contrast medium in the renal pelvis by means of an ultrasound-guided puncture, thus

BOX 2.1. Excretory urography protocol

Before the urography procedure

- 12-24 hours before: fasting and mild laxative.
- 2 hours before: enema to empty the colon.
- Plain L and VD radiographs.
- Injection of air into the bladder (if the ureters are to be assessed).

Administration of the contrast medium

- 600-800 mg I/kg in an intravenous bolus.

Sequence of radiographs

- 10-20 seconds: VD.
- 1-2 minutes: VD.
- 5 minutes: VD and L (+ oblique is the ureters are to be assessed).
- 20 minutes*: VD and L (+ oblique is the ureters are to be assessed).
- 40 minutes: VD and L to assess the bladder.
- Additional radiographs may be necessary if no conclusive results have been obtained.

* The ureters are best seen between 5 and 20 minutes after the administration of the contrast medium and additional radiographs may therefore be taken during this interval to evaluate their image more precisely.

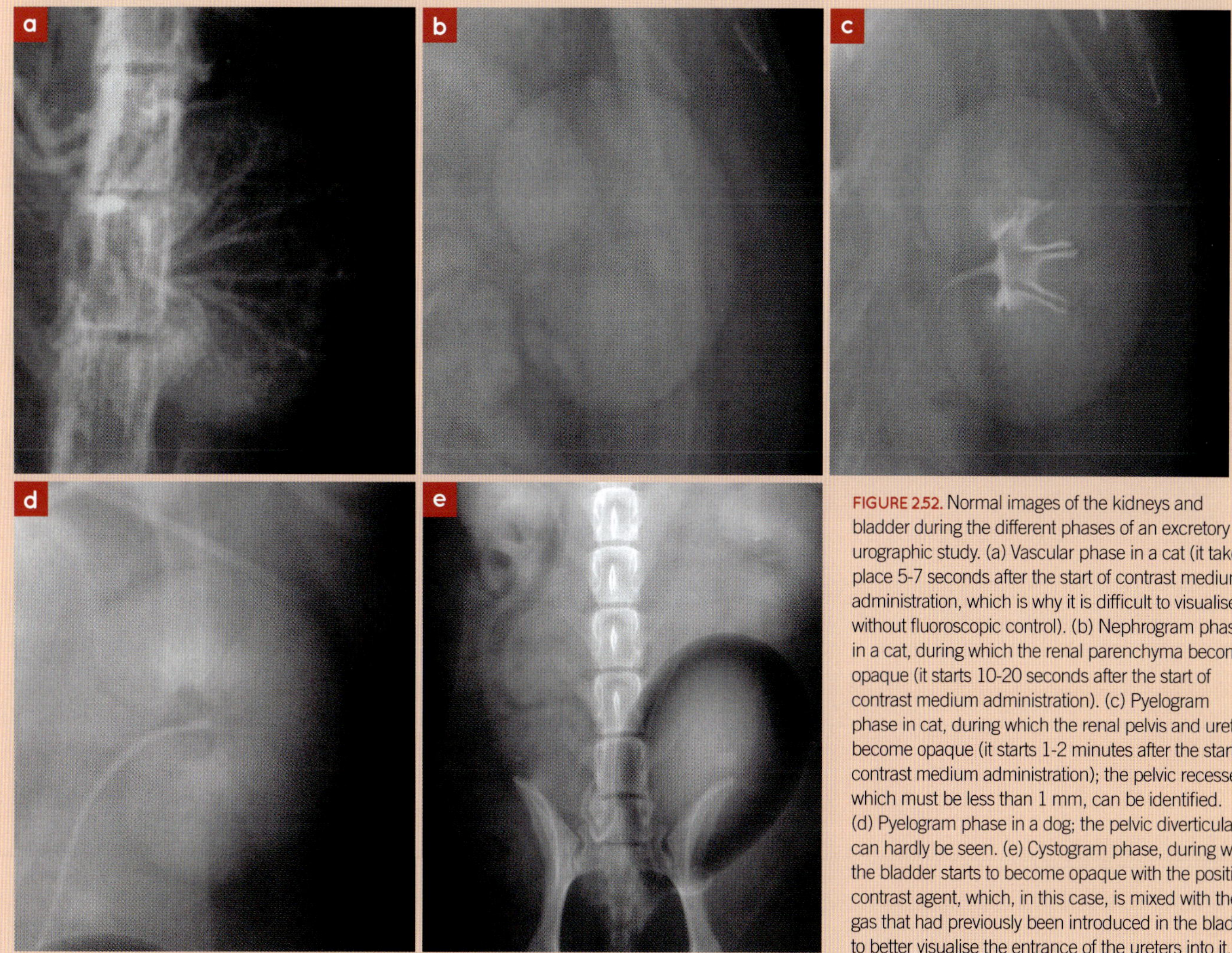

FIGURE 2.52. Normal images of the kidneys and bladder during the different phases of an excretory urographic study. (a) Vascular phase in a cat (it takes place 5-7 seconds after the start of contrast medium administration, which is why it is difficult to visualise without fluoroscopic control). (b) Nephrogram phase in a cat, during which the renal parenchyma becomes opaque (it starts 10-20 seconds after the start of contrast medium administration). (c) Pyelogram phase in cat, during which the renal pelvis and ureters become opaque (it starts 1-2 minutes after the start of contrast medium administration); the pelvic recesses, which must be less than 1 mm, can be identified. (d) Pyelogram phase in a dog; the pelvic diverticula can hardly be seen. (e) Cystogram phase, during which the bladder starts to become opaque with the positive contrast agent, which, in this case, is mixed with the gas that had previously been introduced in the bladder to better visualise the entrance of the ureters into it.

avoiding the adverse effects of intravenous administration. The contrast medium is not diluted and its excretion does not depend on renal function. The main indication of this procedure is the assessment of a ureteral obstruction. The most important potential risk of this test is the possibility of causing haemorrhage in the kidney. It may also cause extravasation of the contrast medium to the peritoneal space, which has no clinical significance, but makes the interpretation of the images difficult. Once the ultrasound-guided puncture has been performed, 1–2 ml of urine first have to be aspirated so as to slowly introduce the same volume of contrast medium, under ultrasound or fluoroscopic control.

Ureters

Normal ureters are not usually identified on a plain radiograph. However, the excellent contrast resolution offered by digital radiography allows, in some

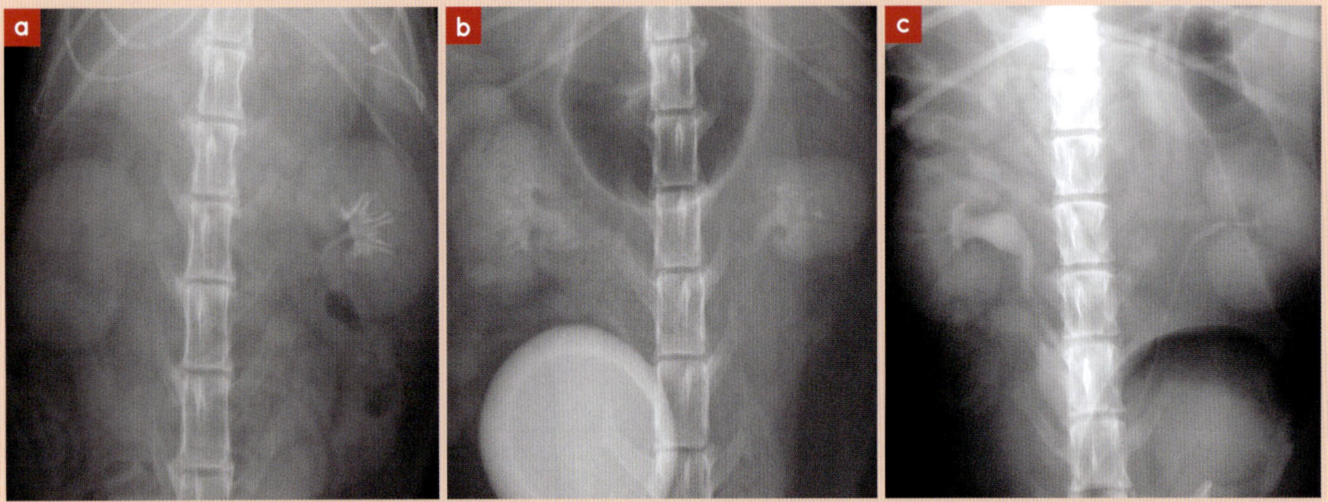

FIGURE 2.53. Abnormal patterns on excretory urograms. (a) Absence of pyelogram in the right kidney 10 minutes after the contrast medium injection, indicative of a marked delay in glomerular filtration. (b) The contrast agent improves the visualisation of the alteration in the outline of both kidneys, the decrease in size of the left kidney and the mild proximal dilatation of the left ureter and moderate dilatation of the right one. (c) Mild dilatation of the renal pelvis and moderate dilatation of the proximal part of the right ureter, which could be due to pyelonephritis or to an obstructive condition of the ureter.

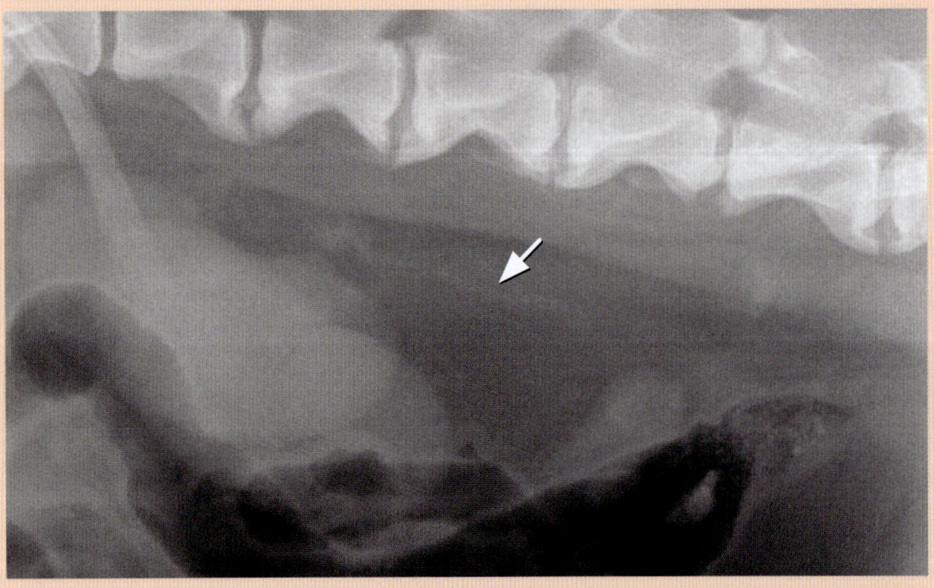

FIGURE 2.54. Enlarged image of a lateral radiograph showing the retroperitoneal region of the abdomen of a healthy dog. The large amount of retroperitoneal fat allows the visualisation in this case of one of the ureters (arrow). This finding is more frequent on digital radiographs, thanks to the greater contrast resolution they have when compared with conventional radiographs.

cases, the partial visualisation of one or the two ureters in animals with a large amount of retroperitoneal fat (fig. 2.54).

Ultrasonography is of limited use for the examination of the ureters, as it is very complicated to identify their whole course owing to their small diameter and the presence of gas. Visualising the ureteral jet that causes the entry of urine into the bladder, which can be identified with B-mode or Doppler ultrasonography, helps to assess ureteral permeability and locate the vesicoureteral junction.

Conventional excretory urography is the technique of choice to evaluate these structures, due to its low cost and high availability. However, a urographic contrast study using computed tomography is excellent to diagnose any ureteral alteration, since it avoids the loss of information due to the superimposition of structures (it does not require the previous emptying of the colon by means of laxatives and an enema) and images with great spatial resolution of small regions can be obtained. The disadvantages of computed tomography are the low availability of equipment and the high cost of the study.

Excretory urography allows the evaluation of the location, diameter, permeability and integrity of the ureters. With this technique, it is possible to observe tubular structures with a diameter of 2–3 mm, which extend from the renal sinus to the vesical trigone. It is usual not to be able to visualise the whole course of the ureter in one single image due to peristalsis (fig. 2.55). The area of opening of the ureters is better observed if gas is injected into the bladder immediately before the urogram, since the gas that is introduced in the bladder contrasts better with the ureters when they are subsequently filled with a positive contrast agent. Oblique lateral views are very useful to differentiate one ureter from the other with certainty in the image (fig. 2.56).

On a plain radiograph it is possible to detect mineral density structures compatible with radiopaque calculi in the area of the ureters (fig. 2.57). However, excretory urography will be necessary to confirm the diagnosis, as we may confuse these structures with calcifications of other tissues or with foreign bodies with mineral density on a plain radiograph.

Exceptionally, it may be possible to identify a ureteral dilatation on plain radiographs, in animals

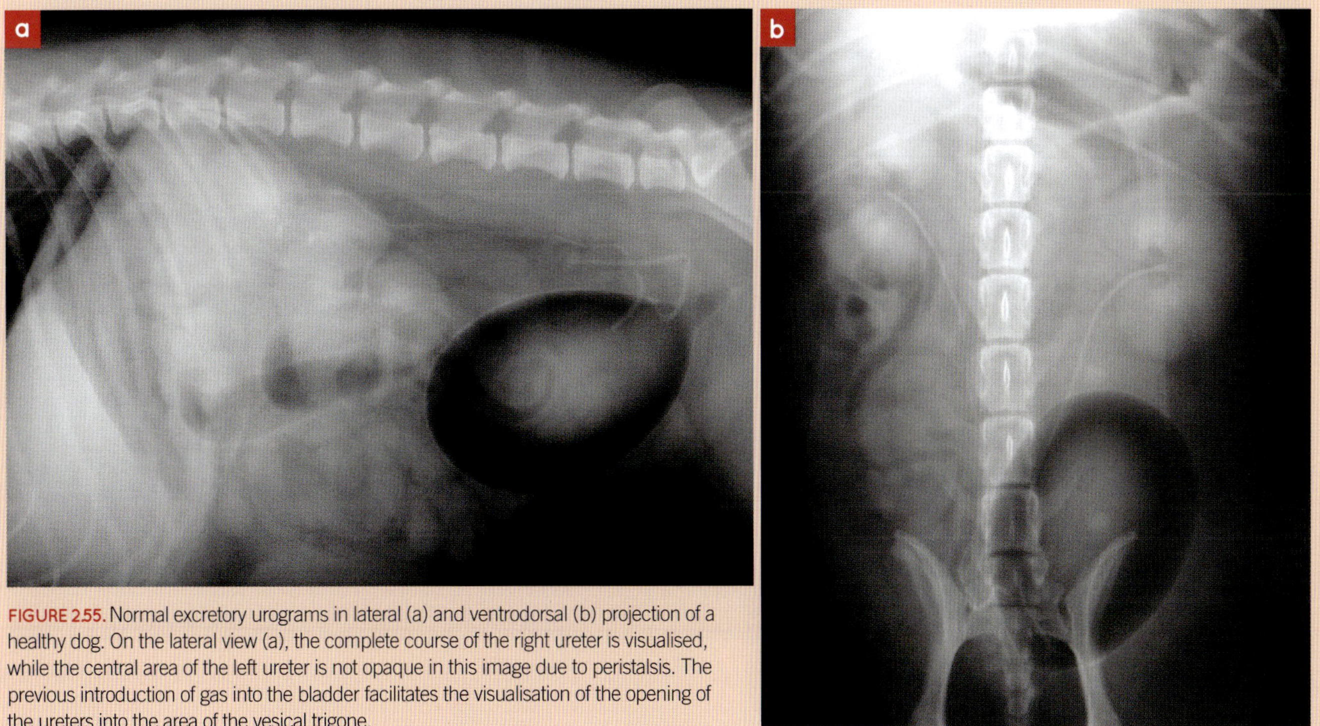

FIGURE 2.55. Normal excretory urograms in lateral (a) and ventrodorsal (b) projection of a healthy dog. On the lateral view (a), the complete course of the right ureter is visualised, while the central area of the left ureter is not opaque in this image due to peristalsis. The previous introduction of gas into the bladder facilitates the visualisation of the opening of the ureters into the area of the vesical trigone.

with a large amount of retroperitoneal fat (fig. 2.58), although excretory urography is usually required to establish this diagnosis. The dilatation of the ureters makes their ultrasound examination easier, although it may be complicated to follow their whole course. Ureteral dilatations may have a congenital (megaureter) or acquired (hydroureter) origin. Ureteral obstructions, which may be caused by calculi, clots, stenosis or masses, cause dilatation anterior to the site of obstruction (fig. 2.59). When a ureter is accidentally ligated during an ovariohysterectomy, it rapidly dilates and permanent distension, urinary stasis and a tendency to suffer from recurrent infections may occur. Pyelonephritis may also cause dilatation of the proximal part of the ureter, although it is usually mild in comparison with the dilatation caused by obstructions.

An ectopic ureter is a congenital anomaly, which affects dogs more frequently than cats, especially females. The clinical sign shown by affected animals is urinary incontinence, although it does not always occur in males. The caudal end of one or the two ureters does not open into the normal anatomical location, the vesicular trigone (caudodorsal area of the bladder), but into a different location, which is usually the neck of the bladder or urethra (fig. 2.1) (see video 2.1), and less frequently, the vagina, uterus or rectum. Ectopic ureters may have a normal diameter or be dilated and

FIGURE 2.56. Oblique lateral excretory urogram of a healthy dog. This projection facilitates the differentiation of the two ureters in the image, in which the ureter located closest to the cassette will have a more ventral position. This image was obtained in right lateral projection, so that the ureter with a more ventral location is the right one (white arrow) and the ureter in a more dorsal position is the left one (black arrow).

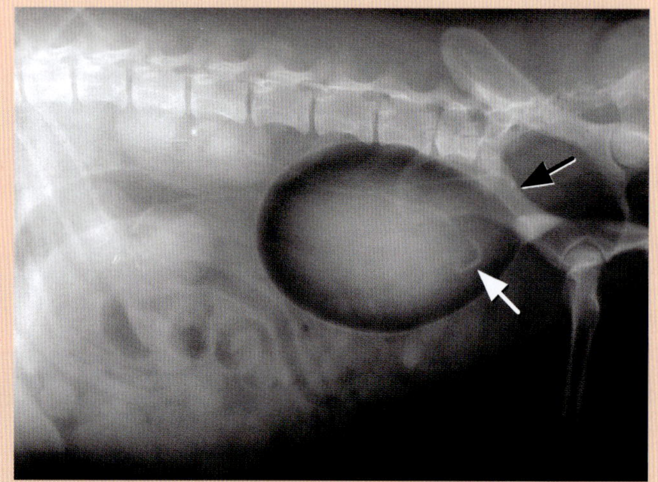

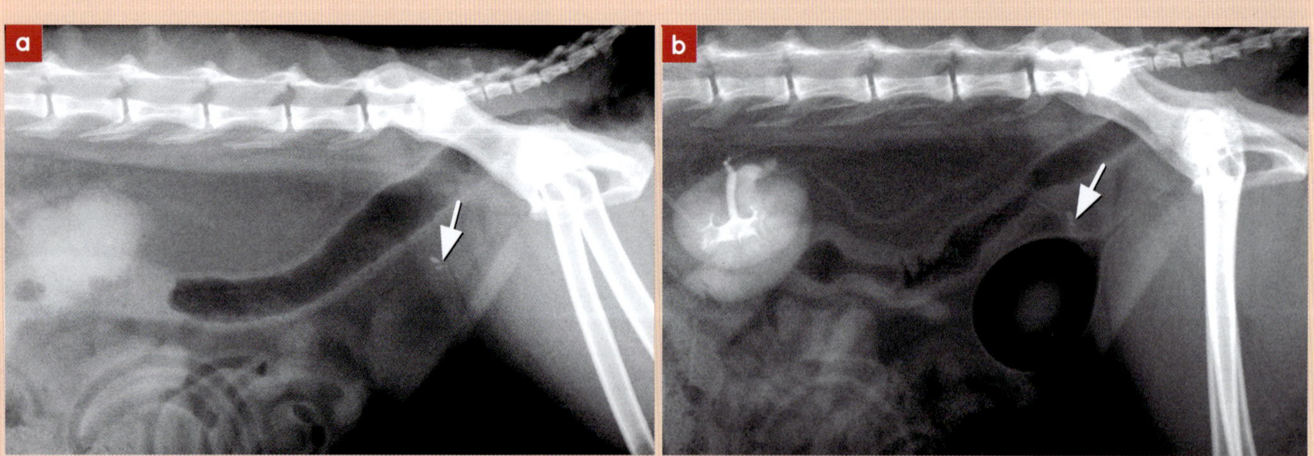

FIGURE 2.57. Plain lateral radiograph (a) and excretory urography (b) of a cat with ureteral calculi (arrow). In the plain radiograph, several small mineral opacity structures can be seen at the ureter insertion area. The urogram confirmed the location of the calculi at the distal end of one of the ureters.

have a relatively tortuous course (fig. 2.61). In some cases, an ectopic ureter enters the area of the vesicular trigone but then has an intraparietal course and opens into an abnormal location, generally the urethra, which can cause confusing images on an excretory urogram,

Video 2.1.
Fluoroscopic excretory urography in patient with ectopic ureter.

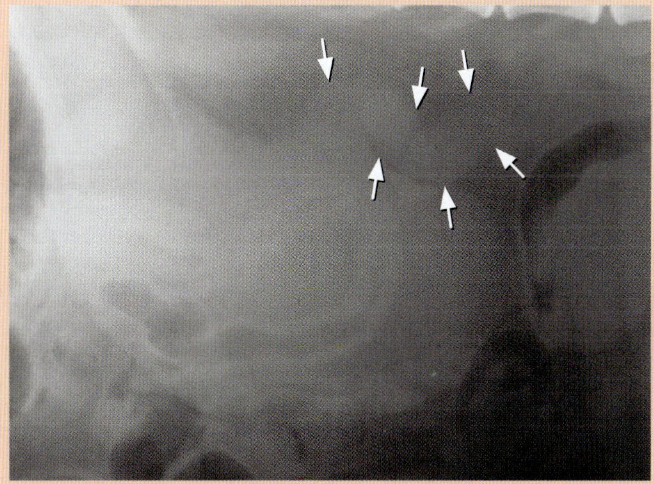

FIGURE 2.58. Enlarged image of the cranial retroperitoneal region on a lateral radiograph of a dog with severe dilatation of the left ureter.
Dilated ureters are not usually differentiated on plain radiographs, but in this case the large amount of retroperitoneal fat made their identification easier.

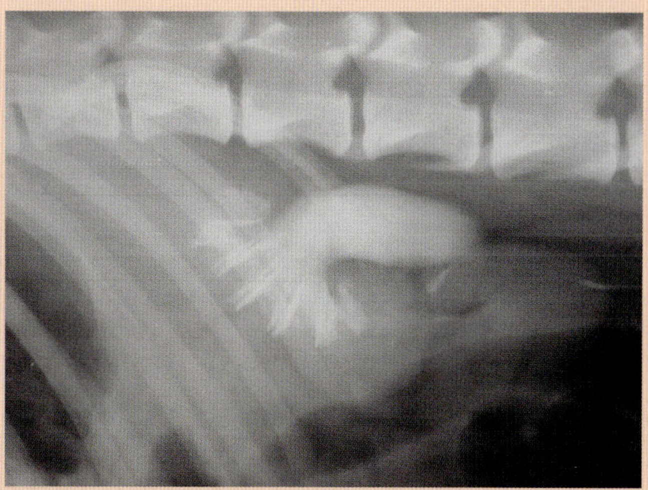

FIGURE 2.59. Enlarged image of a lateral urogram showing the cranial retroperitoneal region of a dog. Severe focal dilatation of the right ureter can be observed. Focal dilatation of the ureters usually occurs as a result of an obstruction caused by calculi, clots, stenosis or masses. Dilatation in these cases is anterior (proximal) to the site of obstruction.

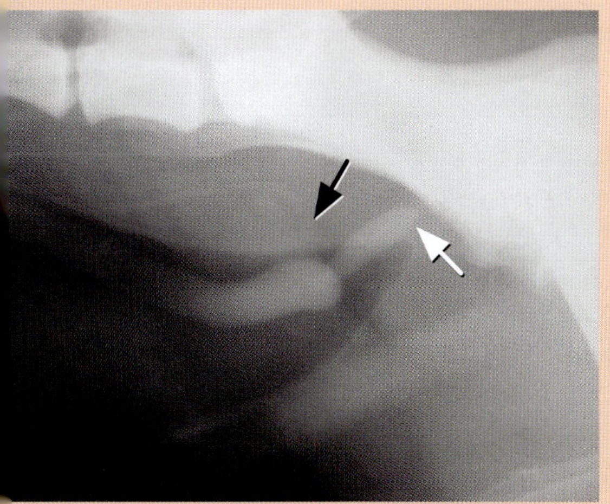

FIGURE 2.60. Enlarged image of a lateral urogram showing the caudal abdomen of a dog, in which a unilateral ectopic ureter may be observed. The ectopic ureter (white arrow) appears dilated and runs beyond the vesical trigone to open into the urethra. The normal ureter (black arrow) has a normal diameter and opens into the vesicular trigone.

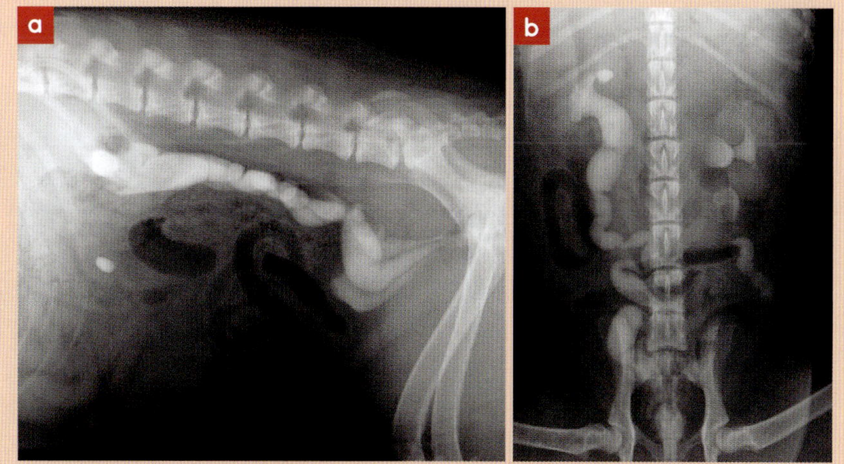

FIGURE 2.61. Lateral (a) and ventrodorsal (b) urograms of a dog, on which a bilateral ectopic ureter is observed. Both ureters appear very dilated, have a tortuous course and open into the area of junction of the neck of the bladder with the urethra, caudal to the vesicular trigone. Both renal pelvises also appear moderately dilated. On the ventrodorsal view (b), it is possible to observe the positive contrast material mixed with gas, as a result of vesicoureteral reflux of the gas introduced into the bladder immediately before the urogram. A small foreign body with mineral density (stone) can be observed in the intestine as an incidental finding.

especially if the ureter is not dilated. This intraparietal course, in which the ectopic ureters usually "leave the bladder out", is more frequent in dogs than in cats. Fluoroscopy and ultrasonography may sometimes help to establish a diagnosis. When the excretory urogram is not conclusive, it should be complemented with a retrograde urethrogram in males and retrograde vaginourethrogram in females.

Ureteroceles are focal cystic dilatations of the submucosa of the ureters and usually form at their distal end, at the vesicoureteral junction or close to it. They may sometimes project towards the lumen of the bladder or urethra. They appear more frequently in ectopic ureters. The excretory urogram shows a focal dilatation with accumulation of contrast where they are located.

Ureteral tumours (fig. 2.62) are uncommon and appear as areas of filling defect on the urogram, accompanied by dilatation anterior to the obstructed site when they cause obstruction. Some bladder tumours may extend to the ureter.

When rupture of a ureter occurs, generally due to trauma, signs of the presence of free fluid may be observed in the retroperitoneal space on plain radiographs and extravasation of the contrast to the peritoneum on the excretory urogram, although the exact site of rupture may be difficult to find. A perirenal or paraureteral urinoma, which consists in a retroperitoneal fibrous sac where extravasated urine accumulates (fig. 2.63), may occasionally form as a consequence of the rupture.

Bladder

Plain radiography allows the observation of the size, shape, location and radiographic density of the bladder, but does not provide any information about its internal structure. The bladder wall and urine have the same radiopacity on radiographs and therefore cannot be differentiated in normal conditions. That is why, as for the assessment of the kidneys, the technique of choice for the study of the bladder is ultrasonography, since it offers detailed information of the bladder wall and content.

Cystography is the contrast technique used to complement the diagnostic information provided by plain radiography. The diagnostic superiority of ultrasonography over cystography is indisputable, but not all veterinary clinics have an ultrasound scanner or enough experience to make a correct ultrasound diagnosis. That is why cystography is still used in those cases for the diagnosis of calculi, inflammations, masses and trauma. It the bladder is ruptured, cystography can provide more precise information than ultrasonography, since ultrasound findings may be uncertain, while the extravasation of the contrast medium to the peritoneal cavity always confirms the diagnosis.

Cystography involves the introduction of a contrast medium (positive, negative or both) in the bladder through a flexible catheter. In order to obtain optimum results, it is important to empty the bladder from urine prior to introducing the contrast material. Sedation or anaesthesia of the patient will facilitate the procedure.

Positive-contrast cystography

Iodinated contrast media, generally diluted at 10 %, are used in doses of 6–12 ml/kg. It is the technique of choice to evaluate anomalous positions of the bladder or a possible rupture of the wall. On the other hand, it may mask small irregularities of the bladder mucosa as well as some abnormal intraluminal contents.

Negative-contrast cystography (pneumocystography)

A negative contrast medium, generally air, is used. When performing this technique, there is a minimal risk of causing gas embolism, which may even lead to the death of the animal. This risk is higher in cats than in dogs and may be reduced by using carbon dioxide or nitrous oxide instead of air, due to the greater solubility of these two substances. Doses of 6–12 ml/kg may be used, or gas may simply be introduced, checking the degree of distension of the bladder by palpation. This is the cheapest and most simple method, but it is the least sensible of the three techniques to detect alterations of the mucosa and small defects in the bladder wall.

Double-contrast cystography

First, a small amount of positive contrast medium is introduced (1–5 ml in dogs and 0.5–1 ml in cats) and then, the bladder is distended with a negative contrast medium. This way, a thin layer of positive contrast material will clearly define the internal margin of the wall. This technique is ideal to examine alterations of the mucosa and the presence of radiolucent calculi in the bladder.

Pathological alterations

On a plain radiograph, the size and the position of the shadow of the bladder vary in function of the amount of urine it contains. The animals that have not urinated for many hours, whether due to pathological causes or not, may have a very distended bladder, which should not be mistaken for an abdominal mass (fig. 2.64). A scarcely distended bladder will be more difficult to identify, especially when it is superimposed with the intestine or when the animal has very little retroperitoneal fat.

The neck of the bladder may appear located cranial to the pubis or in an intrapelvic position in healthy dogs, especially when the bladder is not very distended. However, the position of the bladder is always intra-abdominal in cats.

The alteration of the bladder that is most often diagnosed by means of radiography is lithiasis. Radiopaque calculi (fig. 2.65) are identified on plain radiographs, although they may be masked by other superimposed structures if very small (fig. 2.66). Ultrasonography is required for the diagnosis of radiolucent calculi (generally with ammonium acid urate or cystine) or, alternatively, double-contrast cystography (fig. 2.67). This is because these calculi may be masked by the contrast if positive-contrast cystography is used, particularly if small and few in number. Radiolucent calculi may have a very similar image to that produced by clots or gas bubbles on a double-contrast cystogram. On the other hand, they are easily identified by means of ultrasonography.

Alterations of the radiographic density of the bladder wall may also be detected on plain radiographs. The appearance of calcified areas in the wall is usually due to its dystrophic calcification (fig. 2.68), which is generally associated with chronic inflammatory processes or neoplasms.

The presence of gas in the bladder lumen is usually iatrogenic, when gas is introduced voluntarily or involuntarily when catheterising the patient (fig. 2.69).

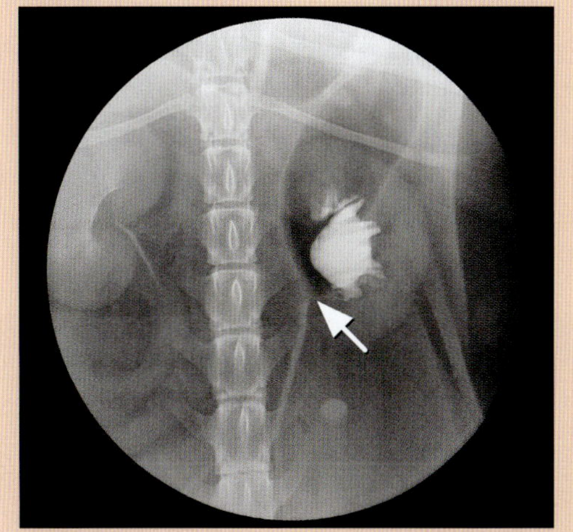

FIGURE 2.62. Enlarged image of a ventrodorsal urogram showing the cranial abdomen of a dog. It is possible to observe a moderate dilatation of the left renal pelvis and a permanent filling defect of the proximal end of the left ureter due to the presence of a ureteral neoplasm in this location.

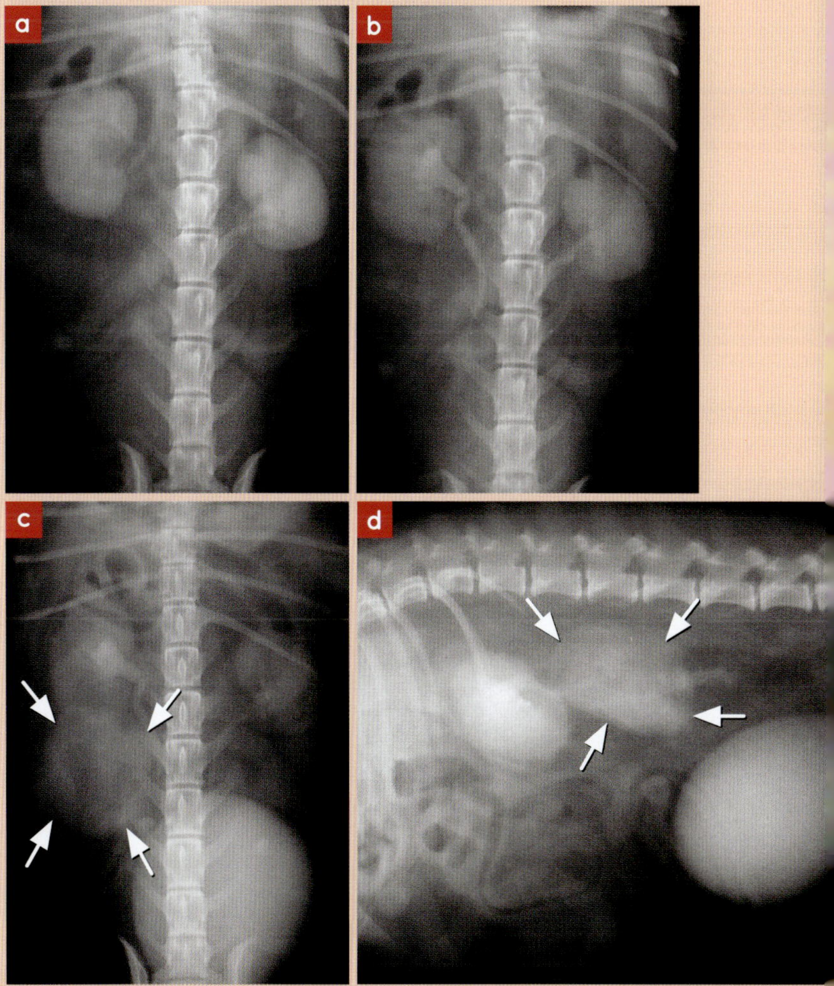

FIGURE 2.63. Ventrodorsal (a, b and c) and lateral (d) urograms showing the cranial abdomen of a dog. A focal accumulation of the constrast medium may be observed in the retroperitoneal space caudal to the right kidney, which also appears enlarged in comparison with the left one, with mild to moderate dilatation of the right renal pelvis and mild to moderate dilatation of the right ureter. The focal accumulation of contrast is due to a paraureteral urinoma (arrows).

In case of emphysematous cystitis, the gas may have an intraparietal (fig. 2.70) or intraluminal location. This type of cystitis is more frequent in diabetic patients, in which the formation of gas is due to microorganisms causing the fermentation of glucose.

The information provided by cystography as regards the thickness of the bladder wall is more limited than that offered by ultrasonography. Double-contrast cystography allows the differentiation of small irregularities of the wall that would otherwise go unnoticed if

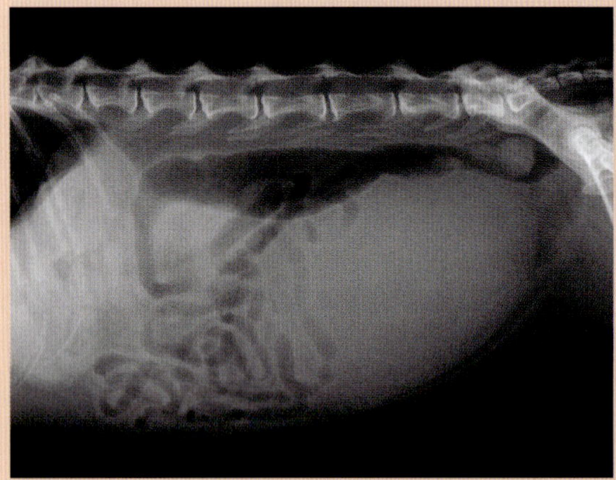

FIGURE 2.64. Lateral radiograph of the abdomen of a cat with severe bladder distension, which causes a dorsal displacement of the colon and a cranial and dorsal displacement of the small intestine.

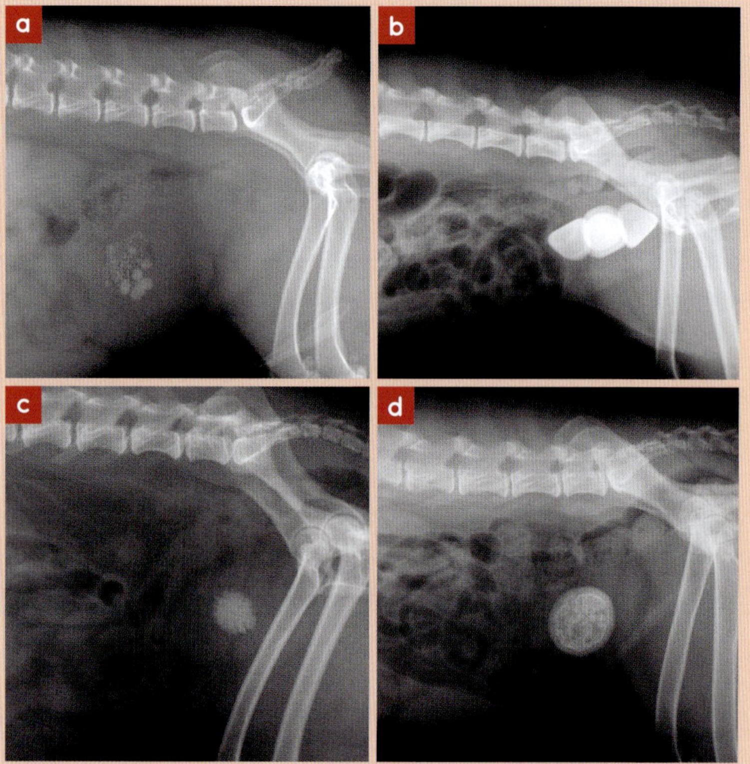

FIGURE 2.65. Enlarged images of the caudal abdomen on lateral radiographs of four dogs with radiopaque calculi in the bladder.

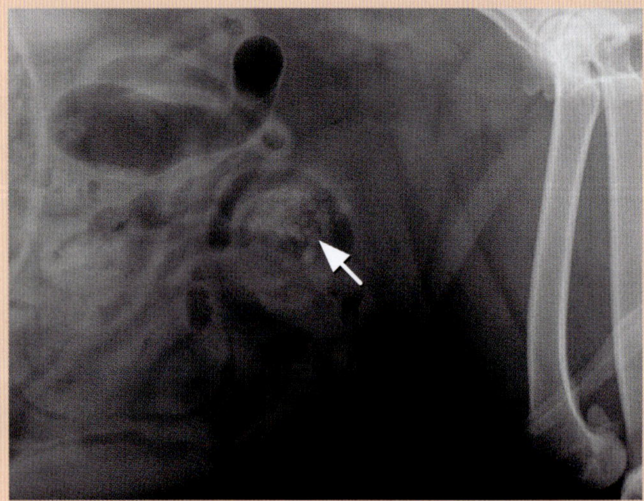

FIGURE 2.66. Enlarged image in lateral projection of the caudal abdomen of a dog with bladder lithiasis. Numerous small-sized calculi are present (arrow), which may go unnoticed due to the superimposition of small intestinal loops.

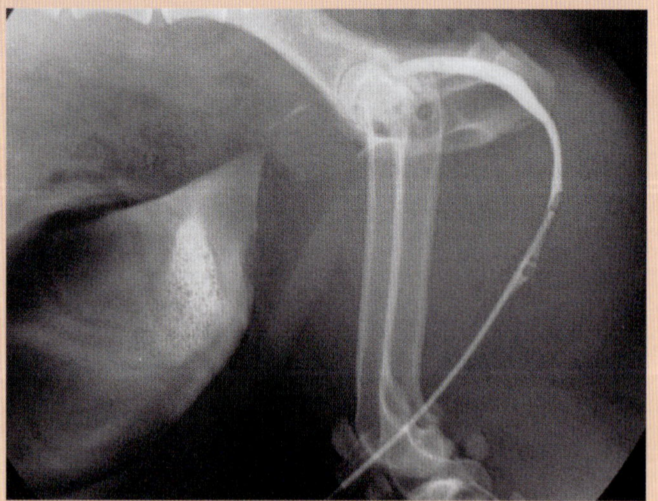

FIGURE 2.67. Enlarged image of a double-contrast cystogram showing the caudal abdomen of a dog. Numerous areas of filling defect compatible with calculi can be observed in the bladder.

a positive contrast medium or gas alone were used (fig. 2.71). If the irregularities of the wall are more marked, for example in the case of tumours or polypoid cystitis, or if the thickness of the wall is significantly increased, even homogeneously, the three techniques provide useful information. However, double-contrast cystography is always the most recommended method for this type of evaluation.

Generalised cystitis is usually caused by a relatively homogeneous increase in the thickness of the bladder wall (fig. 2.72), although the thickening is sometimes more marked in the cranioventral area of the bladder. Tumours, on the other hand, usually cause a more focal and irregular increase in thickness (fig. 2.73), although it may be similar to that caused by localised or polypoid cystitis, or to the image produced by the

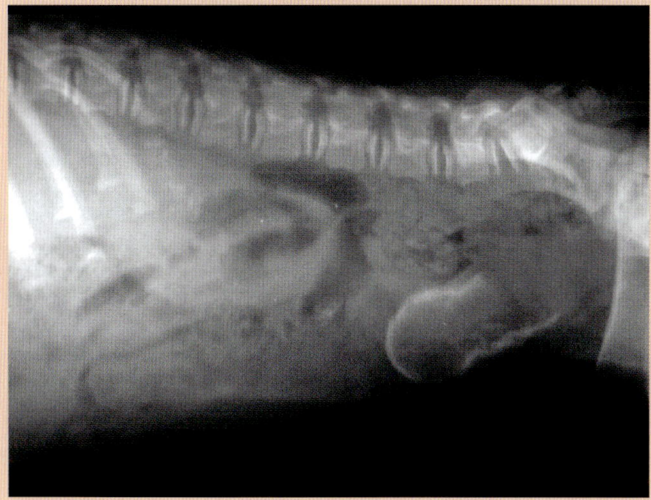

FIGURE 2.68. Lateral radiograph of the abdomen of a young dog with dystrophic calcification of the bladder wall.

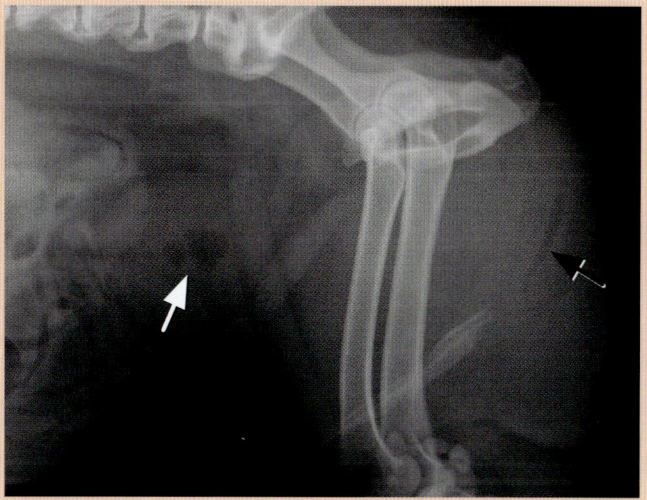

FIGURE 2.69. Enlarged image of the caudal abdomen on a lateral radiograph of a dog with gas in its bladder (white arrow) and urethra (black arrow) due to iatrogenic causes, as a result of a previous catheterisation.

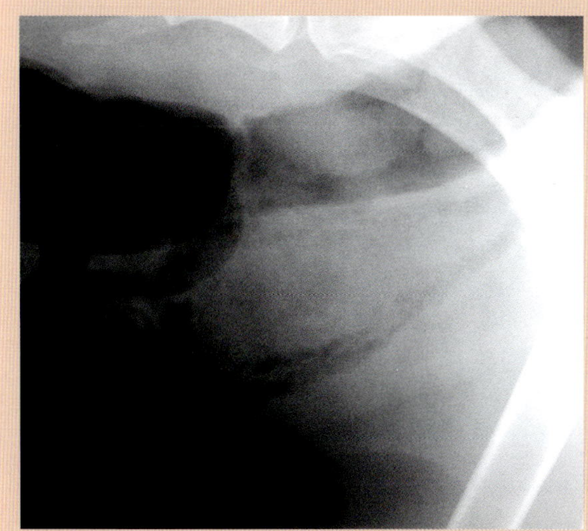

FIGURE 2.70. Enlarged image of the caudal abdomen on a lateral radiograph of a dog with emphysematous cystitis. Areas of gas opacity distributed throughout the bladder wall can be observed. Emphysematous cystitis is more frequent in diabetic patients.

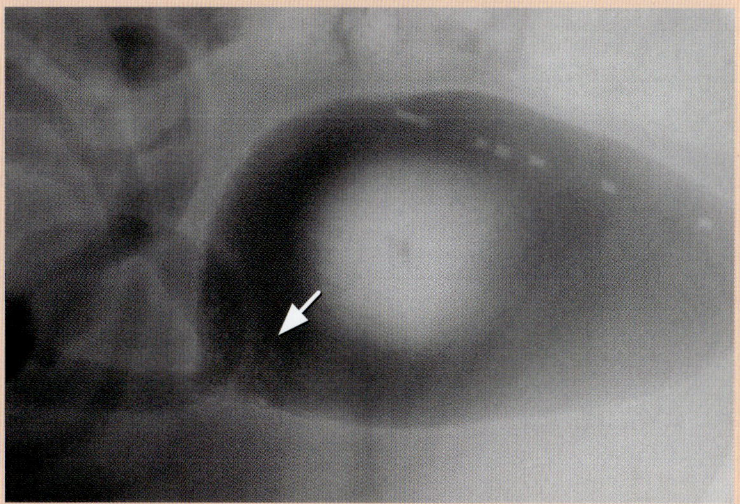

FIGURE 2.71. Enlarged image of a double-contrast cystogram showing the caudal abdomen of a dog. Small areas of accumulation of positive contrast material may be observed in the cranioventral region of the bladder, in addition to a slight deformation of the bladder wall at the same location. These findings are indicative of localised cystitis, although they may also be caused by a tumour (second possible diagnosis).

presence of clots adhered to the bladder wall. Most bladder tumours form in the bladder trigone and usually cause some degree of ureteral or urethral obstruction as they grow. Ultrasonography allows a better definition of the extension of this type of lesions as well as the collection of samples for cytology or biopsies.

If bladder rupture is suspected, either as a consequence of trauma or due to iatrogenic causes, positive-contrast cystography should be chosen (fig. 2.74), even ahead of ultrasonography. The contra17st medium used should be very diluted, as it is irritating for the peritoneum. Although ionic iodinated contrast media may be used for other types of assessments, if a rupture is suspected it is better to choose nonionic iodinated contrast media. Indeed, although all the iodinated contrast agents are absorbed in the peritoneum, ionic contrast agents may worsen a possible bleeding if the lesion is recent. The extravasation of the contrast medium may sometimes not be observed immediately and may appear after 5–10 minutes. The test should therefore not be considered negative until this time has passed. Pneumocystography is not recommended to confirm a bladder rupture, since if this latter is small, the extravasation of the gas to the peritoneum will be slow and may be mistaken for gas contained in the gastrointestinal tract.

Positive-contrast cystography is also more useful than double-contrast cystography to detect anomalous positions of the bladder, for example when it is displaced into a hernial sac or in the case of intrapelvic bladders. In cases of urinary incontinence due to an incompetence of the urethral sphincter mechanism, the animal is able to void its bladder normally, but leaks urine when at rest or during sleep. This anomaly may have a congenital origin in females, which may have a shorter urethra than normal or a bladder with an intrapelvic location (fig. 2.75).

Although they are not very frequent, some anomalies of the urachus may be diagnosed by means of cystography, such as patent urachus (fig. 2.76), patent urachal ligament and urachal diverticula, these latter being more frequent in cats. The animals that suffer from this anomaly of the urachus usually have recurrent bacterial cystitis.

Urethra

A normal urethra is not identified on plain radiographs and ultrasonography is often not useful either for its

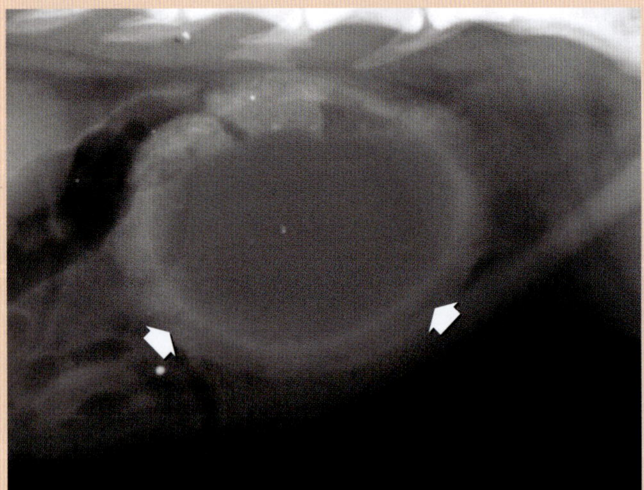

FIGURE 2.72. Enlarged image of a pneumocystogram showing the caudal abdomen of a cat, in which a marked, generalised and regular thickening of the bladder wall can be observed. This image is compatible with generalised cystitis, although it may also be caused by a tumour (second possible diagnosis, although it is unlikely since the tumours that affect the entire bladder wall usually have irregular margins).

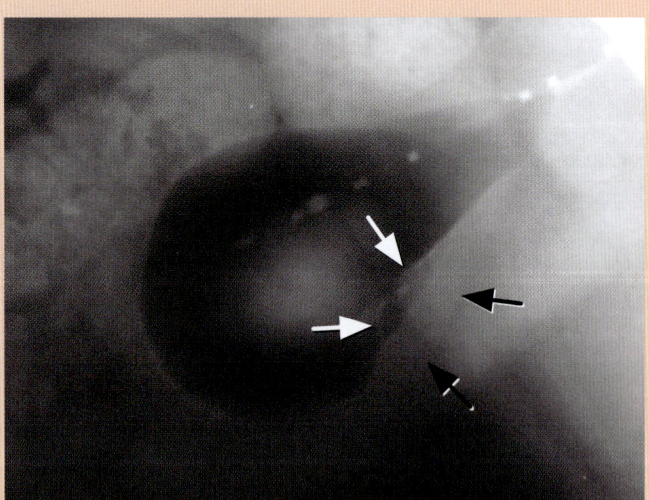

FIGURE 2.73. Enlarged image of a double-contrast cystogram showing the caudal abdomen of a dog, in which a focal thickening of the ventral wall of the bladder can be observed. A thin layer of positive contrast medium clearly delimits the internal margin of the lesion (white arrows). The outer margin is indicated with black arrows. This image is compatible with a bladder neoplasm (other possible diagnoses include localised cystitis and, with much less probability, adhered blood clot).

evaluation. The technique of choice is therefore urethrography. Iodinated contrast media are used and the patient must previously be sedated or anaesthetised.

Fluoroscopy is an excellent technique to provide more accurate diagnostic information when performing an urethrography, allowing real-time visualisation of the dynamic bladder filling processes.

The male urethra is divided into 3 segments: prostatic urethra, membranous urethra and penile or spongy urethra. Together, the prostatic and membranous sections make up the pelvic part of the urethra. The prostatic urethra is completely surrounded by prostatic tissue in dogs, and only dorsolaterally covered in cats. The membranous urethra is covered by cavernous tissue and the urethral muscle. The penile urethra extends from the ischial arch to the tip of the penis and is mostly encased by the erectile tissues of this organ. The female urethra is shorter and wider and entirely pelvic in location. In the cat, the bladder has an intra-abdominal position, so the urethra has a prepelvic segment, proximal to its pelvic segment.

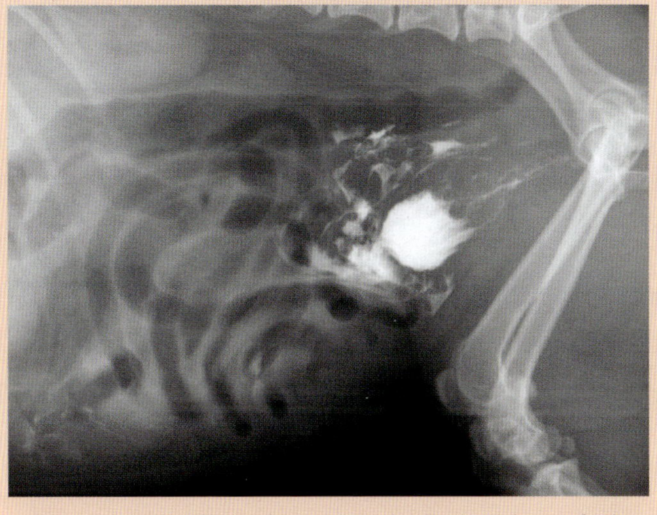

FIGURE 2.74. Lateral positive-contrast urogram showing the abdomen of a dog. Extravasation of the contrast medium to the peritoneal cavity can be observed, which confirms a bladder rupture.

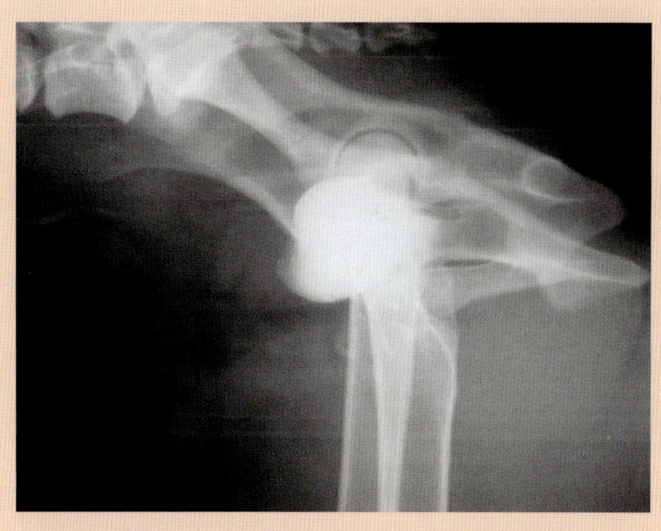

FIGURE 2.75. Enlarged image of the caudal abdomen of a dog after an excretory urogram and positive-contrast cystogram, in which it can be seen that the bladder has an intrapelvic location. This anomaly is a frequent cause of urinary incontinence in young females.

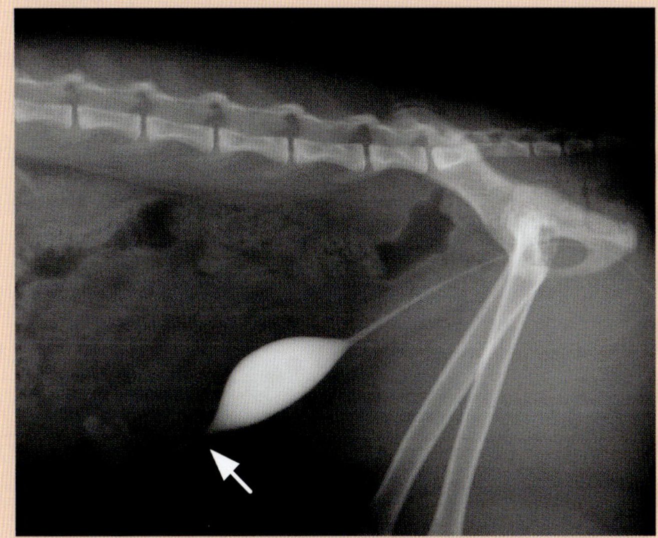

FIGURE 2.76. Lateral positive-contrast cystogram of the abdomen of a cat. The bladder has an ellipsoidal morphology and still has a tube that connects it with the umbilical area (arrow). This image is compatible with patent urachus.

Retrograde urethrography is performed in male animals by inserting a flexible catheter, filled with contrast material (to prevent entry of air bubbles) into the penile urethra (fig. 2.77) (see video 2.2). Tongue forceps can be used to hold the catheter in position and prevent leakage. Next, a small volume of contrast medium (1 ml/kg in dogs and 2–4 ml in total in cats) is introduced without exerting too much pressure, since there is a risk of rupturing the urethra. If fluoroscopy is used, the end of the catheter can be placed in the neck of the bladder to be withdrawn later, at the same time as the contrast medium is injected; this way, the whole course of the urethra is filled and can be visualised in real time on the monitor. The normal urethra has a larger diameter in the pelvis than in the perineal and penile areas. It is normal to observe an area of narrowing at the level of the ichial arch, which should not be mistaken for pathological stenosis.

In females, the urethra is not usually directly catheterised, since the presence of the catheter in the lumen may mask lesions. A retrograde vaginourethrogram under anaesthesia is therefore performed in these patients. A Foley catheter is placed, with its end cut and filled with contrast material, in the vaginal vestibule. The balloon is inflated and the lips of the vulva are closed with forceps, to avoid leakage of the contrast medium at the moment of its injection. As in males, a dose of 1 ml/kg is used. The contrast medium fills the bladder and the urethra at the same time. This procedure is usually performed as a complementary technique to urography when an ectopic ureter is suspected.

Anterograde urethrography is also used for those cases in which the urethra cannot be catheterised. The animal is previously anaesthetised and an iodinated contrast agent is introduced in the bladder by means of bladder puncture or intravenous urography. Next, the bladder is manually compressed to allow the passage of the contrast medium to the urethra at the same time as the radiograph is taken.

Plain radiography allows the detection of radiopaque calculi in the course of the urethra (fig. 2.78). Calculi are most commonly found in males around the ischial arch and at the base of the os penis, because these are areas of natural narrowing. In male cats, calculi or blockages are usually located in the penile urethra, although their radiopacity is often insufficient for them to be detected on a radiograph. Urethral lithiasis is much less frequent in female dogs and cats. In urethrography, calculi will produce images of filling defects in the contrast column (fig. 2.79), which are easily misinterpreted as gas bubbles introduced as a result of catheterisation. The os penis sometimes has a separate centre of ossification at its distal end, which should not be confused with a urethral calculus.

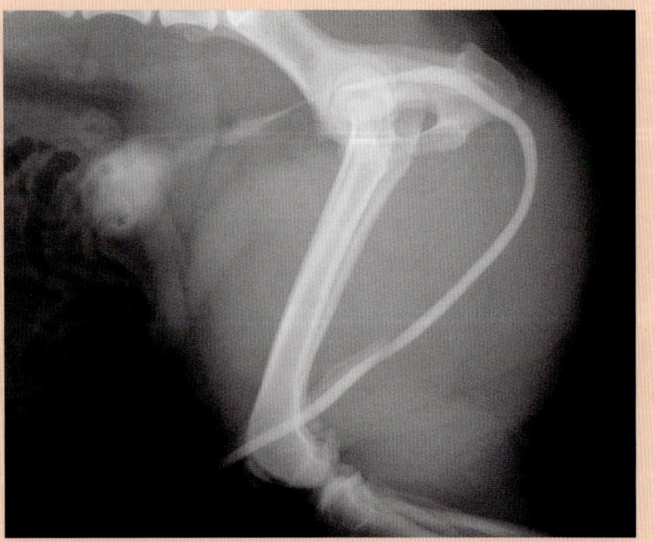

Video 2.2.
Dynamic urethrography in a healthy male.

FIGURE 2.77. Enlarged lateral retrograde urethrogram showing the caudal abdomen and perineal region of a healthy dog, with the limbs extended in cranial direction.

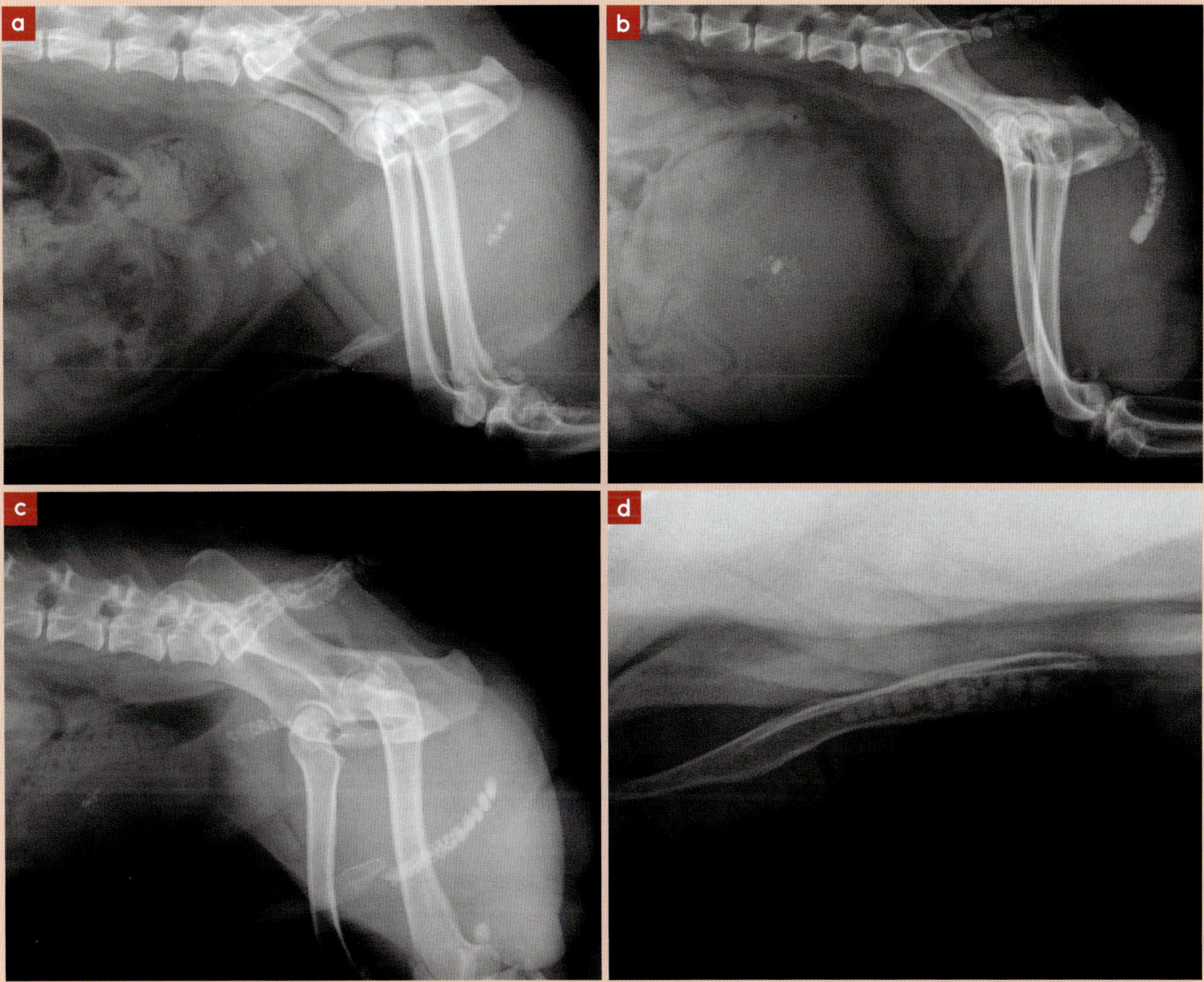

FIGURE 2.78. Enlarged images in lateral projection of the caudal abdomen and perineal region (a, b and c) and penile region (d) of four dogs with radiopaque urethral calculi. (a) Radiopaque calculi with irregular morphology can be identified in the bladder and at two locations in the penile urethra. (b) It is possible to observe a marked distension of the bladder, which contains numerous small-sized calculi, as well as numerous calculi in the perineal segment of the urethra, some of which are large. (c) A low number of small calculi are present in the bladder and numerous calculi, some large, can be seen in the prostatic and penile urethra. (d) Numerous urethral calculi can be identified in the penile segment of the urethra.

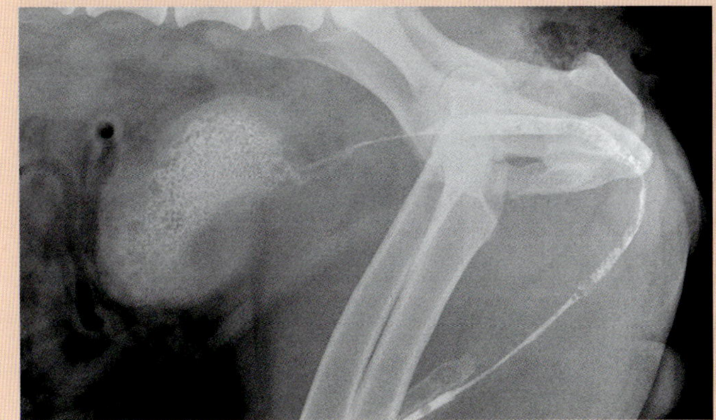

FIGURE 2.79. Enlarged image of urethrogram in lateral projection of male dog with numerous very small radiolucent calculi in bladder and urethra. These stones were not identified on the plain radiography because their opacity is similar to urine and soft tissues. The urethrogram, however, reveals numerous filling defects created by stones located in both the urethra and the bladder.

On a urethrogram, the normal urethra has a tubular morphology and smooth margins. Irregular margins suggest neoplasia or severe inflammation of the urethra (fig. 2.80). Urethral tumours are more frequent in female dogs than in males or cats of both sexes. Computed tomography and magnetic resonance imaging (fig. 2.81) allow a detailed study of the lesion and its possible extension to adjacent tissues or structures.

Stenosis appears as permanent focal narrowings of the urethral diameter. Although they may be associated with tumours or severe inflammation, in many cases they are due to inflammation caused iatrogenically by repeated catheterisation (fig. 2.82) (see video 2.3). Real

Video 2.3.
Fluoroscopic urography in male with urethral strictures.

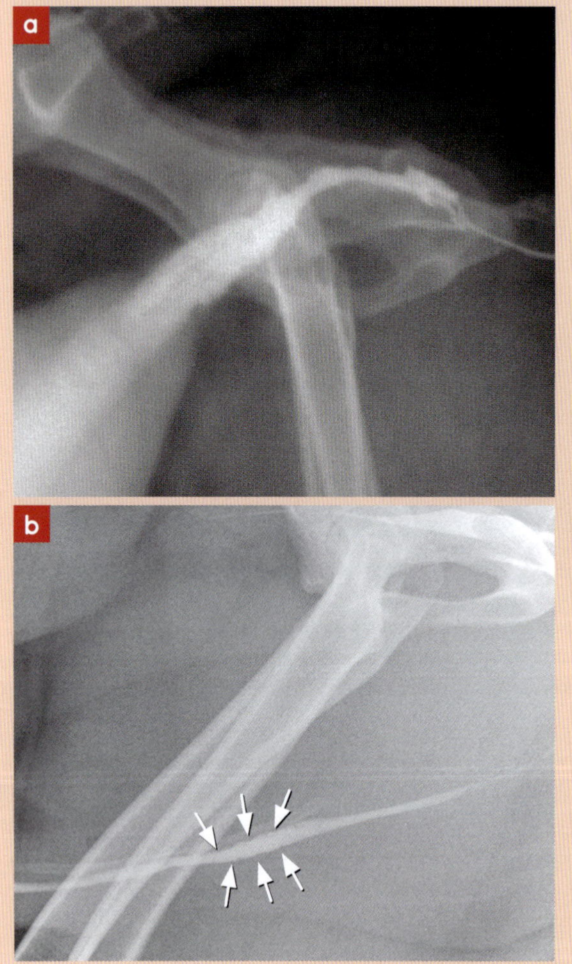

FIGURE 2.80. Magnified images of the pelvic region in lateral view of a female dog (a) and a male dog (b) that underwent retrograde urethrography. Marked irregularity of the contour of the urethrogram due to a urethral neoplasm is observed (a). The arrows mark the irregular contour of a segment of the penile urethra, caused by iatrogenic urethritis due to repeated catheterisation (b).

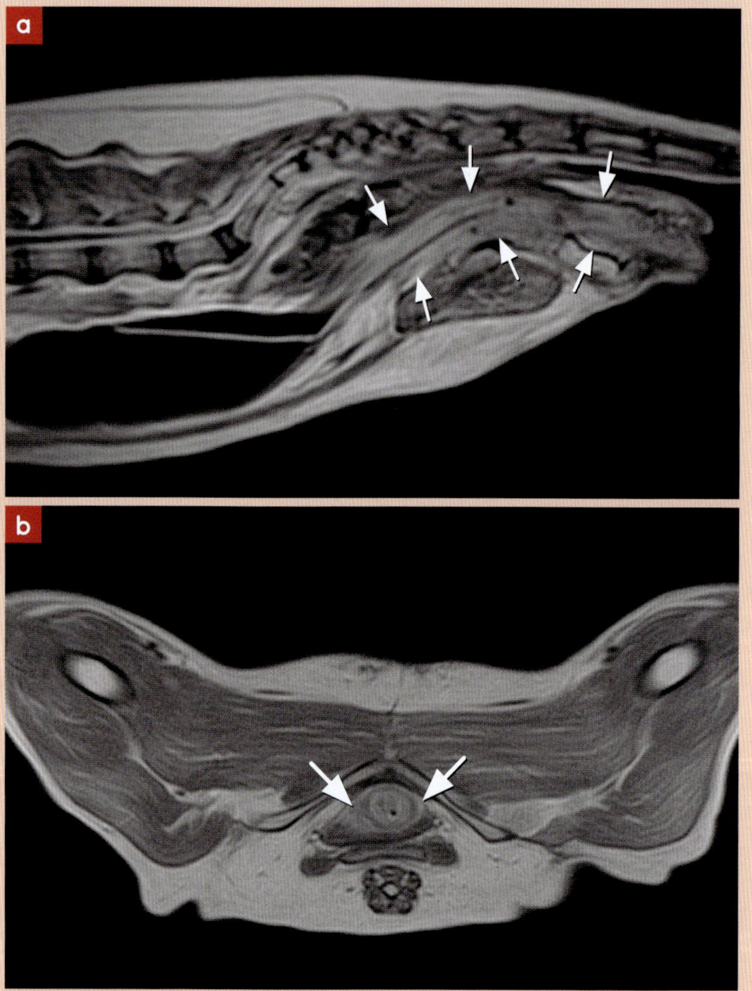

FIGURE 2.81. Post-contrast magnetic resonances images in sagittal (a) and transverse (b) plane of the pelvic region of a dog with a urethral tumour. The urethral wall shows a marked and generalised thickening and is enhanced after the administration of gadolinium. The external limits of the urethral wall are indicated with arrows in both images. Magnetic resonance imaging is an excellent technique for the evaluation of intrapelvic diseases and diseases of the perineal region.

urethral strictures can be confused with inadequate urethral distension or urethral spasms. Real strictures remain unchanged in repeated images and may be accompanied by focal irregularity of the urethral wall, as well as luminal dilatation proximal to the stricture point.

Urethral ruptures can cause urine to leak into the peritoneal cavity, the pelvic cavity or the peri-penile tissues, depending on the location of the rupture or perforation. This is confirmed if extravasation of the contrast medium is noted when conducting the urethrography. Urethral rupture should be suspected in patients with a hip fracture and dysuria or anuria (fig. 2.83). An iatrogenic origin is also common, after repeated catheterisation, especially in patients with recurrent urethral obstructions (fig. 2.84), or in cases of erosion of the wall due to severe inflammation or neoplasia.

Urethral ruptures can provoke fistulas that communicate with the lumen of nearby organs, such as the vagina or the rectum (fig. 2.85). In young animals, urethral fistulas are usually due to congenital defects.

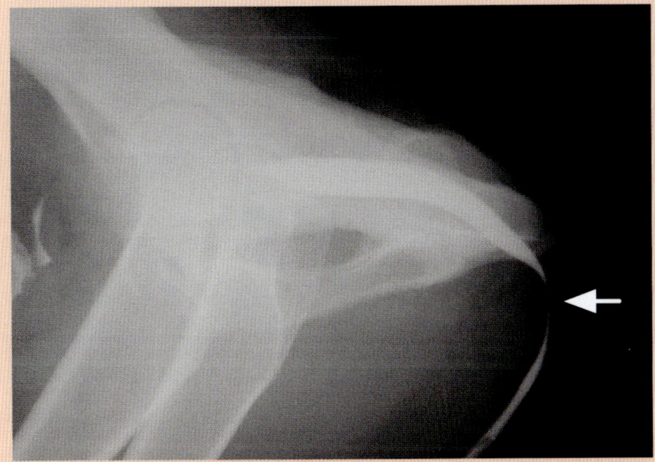

FIGURE 2.82. Enlarged image of a lateral retrograde urogram showing the pelvic region of a male dog, in which it is possible to observe an area of stenosis in the proximal penile segment of the urethra, secondary to focal urethritis caused by repeated catheterisation.

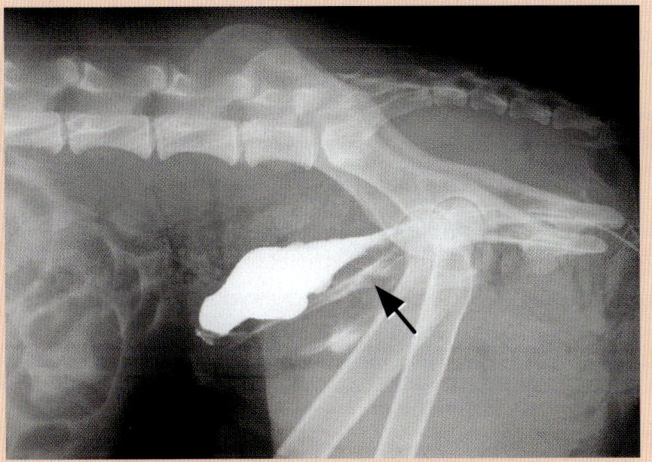

FIGURE 2.83. Lateral retrograde urethrogram showing the caudal abdomen of a female dog with a urethral rupture. The black arrow indicates the extravasation of the contrast medium.

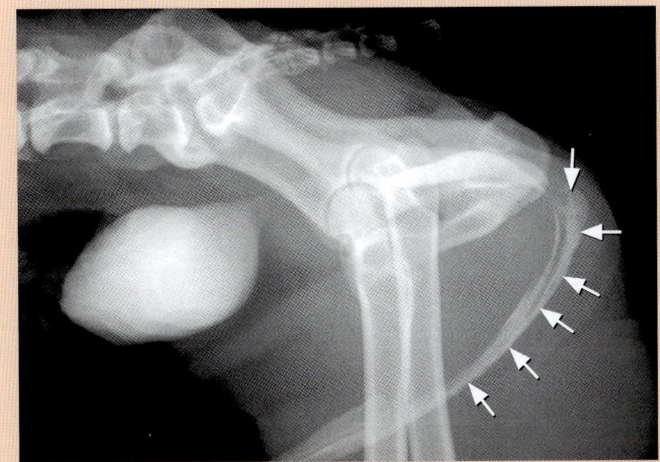

FIGURE 2.84. Enlarged image of a lateral retrograde urogram showing the pelvic region of a male dog. Arrows point to extravasated contrast medium into peri-penile tissues due to urethral perforation.

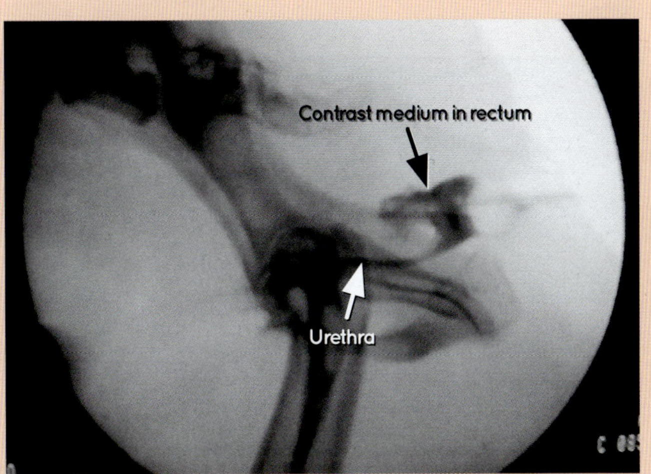

FIGURE 2.85. Frame of a fluoroscopic image in female dog that underwent urethrography to confirm the presence of a rectourethral fistula. The patient presented urine leakage through the anus.

Genital system

Genital system of the female

The normal genital system of a female is not identified on a plain radiograph, with the exception of the uterus during the second half of gestation. Ultrasonography is the technique of choice to assess a normal uterus and ovaries, as well as to identify any pathological changes in these structures. However, the number of foetuses and the relationship between the diameter of the foetal head and that of the pelvic canal in term pregnancies are assessed by means of plain radiography, since ultrasonography does not provide precise information in those cases. Retrograde vaginourethrography, which has previously been described (see Urethra section), allows the radiological examination of the morphology of the vagina and vaginal vestibule.

The normal pregnant uterus can be identified on a plain radiograph from day 30 of pregnancy in the dog and between days 25 and 35 in the cat (fig. 2.86), but it will not be possible to differentiate this image from that produced by a pathological distension of the uterus until bone mineralisation can be detected, that is to say at day 45 of pregnancy in the dog and between days 36 and 45 in the cat. It is necessary to bear in mind that these data refer to the days of pregnancy, which do not necessarily coincide with the days that have passed since the time of breeding in the dog, since sperm may remain viable in the uterus up to 7 days before fertilisation. This means that an absence of foetal bone mineralisation on day 45 post-breeding does not necessarily imply a negative pregnancy diagnosis. However, ultrasonography is much more precise to diagnose a pregnancy, since it is possible to identify the embryonic vesicles from days 18 to 20 of pregnancy in the dog and 15 to 17 in the cat, although it is recommended to confirm the diagnosis a few days later (from day 23), when the heartbeat can be observed.

Ultrasound examinations may however be less precise than radiographs when it comes to counting the number of foetuses. In order to carry out this assessment, it is recommended to take lateral and ventrodorsal radiographs of the abdomen at the end of pregnancy. In order to improve the precision of the diagnosis, the number of heads and that of spines should be counted on both projections, since the superimposition of the foetuses with each other and with other structures may lead to diagnostic errors, especially when there are many of them (fig. 2.87).

Ultrasonography does not enable a precise assessment of the relationship between the size of the foetus and the diameter of the pelvic canal. This measurement should be made using radiography (fig. 2.88). If the cranial diameter of the foetus clearly exceeds the width of the canal on the radiograph, this is considered

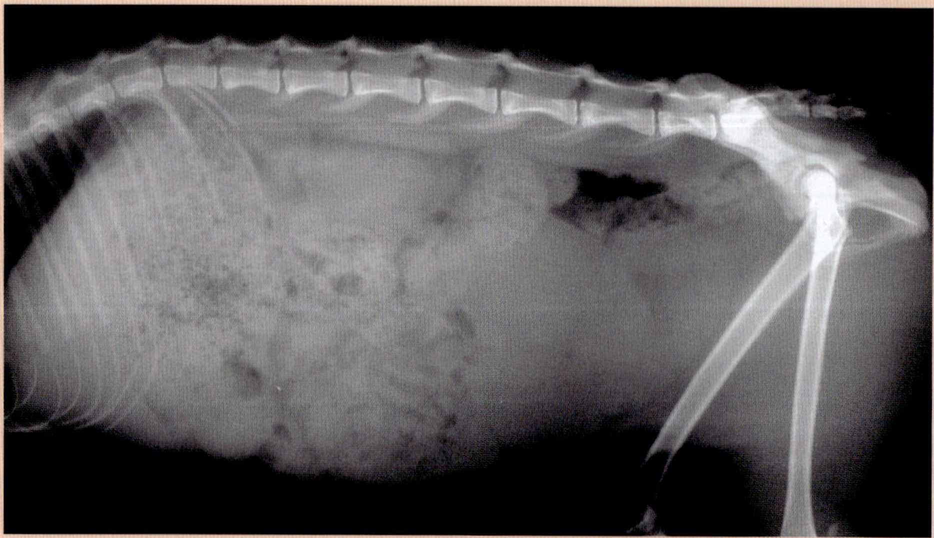

FIGURE 2.86. Lateral radiograph of the abdomen of a cat on day 30 of pregnancy. The dilated uterus appears cranial to the bladder, displacing the colon in dorsal direction and the small intestine in cranial direction. As the bones of the foetuses are not mineralised yet, this image may be confused with dilatation of the uterus due to pathological causes. A fracture of the ischion can also be identified.

as an evident sign of dystocia. This usually occurs when the size of the male is much greater than that of the female, especially in pregnancies of one or two foetuses, or in brachycephalic breeds, in which the size of the skull is proportionally greater and the morphology of the maternal pelvis is flatter. Other causes of dystocia observable by means of radiography include morphological alterations of the bony pelvis (fractures of traumatic origin, which can cause a more or less marked narrowing of the pelvic canal, are the most common) or poor foetal position at the time of birth. Radiography allows the observation of the normal uterus after birth, due to its increased size until day 12 postpartum in the dog and day 6 postpartum in the cat. It will also be useful to detect any retained foetuses once the birth is over.

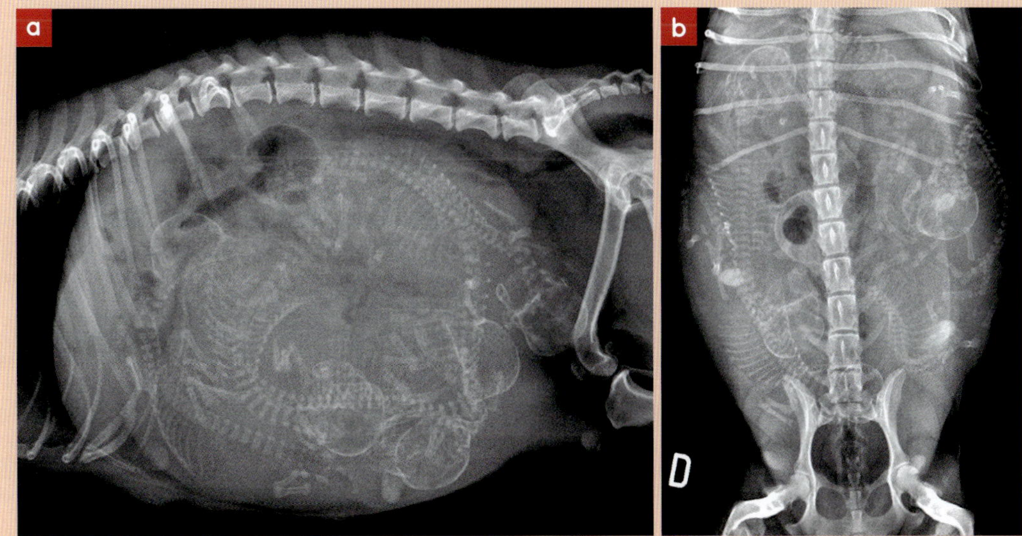

FIGURE 2.87. Lateral (a) and ventrodorsal (b) radiographs of the abdomen of a dog on day 60 of pregnancy with five foetuses. Radiography is the most precise technique to count the number of foetuses, although the radiographs must be taken on the last days of pregnancy so as to minimise the damage that radiation may cause to the foetuses (the risk is higher during the first third of pregnancy, during the period of organogenesis).

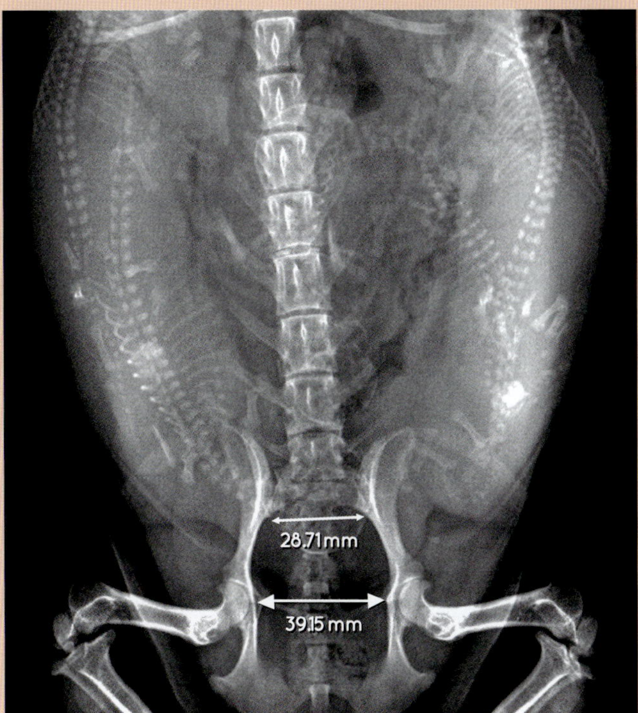

FIGURE 2.88. Ventrodorsal abdominal radiograph of female dog at day 62 of pregnancy. With a ventrodorsal radiograph, the cranial diameter (28.71 mm) can be compared with the width of the pelvic canal (39.15 mm) to prevent possible dystocia due to excessive foetal size.

Although ultrasound examinations are much more appropriate to assess a possible foetal death, some signs suggesting this diagnosis may be detected on the radiograph:

- Presence of gas in the foetus or in the lumen of the pregnant uterus (fig. 2.89).
- Anomalous position of the mineralised foetal structures.
- Evident signs of delay in foetal growth (fig. 2.90).

Those cases of endometrial hyperplasia and endometritis that are not accompanied by a great accumulation of fluid in the lumen of the uterus are easily identified on an ultrasound scan, but are not usually detectable on a plain radiograph. However, marked dilatations of the uterus, generally due to pyometra and, on a less frequent basis, to hydrometra, mucometra or haematometra, are easily identified on radiographs. They appear as tubular structures with soft tissue

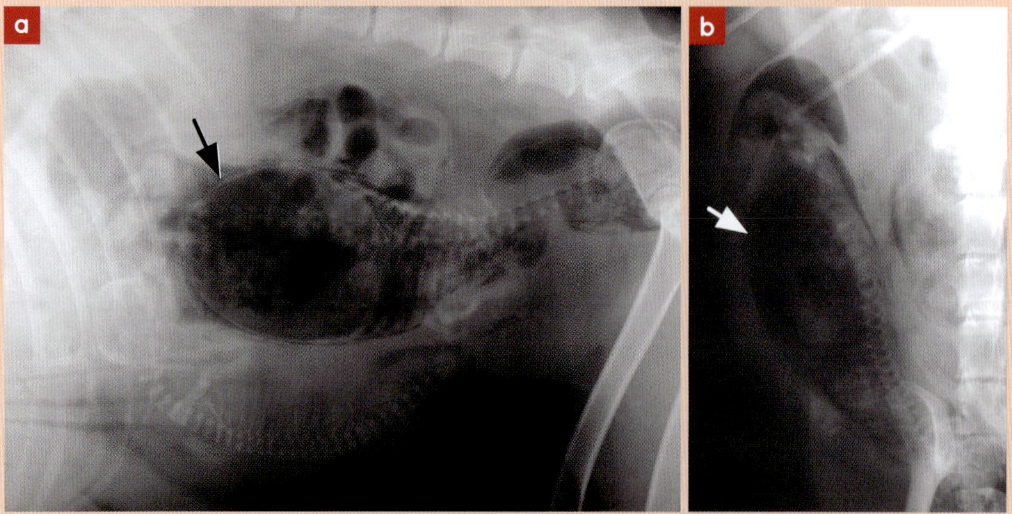

FIGURE 2.89. Enlarged images of the abdomen on lateral (a) and ventrodorsal (b) radiographs of a bitch on day 64 of pregnancy with two foetuses. Intrafoetal and intrauterine gas may be observed and are both indicative of foetal death. The foetal abdominal wall (arrows) may be identified as there is gas on both sides of it.

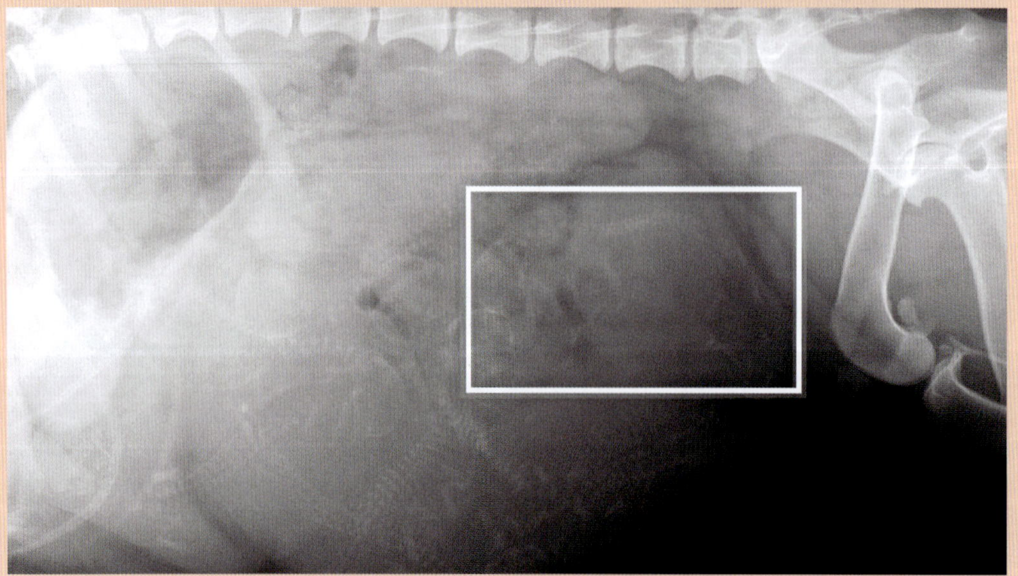

FIGURE 2.90. Lateral radiograph of the abdomen of a bitch on day 50 of pregnancy with seven foetuses. The foetus shown in the rectangle is smaller and the degree of mineralisation is lower compared with other foetuses. This finding may be due to foetal death, although it should be confirmed by means of an ultrasound examination.

opacity, in many cases with a tortuous course, which occupy the central and caudal part of the abdomen (fig. 2.91). In some cases, the dilatation only affects one or two uterine horns, so the changes may only be observed in one of the sides of the abdomen on ventrodorsal radiographs.

Uterine stump abscesses or granulomas, which may appear as a complication of an ovariohysterectomy, are not usually detected on radiographs, unless they reach a size that is sufficiently large to produce a clear "mass effect" between the bladder and the colon.

Uterine neoplasms are very uncommon and cannot normally be differentiated from masses of another origin on radiographs of the abdomen. Ovarian neoplasms also have a low incidence in small animals. These latter may be uni- or bilateral and are sometimes accompanied by free peritoneal fluid and carcinomatosis, which may mask the image of the mass or masses on the radiograph. They are located caudal to the kidneys and may displace these latter in cranial direction and the intestine in ventral direction if they reach a large size (fig. 2.92). Some ovarian tumours (teratomas and teratocarcinomas) may appear calcified.

When a vaginourethrogram is performed, it is important to keep the end of the Foley catheter in the vaginal vestibule and not to introduce it in the vagina, as a vaginal rupture may occur when inflating the balloon. The normal vagina has a spindle-shaped morphology and it is common to see a small amount of contrast medium passing to the body of the uterus during oestrus. The vestibulovaginal junction appears as an area of narrowing between the vagina and the vestibule (fig. 2.93). Vaginal masses (neoplasms, polyps, abscesses, haematomas, infiltration secondary to a urethral tumour) may create filling defects on the vaginogram. Vaginal hypertrophy, more common in brachycephalic breeds, and tumours can cause marked irregularity in the margins of the vagina (fig. 2.94).

Ectopic ureters that open into the vagina may be filled with contrast medium during a retrograde vaginourethrography study, although it is recommended to combine this technique with excretory urography for a more precise evaluation of this anomaly.

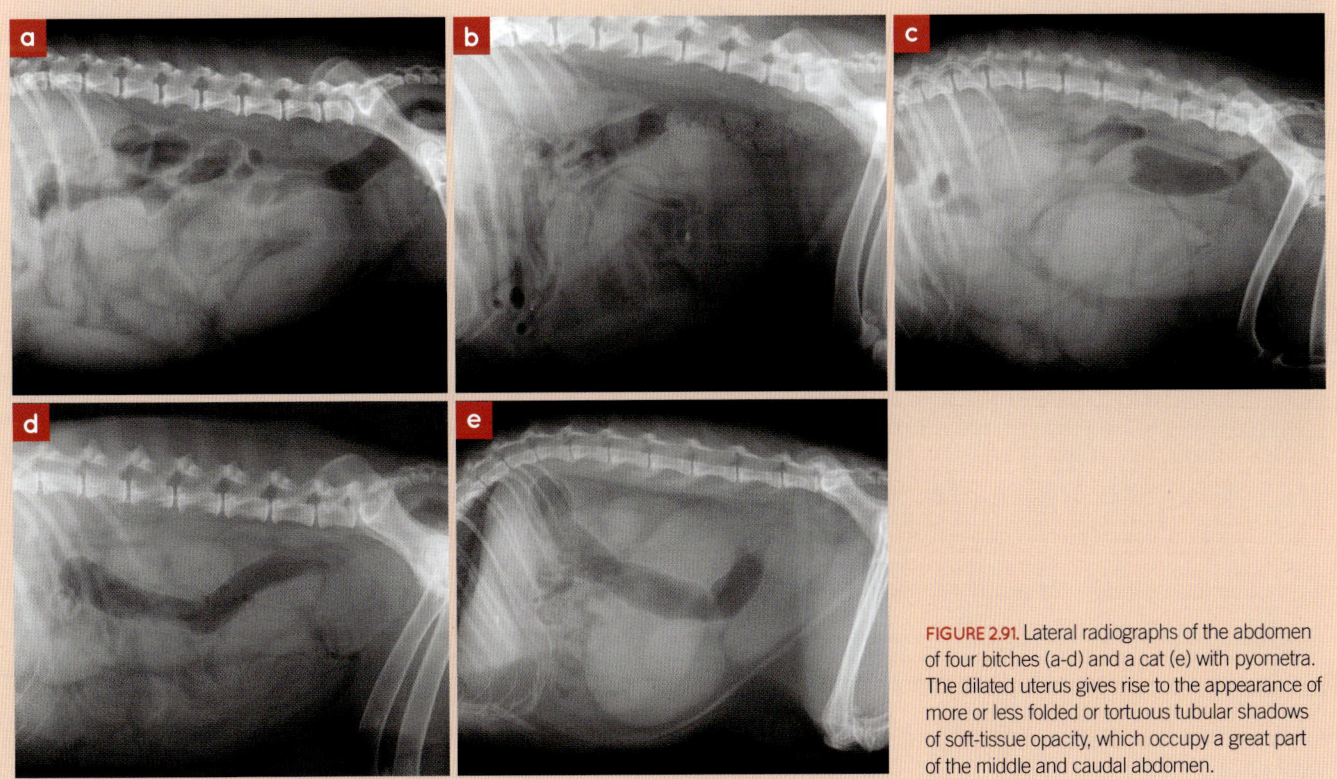

FIGURE 2.91. Lateral radiographs of the abdomen of four bitches (a-d) and a cat (e) with pyometra. The dilated uterus gives rise to the appearance of more or less folded or tortuous tubular shadows of soft-tissue opacity, which occupy a great part of the middle and caudal abdomen.

Vestibulovaginal stenosis is the abnormal narrowing of the vestibulovaginal junction (fig. 2.95), which may be asymptomatic or predispose affected females to recurrent urinary and genital infections. Although it has traditionally been considered that if the height of the vestibulovaginal junction is lower than a third of the height of the vagina on lateral radiographs, this is indicative of stenosis, some research studies suggest that this finding may be incidental in healthy animals.

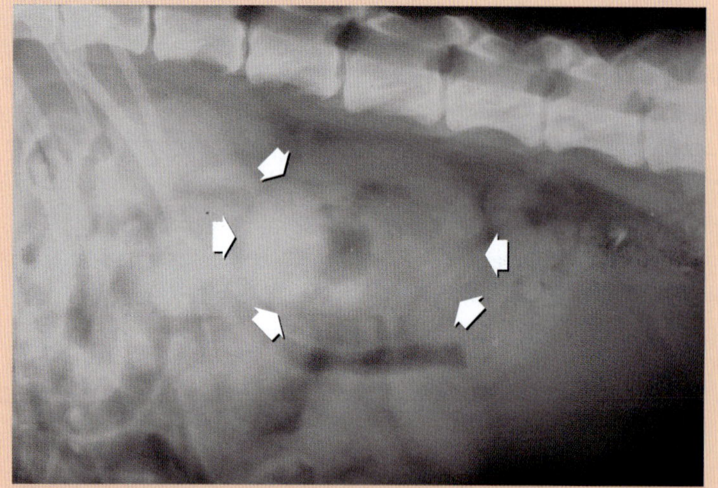

FIGURE 2.92. Enlarged image of the central region of the abdomen on a lateral radiograph of a dog with an ovarian neoplasm. The mass (arrows) is located caudal to the kidneys and displaces the colon in ventral direction.

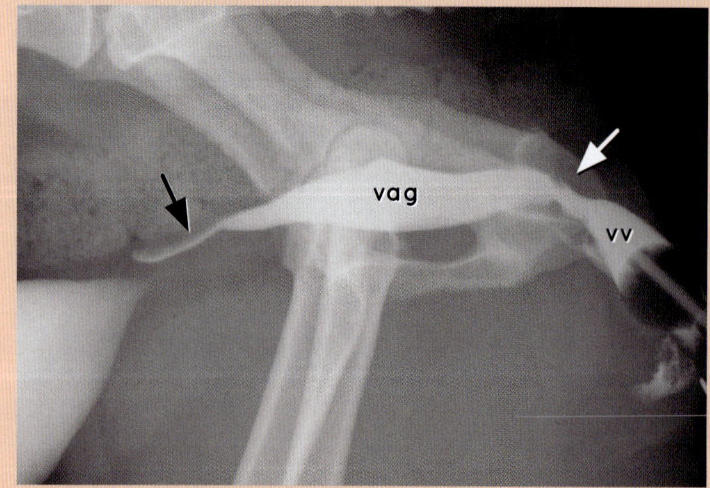

FIGURE 2.93. Normal vaginogram in a dog. The vestibulovaginal junction (white arrow) has a smaller diameter than the vaginal vestibule (vv) and the vagina (vag.). During oestrus, it is normal for a small amount of contrast medium to pass into the uterus (black arrow).

Genital system of the male

Ultrasonography is the technique of choice to examine the prostate and testicles. The information provided by a radiograph is much more limited.

In dogs, the prostate is located immediately caudal to the neck of the bladder. Its normal position is intrapelvic, so its shadow is usually completely or partially masked by the bony pelvis on radiographs of the abdomen.

In cats, the prostate has a more caudal anatomical position than in dogs and its size is very small, which is why it is not identified on radiographs. In addition, prostatic diseases are extremely rare in cats, so we will only refer to dogs from this point on.

The triangle of fat that accumulates between the caudoventral margin of the bladder and the cranioventral margin of the prostate, which is visible on lateral radiographs, helps to identify the image of this gland on the radiograph (fig. 2.96). The normal prostate is sometimes slightly displaced in cranial direction, especially if the bladder is very distended, which facilitates its evaluation. It is considered that the height of the prostatic shadow in non-neutered healthy males does not exceed 70 % of the distance between the promontory of the sacrum and the pubis on lateral radiographs. In some breeds, such as the Scottish Terrier, the normal prostate may exceed this limit.

Retrograde urethrography enables the evaluation of the image of the prostatic urethra and sometimes provides additional information on the prostatic parenchyma. In a healthy dog, the prostatic urethra has a more or less homogeneous diameter and smooth margins. It is sometimes possible to observe the passage of contrast medium to the normal prostatic parenchyma, when the prostatic ducts are partially filled.

The most frequent cause of an increase in the size of the prostate is benign hyperplasia, which is very common in non-neutered males from 5 years of age. Prostatitis, prostatic abscesses and neoplasms may also cause a more or less marked increase in the size of the gland (fig. 2.97). In some cases, prostate enlargement is accompanied by the cranial displacement of the gland towards the abdomen. If the increase in size is marked, this usually causes compression or dorsal displacement of the rectum, which may be the only evident radiological sign of prostatomegaly if the gland maintains its intrapelvic position (fig. 2.98). When the height of the shadow exceeds 90 % of the distance between the promontory of the sacrum and the pubis, this finding is considered indicative of a mass-type lesion (tumour, abscess, large-sized cyst). If the increase in size is significant, a mass in the caudal abdomen that displaces the adjacent structures in cranial and dorsal direction (fig. 2.99) will appear on the radiograph. When the diameter of the urethra is very reduced as a consequence of a prostatic disease, the bladder may appear very distended.

In the case of prostatic neoplasms, the outline of the gland may be irregular or appear poorly defined in the image, even if there is sufficient fat surrounding it. As associated findings, it is possible to observe images indicative of an increase in the size of the sublumbar lymph nodes ("mass effect" located ventral to L5-L6-L7) and lesions in the closest bony structures, which suggest metastasis. Bone metastases from prostatic tumours usually appear as proliferative lesions in the ventral margin of the lumbar vertebrae and, in a less frequent manner, in the margin of the sacrum, wings of the ilium and femur. At more advanced stages, they may metastasise to the lungs and other long bones. The appearance of areas of calcification in the prostatic parenchyma is very suggestive of neoplasia (fig. 2.100), although they may also appear in severe chronic prostatitis.

Paraprostatic cysts can reach a large size and are identified on plain radiographs as soft-tissue opacity masses located in the caudal area of the abdomen. Calcification of the wall is sometimes observed. An ultrasound scan or alternatively a cystogram will allow the differentiation of the bladder from masses with an origin located in other abdominal organs (fig. 2.101).

Neutered dogs show prostatic atrophy secondary to orchiectomy, so the identification of the shadow of the prostate on radiographs will be difficult. The same may occur in patients with Sertoli-cell testicular tumour or in those that receive oestrogen therapy.

If the prostatic shadow is large and the urethra appears displaced within it, this finding will be indicative of the presence of a mass-type lesion in the parenchyma of the gland, while if the image of the prostatic urethra shows a marked narrowing or irregularity in its margins (fig. 2.102), this will indicate aggressive disease of the prostate or urethra. The contrast medium

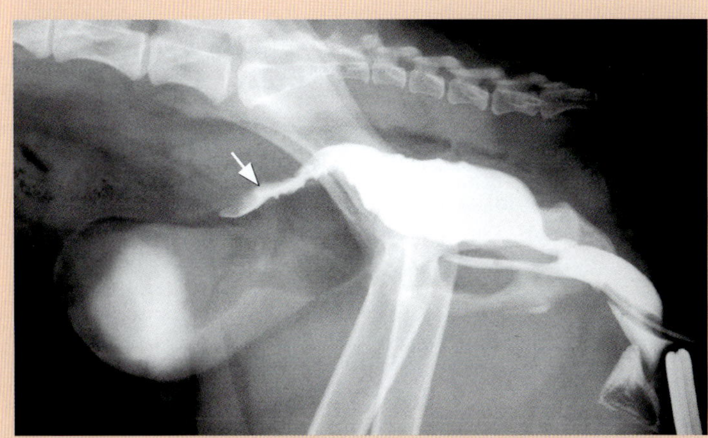

FIGURE 2.94. Enlarged image of the pelvic region in lateral view of a female dog that underwent retrograde vaginourethrography. The vaginogram reveals irregular margins as well as the opacified part of the uterine body (arrow). This finding is indicative of chronic inflammation, hyperplasia or neoplasia.

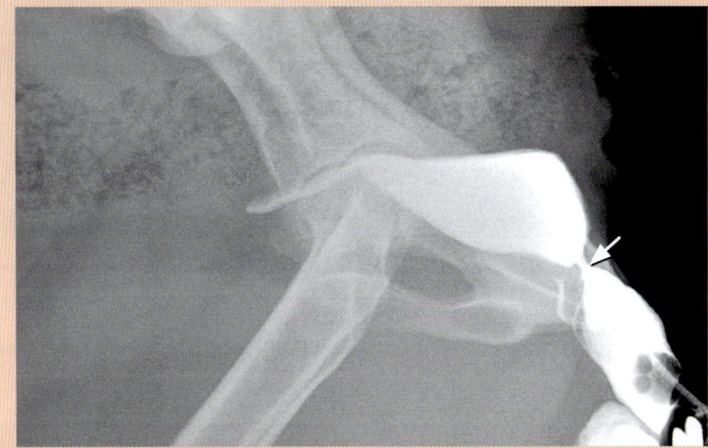

FIGURE 2.95. Enlarged image of lateral pelvic radiograph in female dog that underwent retrograde vaginourethrography. The findings are consistent with vestibulovaginal stenosis (arrow) with a maximum vaginal height:vestibulovaginal junction height ratio of 0.09 (values less than 0.33 suggest stenosis).

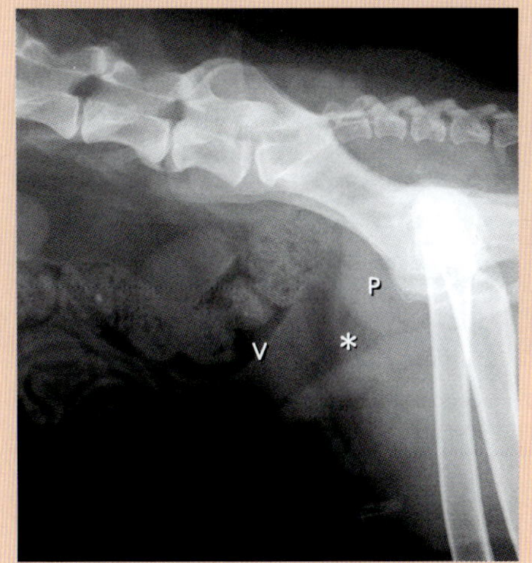

FIGURE 2.96. Enlarged image of caudal abdomen on lateral radiograph of male dog in which a normal prostate is partially visualised. The triangular region of fat (asterisk) between the caudoventral border of the bladder (B) and the cranioventral border of the prostate (P) helps with the identification of the prostate on radiograms.

may extravasate into cavitary lesions of the prostatic parenchyma that are communicated with the urethra (fig. 2.103). If the morphology of these lesions is very irregular, this is considered compatible with neoplasia.

Radiography provides very limited information about the testicles, scrotum or penis. The only detectable testicular disease would be a mass caused by a very enlarged testicle with an abdominal or inguinal location. In the case of the scrotum, it may be possible to identify the presence of intestinal loops with gas in a scrotal hernia. Deformations, fractures and osteomyelitis of the os penis (fig. 2.104) have also been described.

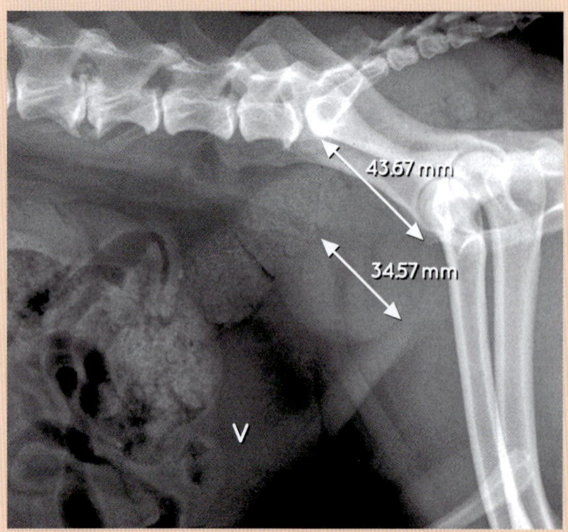

FIGURE 2.97. Enlarged image of the caudal abdomen on a lateral radiograph of a male dog with prostate enlargement. The height of the prostate shadow (34.57 mm) is 79 % the distance between the sacral promontory and the pubis (43.67 mm) in this radiograph. B: bladder.

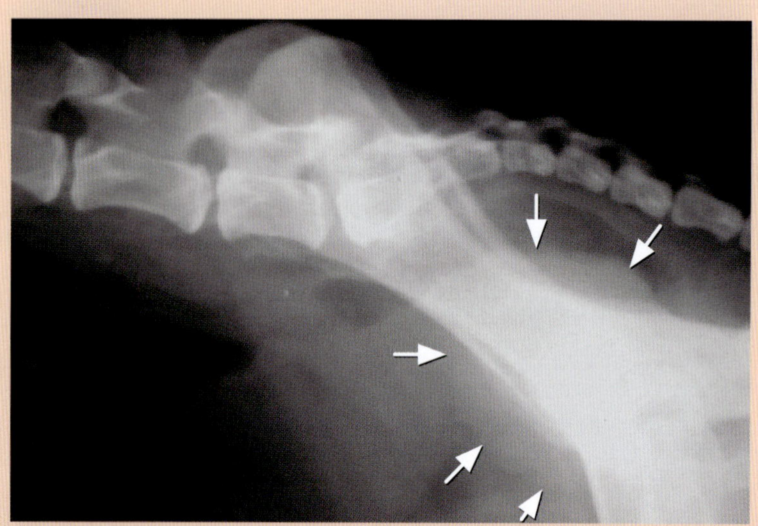

FIGURE 2.98. Enlarged image of the pelvic region on a lateral radiograph of a dog with prostatomegaly. The prostate (arrows) maintains its intrapelvic location. However, a dorsal displacement of the rectum is clearly observed, which is indicative of marked prostatomegaly.

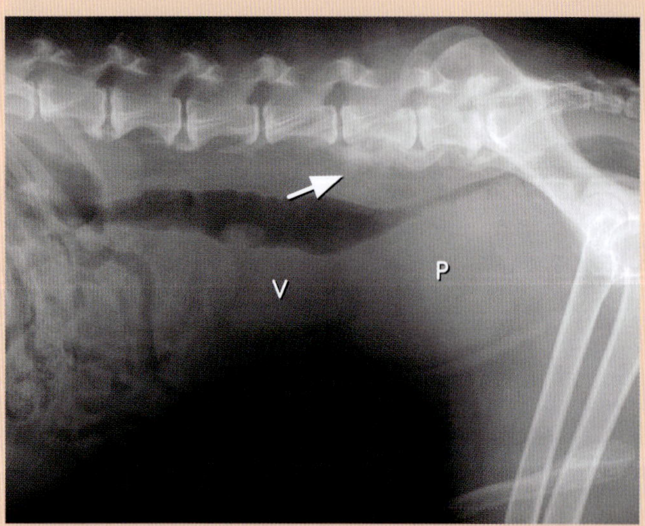

FIGURE 2.99. Lateral radiograph of the abdomen of a dog with a prostatic neoplasm. The prostate (P) is very enlarged in size and occupies a great part of the caudal abdomen, compressing the caudal third of the descending colon. The bladder (B) appears cranial to the prostatic mass. Irregular osteoproliferative lesions (arrow) compatible with bone metastases of the prostatic tumour can be observed in the ventral margin of the L6 and L7 vertebrae.

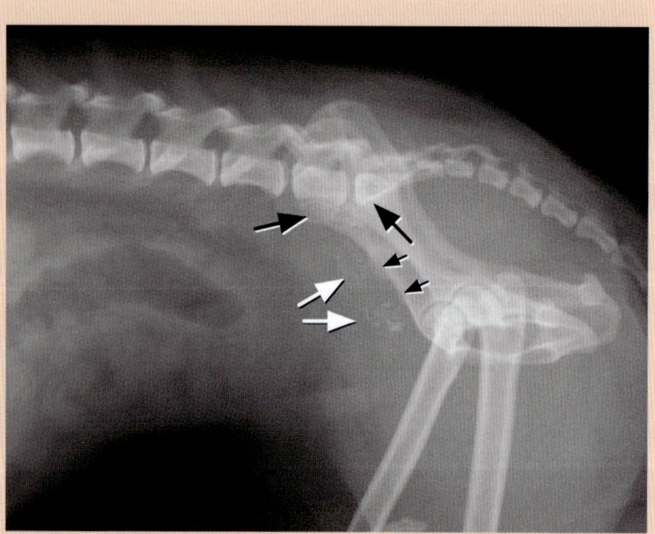

FIGURE 2.100. Lateral radiograph of the abdomen of a dog with a prostatic neoplasm. In the area where the prostate is located, areas of calcification of the soft tissues are observed (white arrows). The outline of the gland is not clearly identified. Irregular bony overgrowths compatible with metastases of the prostatic tumour can be observed in the area ventral to L7, sacrum and cranial margin of one of the wings of the ilium (black arrows).

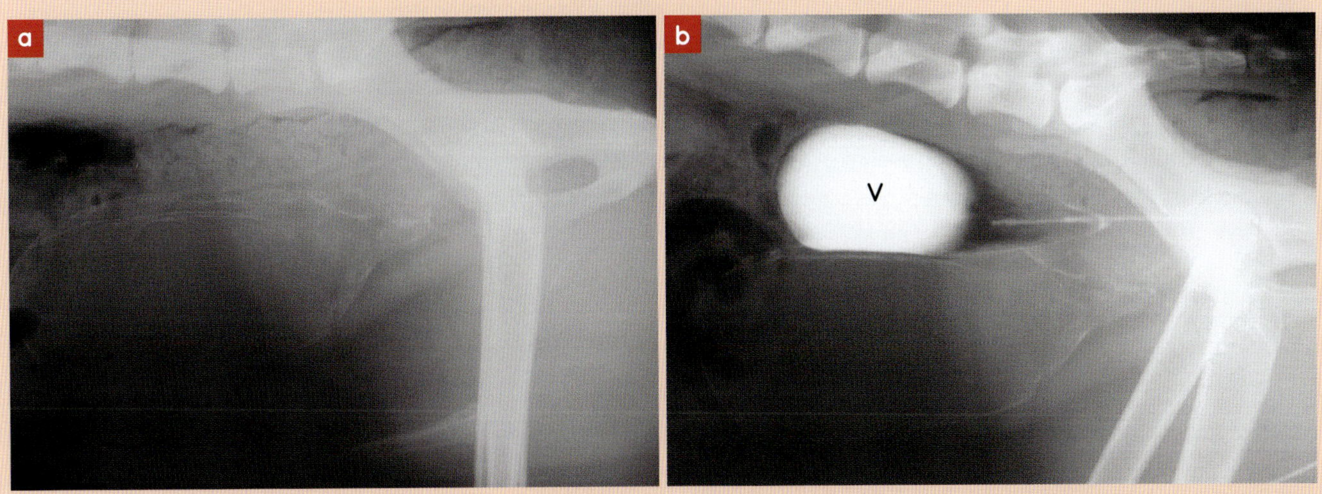

FIGURE 2.101. Enlarged images of the caudal abdomen on lateral radiographs of a dog with a large paraprostatic cyst with calcified walls, before (a) and after (b) introducing a double contrast medium into the bladder to identify its position (B) in relation to this structure.

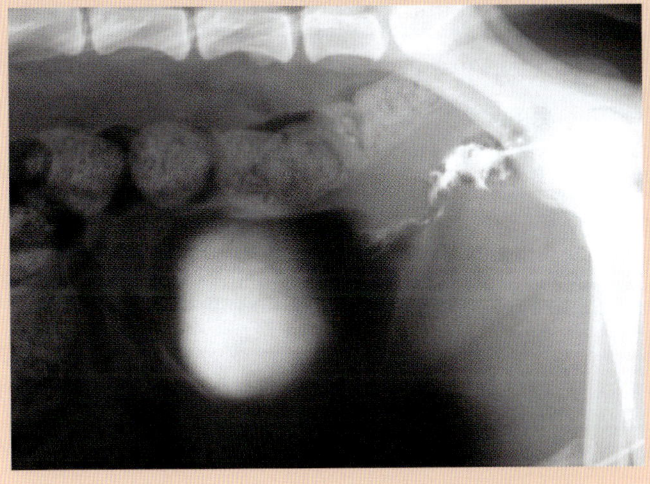

FIGURE 2.102. Enlarged image of a lateral double-contrast cystogram in a dog. It is possible to observe a reflux of positive contrast medium and gas into the prostatic urethra, which has very irregular margins. This indicates aggressive disease of the prostate and urethra. Final diagnosis: prostatic neoplasm.

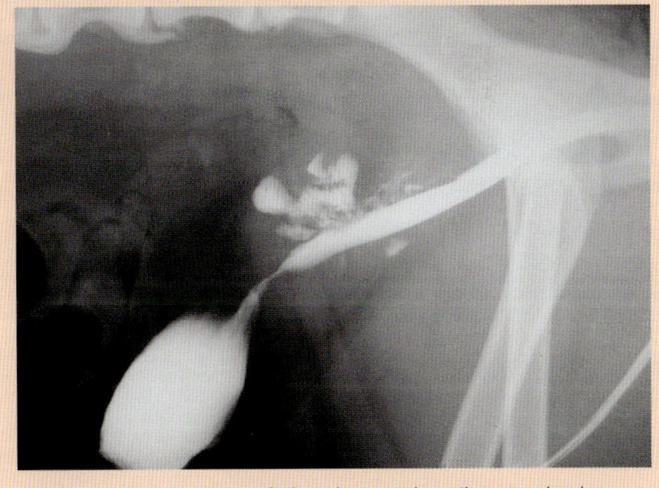

FIGURE 2.103. Enlarged image of a lateral retrograde urethrogram showing the caudal abdomen of a dog. An extravasation of the contrast medium into cavitary areas with an irregular morphology is observed, which is considered indicative of a prostatic neoplasm.

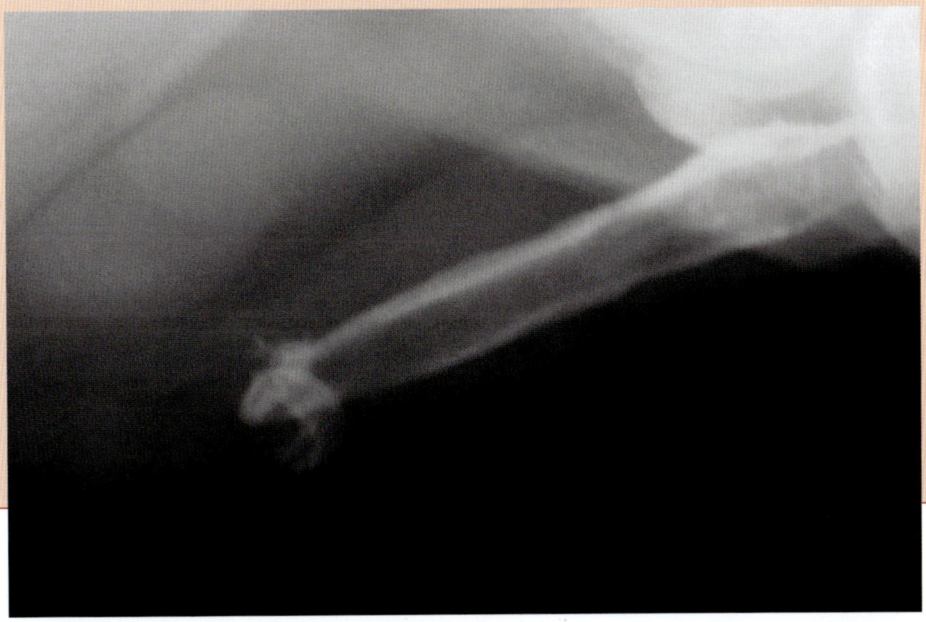

FIGURE 2.104. Enlarged image of the area of the prepuce on a lateral radiograph of a dog with a fracture of the os penis.

Stomach

Although plain radiography and contrast radiography have traditionally been considered the techniques of choice for the asessment of the stomach and intestine, the now almost daily use of ultrasonography as a diagnostic tool perfectly complements the information provided by plain radiographs and drastically reduces the need to perform other contrast techniques to examine the gastrointestinal tract in small animals.

The stomach is divided into a cardiac part, a fundus, a body and a pyloric part (pyloric antrum and canal). In the dog, the body of the stomach has a central position and the pyloric antrum is located in the right side. In the cat, the stomach is located mainly in the left side, with the pyloric antrum on the median line.

The image of the stomach depends on its content (fig. 2.105) and on the radiographic projection used. When the patient has not eaten for some time, the stomach usually contains a variable amount of gas and fluid/mucus. In healthy dogs and cats, the stomach with no food usually appears cranial to the last pair of ribs, although it may also extend slightly beyond them, occupying approximately two intercostal spaces. When it contains food, this latter appears as radiopaque material with a granular aspect, and the size of the stomach may double or triple in normal conditions. On lateral radiographs, the axis of the stomach lies perpendicular to the spine, parallel to the ribs or at an intermediate point between these two positions.

One of the most important factors that affect the image of the stomach is the position of the patient when taking the radiograph. The relationship between the position of the stomach and its radiographic image is an important concept that should be borne in mind to interpret radiographs correctly and identify certain gastric lesions. The variation in the image of the stomach is due to changes in the distribution of the fluid and gas that can be found in its lumen: the fluid content is deposited on the inclined area as a result of gravity and the gas is displaced towards the uppermost area of the lumen of the stomach (fig. 2.106).

It is important to know how to make the most of the displacements of fluid and gas in the stomach to visualise some of its parts with more clarity (fig. 2.107).

It is not possible to appropriately evaluate the thickness of the wall or its folds by means of plain radiography, since the wall and the gastric fluid/mucous content have the same radiographic density and cannot be distinguished in the image (that is to say, we can think that a wall is thickened, when in fact what we see is the image of the wall plus the fluid in the lumen (fig. 2.108).

Different contrast techniques may be used to assess the stomach:

- Conventional gastrography with barium sulphate.
- Gastrography with iodinated contrast media.
- Pneumogastrography.
- Double-contrast gastrography.
- Gastric emptying studies using food mixed with barium or with radiopaque markers.

Peristalsis and gastric emptying can be observed in real time using fluoroscopy and a positive contrast medium.

Before performing a contrast study of the stomach, the patient must not eat for 12 to 24 hours. The study should start by taking plain radiographs to confirm the need to carry out the examination with a contrast medium, ensure the correct preparation of the patient and adjust the exposure values. If sedation of the animal is necessary, acepromazine or ketamine may be used, since those drugs almost do not affect gastric motility.

Gastrography using barium sulphate

To perform a conventional gastrogram using barium sulphate, this latter is administered in a liquid preparation, preferably at a concentration of 30 % and at doses of 7–15 ml/kg (7–8 ml/kg in large breed dogs and 10–15 ml/kg in small breed dogs and cats). Although it is easier to administer the contrast medium by oral route using a syringe, this method involves some risk of aspirating the contrast medium, which could lead to the development of aspiration pneumonia (fig. 2.109). As an alternative, it is possible to administer the contrast material through an orogastric tube. Nowadays, this technique is almost only used to carry out gastric emptying studies.

Gastric emptying is a complex phenomenon, which depends on various factors, such as the type of contrast medium used, the volume administered and the use of certain drugs. The greater the volume of intraluminal content, the faster the stomach will empty; it is therefore important to use the standard dose of the contrast medium. In normal conditions, gastric emptying usually starts in the first 15 minutes after the administration of barium, although in nervous animals it may be delayed until 30–45 minutes. The stomach usually completely empties in 1 to 4 hours in the dog. Minimal significance should be given to abnormally fast gastric emptying. On the other hand, a delay in gastric emptying is more significant. If the administered dose of barium is low, a delay in gastric emptying may be observed, which may lead to a false diagnosis of pyloric obstruction. If the administered dose is high, gastric emptying may be faster than normal.

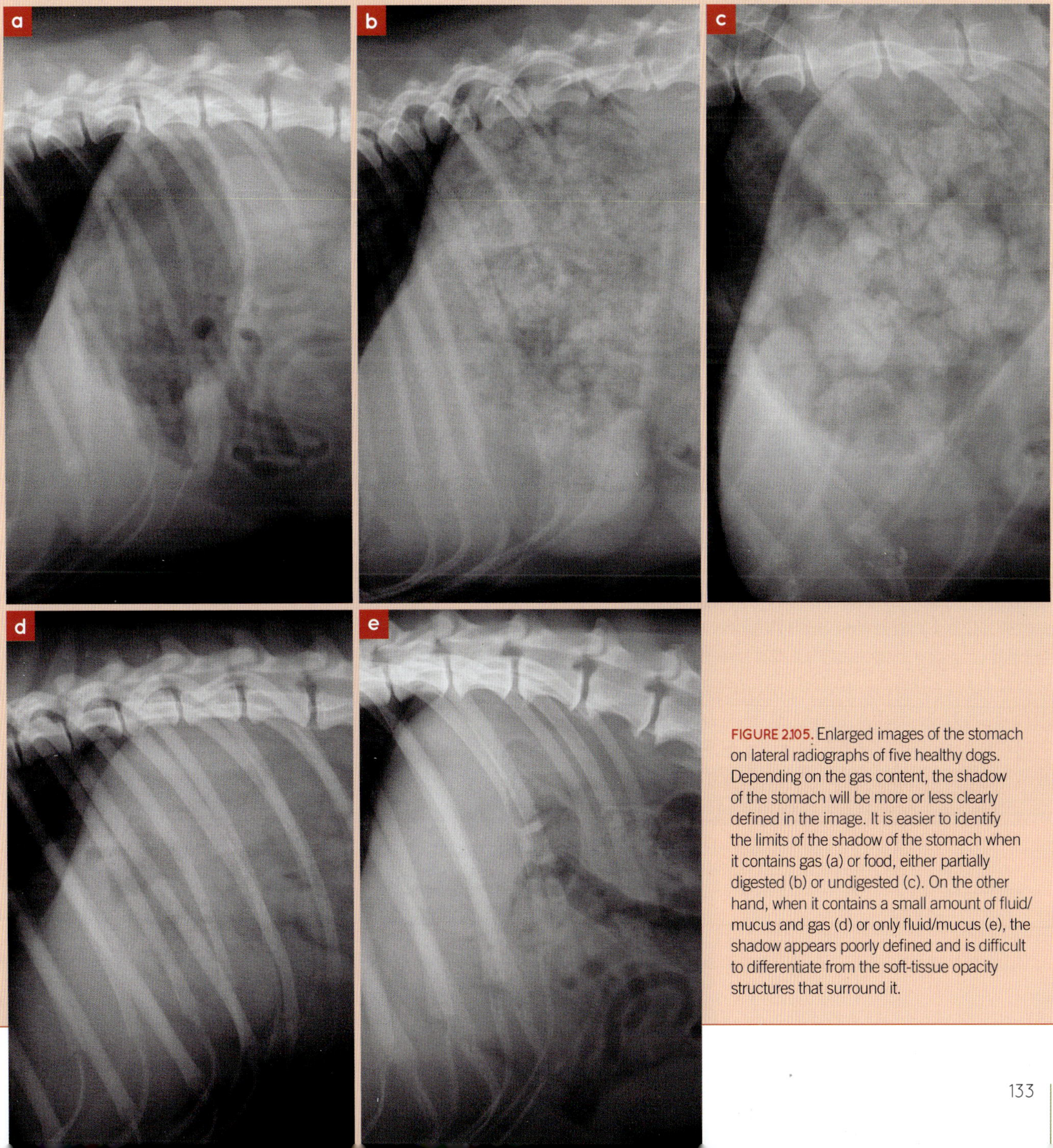

FIGURE 2.105. Enlarged images of the stomach on lateral radiographs of five healthy dogs. Depending on the gas content, the shadow of the stomach will be more or less clearly defined in the image. It is easier to identify the limits of the shadow of the stomach when it contains gas (a) or food, either partially digested (b) or undigested (c). On the other hand, when it contains a small amount of fluid/mucus and gas (d) or only fluid/mucus (e), the shadow appears poorly defined and is difficult to differentiate from the soft-tissue opacity structures that surround it.

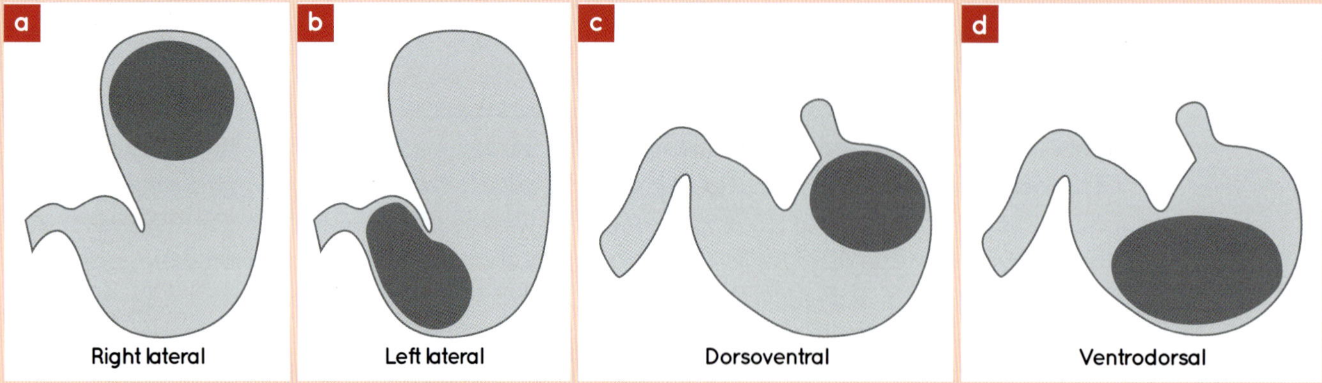

FIGURE 2.106. Representation of the variation of the radiographic image of the stomach due to the changes in the distribution of the fluid content and gas in function of the radiographic projection used. This diagram is only true when the stomach has a moderate amount of gas and fluid/mucus in its lumen.

The differences depending on the projection are:

- **a** On **right lateral views,** the gas is located in the fundus and body of the stomach, since they are located in the left side of the patient and therefore represent the uppermost area in this position. The fluid content is deposited on the inclined area and fills the pyloric part. The fundus and body are identified immediately caudal to the left crus of the diaphragm (in the cranial and dorsal part of the abdomen). The pyloric part appears as a soft-tissue density shadow, located in ventral position immediately caudal to the liver. The shadow of the pyloric part sometimes has a rounded shape and may be mistaken for a mass or a rounded foreign body.
- **b** On **left lateral views**, the gas is displaced to the pyloric part of the stomach, which is located in the right side of the patient and represents the uppermost part of the stomach in this position. The fluid content is deposited in the gastric fundus and body, which makes their identification difficult.
- **c** On **ventrodorsal views**, the gas is located in the cardial part, fundus and part of the body of the stomach, while the fluid content is deposited on the ventral area of the body of the stomach and in the pyloric part.
- **d** On **ventrodorsal views**, the gas is located in the pyloric part and in the ventral area of the body of the stomach. The fluid content fills the fundus and the rest of the body of the stomach. If they are completely empty, the fundus and body may appear as homogeneous soft-tissue density shadows.

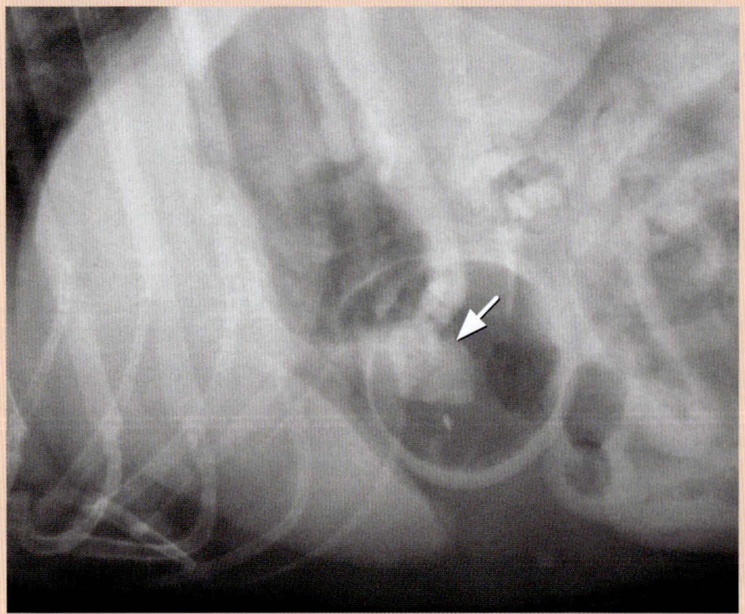

FIGURE 2.107. Enlarged image of the cranial abdomen on a lateral radiograph of a dog with a radiolucent foreign body in the pyloric antrum. When taking a left lateral radiograph, the gas is displaced to the antrum and surrounds the object (arrow), which allows its identification in the image.

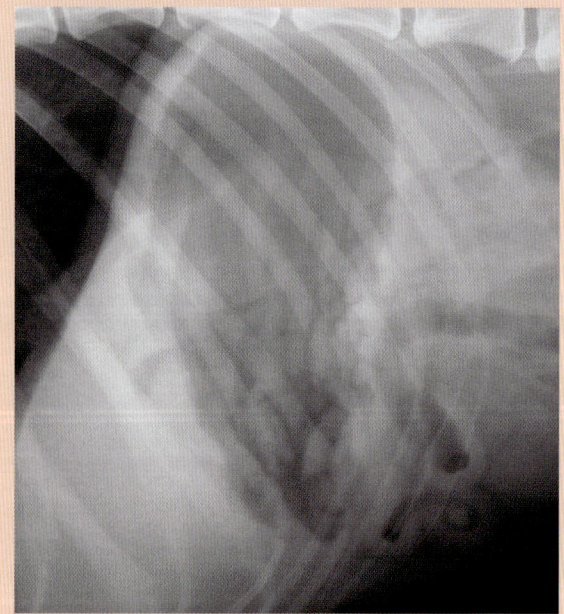

FIGURE 2.108. Enlarged image of the cranial abdomen on a lateral radiograph of a dog, in which prominent gastric folds are observed. This radiological finding may appear in cases of gastritis, but this diagnosis should never be confirmed only by means of radiography, since the presence of fluid or mucus between the folds of a normal gastric wall may create the same image. An ultrasound scan must be performed for a precise assessment of the thickness of the gastric wall.

Some gastric emptying studies have been performed using food mixed with barium, but this is not considered useful since the range of normality for the empyting time is very wide (from 7 to 15 hours). Radiopaque barium-impregnated polyethylene spheres (BIPS) have also been used mixed with food. The number and size of the spheres, the type and amount of food with which they are mixed and the amount of time without eating should be strictly adjusted to a standardised protocol, or else the results will be difficult to interpret. A disadvantage of this technique is that the time of examination may be very long (up to 10 hours), so it is not used in practice.

Positive-contrast gastrography using iodinated contrast media

Positive-contrast gastrography using iodinated contrast media is recommended only when a rupture or perforation of the stomach (or the intestine) is suspected. These contrast media are diluted in the gastrointestinal tract, so the quality of the contrast study is lower in comparison with that of the studies performed with barium, but they will be absorbed in the peritoneal cavity if they extravasate. Their use is contraindicated in dehydrated patients. Although hyperosmotic iodinated contrast media can be used at doses of 7 ml/kg, low-osmolarity nonionic iodinated contrast media such as iohexol and iopamidol, which can be administered diluted at 33 % in doses of 8 ml/kg, are more recommended.

Negative-contrast gastrography

Negative-contrast gastrography is performed by introducing air (20 ml/kg) in the stomach through a gastric tube. It is essential that the animal does not eat for 12–24 hours prior to the study so as to avoid the presence of food in the stomach at the time of examination. It is a relatively simple technique, which can improve the visualisation of certain radiolucent foreign bodies and intraparietal masses. However, it is hardly ever used nowadays, firstly, because double-contrast gastrography would provide more information in these cases and secondly, because the combination of plain radiography and ultrasonography frequently allows the establishment of these diagnoses without the need to sedate the patient or administer contrast media.

Double-contrast gastrography

Double-contrast gastrography would be the most appropriate contrast technique to evaluate the mucosa and folds of the stomach, although we should bear in mind that an ultrasound examination is preferable, since it provides direct information about the thickness, differentiation of the layers and peristalsis of the stomach wall.

In order to perform a double-contrast gastrogram, non-diluted liquid barium sulphate (3–5 ml/kg) is administered first by means of an orogastric tube, followed by air (10–20 ml/kg or simply the sufficient amount to achieve an appropriate distension of the organ).

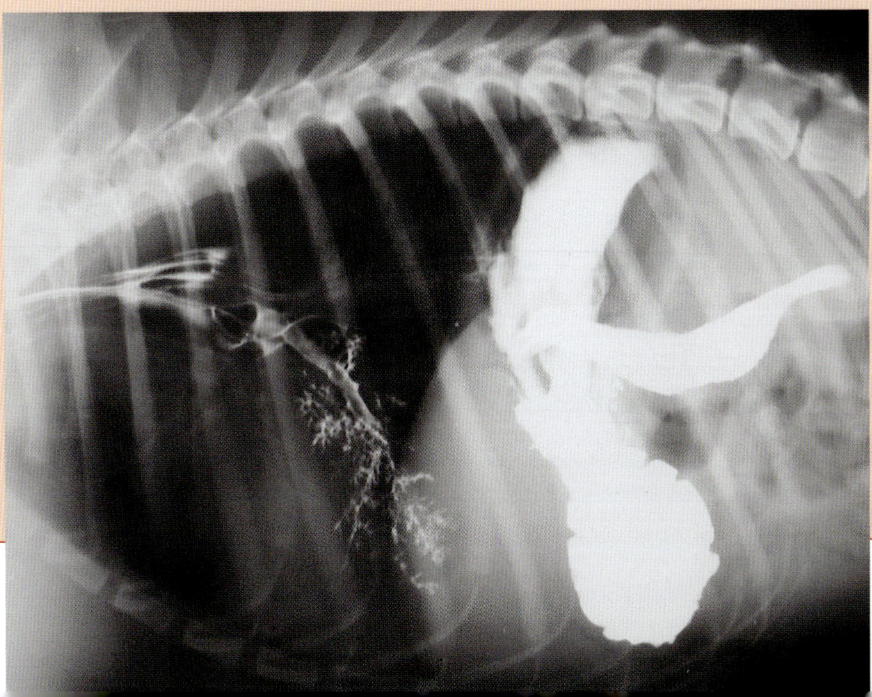

FIGURE 2.109. Lateral radiograph of the thorax and cranial abdomen of a dog with barium aspiration in the airways after its administration by oral route with a syringe. The aspiration of a small or moderate amount of barium is usually well tolerated by the patient, although its reabsorption through the lymphatic system may last months or years, and it may remain visible on radiographs of the thorax during this period of time.

This technique limits the study to the stomach since it is does not allow a correct assessment of gastric emptying or of the intestine.

Pathological alterations

The most common indication for a plain radiograph of the stomach is the suspicion of a **foreign body**. It is easy to visualise objects with a higher radiopacity than that of soft tissues and fluids (radiopaque foreign bodies), as there is a clear difference between these and the wall of the stomach and fluid or mucous content in its lumen (fig. 2.110). Diagnostic interpretation may be more difficult when these objects are surrounded by food, which has a heterogeneous opacity that may be confused with that of other objects, especially if these are small.

When foreign bodies have a similar radiopacity to that of soft tissues or fluids (radiolucent foreign bodies), their radiographic identification is much more complicated. Indeed, if they are surrounded by fluid or mucus, or adjacent to the gastric wall, it will often be impossible to distinguish them on plain radiographs (fig. 2.111), unless they have a characteristic morphology (e.g. some types of balls) (fig. 2.112).

Contrast techniques may help to confirm the presence of an object in the stomach, but it is worth trying to identify it by means of an ultrasound examination, although it will provide a limited amount of information when the foreign body is surrounded by gas. If gastrography is used, foreign bodies are usually easier to diagnose when a small amount of barium is administered, or with double-contrast gastrography instead of barium gastrography with the standard dose, since the administration of a large volume of positive contrast agent may lead to the object being masked in the image.

The aspect of foreign bodies on a contrast radiograph of the stomach depends on their characteristics. Some objects such as balls, wood, fruit stones, plastic, etc., produce well-defined and delimited filling defects. On the other hand, objects with an absorbent surface such as fabrics or sponges may not initially create a filling defect image, as they absorb the contrast medium and are better visualised when most of the contrast material has passed from the stomach to the duodenum (fig. 101).

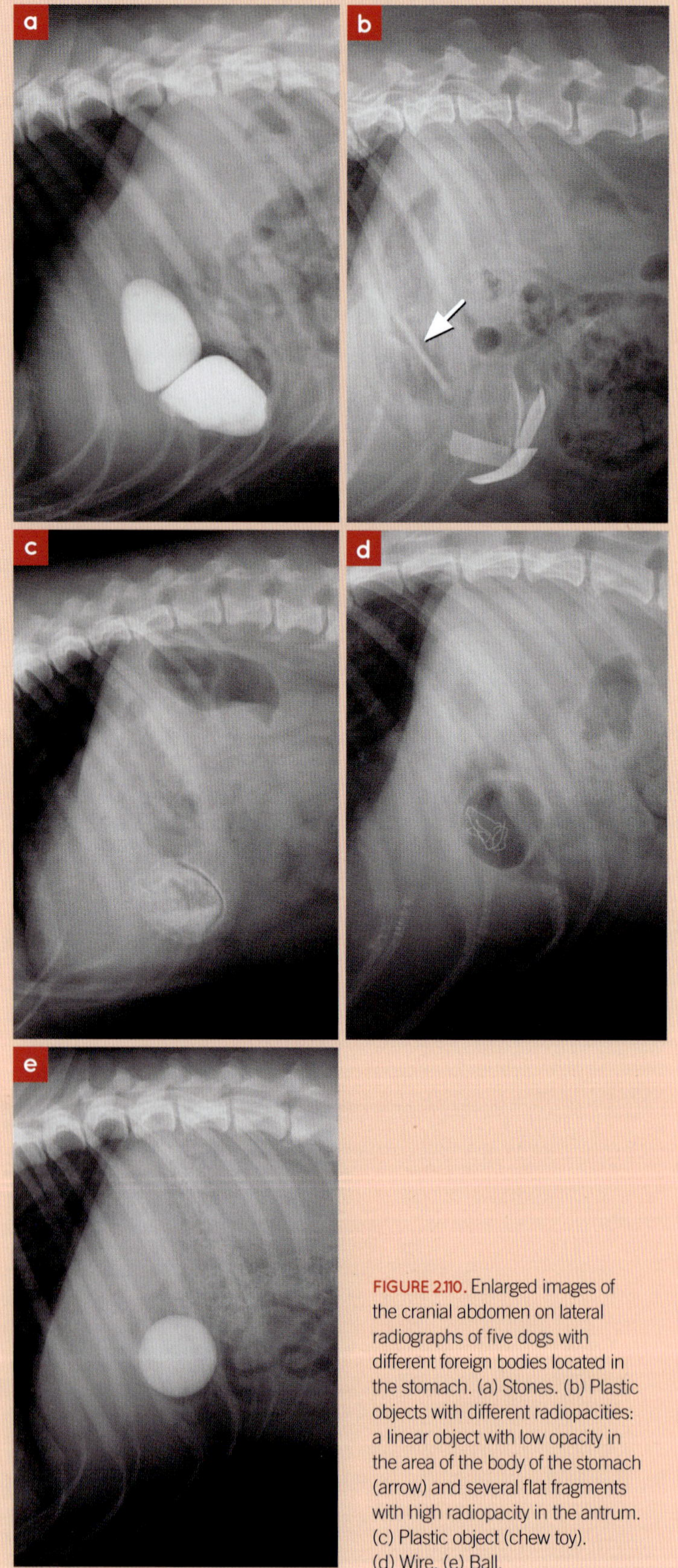

FIGURE 2.110. Enlarged images of the cranial abdomen on lateral radiographs of five dogs with different foreign bodies located in the stomach. (a) Stones. (b) Plastic objects with different radiopacities: a linear object with low opacity in the area of the body of the stomach (arrow) and several flat fragments with high radiopacity in the antrum. (c) Plastic object (chew toy). (d) Wire. (e) Ball.

Another diagnosis that is usually made by means of radiographic studies is **pyloric obstruction**, which can be acute or chronic. An acute obstruction may be due to a gastric volvulus or to the presence of foreign bodies. Chronic pyloric obstruction is generally due to a narrowing of the orifice of the pylorus, caused by diseases that affect the wall or block the orifice, such as hypertrophic pyloric stenosis, pyloric spasm, inflammation, fibrosis, neoplasia or hypertrophy of the mucosa of the antrum. On a plain radiograph, obstructive diseases of the pylorus may be visualised as a stomach increased in size, depending on the severity and duration of the obstruction. An accumulation of mineral opacity material located proximal to a point

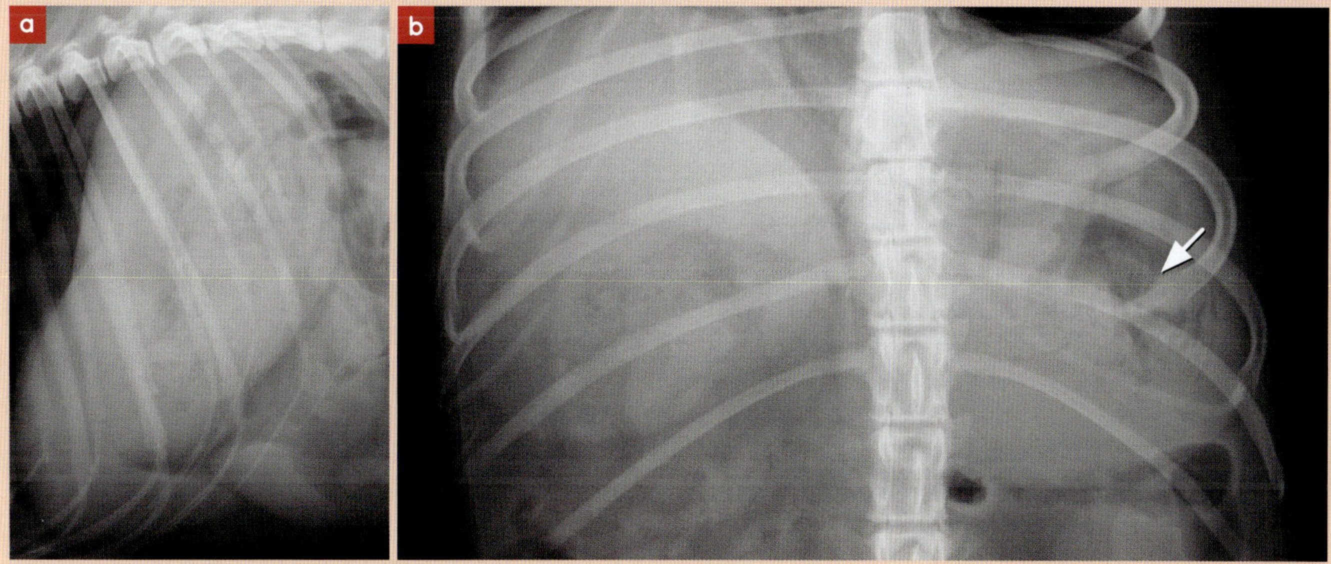

FIGURE 2.111. Enlarged images of the cranial abdomen on lateral (a) and ventrodorsal (b) radiographs of a dog with a radiolucent foreign body in the stomach. On the lateral view, the object (a piece of fabric) may be mistaken for normal gastric content, although on the ventrodorsal projection, the presence of parallel bands of gas density in the fundus (arrow) suggests the presence of a foreign body.

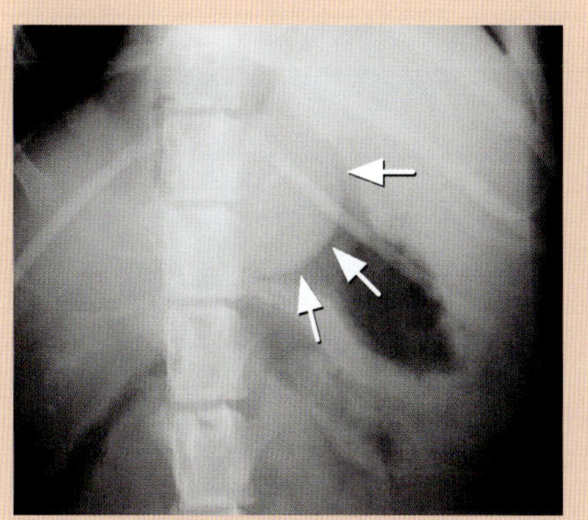

FIGURE 2.112. Enlarged image of the abdomen on a ventrodorsal radiograph of a dog with a ball (arrows) in the body of the stomach. The ball has a very similar radiopacity to that of the gastric wall and fluid/mucous content, but its characteristic round edge allows its identification in the image.

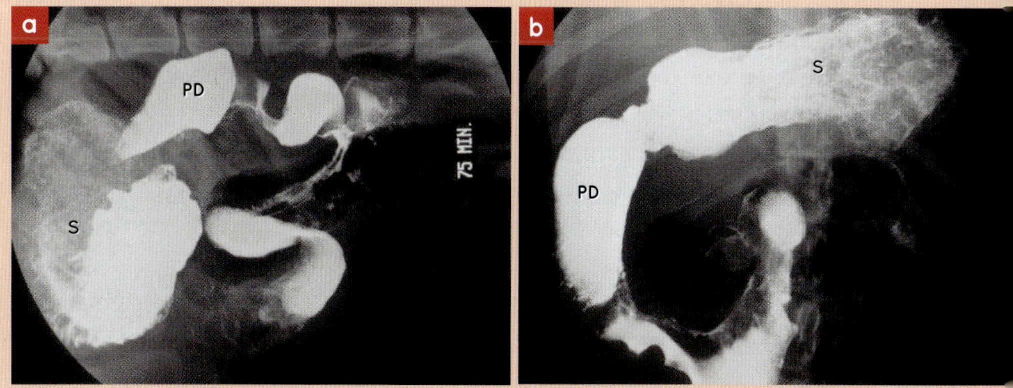

FIGURE 2.113. Enlarged images of the cranial abdomen on lateral (a) and ventrodorsal (b) radiographs of a dog, 75 minutes after the administration of barium. An accumulation of the contrast material can be observed mainly in the stomach (S) and proximal duodenum (PD), due to the presence of a foreign body that retains a great part of the contrast agent (plastic grid).

of gastrointestinal obstruction (stomach or intestine), which has been termed "gravel sign", is sometimes observed (fig. 2.114). This sign usually appears associated with chronic digestive obstructions.

In contrast studies, the main finding in cases of pyloric obstructions is delayed gastric emptying. A delayed gastric emptying should be considered significant when only a small amount of contrast material has passed to the duodenum after several hours. The retention of most of the barium in the stomach 3 to 4 hours after its administration is indicative of an obstructive pyloric disease.

A pyloric spasm may occur when the contrast study is performed if the animal is nervous. That is why it is useful to keep the animal in a quiet place for 30 minutes and repeat the radiograph after this period of time. A sedative or spasmolytic drug may also be administered. If the passage of the barium to the duodenum is delayed more than one hour even though the animal has been kept in a quiet place and has been administered a spasmolytic drug, the possibility of a pyloric dysfunction should be considered (2.115).

Gastric dilatation and torsion or volvulus are diagnosed by means of plain radiography. Acute **dilatation** of the stomach may be due to a complex variety of causes. The stomach will maintain its normal position and anatomical relationships, but will appear increased in size and filled mainly with gas in the image (fig. 2.116). The dilatation of the stomach may be caused by an obstruction of the pyloric canal or by atony of the gastric wall, but it may also appear due to aerophagy.

Acute dilatation may or not be followed by a gastric **torsion**. Gastric torsion or volvulus can be differentiated from simple acute dilatation because the stomach is rotated. The radiographic image of the stomach varies depending on the type and degree of rotation, on the one hand, and on the degree of distension, on the other (fig. 105). As the stomach dilates, the greater curvature turns in ventral direction and to the right, and is located along the ventral abdominal wall. The pylorus is displaced in dorsal and cranial direction and to the left. Rotation in the opposite direction is uncommon. In case of doubt, taking radiographs in the four standard radiographic projections (right lateral, left lateral, ventrodorsal and dorsoventral) may provide more precise information (fig. 2.118).

Apart from the distension and displacement of the stomach, a typical radiographic finding in case of torsion is the image of compartments, or "double bubble" sign. This image is created by bands of soft -tissue density projected through the stomach lumen, which is filled with gas (they appear because the stomach folds in on itself and the folded wall is projected towards its lumen and is thus outlined by the intraluminal gas that surrounds it).

Gastric torsion can also affect the image of other organs, such as the spleen, which may appear enlarged and displaced from its normal position. Radiographic signs of reflex paralytic ileus, dilatation of the oesophagus due to an obstruction at the level of the gastroesophageal junction and pulmonary hypovolaemia and microcardia may also be visualised.

At the initial stages of **gastric perforation**, the findings on a plain radiograph may be difficult to interpret. Depending on the size of the perforation or rupture, a variable amount of stomach content will pass to the peritoneal cavity. This causes an initially focal peritonitis, which is easily detected with an ultrasound scan, but can be more difficult to detect on radiographs. The most significant radiological finding is the detection of free gas in the peritoneal cavity. When the amount of gas is small, the sign that is easiest to recognise is the visualisation of the diaphragm when gas accumulates between this structure and the liver (fig. 2.119) (see Peritoneal cavity and retroperitoneal space).

It may be difficult to identify the area of perforation or rupture of the gastric wall with an ultrasound examination, which is why in almost all the cases in which a gastric perforation is suspected, the use of positive-contrast gastrography with iodinated contrast media will be recommended, since these latter are absorbed in the peritoneum if they are extravasated, while barium is not.

Barium extravasation into the peritoneal cavity is a serious complication that requires urgent treatment, if possible within 2 hours. A thorough lavage of the peritoneal cavity, with copious irrigation and wiping up of any barium traces with gauze or sponge is required. It may, however, be difficult to remove all barium residues from the cavity. An omentectomy is recommended, if deemed necessary. Patients should be monitored for the following two weeks, as mortality rates are higher during this time.

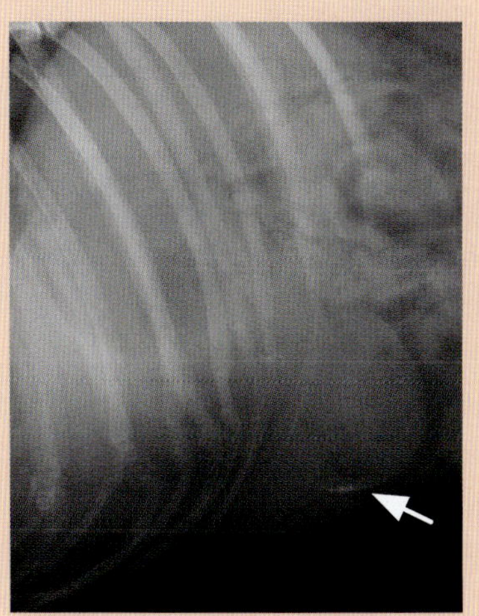

FIGURE 2.114. Enlarged image of the cranial abdomen on a lateral radiograph of a dog with a persistent accumulation of radiopaque material ("gravel sign") in the pyloric antrum (arrow). This finding may be indicative of an obstructive process, in this case in the pylorus.

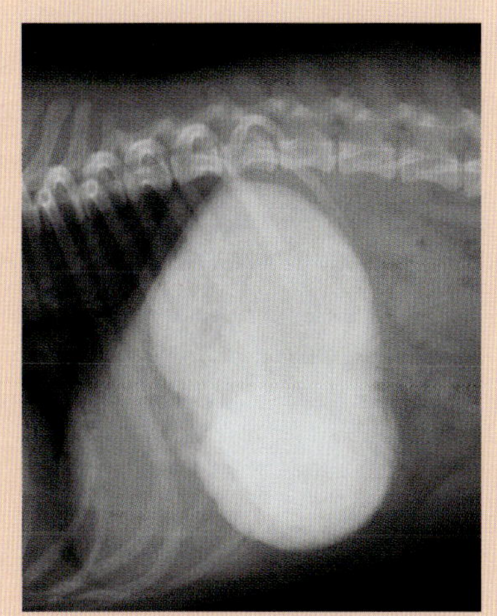

FIGURE 2.115. Enlarged image of the cranial abdomen on a lateral radiograph of a dog after receiving a standard dose of barium 70 minutes before the radiograph was taken. Limited passage of contrast material to the duodenum one hour after the administration of barium is indicative of pyloric dysfunction.

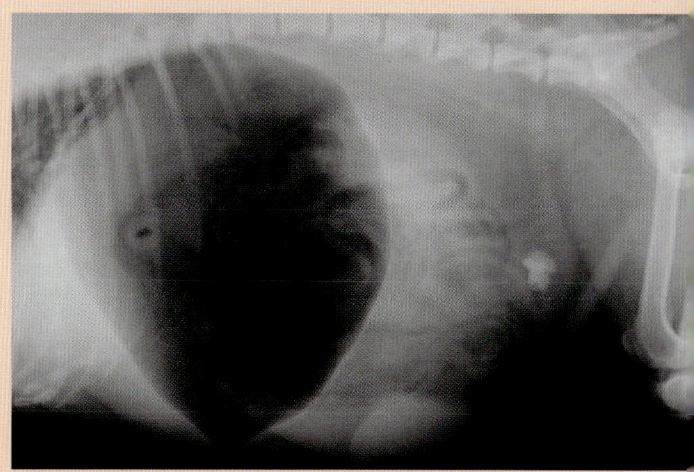

FIGURE 2.116. Lateral radiograph of the abdomen of a dog with severe gastric dilatation. No signs of rotation of the stomach are observed.

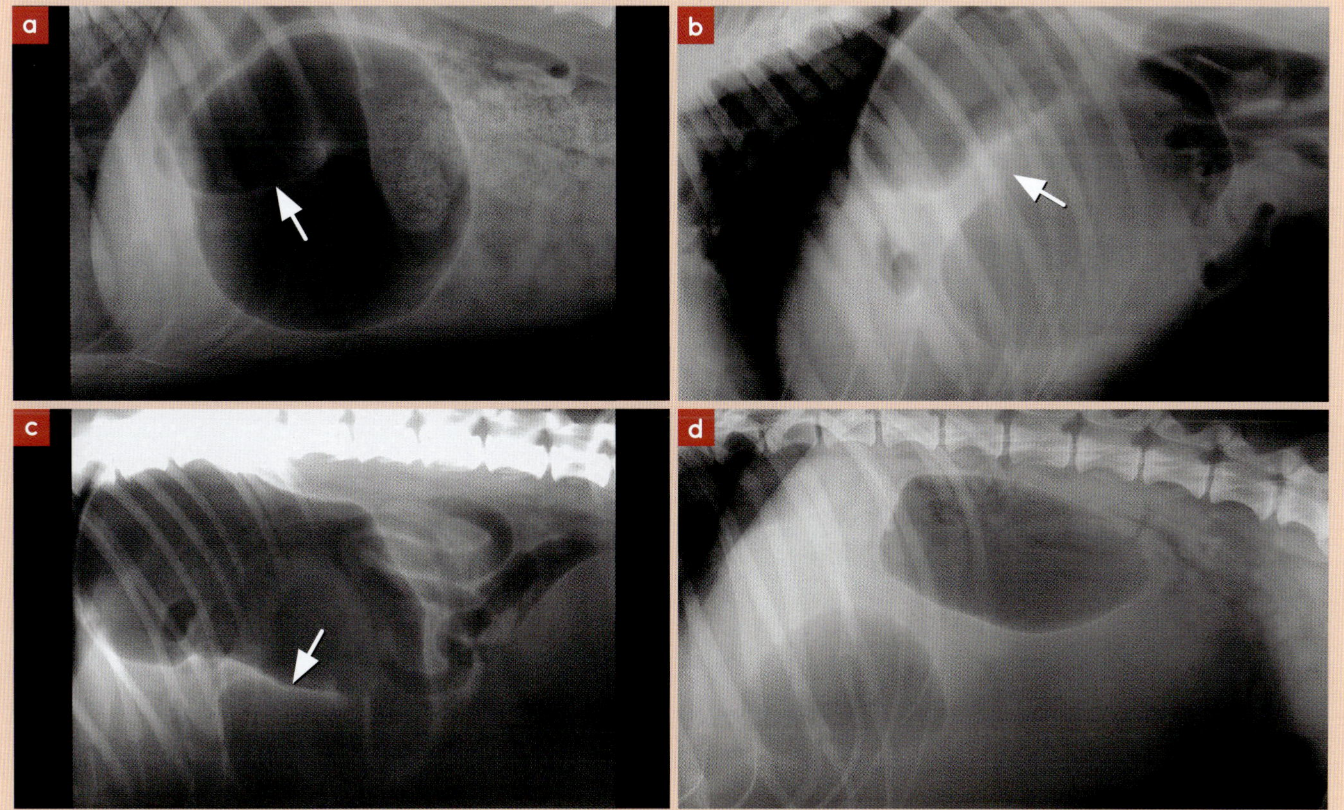

FIGURE 2.117. Lateral radiographs of the abdomen of four dogs with gastric torsion (gastric volvulus). (a) Marked dilatation of the stomach with 180-degree rotation. A soft-tissue density band is projected through the lumen filled with gas, creating an image of compartments or "double bubble" sign (arrows in images a, b and c). (b) Similar image to the previous one, although in this case the radiopacity of the stomach is greater because it contains fluid and gas. (c) Marked gastric dilatation with a rotation of less than 180º, the stomach essentially contains gas. (d) Extreme gastric dilatation with mainly fluid content and a moderate amount of gas, which makes the identification of the rotation of the stomach difficult.

Although an ultrasound scan should always be performed in case of suspicion of a gastric neoplasm, radiography can also provide useful information, especially if no ultrasound scanner is available or we do not have enough experience to establish a precise ultrasound diagnosis. The radiographic image of a gastric neoplasm may vary depending on its size, shape and location. On a plain radiograph, it may be possible or not to observe a more or less evident "mass effect". In contrast studies, the main radiographic finding is the visualisation of a mass-type lesion that is projected towards to the lumen of the stomach, thus creating an image of filling defect on the gastrogram (fig. 2.120). Small masses may be completely masked when a relatively large amount of barium is used.

Diffuses diseases of the stomach include those producing inflammation, hypertrophy or atrophy of the wall. These processes generally do not cause any evident alteration in the radiographic image of the stomach and ultrasonography or endoscopy are more

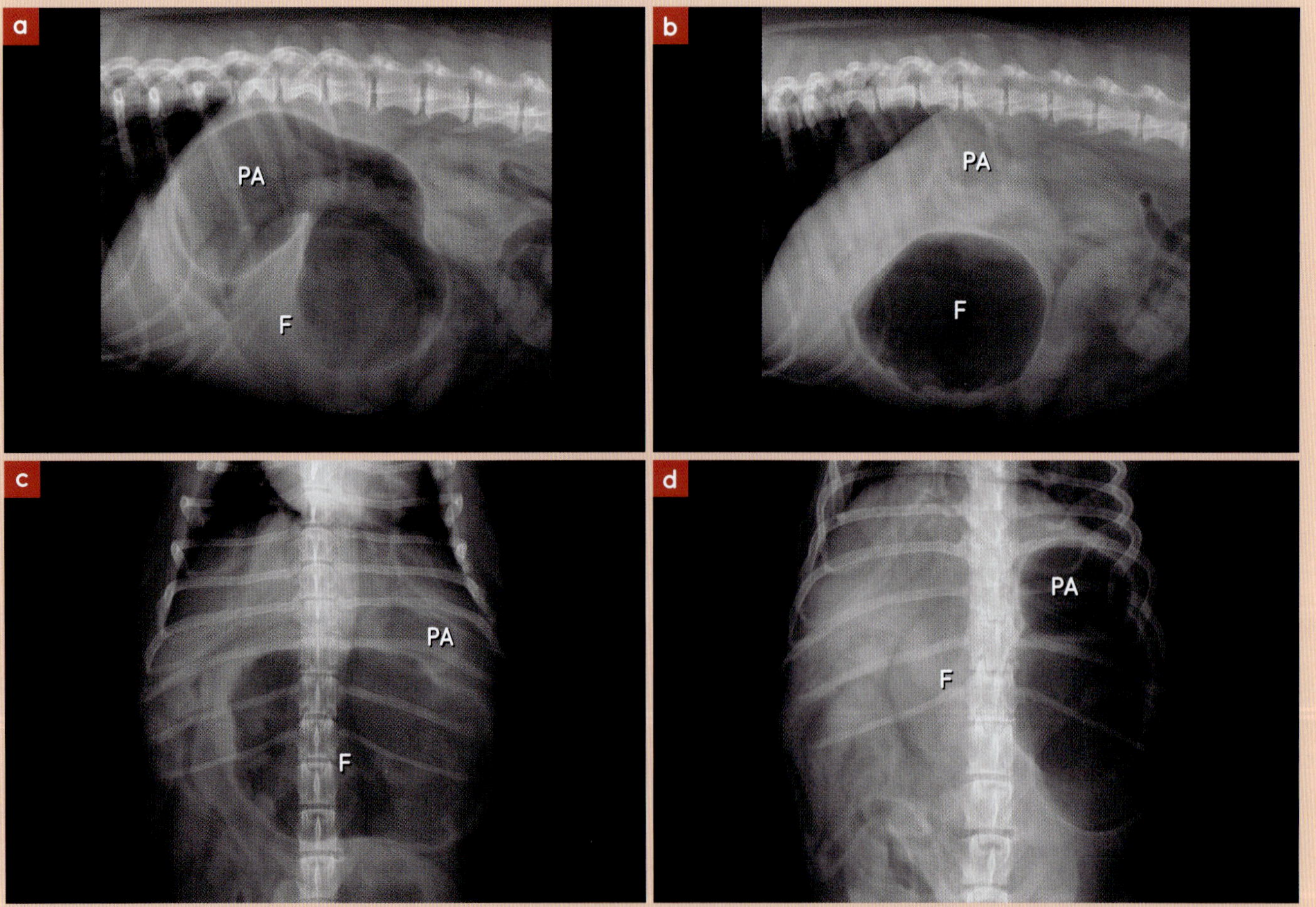

FIGURE 2.118. Enlarged images of the cranial abdomen on right lateral (a), left lateral (b), ventrodorsal (c) and dorsoventral (d) radiographs of a dog with gastric torsion. On the lateral views, the pyloric antrum (PA) is located dorsal and the fundus (F) ventral, and on the ventrodorsal and dorsoventral views the pyloric antrum is located on the left and the fundus on the right, as opposed to what occurs in normal conditions. In a healthy dog, the gas is displaced to the fundus and the fluid content to the pyloric antrum on right lateral views, while on left lateral views the gas accumulates in the antrum and the fluids do so in the fundus. The opposite occurs in this patient due to gastric rotation. In a similar way, when the stomach has a normal position, the gas accumulates in the antrum and part of the body of the stomach and the fluids are displaced towards the fundus on ventrodorsal views, while on dorsoventral views, the gas would be located in the fundus and the fluids in part of the body of the stomach and antrum. In this patient, these relationships are inverted due to the torsion.

useful diagnostic techniques. We should insist on the fact that an image with prominent gastric folds does not necessarily indicate inflammation of the wall, since the same image may be observed in a healthy animal due to the presence of fluid or mucus between the folds of the stomach. In uraemic gastritis, calcification of the gastric mucosa, which is sometimes radiographically identified, may occur (fig. 2.121).

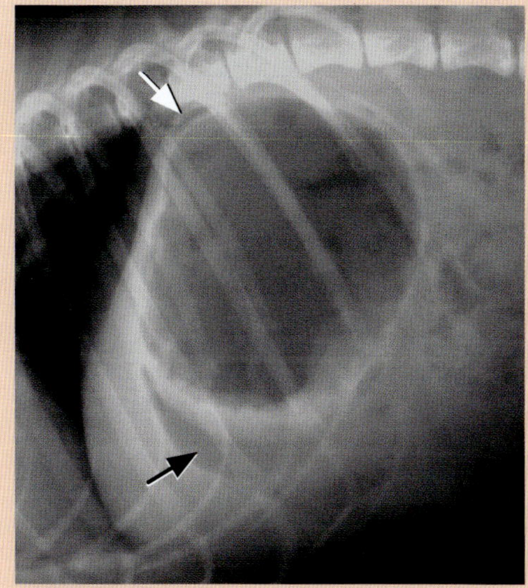

◀ FIGURE 2.119. Enlarged image of the cranial abdomen on a lateral radiograph of a dog with gastric perforation. The amount of free peritoneal gas is small and this essentially accumulates in the area ventral to the stomach (black arrow), which may be mistaken for an accumulation of fat. The identification of the diaphragm (white arrow), which is possible due to the presence of a minimal amount of gas between the diaphragm and the liver, confirms the diagnosis of pneumoperitoneum. A gastrogram with iodinated contrast media is necessary to confirm that this gas comes from the stomach.

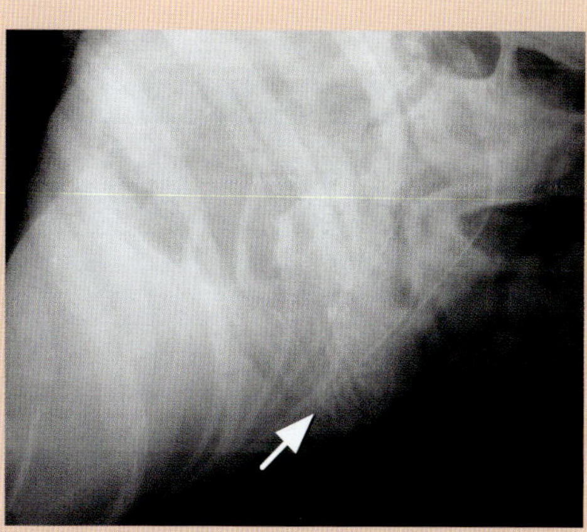

FIGURE 2.121. Enlarged image in lateral projection of the cranial abdomen of a dog with calcification of the gastric mucosa in the area of the pyloric antrum (arrow). This finding often appears associated to uraemic gastritis.

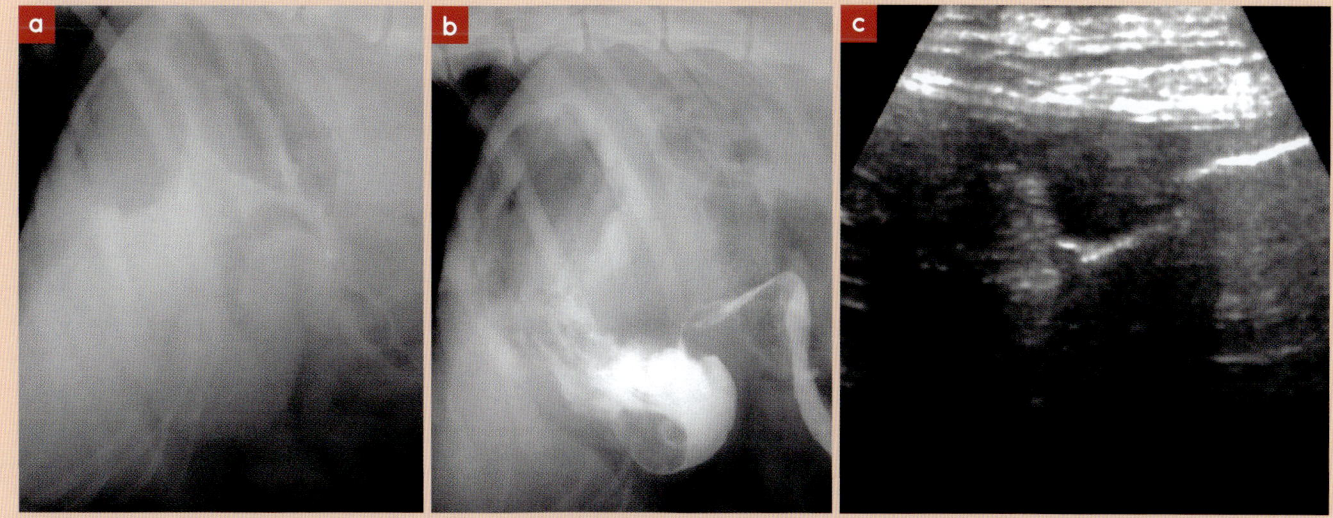

FIGURE 2.120. Enlarged images of the cranial abdomen on lateral radiographs, before (a) and after (b) the administration of barium (lower dose than the standard one so as not to mask the lesion) to a dog with a gastric neoplasm. The mass creates a filling defect in the pyloric antrum. (c) Ultrasound image of the mass.

Small intestine

Plain radiographs allow the assessment of the outline, size, position, shape and radiopacity of the intestine, but contrast studies or ultrasound scans are required to examine the alterations of the wall, as well as peristalsis or abnormal transit times.

Various references for the normal diameter of the small intestine in dogs have been published (fig. 2.122):

- It should not exceed twice the width of a rib.
- It should not exceed the height of the central part of the body of L2.
- The ratio between the maximum diameter of the small intestine and the minimum height of the body of L5 should not exceed 1.6.

In cats, the small intestine diameter should not exceed 12 mm or twice the L2 vertebral height (fig. 2.123).

The width of the duodenum may slightly exceed these limits in normal conditions, since its diameter is slightly greater than that of the jejunum and ileum.

It is not possible to appropriately evaluate the thickness of the intestinal wall on a plain radiograph, as we may mistake it for the wall plus intraluminal fluid/

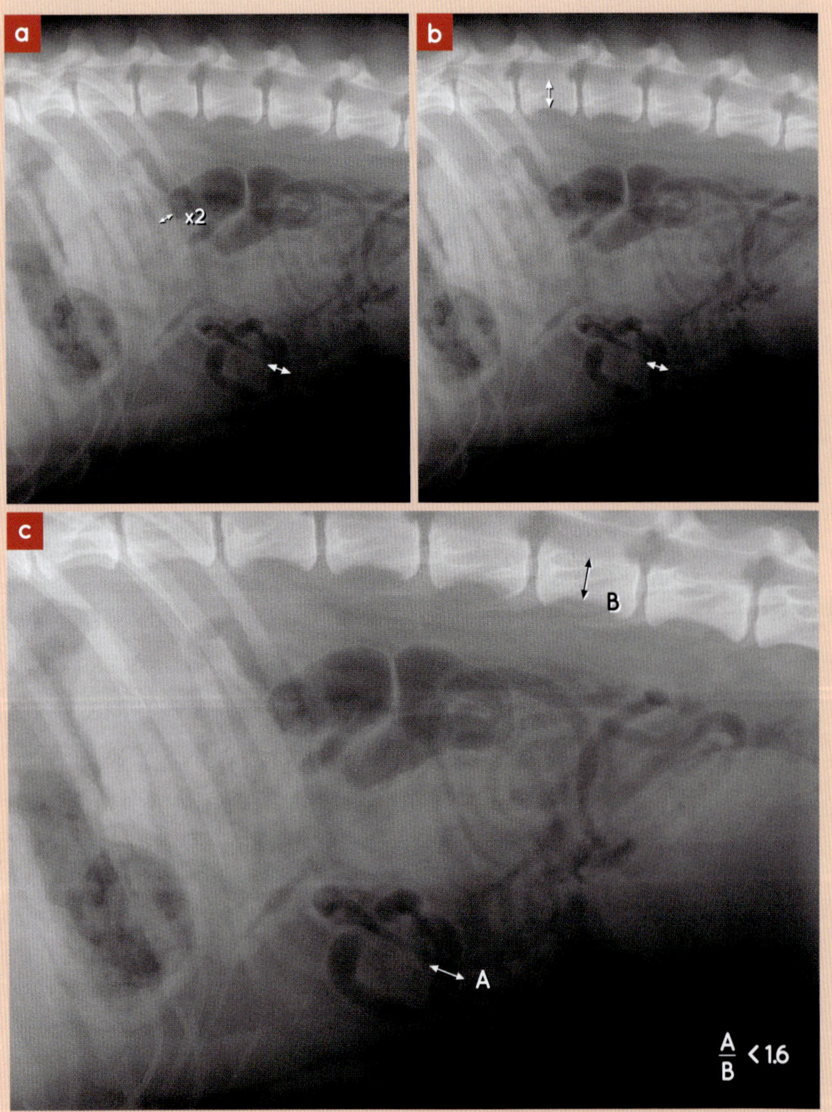

FIGURE 2.122. References of the normal diameter of the small intestine on lateral radiographs of the abdomen in the dog: it should not exceed the width of a rib (a); it should not exceed the height of the central part of the body of L2 (b); the ratio between the maximum diameter of the small intestine (A) and the minimum height of the body of L5 (B) should not exceed 1.6 (c).

mucus (fig. 2.124), which may lead to an incorrect diagnosis of increased thickness (fig. 2.125). The real thickness of the intestinal wall is best observed directly by means of ultrasonography.

Nowadays, the administration of a contrast medium will be necessary to evaluate the intestines only on a few occasions. It is recommended to prepare the animal prior to the contrast study (no food for 24 hours and administration of an enema 2 to 4 hours before the test). Barium sulphate in suspension (in the form of micropulverised or liquid preparations) is the contrast medium of choice in most cases. A dose of 6–12 ml/kg at a concentration of 20 % in dogs and 12–16 ml/kg in cats is recommended. The administration of an inappropriate dose is one of the most common cases of non-diagnostic contrast studies.

Lateral and ventrodorsal radiographs are taken every 10 to 30 minutes, depending on the speed of transit of the contrast medium, until this latter reaches the colon. It is convenient to take a radiograph 24 hours later to rule out any abnormal retentions of the contrast material in the small intestine. The normal transit time varies from 2 to 4 hours in dogs and is approximately 1 hour in cats.

Iodinated contrast media are usually used when a perforation is suspected or when a faster transit time is required. Hyperosmotic contrast agents attract fluids towards the lumen of the intestine, are diluted and progress faster than barium, but offer images with a poorer diagnostic quality (fig. 2.126) and may cause transient dehydration of the patient. They are administered in doses of 2–3 ml/kg in dogs and 2 ml/kg in cats. Low-osmolarity iodinated contrast agents, such as iohexol or iopamidol, also progress faster through the intestine, but attract fewer fluids to the lumen. The diagnostic quality of the study is therefore improved (although it cannot be compared to that of barium studies) and their use is more recommended in very sick animals. They may be diluted at 1:2 in water and 10 ml/kg of the mixture may be administered both in dogs and cats.

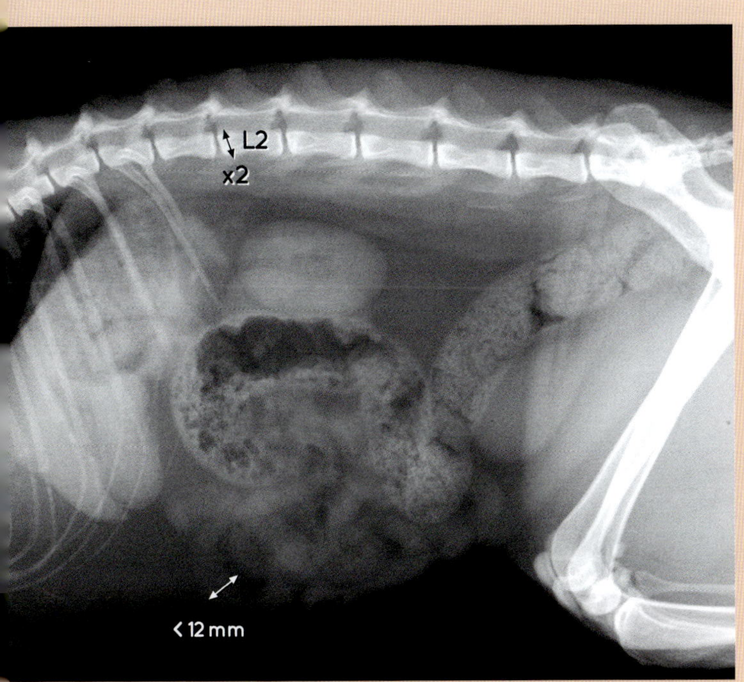

FIGURE 2.123. References for normal small intestine diameters in lateral abdominal radiograph in the cat: measuring less than 12 mm in the image or does not exceed 2 times the caudal or cranial height of L2.

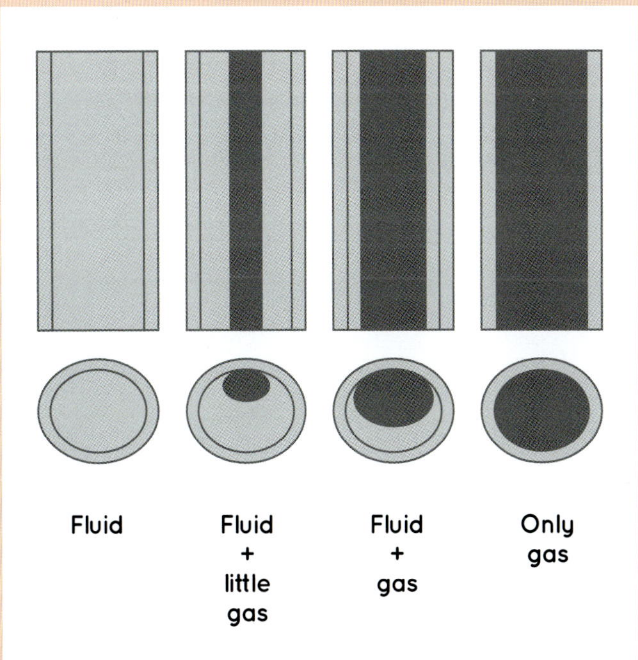

FIGURE 2.124. Diagram representing the radiographic image of the small intestine depending on its intraluminal content. It is not possible to evaluate the thickness of the intestinal wall on a radiograph, since the fluid/mucous content has the same radiopacity and cannot be differentiated from the wall, thus creating a false appearance of increased thickness of the wall.

The use of barium-impregnated polyethylene spheres to detect alterations of the intestinal transit has also been described. They are presented in two sizes: 1.5 mm and 5 mm of diameter. The smaller ones have a similar intestinal transit time to that of food, while the larger ones are designed to remain trapped in the area immediately anterior to an obstructive lesion.

The lack of passage of luminal content through the intestinal tract is termed **ileus**, and is radiographically characterised by an image of intestinal dilatation. Different patterns of intestinal dilatation may be observed:

- **Mild focal dilatation**: 1 to 3 affected loops and luminal distension of 1.5 to 2 times the normal diameter (fig. 2.127).
- **Severe focal dilatation**: 1 to 3 affected loops and luminal distension greater than twice the normal diameter (fig. 2.128).
- **Mild generalised dilatation**: great number of affected loops and luminal distension of 1.5 to 2 times the normal diameter (fig. 2.129).
- **Severe generalised dilatation:** great number of affected loops and luminal distension greater than twice the normal diameter (fig. 2.130).

An ileus may be mechanical, when it is due to a physical obstruction of the lumen of the intestine, or functional (paralytic ileus), when the peristaltic contractions of the intestine stop due to vascular or neuromuscular anomalies in the intestinal wall.

In a mechanical ileus, the physical obstruction of the intestinal lumen may be complete or partial. The most common causes of obstruction are large foreign bodies, intussusceptions and intestinal masses. A lesion that is extrinsic to the intestine may also cause a mechanical obstruction by external compression of an intestinal loop; adherences due to previous surgeries, hernias of the abdominal wall and, occasionally, masses that originated in other abdominal organs are included in the category.

The most indicative radiographic sign of mechanical obstruction is the dilatation of the intestinal loops

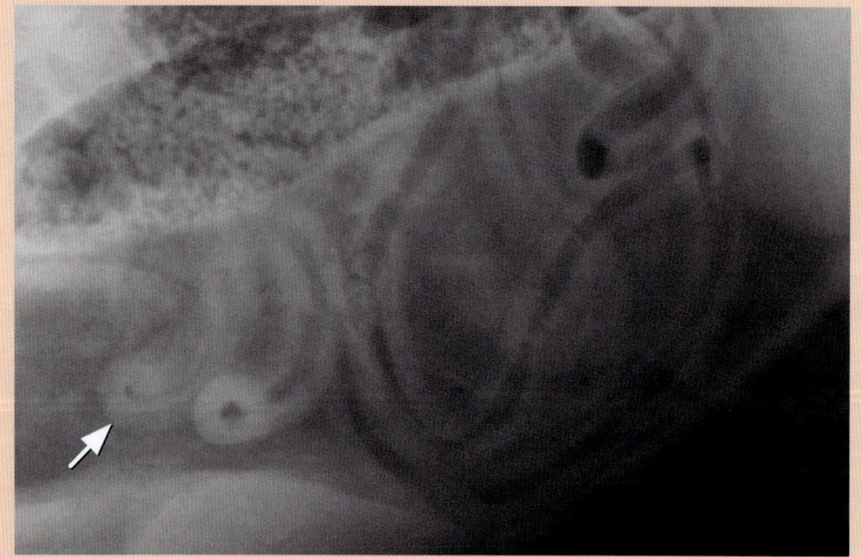

FIGURE 2.125. Very enlarged image of the central area of the abdomen on a lateral radiograph of a healthy dog. The intestinal segments that have a small amount of gas or a large amount of fluid/mucus in the lumen (arrow) have a false appearance of "thickened intestinal wall" on the radiograph. An ultrasound scan, on the other hand, does allow the examination of the real thickness of the wall.

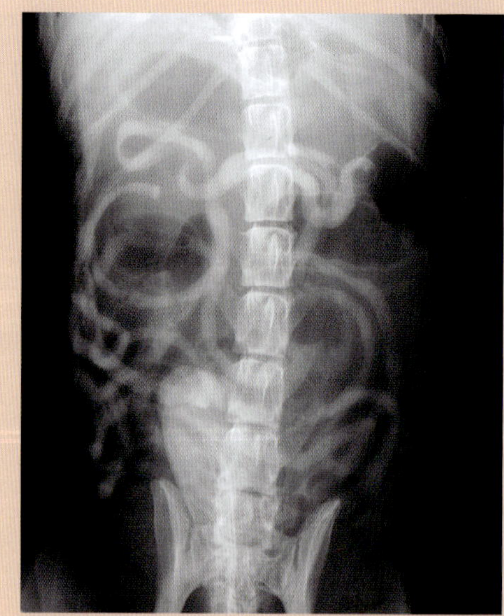

FIGURE 2.126. Ventrodorsal radiograph of the abdomen of a dog 45 minutes after the administration of an iodinated contrast medium by oral route. These contrast media are diluted with the fluid content of the small intestine and progress through it faster than barium. They are therefore only used when a perforation is suspected or when there is a real interest in a faster transit, although a good detailed image of the intestinal mucosa is not obtained.

anterior to the obstruction. The degree of dilatation of the loops is variable. The more complete an obstruction is, and the longer it lasts, the greater the degree of dilatation of the loops will be (fig. 2.131). The more distal (along the small intestine) the obstruction is, and the more complete, the greater the number of dilated loops there will be. Thus, partial obstructions create less evident alterations on plain radiographs (fig. 2.132), especially if they are recent or if they are located in proximal segments of the small intestine. The "gravel sign" may appear due to an accumulation of granular material at a site anterior to a point of obstruction. When the obstruction is complete, the segment of small intestine that is distal to the point of obstruction is usually empty.

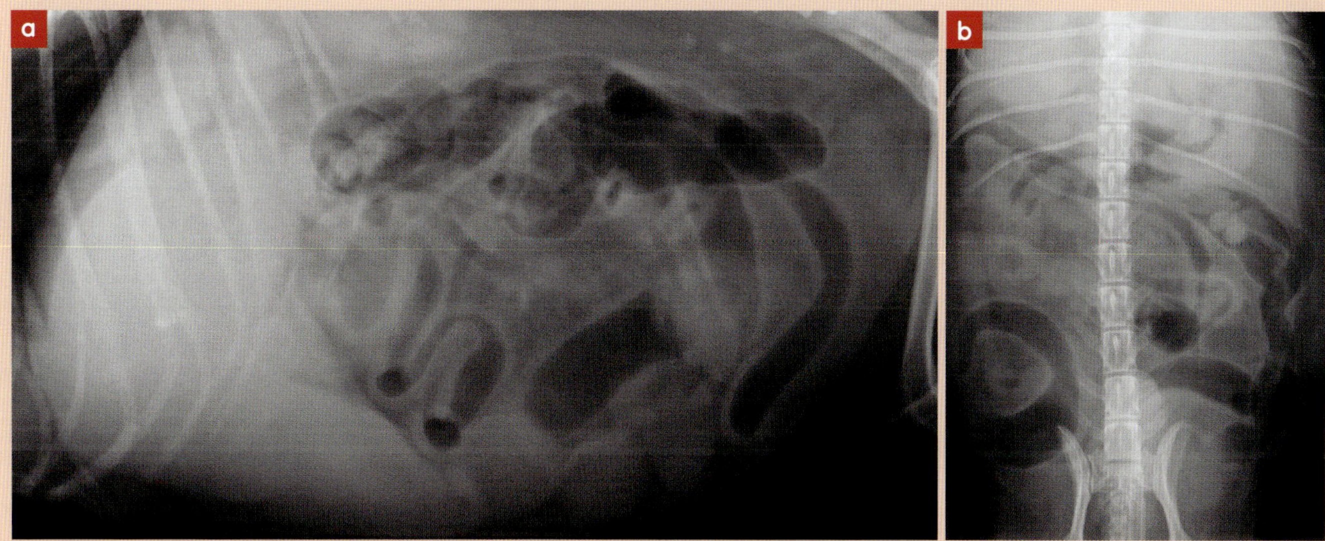

FIGURE 2.127. Lateral (a) and ventrodorsal (b) radiographs of the abdomen of a dog with a mild (1.5 to 2 times the normal diameter) focal intestinal dilatation (1 to 3 dilated loops). This pattern is indicative of a partial obstruction or of a recent complete obstruction in proximal segments of the small intestine.

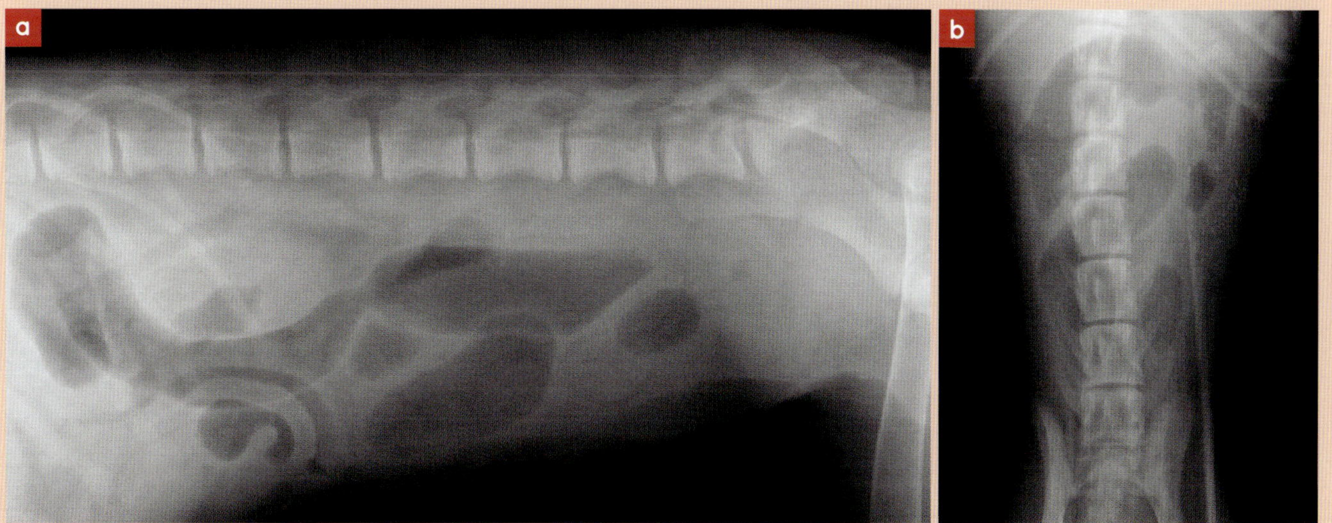

FIGURE 2.128. Lateral (a) and ventrodorsal (b) radiographs of the abdomen of a dog with a severe (more than twice the normal diameter) focal intestinal dilatation (1 to 3 dilated loops). This pattern is indicative of a complete obstruction in proximal segments of the small intestine, recent complete obstruction in any segment of the intestine, or chronic partial obstruction.

As a reference to assess a possible obstruction, it is considered that a value above 1.6 times the ratio between the diameter of the intestine and the minimum height of the body of the L5 vertebra is indicative of an intestinal obstruction in dogs.

When the clinical and radiographic findings are indicative of a mechanical obstruction of the intestine, it is recommended to carry out an ultrasound study of the abdomen, since it will often allow the determination of the cause of the obstruction. If the ultrasound scan is not conclusive and the suspicion is maintained, a contrast study or an exploratory laparotomy will then be indicated.

In a functional ileus, the peristaltic contractions of the intestine stop due to vascular or neuromuscular anomalies and the lumen dilates, although it is still permeable.

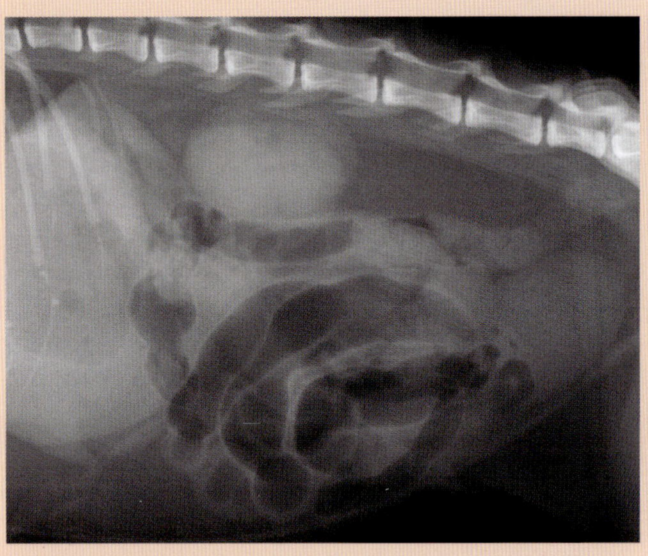

FIGURE 2.129. Lateral radiograph of the abdomen of a cat with mild (1.5 to 2 times the normal diameter) generalised intestinal dilatation (elevated number of dilated loops). This pattern is indicative of a partial or recent complete obstruction in distal segments of the small intestine or functional ileus.

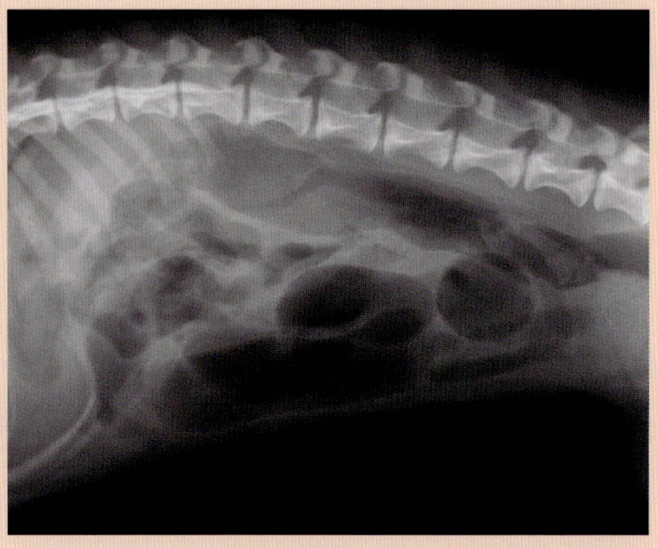

FIGURE 2.130. Lateral radiograph of the abdomen of a dog with severe (more than twice the normal diameter) generalised intestinal dilatation (elevated number of dilated loops). This pattern is indicative of a complete or chronic partial obstruction in distal segments of the small intestine.

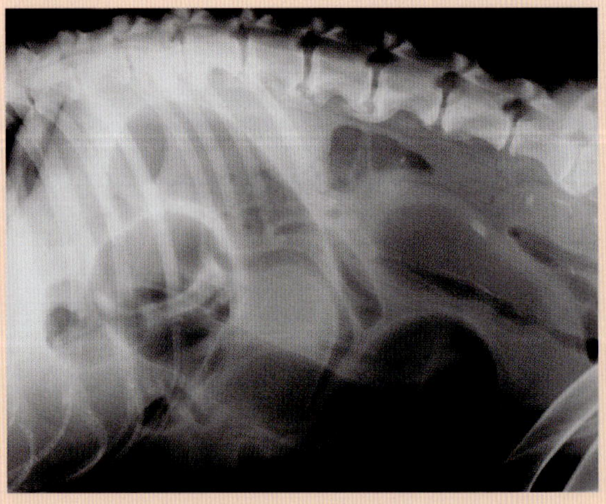

FIGURE 2.131. Lateral radiograph of the abdomen of a dog with a complete obstruction of the small intestine after several days of evolution.

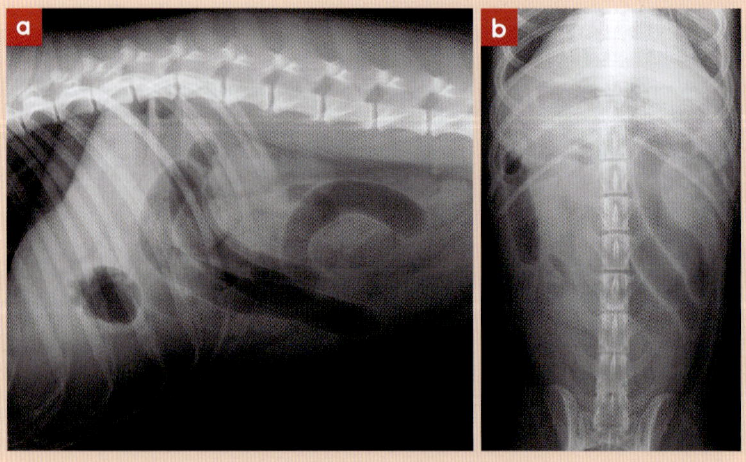

FIGURE 2.132. Lateral (a) and ventrodorsal (b) radiographs of the abdomen of a dog with a chronic partial obstruction in distal segments of the small intestine.

A functional ileus may be secondary to different processes, such as peritonitis, pancreatitis, a recent abdominal surgery, severe viral enteritis and diseases of the autonomic nervous system, among others (fig. 2.133).

It is often not possible to differentiate intestinal dilatation caused by a functional ileus from that caused by a mechanical ileus on plain radiographs. The affected length of the intestine may provide some information in this sense, since localised dilatations are more likely to be due to mechanical causes while generalised dilatations are more likely to be caused by a functional ileus, although it is not always the case. In fact, moderate to severe chronic mechanical obstructions may lead to a functional ileus.

Radiopaque **foreign bodies** are easily recognised on plain radiographs (fig. 2.134). On the other hand, those objects with a similar radiopacity to that of fluid/mucus and soft tissues (radiolucent) may not be identified on plain radiographs, although intestinal dilatation will be observed depending on the degree of mechanical obstruction they cause. Ultrasound examinations or contrast studies may offer a more precise diagnosis in this aspect. If the foreign body is fenestrated or absorbent, barium may go through it or be retained, thus causing a mottled or linear pattern of opacification (fig. 2.135). If it is not fenestrated or absorbent, the object may stop the transit of barium (fig. 2.136) or create a filling defect in the contrast column.

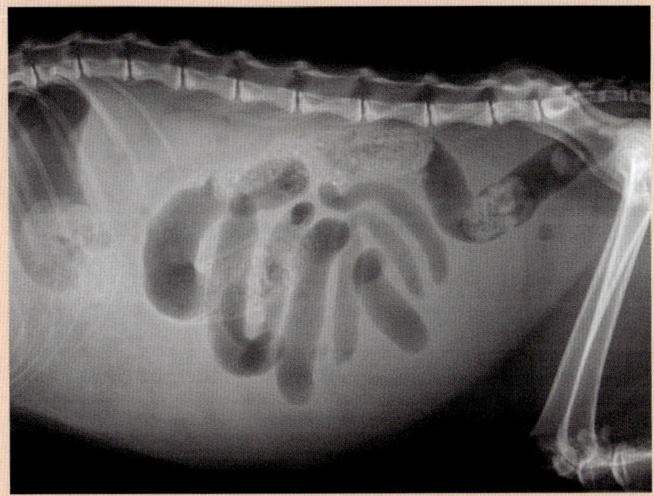

FIGURE 2.133. Lateral radiograph of the abdomen of a cat with a functional ileus secondary to a peritonitis.

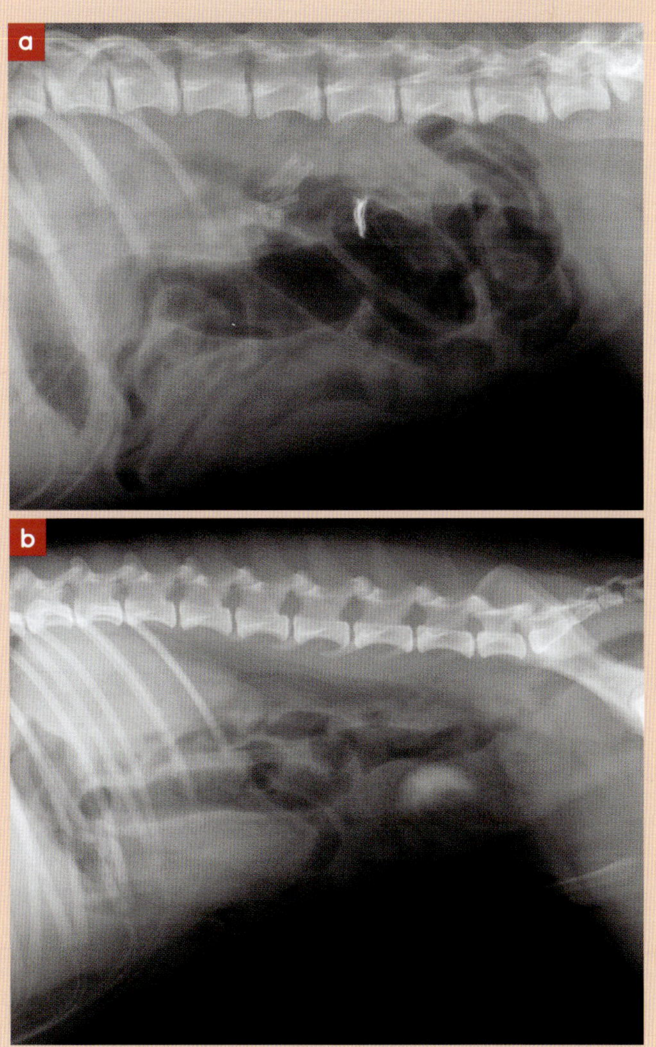

FIGURE 2.134. Lateral radiographs of the abdomen of two dogs with radiopaque foreign bodies in the small intestine. (a) Remnants of plastic tubes. (b) Crushed ball. Signs of intestinal obstruction are observed in both cases.

Linear foreign bodies (e.g. shoelaces, threads, etc.) create a relatively characteristic radiographic image. Part of the object often remains in the stomach (or even in the oesophagus or mouth) while the rest is located in the small intestine. This latter appears pleated in the image, with focal retention of small amounts of gas (gas pockets) between the folds (fig. 2.137). The image of intestinal pleating may be more evident in the contrast study (fig. 2.138) and is also observed by means of ultrasonography.

Invaginations or intussusceptions usually cause severe intestinal dilatation, although in most patients it is not possible to differentiate an invagination from other causes of mechanical obstruction (fig. 2.139) only with plain radiography. The ultrasound diagnosis of an invagination is relatively easy and in most cases, radiographic contrast studies are excluded, as the image may vary in function of the degree of permeability of the intussusceptum (invaginated part of the intestine), and of the space between the intussusceptum and the intussuscipiens (part of the intestine containing the invaginated part).

The **masses** that originate on the intestinal wall include tumours, polyps or granulomatous infiltrates. The development of an obstructive intestinal pattern due to these lesions depends on their size, of whether

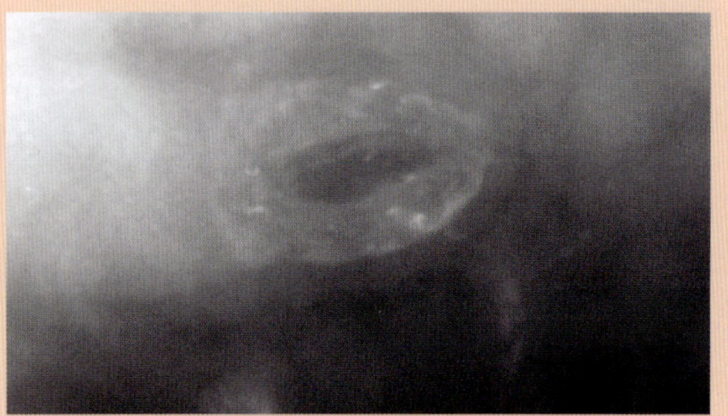

FIGURE 2.135. Enlarged radiographic image of a peach stone with remnants of barium in its structure.

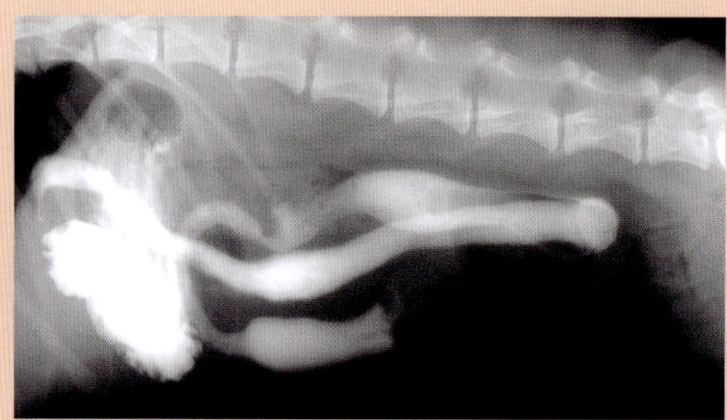

FIGURE 2.136. Lateral abdominal radiograph of a dog with a complete obstruction caused by a foreign body, 30 minutes after the administration of barium. The object causes a sudden interruption of the contrast column.

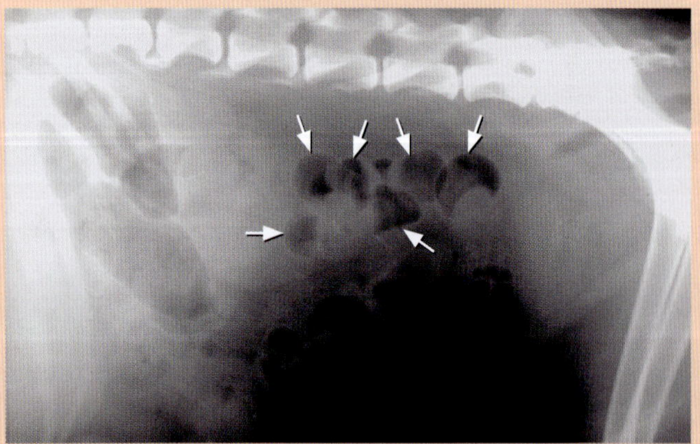

FIGURE 2.137. Lateral abdominal radiograph of a dog with a linear foreign body in the small intestine. The folded intestinal wall causes the retention of gas between the folds (gas pockets, arrows). Bladder lithiasis is also observed.

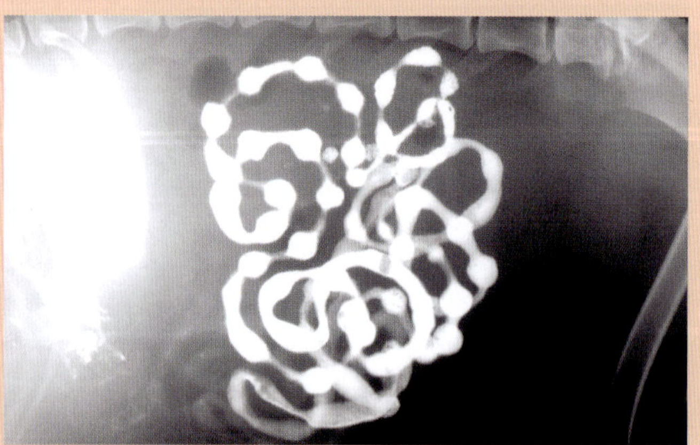

FIGURE 2.138. Lateral abdominal radiograph of a dog, with a linear foreign body in the small intestine, 45 minutes after the administration of barium. The folded intestinal wall causes a "string of pearls" appearance. This type of image may also be found in the duodenum of healthy cats due to peristaltic waves (see chapter Most common diagnostic errors).

they grow towards the lumen of the intestine or outside it (fig. 2.140). With time, most of them, which initially do not cause any obstruction, evolve and cause a partial and then complete obstruction. They are usually detected clinically in the phase of partial obstruction, with mild to severe focal distension. These lesions are better identified if an ultrasound scan is performed or, alternatively, a contrast study, in which an image of a filling defect or luminal narrowing associated or not with multiple marks in the barium column ("apple core" appearance) may appear.

Diffuse infiltrative diseases of the intestinal wall (intestinal inflammatory disease, inflammation of infectious origin and some types of neoplasia) may cause an abnormal gas density pattern with or without intestinal dilatation, although radiography will often not reveal any significant findings. An ultrasound examination is much more appropriate to evaluate this type of disease.

Large intestine

Plain and contrast radiographs have traditionally been used to evaluate the diseases of the large intestine. Nowadays, endoscopy has replaced contrast radiography of the colon to a large extent, especially when a flexible endoscope, which can reach the transverse colon, ascending colon and caecum, is available. Ultrasonography also provides useful diagnostic information, in particular regarding alterations of the wall, excluding the rectum due to its intrapelvic location. Computed tomography and magnetic resonance imaging may have a great interest for the examination of rectal diseases, since they offer images with excellent anatomical detail of the whole pelvic region.

The large intestine is easily identified on plain radiographs because it usually contains faeces and gas, which have a radiographic density that contrasts with the surrounding structures. The colon has a similar shape to that of a question mark (fig. 2.141). The canine caecum is semicircular ("C" or spiral shape), is compartmented and usually contains a certain amount of intraluminal gas. This gas and its characteristic shape make the caecum easy to recognise in the right middle abdomen on most plain radiographs (fig. 2.142). The feline caecum is a short diverticulum,

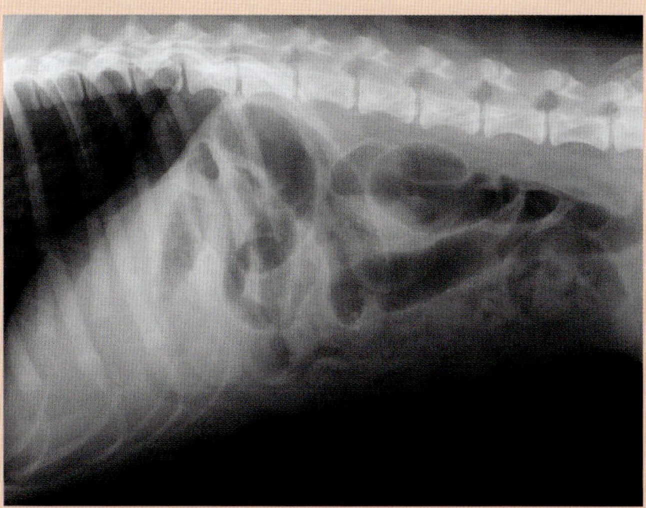

FIGURE 2.139. Lateral radiograph of the abdomen of a dog with an invagination in the small intestine. A pattern of severe focal intestinal dilatation may be observed.

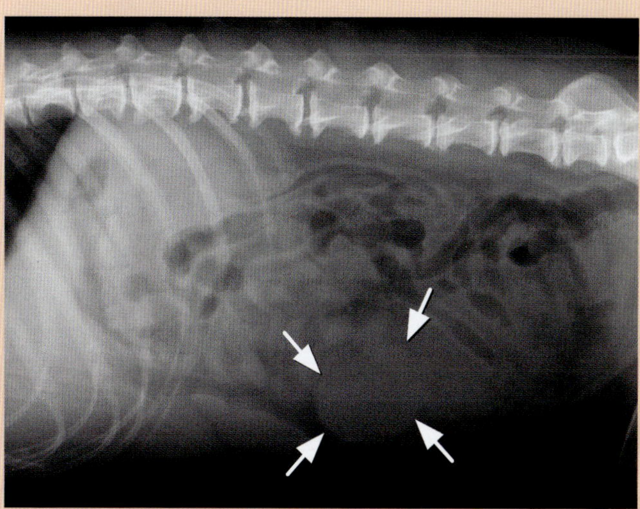

FIGURE 2.140. Lateral radiograph of the abdomen of a dog with a small-intestinal neoplasm (arrows).

with no compartments, which rarely contains gas, so it is not usually identified on radiographs.

The diameter of the normal colon varies depending on the amount of faeces it contains and on the defecation habits of each individual. As a general rule, the normal colonic diameter should not exceed the length of L7 in dogs, while in cats, the maximum diameter of the colon should not exceed 2.2 times the diameter of the small intestine, 2.8 times the height of the cranial end of the body of L2 or 1.3 times the length of the body of L5. These measures are nonetheless indicative. Any slight increase in the diameter should always be correlated with the rest of the patient's clinical data.

The position of the midportion of the descending colon can vary in the caudal left abdomen. In some dogs, it is positioned along or even slightly right to the median axis, depending on the amount of content in the bowel, the amount and distribution of intra-abdominal fat and the degree of bladder distension.

Some dogs may have a longer length than usual, which is called "*redundant colon*". This is considered an anatomical variation without any clinical significance.

A more exhaustive assessment of the large intestine requires a contrast study using barium sulphate in suspension (barium enema), gas (pneumocolon) or a combination of both (double-contrast enema). The most commonly used technique is barium enema. Nowadays, a barium enema would be indicated in the following cases:

- When a narrowing of the lumen hinders the passage of an endoscope.
- If the limitations of the endoscope itself do not allow a complete examination of the colon and caecum.
- When a parietal or extraparietal lesion is suspected and the mucosa has a normal aspect in the endoscopic examination.

The animal that is going to undergo a contrast enema must not eat for 24 to 36 hours and should be administered laxatives by oral route and hot water enemas prior to the study. Plain radiographs will be taken before administering the contrast agent to adjust the exposure values and confirm that the patient has been properly prepared.

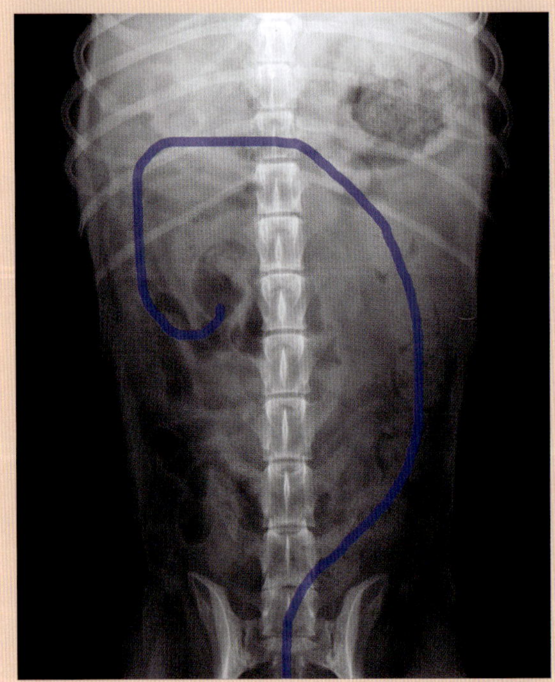

FIGURE 2.141. Ventrodorsal radiograph of the abdomen of a healthy dog. The large intestine has the shape of a question mark on this view.

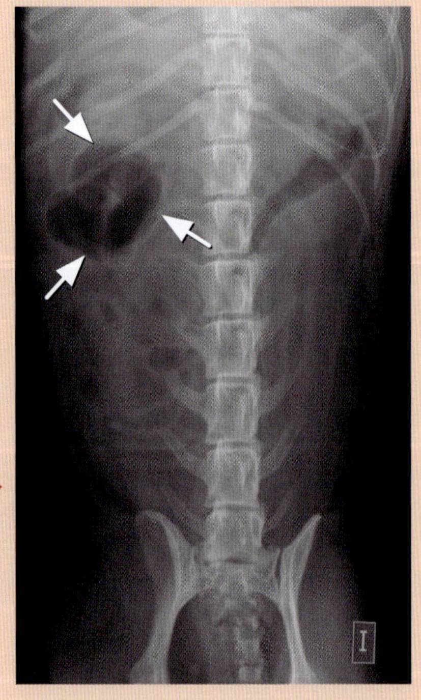

FIGURE 2.142. Ventrodorsal radiograph of the abdomen of a healthy dog. The caecum (arrows) often appears as a curved tubular structure filled with gas in the right cranial abdomen on radiographs. We should not confuse this image with an abnormal dilatation of the small intestine.

After anaesthetising the patient, barium is administered at room temperature through a catheter with an inflatable balloon, which is placed in the distal part of the rectum to avoid leakage of the contrast agent. Doses of 7 to 15 ml/kg of barium sulphate in suspension at a concentration of 20 % are usually used. If a perforation of the colon is suspected, barium should be replaced by an iodinated contrast medium, preferably of low osmolarity, at a concentration of 15 to 20 %, although the amount of detail of the mucosa will be significantly reduced.

The persistence of faecal material in the colon and rectum is termed faecal retention (fig. 2.143). If there is an accumulation of a great amount of faeces that acquire a very high radiopacity due to the continuous absorption of water from the content of the colon, we are dealing with a case of faecal **impaction** (fig. 2.144). A chronic impaction may cause a generalised increase of the size of the colon.

The presence of **foreign bodies** in the large intestine has a limited significance, since they rarely cause problems if they have not caused any when progressing through the small intestine (fig. 2.145). However, importance should be given to those that are sharp and may seriously damage the wall.

Inflammatory processes do not usually cause any radiographic alterations. They can usually be properly evaluated by means of ultrasonography, with the exception of the rectum due to its intrapelvic location. In case of severe colitis (fig. 2.146), contrast studies may show irregularity and localised or generalised ulceration of the mucosa, narrowing of the lumen, thickening of the folds of the wall, diverticula and adherences.

Localised **dilatations** of the colon are usually due to faecal impactions (fig. 2.147.) or mechanical obstructions, caused for example by caecocolic or ileocolic intussusceptions, narrowing of the pelvic canal due to fractures, tumours of the colon or foreign bodies.

The colon may be generally dilated due to an excess of faecal content. If the dilatation is associated with hypomotility of the wall, it is then called megacolon. The most common causes of megacolon include chronic constipation and alterations of nutritional, metabolic, neurological or mechanical origin (foreign bodies, anorectal anomalies, perineal hernias, intrapelvic masses, etc.). Idiopathic megacolon, which is more frequent in cats (fig. 2.148), has also been described. To distinguish permanent and irreversible megacolon in cats from colon dilation due to excess faecal content, the colon diameter:L5 length ratio can be used. A ratio over 1.5 is considered suggestive of megacolon.

A localised **narrowing** of the lumen of the large intestine can be due to a spasm or stenosis caused by a neoplasm, chronic inflammation or scar tissue.

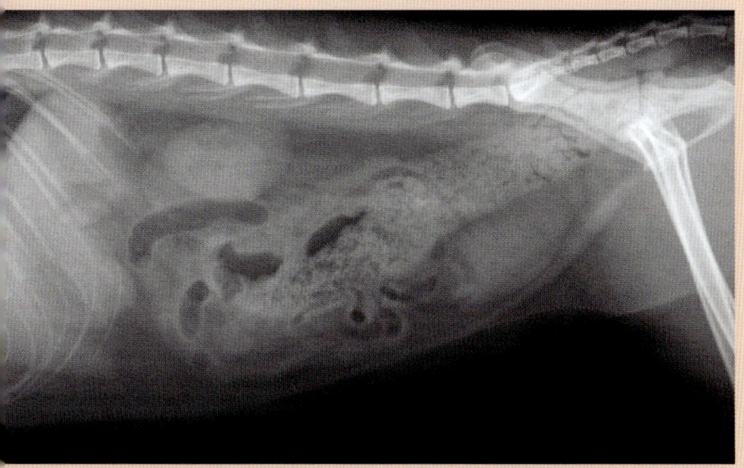

FIGURE 2.143. Lateral radiograph of the abdomen of a cat with faecal retention due to constipation.

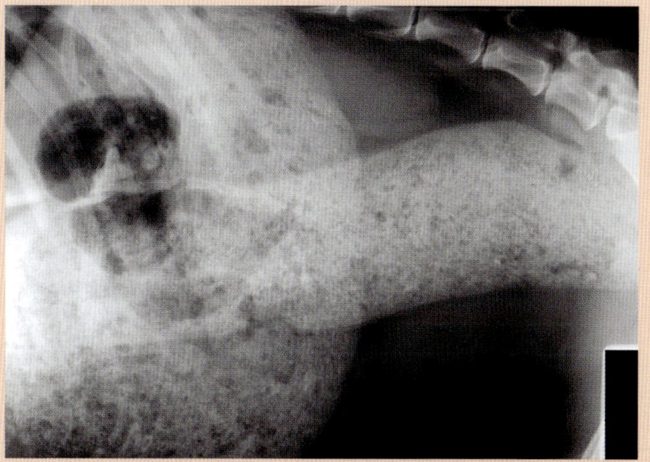

FIGURE 2.144. Lateral radiograph of the abdomen of a dog with faecal impaction. The large intestine appears very dilated (it occupies a great part of the abdomen) and filled with faecal material with a high radiopacity.

As opposed to stenosis, a spasm is transient and is usually caused by an incorrect technique when performing the barium enema. Most cases of stenosis are caused by neoplasms (fig. 2.149), although adenomas, ulcerative colitis and eosinophilic colitis may show similar radiographic findings.

Colorectal diverticula are not very frequent and usually appear in senior male dogs with prostatic alteration and chronic constipation, or associated with perineal hernias. A localised accumulation of faeces may be observed on plain radiographs, while in contrast studies the contrast medium accumulates in a structure with a saccular morphology and smooth margin (fig. 2.150).

Vaginorectal, urethrorectal and rectocutaneous **fistulas**, which may have a congenital or acquired origin, have been described. If this type of lesions is suspected, it is recommended to perform the positive-contrast enema with iodinated contrast agents, which may show the communication between the colon and the vagina, urethra or skin.

Colonic **torsion** is a serious but uncommon disease in small animals. It causes ischaemia and necrosis of the affected intestinal segment, which lead to sepsis, circulatory shock and, ultimately, the death of the patient. The clinical signs are non-specific and, often, not representative of the degree of torsion. The plain radiograph can show marked focal segmental distension of the colon, significant focal narrowing and/or displacement of cecum or descending colon, generally with mild or no small intestine distension. These findings are inconclusive so a barium enema is recommended when colonic torsion is suspected. This would usually show focal narrowing of the affected colon segment and longitudinal striations of the wall that course in a helical pattern, which is considered a very indicative sign of colon torsion. It is important to remember that displacement of the cecum or descending colon may be incidental findings in the plain radiograph without pathological significance. Such findings must be correlated with the clinical history, other additional findings in the plain radiographs and, above all, with barium enema results in order to grant them clinical significance.

The spontaneous appearance of gas in the colonic wall has been described, which is called ***pneumatosis coli***. It is characterised by the visualisation of thin bands of gas opacity in the colonic wall (submucosal or subserosal emphysema). This may be an incidental finding, but it has also been associated with various pathological situations, some serious such as intestinal infarction. Possible causes should always be investigated. It can lead to a secondary pneumoperitoneum.

Congenital anomalies of the large intestine are uncommon in dogs and cats. Anal perforation (fig. 2.151), atresia of the rectum, atresia of the colon, fistulas, diverticula, duplication of the large intestine or rectum, and a short colon and rectum with the caecum in the left hemiabdomen have been described.

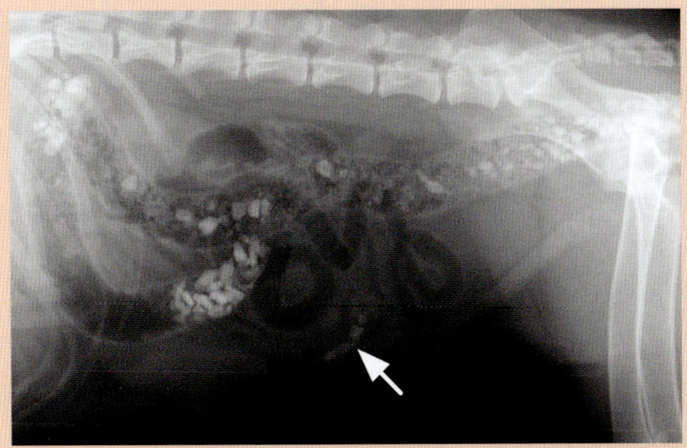

FIGURE 2.145. Lateral radiograph of the abdomen of a dog with foreign bodies (stones) in the large intestine. Most of the stones appear in different segments of the colon and a much more reduced number can be observed in the small intestine (arrow).

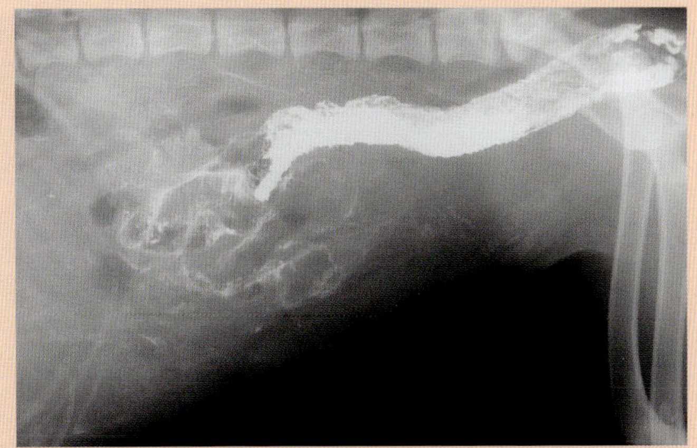

FIGURE 2.146. Lateral radiograph of the abdomen of a dog with severe colitis and peritonitis due to a perforation of the wall of the colon, after an enema with an iodinated contrast medium, which reveals its extravasation to the peritoneal cavity.

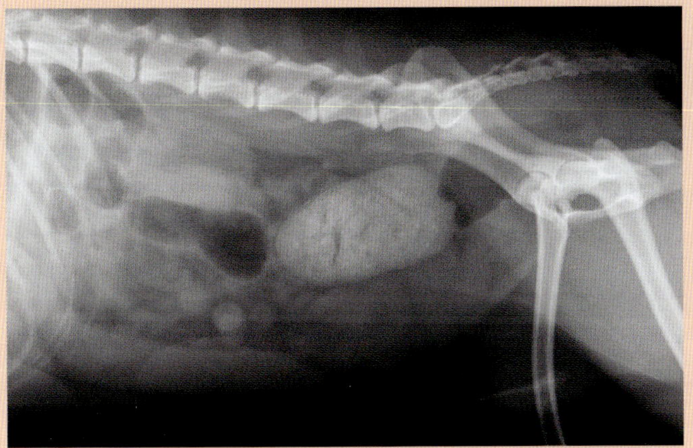

FIGURE 2.147. Lateral radiograph of the abdomen of a dog with focal dilatation of the central area of the descending colon due to the presence of a faecaloma.

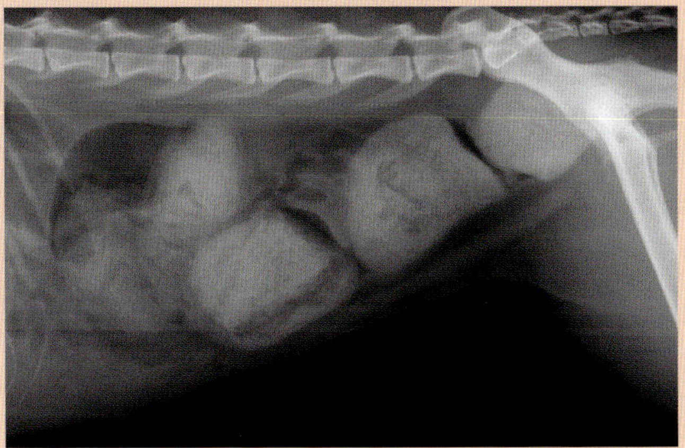

FIGURE 2.148. Lateral radiograph of the abdomen of a cat with megacolon. The colon is very dilated and accumulates a large amount of faeces with high radiopacity.

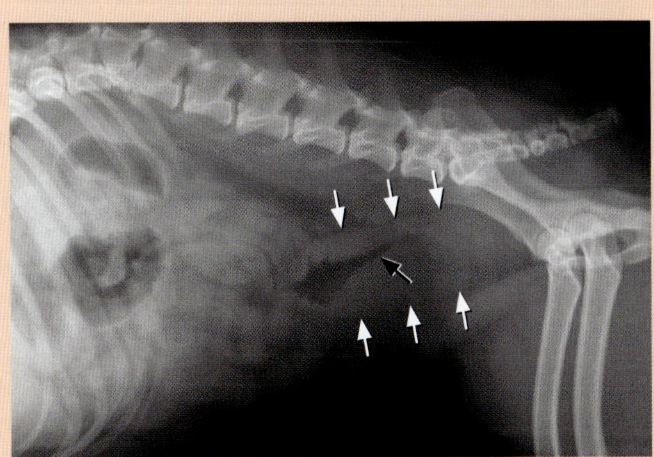

FIGURE 2.149. Lateral radiograph of the abdomen of a dog with a neoplasm of the colon. The external limits of the site of the tumour are marked with white arrows. The pattern of intraluminal gas (back arrow) is indicative of stenosis.

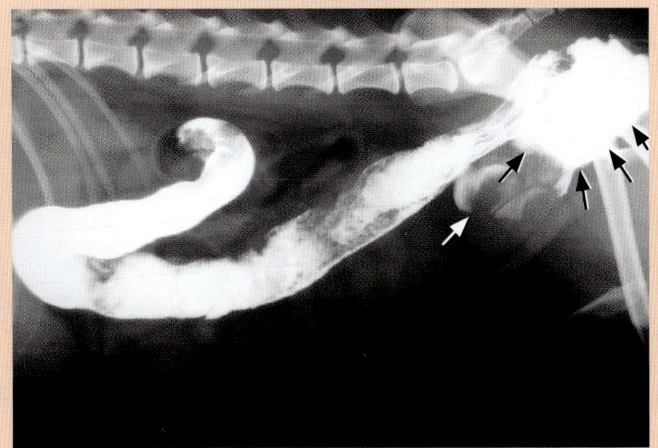

FIGURE 2.150. Lateral radiograph of the abdomen of a dog with a perforated rectal diverticulum (black arrows) after an enema with an iodinated contrast medium, which reveals its extravasation (white arrow) to the peritoneal cavity.

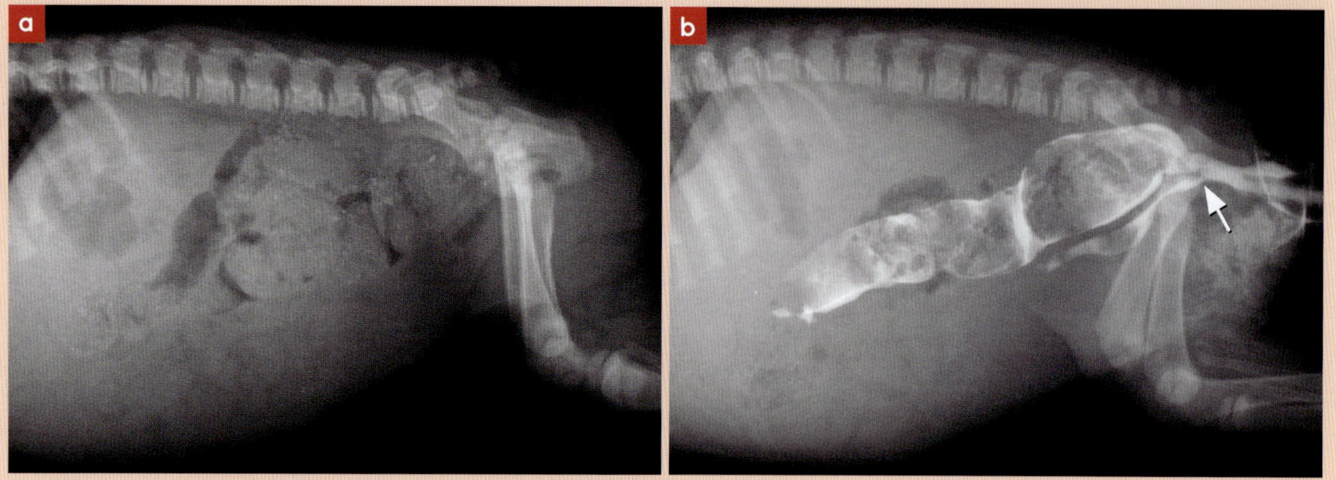

FIGURE 2.151. Lateral radiograph of the abdomen of a 1.5 month-old dog with anal atresia and a congenital rectovaginal fistula, before (a) and after (b) an enema with an iodinated contrast agent, which reveals the communication (arrow) between the vagina and the rectum.

Cases for **self-assessment**

Case 2.1.

Presentation | Explanation

Case 2.2.

Presentation | Explanation

Neck and thorax

3

Normal radiographic anatomy of the neck and thorax
https://goo.by/SoZuL

Principles of interpretation

Neck

Except in the case of the cervical spine, which is reviewed in Chapter 5, radiographs of the neck provide a limited amount of information on the anatomical structures that form this part of the body. In normal conditions, it is possible identify the pharynx, larynx, cervical trachea, soft palate, epiglottis and hyoid bone. The other soft tissues (oesophagus, blood vessels, lymph nodes, muscles, salivary glands and thyroid and parathyroid glands) are not identified in normal radiographic images. The presence of a very small amount of air in the lumen of the cervical oesophagus is usually an incidental finding associated with aerophagia, although the persistence of this finding in repeated studies may be due to pathological alterations. The partial calcification of the cartilages of the larynx is very common and usually takes place at 2–3 years of age.

Lateral radiographs are most appropriate for the examination of soft tissues in the neck, since most of the identifiable structures are superimposed with the cervical spine on ventrodorsal and dorsoventral radiographs. However, it will sometimes be necessary to take two orthogonal radiographs, for example when a foreign body is identified on the lateral projection, since its exact location cannot be confirmed in any other way.

Other diagnostic techniques may provide much more information about this anatomical region. Ultrasound scans may be very useful for the assessment of the thyroid and parathyroid glands, larynx, salivary glands and masses in general, and they also allow the collection of samples for cytology or biopsy. Computed tomography and magnetic resonance imaging (MRI) are excellent for the examination of this region, although MRI is somewhat better than tomography due to its better definition of soft tissues.

While offering real-time radiographic images with somewhat decreased anatomical detail, fluoroscopy does not provide any morphological information comparable to that provided by other diagnostic imaging techniques. Nevertheless, it has a significant advantage over them when assessing swallowing alterations, as it enables the direct visualisation of the passage of food from the mouth to the oropharynx and then to the esophagus.

Thorax

Radiographs of the thorax are essential for the diagnosis of most of the diseases that affect this region. Although radiographic findings are often sufficient to establish a fairly precise diagnosis, the combination of radiography with other diagnostic imaging techniques, such as ultrasonography or computed tomography, guarantees in most cases an accurate diagnosis of the patient with a thoracic condition.

The main limiting factors in the interpretation of radiographs of the thorax are:

- The loss of information due to the superimposition of structures.
- The wide variety of anatomical conformations and physiological changes that affect the image of the thorax.
- The similarity between physiological and pathological images in some cases.
- The same appearance that very different diseases have on radiographs.

In dogs, the cardiac silhouette and the shadows of the mediastinum and diaphragm may greatly vary depending on the conformation of the thorax. Three types of conformation are basically identified (fig. 3.1):

- Deep, narrow chest (e.g. Greyhound, Doberman, Collie).
- Intermediate (e.g. German Shepherd, Labrador, Poodle).
- Wide and shallow chest (e.g. Bulldog, Dachshund, Basset Hound).

The conformation of the thorax is quite constant in cats and is similar to the intermediate conformation in dogs.

The thoracic vertebrae, thoracic inlet, sternum and shadow of the diaphragm should be included when taking a radiograph of the thorax. Apart from these structures, the trachea, mediastinum, aorta, caudal vena cava, cardiac silhouette and lung fields may also be visualised in the image. It is recommended to follow a systemic order of assessment and, whenever possible, to carefully examine each of these elements in two orthogonal views, which should include a lateral view and a dorsoventral or ventrodorsal view.

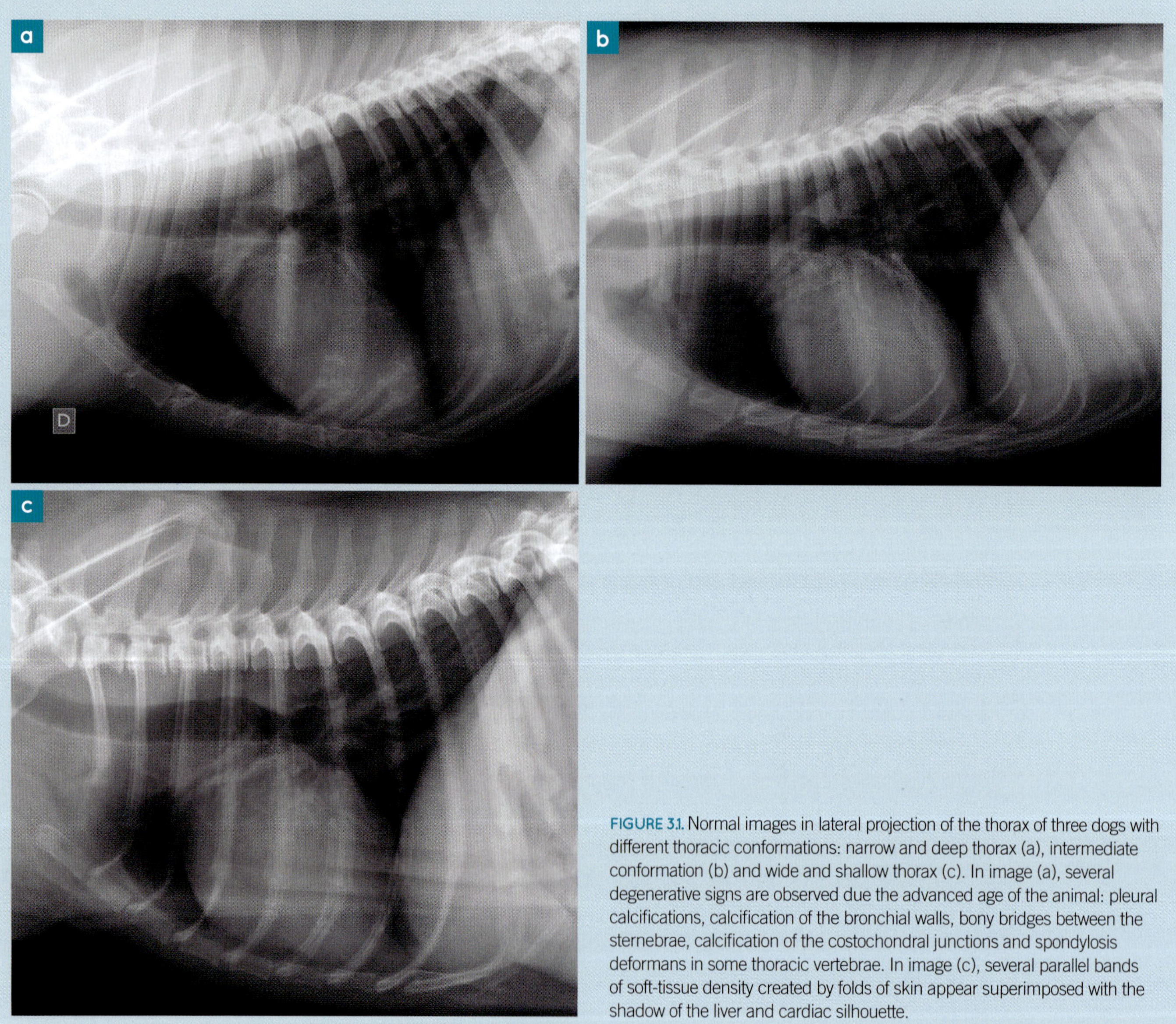

FIGURE 3.1. Normal images in lateral projection of the thorax of three dogs with different thoracic conformations: narrow and deep thorax (a), intermediate conformation (b) and wide and shallow thorax (c). In image (a), several degenerative signs are observed due the advanced age of the animal: pleural calcifications, calcification of the bronchial walls, bony bridges between the sternebrae, calcification of the costochondral junctions and spondylosis deformans in some thoracic vertebrae. In image (c), several parallel bands of soft-tissue density created by folds of skin appear superimposed with the shadow of the liver and cardiac silhouette.

Depending on the reason why the radiographic study is carried out, the projections should be chosen taking the following criteria into account:

- **Assessment of the cardiac silhouette:** the right lateral and dorsoventral projections are used, since they provide a more real image of the silhouette. In the left lateral projection, the silhouette appears more rounded (fig. 3.2); in the ventrodorsal view, the heart is positioned farther away from the cassette than in the dorsoventral view, causing the silhouette to appear slightly magnified (fig. 3.3).
- **Assessment of the lungs:** lateral (generally right) and ventrodorsal projections are used. In order to correctly assess the lung parenchyma, it is better if this is filled with as much air as possible (there will be a greater contrast with the structures that have different radiographic densities), so we will preferably take a ventrodorsal radiograph, as the capacity of distension of the lungs is greater when the animal is placed in dorsal recumbency than in sternal recumbency.
- **Assessment of pulmonary metastases:** the two lateral projections, right and left, are used. When

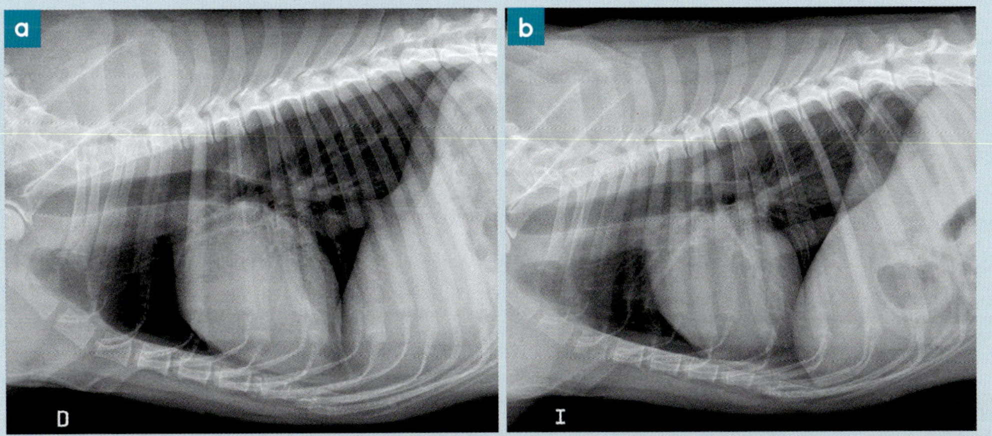

FIGURE 3.2. Right (a) and left (b) lateral projections of the chest of a healthy dog. The shape of the cardiac silhouette is more rounded on the left lateral X-ray, which could lead to a misdiagnosis of cardiomegaly.

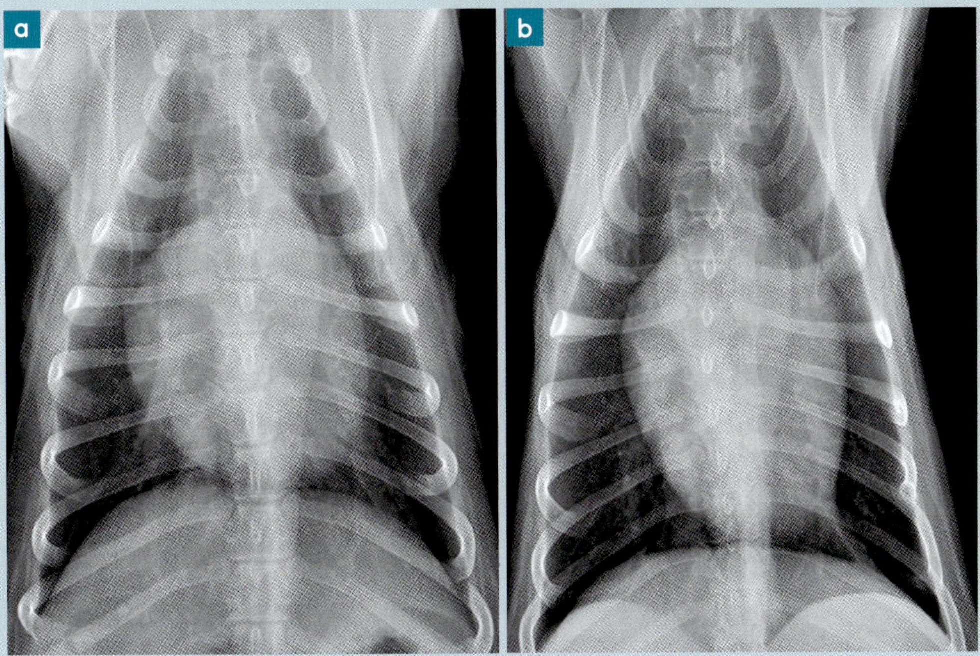

FIGURE 3.3. Dorsoventral (a) and ventrodorsal (b) projections of the chest of a healthy dog. The shape of the cardiac silhouette changes from one projection to another. It appears magnified in the ventrodorsal view because the patient is in dorsal recumbency, and this means that the distance from the heart to the cassette/detector is longer.

placing the animal in lateral recumbency, the lung that is lower (closer to the cassette) is partially collapsed, as its expansion capacity is limited. On the other hand, the other lung is normally filled with air. If soft-tissue density nodules appear in the lung parenchyma, these would be easier to differentiate in a fully distended lung than in a slightly collapsed lung. That is why the presence of metastases is assessed with a right lateral radiograph, which offers a better image of the left lung, and a left lateral radiograph, which allows a better examination of the right lung. When suspicious images appear on these projections, it is recommended to complete the study with a ventrodorsal radiograph.

- If the animal presents with **severe dyspnoea**, taking standard radiographs may lead to significant respiratory distress. In these cases, it would be recommendable to take radiographs with the animal standing, although not all machines allow the placement of the X-ray tube in horizontal position so as to take this type of radiographs. If this cannot be done, the dorsoventral projection should be chosen ahead of the ventrodorsal and lateral ones, as there is a smaller risk of respiratory distress for the animal.
- Oblique radiographs centred on the lesion may be useful to evaluate **lesions of the thoracic wall**, e.g. rib tumours.

It is very important to pay maximum attention to the technical quality of radiographs of the thoracic wall. The use of incorrect exposure values, improper patient positioning, poor developing technique or incorrect digital post-processing can greatly affect the interpretation of the images.

Generally, a high kilovoltage and low milliamperage should be used so as to reduce the time of exposure and minimise the influence of respiratory movements on the images. If exposure values are too low (resulting in underexposed X-rays), the image will appear lighter than expected in analog radiography, while noise artifacts may appear in digital radiography. On the other hand, if the exposure values used are too high (resulting in overexposed radiography), the entire image will appear darker in analog radiography, and black focal areas will be noticeable in digital radiography, as explained in Chapter 1. In both cases the image of the lung will be particularly affected and these variations may even be mistaken for pathological alterations. Generally, the use of an anti-scatter grid (either stationary or Potter-Bucky) is necessary when the thickness of the thorax, once placed on the cassette, exceeds 10 cm. However, high-quality direct digital detector panels can provide excellent images of the thorax and other anatomical regions with a thickness greater than 10 cm without the need for a grid. This allows for a large reduction in milliamperage per second, which in turn significantly reduces the amount of scatter radiation produced.

Although it is difficult in practice, chest radiographs should ideally be taken at maximum inspiration. The greater the amount of air in the lungs, the easier it will be to identify small lesions in these organs radiographically. If the X-ray is taken during exhalation, the cardiac silhouette will appear larger and may come into contact with or overlap with the shadow of the diaphragm, and the lungs will exhibit higher radiographic density.

As regards the position of the patient, special attention should be paid to the position of the forelimbs, which must be correctly extended so they are not superimposed with the cranial part of the thoracic cavity. In addition, when a radiograph is taken in lateral recumbency, the median plane of the thorax is usually inclined on the cassette rather than being parallel to it, due to the relatively triangular morphology of this anatomical region. A radiolucent wedge should therefore be placed under the sternum in order to correct the position. When observing a lateral radiograph, we will know that the thorax was correctly placed when the costochondral junctions of both sides appear practically at the same level. If they appear widely separated in the image, this finding will indicate that the median plane is not parallel to the X-ray table, affecting the image of the cardiac silhouette and the trachea. As a result, the cardiac silhouette appears more supported on the sternum and the trachea appears falsely elevated (fig. 3.4). It is quite important not to mix up these findings caused by an incorrect positioning with real pathological alterations. The rotation of the thorax at the time of taking a dorsoventral or ventrodorsal radiograph will be identified in the images by the lack of superimposition of the sternum and thoracic spine, and will particularly affect the cardiac silhouette, which will appear falsely deformed (fig. 3.5).

Digital radiographs offer a better contrast resolution than conventional radiographs, which translates into a better definition of some structures, especially in the thorax, such as the pulmonary vessels or the walls of larger bronchi. Lungs appear less radiolucent than in analog radiographs, which may lead to an incorrect diagnosis of a pathological increase in lung opacity.

In comparison with dogs, the thorax of cats has a more triangular morphology, the cardiac silhouette is of a smaller craniocaudal diameter (2 intercostal spaces compared to 2.5 to 3.5 intercostal spaces in dogs) and the dorsocaudal margin of the caudal lung lobes may appear slightly separated from the spine in lateral projections in healthy animals. This latter finding would raise suspicion of mild pleural effusion in the case of dogs (fig. 3.6).

In young animals, it is possible to identify the shadow of the thymus until approximately 6 months of age. After that, the shadow cannot be differentiated from the rest of the structures contained in the cranial mediastinal space. Due to the typical organomegaly observed in young animals, the cardiac silhouette may also appear larger in comparison with adult animals.

Degenerative changes can frequently be observed in older animals, such as spondylosis deformans in the thoracic vertebrae, formation of bony bridges between the sternebrae, calcification of the costochondral junctions, calcification of the tracheal rings and bronchial walls, formation of pulmonary osteomas, calcified pleural plaques, thickening of the pleura and a diffuse interstitial lung pattern associated with fibrosis. In older cats, the heart tends to lie more on the sternum due to an elongation of the aorta, which may increase the curvature of the aortic arch and cause a marked undulation of the descending aorta.

The superimposition of subcutaneous fat in obese animals may significantly worsen the quality of the images of the thorax and especially affects the assessment of the lungs. The mediastinum and cardiac silhouette may also appear enlarged in obese patients and the lung margin may be slightly separated from the thoracic wall, which could be confused with a mild pleural effusion.

The combination of radiography and echocardiography offers very complete information about the diseases that affect the heart and great vessels. Non-cardiac thoracic ultrasonography is also useful to obtain complementary information in cases of pleural or mediastinal effusion, assess thoracic masses that are not surrounded by air, pulmonary consolidation and diaphragmatic hernias, and collect samples or perform thoracic drainage under ultrasound guidance.

Fluoroscopy allows real-time evaluation of peristalsis of the oesophagus and of the passage of food or contrast medium through it. It is very useful for the diagnosis of tracheal, bronchial or laryngeal collapse, diaphragmatic paralysis and sliding hiatal hernias. this also allows samples to be collected for cytology and biopsy of thoracic lesions not detectable by ultrasound, as well as angiography studies. Some state-of-the-art X-ray machines come with the option of dynamic digital radiography (DDR), which is based on the rapid acquisition of radiographic series. This technique may serve as an alternative to fluoroscopy in some cases, especially when the examination time is relatively short, as DDR may result in a significant increase in exposure compared to fluoroscopy. Reducing the exposure dose and, therefore, the resolution of dynamic radiographic images to the minimum required may make this an appropriate alternative for some dynamic radiological studies in veterinary medicine.

Among advanced imaging techniques, computed tomography is generally more appropriate to examine the thorax than magnetic resonance imaging. A computed tomography examination can be performed in a few seconds, which allows the use of techniques of apnoeic anaesthesia to avoid the influence of respiratory movements on the images. Conversely, several minutes are usually necessary for an examination with conventional magnetic resonance imaging equipment. Such prolonged apnoea cannot be maintained and the artefacts due to respiratory and cardiac movements significantly affect the quality of chest images. Computed tomography is particularly indicated for the assessment of pneumothoraces or persistent and recurrent pleural effusions, localised lesions in the mediastinum, tracheal collapse and bronchial obstruction. It is also useful for the detection of pulmonary metastases and

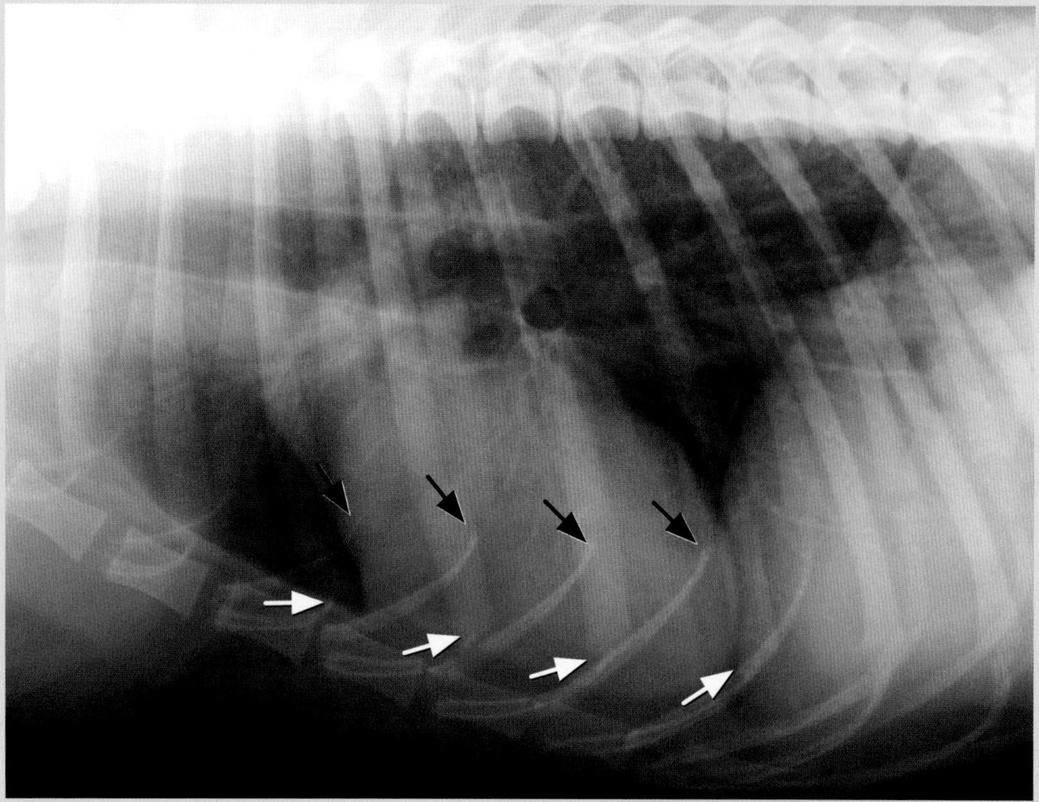

FIGURE 3.4. Lateral radiograph of the thorax of a healthy dog, in which there is a wide separation between the costochondral junctions of both sides (shown by black arrows on one side and white arrows on the other), due to the rotation of the thorax along its longitudinal axis. This rotation is corrected by slightly elevating the sternum with a radiolucent block until the median plane of the thorax is approximately parallel to the cassette. As a consequence of the incorrect position, the contact of the cardiac silhouette on the sternum is falsely increased and the trachea appears falsely elevated.

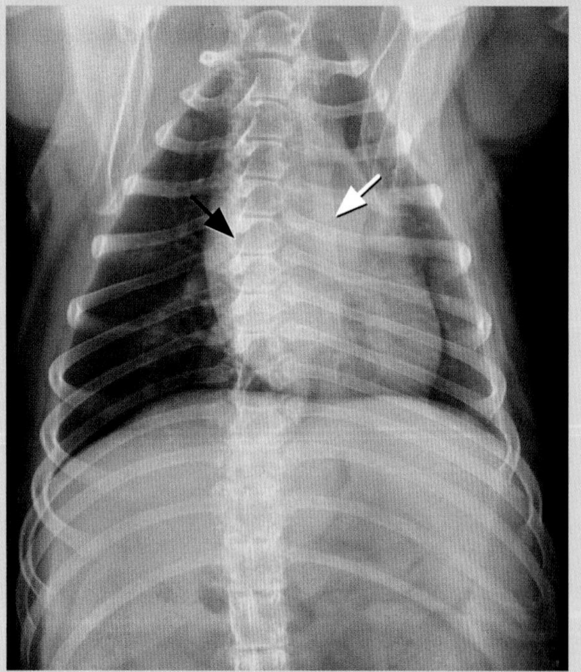

FIGURE 3.5. Dorsoventral radiograph of the thorax of a healthy dog, in which the thoracic spine (black arrow) and the sternum (white arrow) appear separated due to a rotation of the thorax along its longitudinal axis. As a consequence of the incorrect position, most of the cardiac silhouette appears falsely located in the left hemithorax.

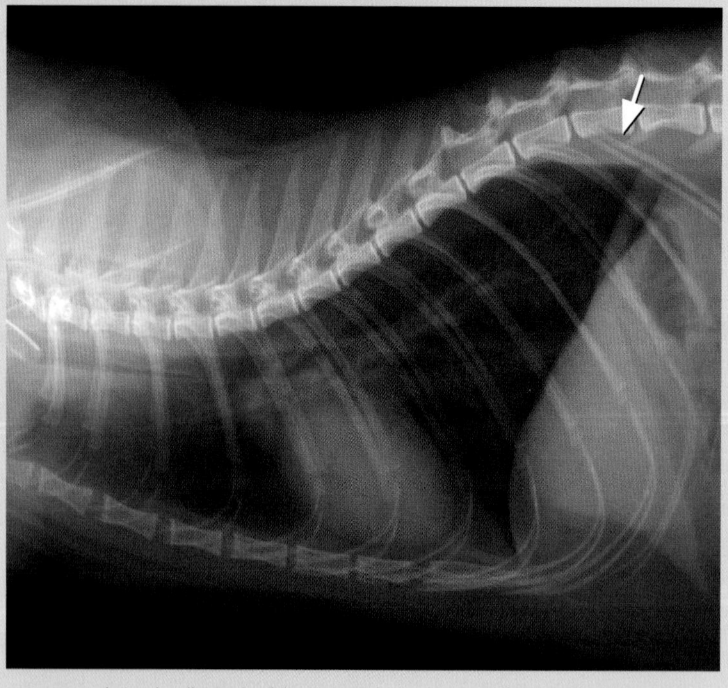

FIGURE 3.6. Lateral radiograph of the thorax of a healthy cat. Compared with that of a dog, the thorax of a cat has a more triangular morphology, the cardiac silhouette has a smaller craniocaudal diameter (2 intercostal spaces) and the caudodorsal margin of the caudal pulmonary lobes may appear slightly separated from the spine in normal conditions (arrows). This latter finding would make us suspect a mild pleural effusion in the case of dogs.

lymphadenopathies, thomboembolism, pulmonary torsion, infiltrative interstitial lung disease, as well as to differentiate between consolidation and atelectasis and assess thoracic masses in general. Magnetic resonance may also be of interest for the pre-surgical examination of the thoracic wall and pleural and mediastinal masses, essentially.

Thoracic wall

The thoracic wall is formed by the thoracic spine (see chapter 5), the sternum, the diaphragm (see chapter 2), the ribs, costal cartilages and intercostal spaces.

Ribs

In normal conditions, the ribs are symmetrical, have a homogeneous density and smooth borders. The space between them must be regular. However, congenital anomalies, hypoplasia or aplasia, which are uni- or bilateral, are often seen in the thirteenth pair of ribs. The C7 and L1 vertebrae may also have rudimentary ribs when they are transitional.

In the first weeks of life, costal cartilages cannot be identified on radiographs as they have soft-tissue opacity. They become apparent as they start calcifying. In older cats, segments of the costal cartilages may appear markedly calcified, thus having an appearance of ruptures. In older dogs and cats, calcifications with an irregular morphology may be observed in the costochondral junctions, and these may even be mistaken for intrathoracic lesions. In chondrodystrophic breeds, especially in the Teckel and Basset Hounds, the ribs have a peculiar curvature, which may create a similar image to that of a mild pleural effusion on dorsoventral and ventrodorsal radiographs (fig. 3.7).

There may be a generalised increase of the intercostal space in conditions that cause an excessive expansion of the thorax, for example, in severe cases of pleural effusion, pneumothorax or emphysema.

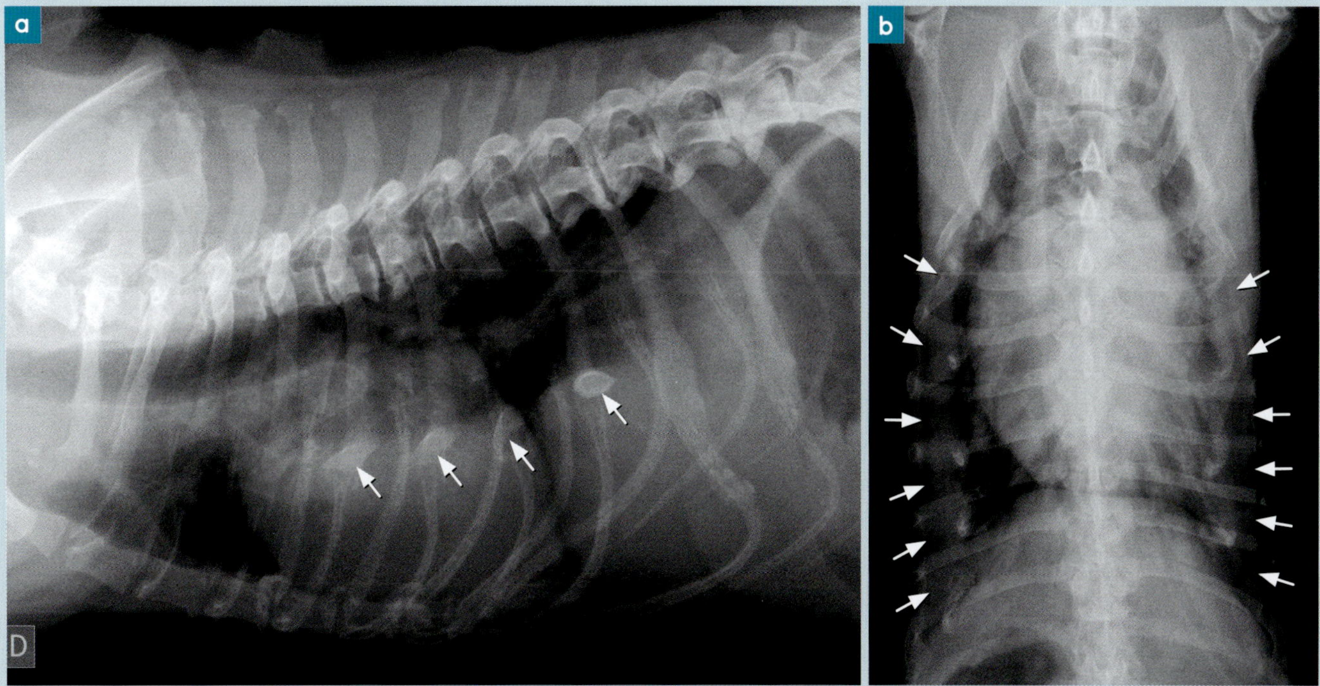

FIGURE 3.7. Right lateral (a) and dorsoventral (b) projections of the chest of a Basset Hound with no significant abnormalities in the thoracic image. The left lung is less distended due to atelectasis brought about by prolonged left lateral recumbency. In image (a) the arrows indicate the relatively high position of the costochondral joints in this breed. In the dorsoventral projection, the peculiar morphology of the ribs results in (b) the visualisation of soft tissue density bands (arrows) in the lateral areas of the chest, which could be mistaken for pleural effusion.

Rib **fractures** are more or less easily identified depending on their location and the degree of displacement of the fragments (fig. 3.8). When dealing with thoracic trauma, a thorough examination of each pair of ribs is advised and should be performed on two orthogonal radiographs whenever possible. The early detection of rib fractures after a trauma is considered to be indicative of possible lung trauma, although the radiographic image of a contusion in the lung may be undetectable until 6 hours after the trauma occurred. A patient with a rib fracture may present with paradoxical motion of the affected region of the thorax: outward motion during expiration and inward motion during inspiration. Fractures are usually transverse and generally affect more than one rib. They are often associated with a pneumothorax or subcutaneous emphysema. Although their most frequent cause is thoracic trauma, pathological fractures may appear secondary to a neoplasm or to conditions that cause severe osteopenia (e.g. secondary renal hyperparathyroidism). They may also be caused by sustained or repetitive stress in cases of feline asthma, chronic bronchial disease or lobular emphysema. Old fractures may appear as incidental findings on chest radiographs.

The most frequent primary **neoplasms** of the ribs are osteosarcomas and chondrosarcomas. Their image is usually that of a mixed aggressive bone lesion, which is both osteolytic and osteoproliferative, with

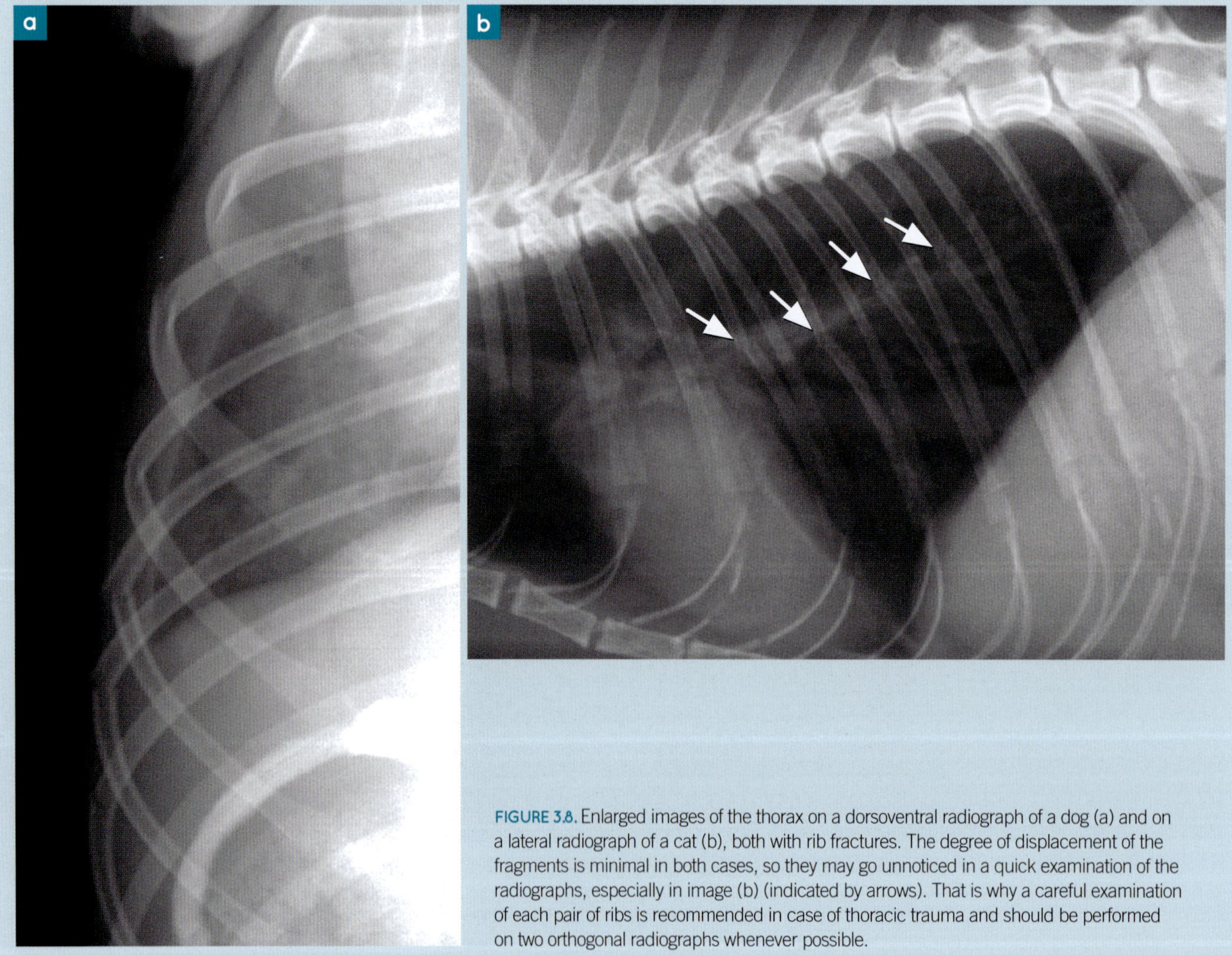

FIGURE 3.8. Enlarged images of the thorax on a dorsoventral radiograph of a dog (a) and on a lateral radiograph of a cat (b), both with rib fractures. The degree of displacement of the fragments is minimal in both cases, so they may go unnoticed in a quick examination of the radiographs, especially in image (b) (indicated by arrows). That is why a careful examination of each pair of ribs is recommended in case of thoracic trauma and should be performed on two orthogonal radiographs whenever possible.

marked inflammation of soft tissues. They may cause a displacement of the adjacent ribs and a secondary involvement of these. They usually originate what is termed the **extrapleural sign**, which refers to a focal displacement of the pleura and lung to the inside of the thorax caused by masses in the thoracic wall, either of costal or soft-tissue origin (it is an adaptation of the general term "mass effect"). Many rib tumours are diagnosed at an advanced stage because their growth is greater towards the inside of the thorax than towards the outside. They are sometimes associated with pleural effusion (fig. 3.9), which may make the radiographic detection of the primary lesion more difficult. In cases of multiple myeloma, ribs and bone metastases in this location may have a multiple osteolytic pattern. Benign neoplasms (osteomas, chondromas and osteochondromatosis) are uncommon and usually appear as osteoproliferative, non-aggressive lesions.

On occasions, we may find soft-tissue tumours that affect the ribs in a secondary manner (e.g. mesotheliomas) and have a similar image to that of primary tumours. In both cases, the differential diagnosis should include osteomyelitis.

Computed tomography and magnetic resonance imaging allow a very accurate assessment of any mass affecting the costal wall, the extension of the lesion and the degree of infiltration in adjacent tissues, although computed tomography is preferred to examine the lung when there is a suspicion of metastasis.

Sternum

Variations in its size, morphology or in the number of sternebrae that have no clinical significance are frequently observed. Cats often have a ventral displacement of the xyphoid process, which sometimes causes pain. In geriatric animals, it is usual to find **bony overgrowths** that originate from the ends of the sternebrae and tend to form bridges between each other (fig. 3.10). It is considered to be a degenerative sign associated with age and with no clinical significance.

Fractures of the sternebrae are usually incidental findings and rarely cause clinical signs. A poor alignment of the sternum may also be observed, but it should only be considered significant if it is accompanied by inflammation of soft tissues, pleural effusion or associated clinical signs.

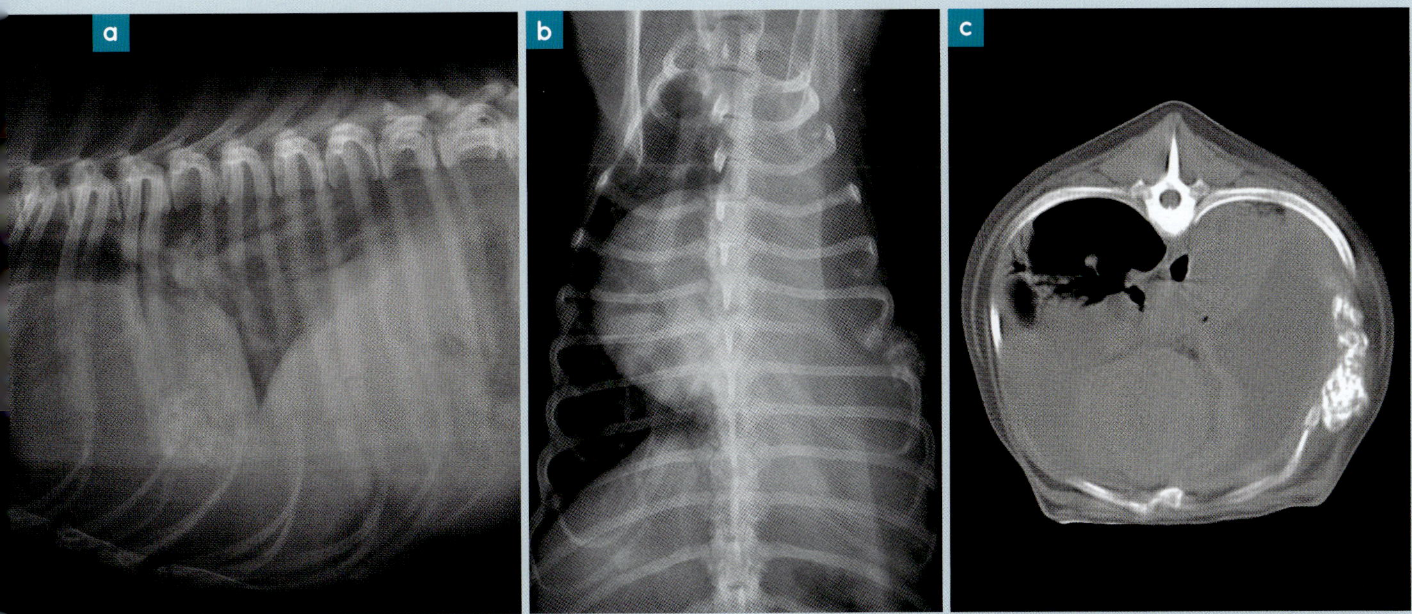

FIGURE 3.9. Lateral (a) and dorsoventral (b) radiographs and computed tomography image of a dog with a primary neoplasm on the seventh left rib. An aggressive osteoproliferative and osteolytic bone lesion is observed, as well as signs of severe pleural effusion in the left hemithorax. In image (b), signs of pleural effusion can be observed in the right hemithorax, while in image (c), obtained several days later, the degree of effusion is moderate.

It is uncommon to find **neoplasms** affecting the sternum. They usually appear as aggressive osteolytic and osteoproliferative lesions and marked inflammation of the adjacent soft tissues. **Osteomyelitis** may have a similar aspect and is usually caused by penetration of foreign bodies or bites in this region.

Pectus excavatum is a congenital deformity of the sternum, which causes it to have a more or less marked abnormal dorsal curvature (fig. 3.11). The ribs appear deformed and the heart and mediastinum are displaced dorsally, and to one side of the thoracic cavity on some occasions. It does not usually cause any clinical symptoms, but it may make breathing more difficult when the deformity is marked. Although it affects both cats and dogs, it is more common in brachycephalic dog breeds. It is sometimes associated with other congenital deformities such as peritoneopericardial hernia, tracheal hypoplasia or defects of the ventricular septum.

Pharynx, larynx and trachea

Pharynx and larynx

The pharynx is a musculomembranous sac that belongs to the digestive and respiratory system. Its cranial part is connected with the mouth and nasal cavity, while its caudal end communicates with the oesophagus and the larynx. This latter connects the pharynx with the trachea. Figure 3.12 shows the radiologically identifiable structures of the pharynx, larynx and trachea.

The larynx contains air and is surrounded by cartilages, which are radiographically identified as soft-tissue opacities. Calcification of these cartilages is a common finding of no clinical significance, which improves visualisation on X-rays.

Radiological examination of the pharynx and larynx is indicated in patients with suspected upper airway obstruction, nausea, ptyalism, dysphagia, dysphonia, palpable mass in the cranial area of the neck or presence of fistulous tracts in the area.

Radiography provides only limited information on the alterations that may occur in the pharynx and larynx, although it can be useful for locating foreign bodies or identifying neoplasms, inflammatory polyps, cysts, stenosis, abscesses, inflammation and functional alterations. Fluoroscopy is preferable for the diagnosis of functional disorders of the pharynx as it provides real-time radiographic images allowing direct visualisation of the passage of the food bolus from the mouth to the oropharynx and from the oropharynx to the oesophagus. Ultrasound could help to more easily diagnose functional disorders of the larynx, such as laryngeal paralysis.

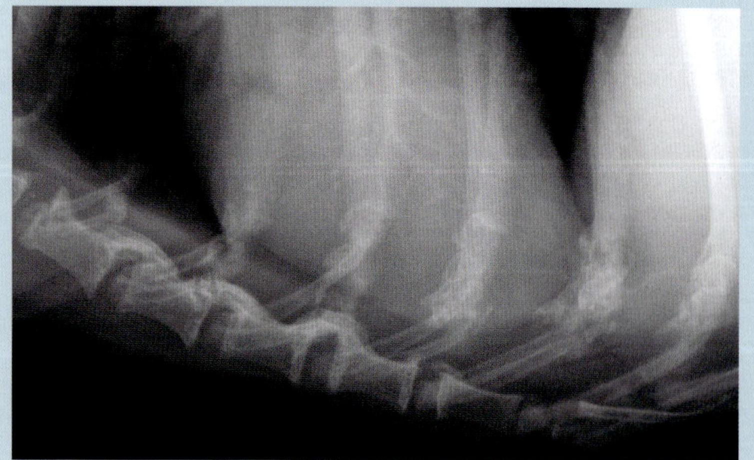

FIGURE 3.10. Enlarged image of the sternal region on a lateral radiograph of an older dog. It is possible to observe bony overgrowths, which tend to connect the ends of the sternebrae, and calcifications with an irregular morphology in the costochondral junctions. Both findings do not have any clinical significance.

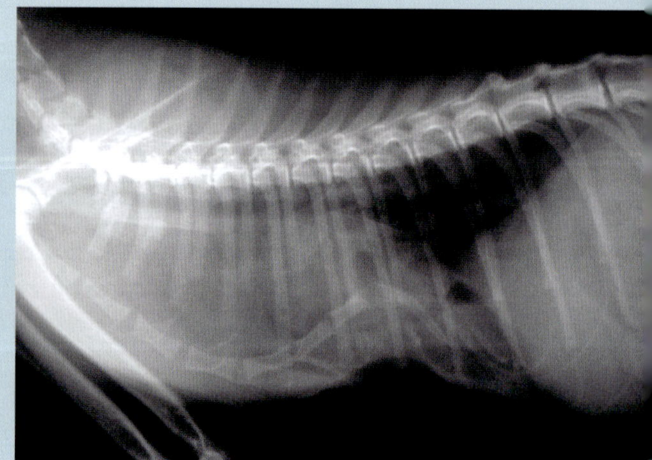

FIGURE 3.11. Lateral radiograph of the thorax of a cat with pectus excavatum. This is a congenital alteration in which the sternum appears deformed and curved in dorsal direction towards the thoracic cavity.

Foreign bodies can be easily identified if their radiopacity is higher than that of soft tissues (fig. 3.13), or if they are surrounded by gas in the pharyngeal or laryngeal lumen. Sharp objects may puncture the wall and cause the formation of abscesses in adjacent areas and/or the appearance of gas in the surrounding soft tissues (fig. 3.14).

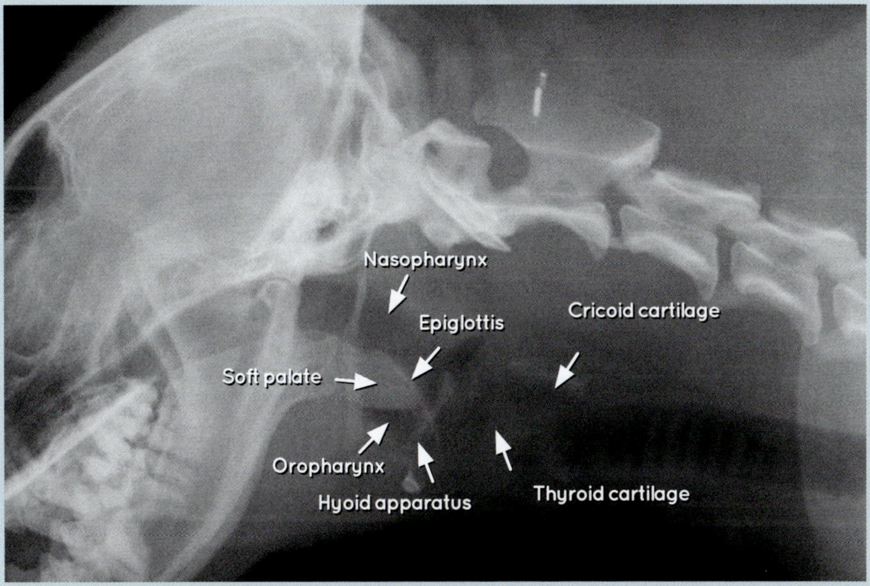

FIGURE 3.12. Radiographic anatomy of the pharynx and larynx of a dog as visualised in the lateral projection.

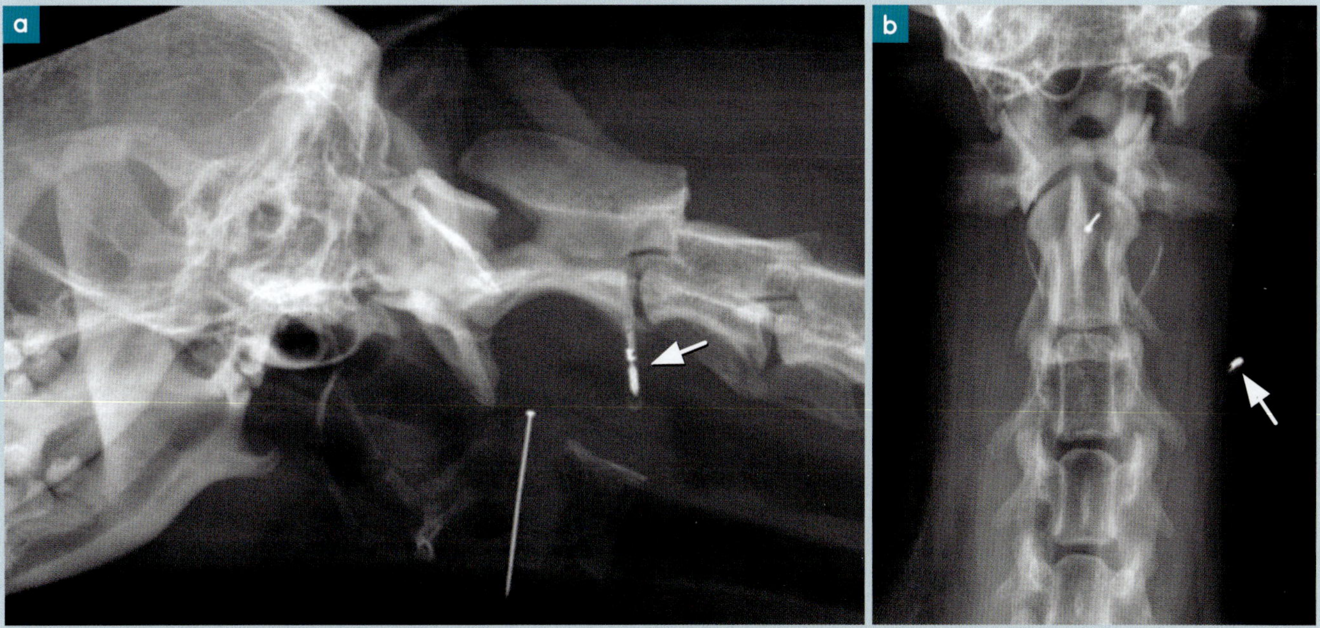

FIGURE 3.13. Lateral (a) and ventrodorsal (b) radiographs of the neck of a dog with a metallic foreign body (nail) in the larynx. It is essential to obtain two orthogonal radiographs to determine the exact location of the object. The identification microchip is shown with an arrow in both images.

Pharyngeal and laryngeal **masses** are generally of neoplastic or inflammatory origin, but benign laryngeal cysts have also been described in dogs and cats. Nasopharyngeal polyps are common in cats (fig. 3.15), often associated with otitis media.

Mass-like lesions (space-occupying lesions) are also common in tissues adjacent to the pharynx or larynx, which may cause displacement or obliteration of the lumen, as occurs in the case of retropharyngeal lymphadenopathy (fig. 3.16) and thyroid tumours (fig. 3.17).

Pharyngeal and **cricopharyngeal dysphagias** may have a congenital origin, especially in Spaniel breeds, or be acquired, generally in older animals, in which they may appear as a sequela of diseases of the central nervous system or neuromuscular diseases. They usually do not cause any significant alterations on radiographs and would require a real-time fluoroscopic study of the patient's swallowing movements (see video 3.1), in which food mixed with barium is administered to the patient, in order to be diagnosed. In cases of dysphagia, it is possible to observe nasal reflux of barium, its accumulation in the pharynx, a failure in the relaxation of the cricopharyngeal sphincter, aspiration of barium into the larynx and pharynx or uncoordinated movements of the pharyngeal muscle. It is important to take chest X-rays when dysphagia is suspected, since it is very common for these patients to suffer from aspiration pneumonia.

The incidence and clinical relevance of **pharyngeal collapse** have recently been studied in small animals, the etiology of which is not yet well defined, although it is most likely multifactorial. Pharyngeal collapse may be partial or total and may result from a dorsal displacement of the soft palate, a ventral deviation of the dorsal pharyngeal wall, or a combination of both. Most patients with pharyngeal collapse have concomitant respiratory diseases, such as tracheal collapse, mainstem bronchial collapse or brachycephalic syndrome. It has been reported that dogs with brachycephalic syndrome (especially English Bulldog, French Bulldog and Pug) are more predisposed to pharyngeal collapse. This may be due to the progressive development of pharyngeal muscle

Video 3.1.
Videofluoroscopic examination of a dog with **cricopharyngeal dysphagia**

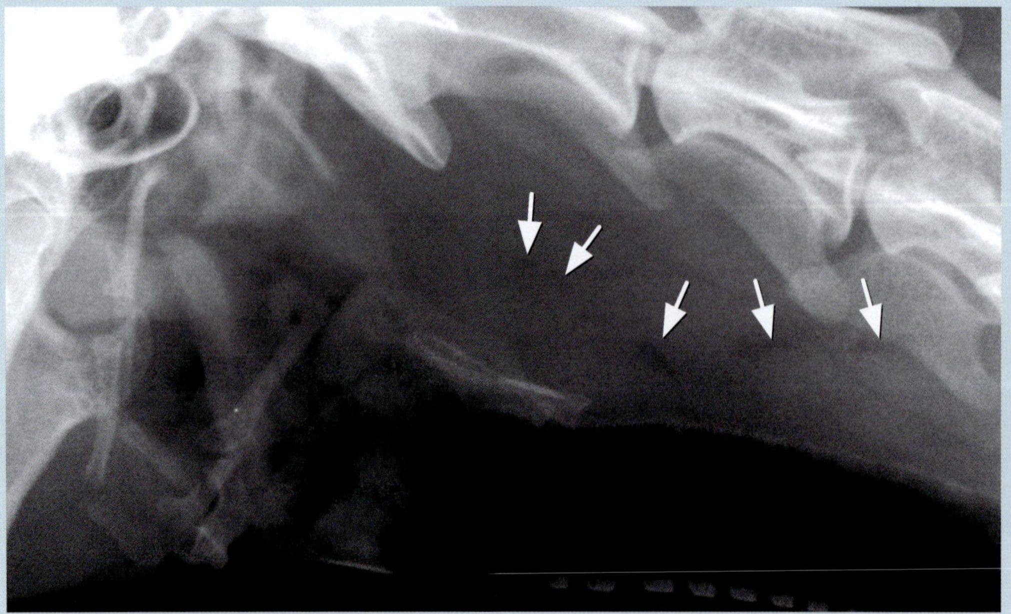

FIGURE 3.14. Enlarged lateral projection of the neck of a dog with foreign body (toothpick with sharp edges) dorsal to the larynx. The foreign body is not identified on the image as it is radiolucent, but areas of gas opacity (arrows) are seen in the surrounding soft tissues.

abnormalities as a result of sustained increase in upper airway resistance in these patients. Conventional X-rays may reveal narrowing of the nasopharynx lumen, but as this is a dynamic process that is not sustained over time, a cervical X-ray may not provide useful diagnostic information if the time at which the static image is captured does not coincide with the time at which the lumen is narrowed. Therefore, the most appropriate radiological technique to confirm the diagnosis of pharyngeal collapse is fluoroscopy, although dynamic digital radiography serve as an alternative (see video 3.2).

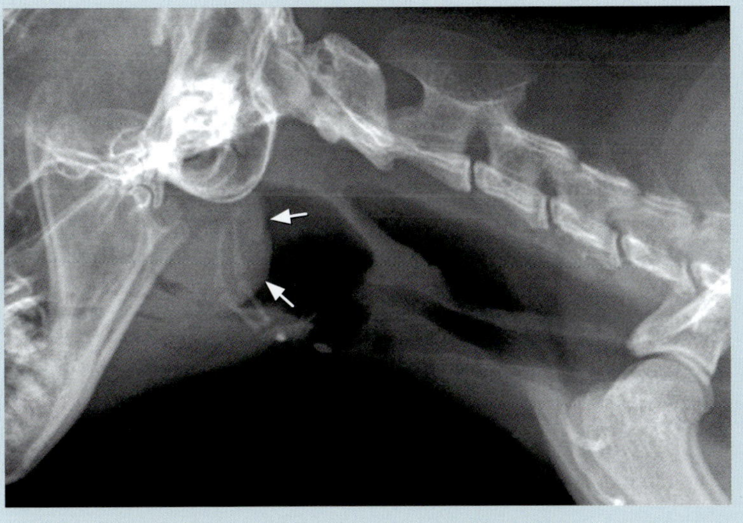

FIGURE 3.15. Lateral projection of the neck of a young cat with a mass located in the nasopharynx (caudal border indicated by arrows). Definitive diagnosis: nasopharyngeal polyp.

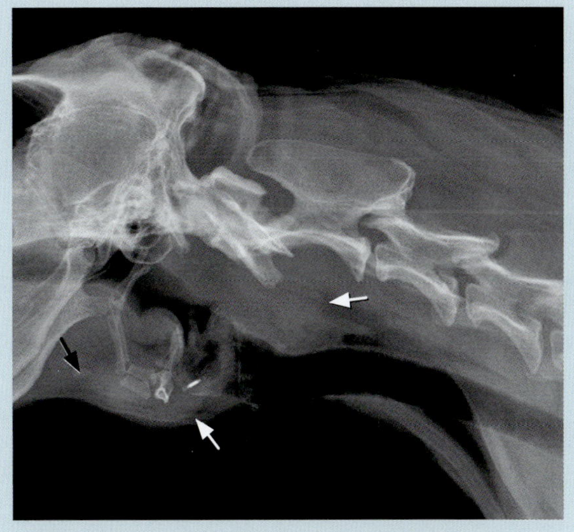

FIGURE 3.16. Lateral projection of the neck of a dog with a "mass effect" dorsal to the larynx and another ventral to the hyoid (white arrows). The first one was identified by ultrasound as a retropharyngeal lymphadenopathy and the second as submandibular lymphadenopathy. The black arrow points to a sialolith of mineral opacity.

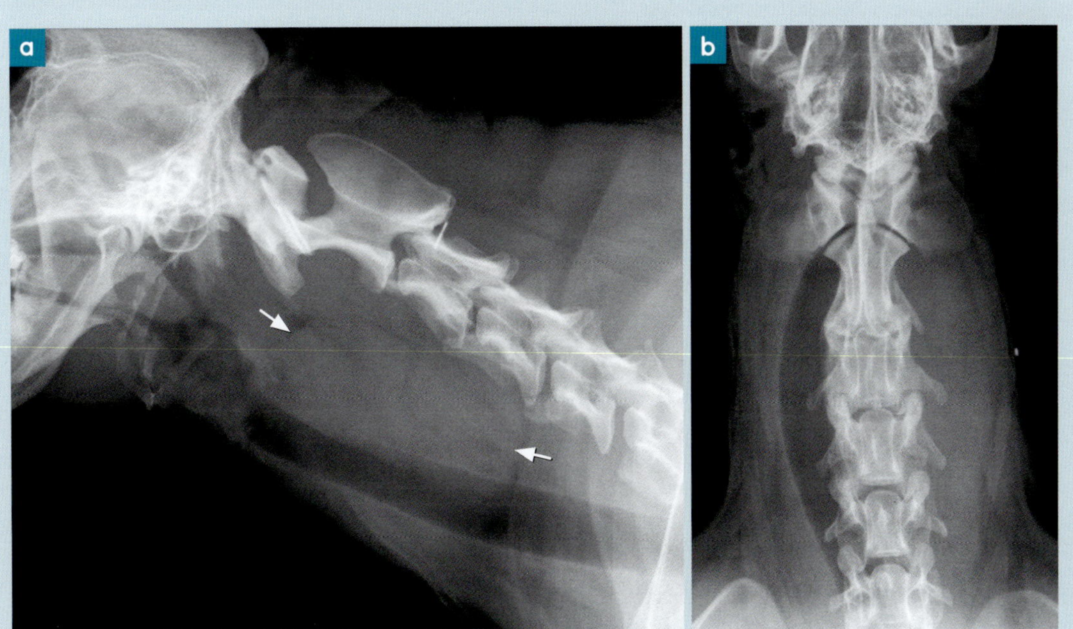

FIGURE 3.17. Lateral (a) and ventrodorsal (b) views of the neck of a dog with a large thyroid tumour. The mass of thyroid origin is indicated by the white arrows (a) and causes marked ventral displacement of the larynx and cranial half of the cervical trachea. Image (b) shows the right lateral displacement and the curvature of the trachea due to the presence of the mass.

Video 3.2.
Dynamic radiography of a dog with **pharyngeal collapse**

Laryngeal collapse may appear as a single pathology or may be associated with laryngeal paralysis, nasal or nasopharyngeal obstruction or trauma. Chronic upper airway obstruction can lead to laryngeal collapse due to fatigue and progressive cartilage degeneration.

Although the neck X-ray does not provide useful information in patients with laryngeal paralysis, a chest X-ray should be included in the diagnostic protocol of these patients, as secondary aspiration pneumonia is common before and after surgical treatment.

In cases of **brachycephalic syndrome**, which is characterised by several anomalies in the upper airways in brachycephalic dog and cat breeds, an anomalous image of the soft palate may be observed in this region. The soft palate may appear fairly elongated (extending beyond the epiglottis) or thickened due to oedema (fig. 3.18). The affected animals sometimes have laryngeal collapse, but it usually occurs in laterolateral direction and is therefore difficult to identify on lateral radiographs, unless it is very severe. Tracheal hypoplasia also commonly appears in these patients.

In cases of **retroversion of the epiglottis**, caused by its excessive mobility, the epiglottis may have a more vertical position than normal.

Trachea

The trachea is a semi-rigid tubular structure that connects the larynx with the bronchi. The carina can be identified in its distal part. On lateral radiographs, it appears as a more radiolucent circular or oval area that is located at the level of the 4th or 5th intercostal space. The tracheal rings have a "C" shape and are dorsally connected by the tracheal muscle and connective tissue.

In order to examine the complete trachea, it is necessary to take a radiograph that includes its cervical and thoracic parts (fig. 3.19). In medium or large-sized dogs, it will be necessary to take two radiographs, one of the neck and another of the thorax, to carry out this assessment. On plain radiographs, the internal aspect of the tracheal wall is easily observed because it contrasts with the intraluminal air. On the other hand, in normal conditions, the external aspect of the wall is difficult to differentiate from the structures of the neck or from the mediastinum that surrounds it.

In general, lateral radiographs are more useful, since the trachea is superimposed with the cervical and thoracic spine on dorsoventral and ventrodorsal radiographs. A craniocaudal tangential radiograph of the trachea may be taken to visualise the tracheal lumen at the level of the thoracic inlet, but it is difficult to place the patient correctly and it rarely provides significant additional information.

In cats and dog breeds with an intermediate conformation, the thoracic trachea forms an acute angle with the spine. This angle is greater in dogs with a narrow

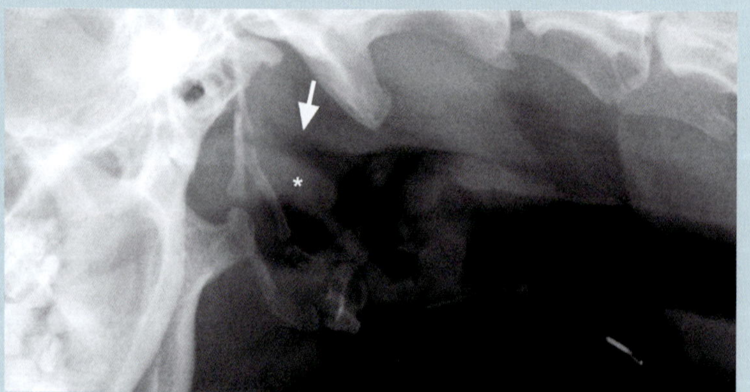

FIGURE 3.18. Enlarged lateral projection of the neck of a dog with soft palate thickening (asterisk) and nasopharynx lumen narrowing (arrow) caused by inflammation of its wall. The soft tissues surrounding the larynx also appear thicker due to the inflammation.

and deep thoracic conformation, while in those with a wide and shallow thorax, the course of the trachea is almost parallel to the vertebrae.

The diameter of the trachea is assessed by dividing its value by the height of the thoracic inlet, which is measured on a lateral projection. The height of the thoracic inlet is measured from the ventral border of the spine at the level of the centre of the most cranial rib, to the dorsal border of the manubrium of the sternum where it is thinnest. The diameter of the trachea is measured between the internal aspect of the dorsal border and the internal aspect of the ventral border of the wall, perpendicularly to the longitudinal axis of the trachea and where the line of measurement of the height of the thoracic inlet crosses the trachea (fig. 3.20). This parameter varies depending on the dog or cat breed (Table 3.1). In young animals (under 1 year of age), the normal value is slightly lower than in adults.

A poor position of the neck or head when taking a lateral radiograph may cause the trachea to be flexed,

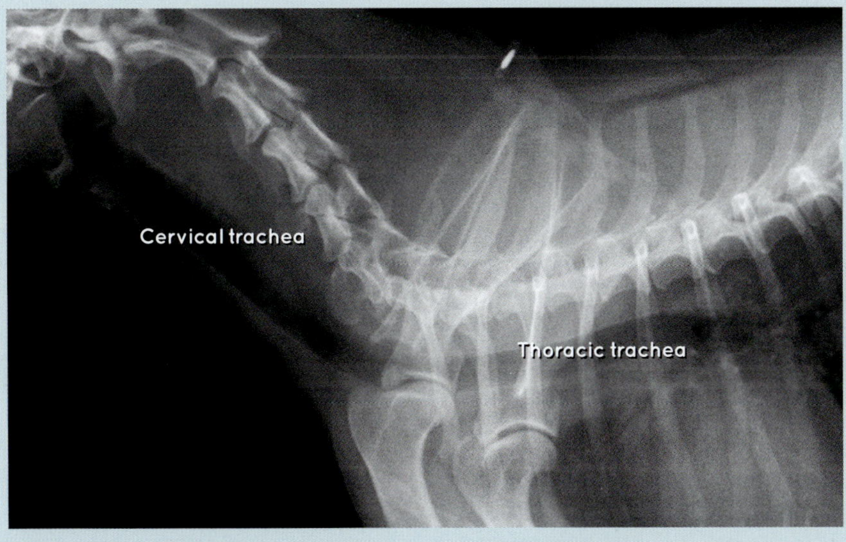

FIGURE 3.19. Normal radiographic image of the trachea of a dog. In order to evaluate its whole course, the cervical and thoracic part should be included in the same image, as long as the size of the patient allows it. In medium and large-sized dogs, radiographs of the two regions have to be taken separately (due to the size of the animal and to differences in exposure values). The identification microchip appears dorsal to the scapulae.

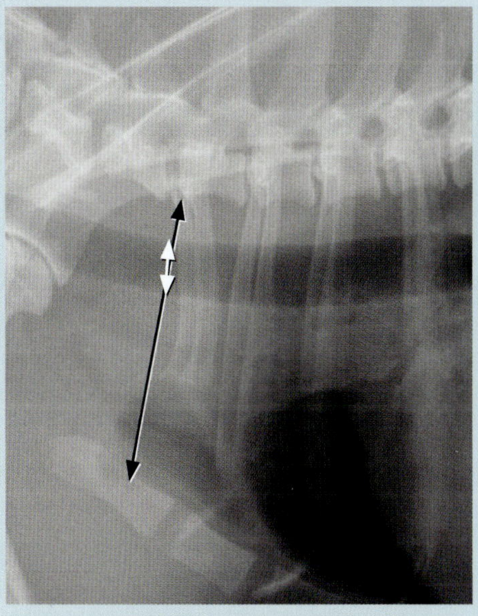

FIGURE 3.20. Enlarged image of the thoracic inlet on a lateral radiograph of a healthy dog. The diameter of the trachea is evaluated using the ratio between the diameter of the trachea (white arrow) and the height of the thoracic inlet (black arrow). The height of the thoracic inlet is measured from the ventral border of the spine at the level of the centre of the most cranial rib, to the dorsal border of the manubrium of the sternum where it is thinnest. The diameter of the trachea is measured between the internal aspect of the dorsal border and the internal aspect of the ventral border of the wall, perpendicularly to the longitudinal axis of the trachea, where the line of measurement of the height of the thoracic inlet crosses the trachea. In dogs, this parameter varies depending on the breed.

TABLA 3.1. Tracheal diameter assessment in certain dog and cat breeds.

	Race and typology	Normal tracheal diameter/height of the thoracic inlet ratio
Dogs	Intermediate conformation or deep and narrow thorax	0.21 ± 0.03
	Bulldog	0.10 ± 0.03
	Other brachycephalic dog breeds	0.16 ± 0.03
Cats	Common European Cat	0.18
	Persian Cat	0.20

which should not be mistaken for a real displacement of this organ caused by adjacent masses. The trachea will also be falsely elevated if the median plane of the thorax is very inclined on the X-ray table when the radiograph is taken. This is corrected by placing a radiolucent wedge underneath the sternum.

An image of apparent tracheal collapse may be seen in obese animals, due to the accumulation of fat around the trachea, especially at the level of the thoracic inlet. On dorsoventral and ventrodorsal radiographs, the trachea appears superimposed with the spine, perfectly centred or slightly to the right of the median line, but never to its left in normal conditions. In obese animals, the trachea may be clearly located on the right side. The tracheobronchial bifurcation, on the other hand, should always be located on the median line.

Calcification of the tracheal rings is frequently observed in older animals and patients with Cushing's syndrome, but this finding alone has no pathological significance.

The most common abnormality affecting the trachea is **tracheal collapse**, defined as the focal narrowing of the windpipe that occurs in relation to the respiratory cycle. This narrowing occurs dorsoventrally, hence only a lateral projection is useful for its diagnosis. Collapse can occur anywhere along the trachea from the middle of the cervical area to the carina. Collapse of the thoracic segment (fig. 3.21) is generally more marked during expiration, while collapse of the cervical part and thoracic inlet (fig. 3.22) is more pronounced during inspiration. Coughing fits can accentuate the collapse of the intrathoracic trachea.

It is usually diagnosed in middle-aged or senior dogs of small and miniature breeds. As this is a dynamic process, fluoroscopy is the most suitable radiological technique for diagnosis (see video 3.3). Failing this, one X-ray (including the cervical and thoracic portions of the trachea) could be performed on inspiration and another on expiration, although in practice it is difficult to adjust the moment of the shot with the respiratory cycle.

It is important to bear in mind that some healthy animals, especially small and miniature breed dogs, may have a slacker dorsal tracheal membrane and thinner tracheal rings, which causes a variation in the tracheal diameter that is manifested in the following way: during inspiration, the diameter of the cervical trachea is slightly reduced and that of the thoracic trachea increases, while during expiration, the diameter of the cervical trachea is slightly reduced and that of the cervical part increases. However, in normal conditions, this variation should be minimal. On radiographs, the collapse may be graded according to whether the reduction of the diameter of the trachea reaches 25 %, 50 %, 75 % or from 90 % to 100 %. This grading scale is similar to that used in bronchoscopy, in which the collapse is classified as grade 1 (mild) when the diameter reduction reaches 25 %, grade 2 (moderate), when it reaches 50 %, grade 3 (severe) with it is reduced by 75 % and grade 4 (total) when it is total. A 25% diameter reduction or less is not considered significant (note that the diameter of the normal trachea may vary slightly between inspiration and expiration). A moderate degree of tracheal collapse is frequently observed in small and miniature breed senior dogs with no evidence of significant clinical signs.

A fluoroscopic examination in patients with suspected tracheal collapse should examine the entire trachea over several respiratory cycles. It is also recommended to induce coughing (e.g. closing the mouth and plugging the nostrils).

In patients with clinical signs suggestive of tracheal collapse, special attention should be paid to the image of the bronchial bifurcation and the larger lobar bronchi, as collapse of these bronchi can occur together with tracheal collapse or as a single alteration. Fluoroscopy is the most suitable technique for evaluating **bronchial collapse** (see video 3.4) with or without associated tracheal collapse. Bronchial collapse can also

Video 3.3.
Dynamic radiography of a dog with **tracheal collapse**

Video 3.4.
Dynamic radiography of a dog with **bronchial collapse**

vary within the respiratory cycle and is usually most evident in fluoroscopy when cough is induced.

Cats rarely suffer from tracheal collapse caused by degeneration of the cartilages. If cervical tracheal collapse is observed in a cat, the possibility of an upper airway obstruction should be considered as this may cause a significant increase in the inspiratory effort and create enough negative intratracheal pressure to collapse the lumen.

Tracheal stenosis is defined as a localised and permanent narrowing of the trachea, not associated with the respiratory cycle, which differentiates it from tracheal collapse. It does not usually cause any clinical signs, unless the reduction of the diameter exceeds 80 %. It usually occurs as a result of previous tracheal lesions, often from bites, foreign bodies or tracheal intubation procedures, although it may also have a congenital aetiology, especially in small breeds.

Focal narrowing of the trachea may also be due to external compression, for example, due to major mediastinal lesions (fig. 3.23). In these cases, narrowing of the lumen is usually accompanied by tracheal displacement.

The presence of a band of soft tissue density in the dorsal area of the trachea, between the middle of the cervical and the middle of the thoracic portion, may be due to the visualisation of the dorsal tracheal membrane, which can be attributed to its redundancy (redundant dorsal tracheal membrane), but also to a contraction or invagination of this membrane. The degree of narrowing may even vary with the respiratory cycle, as in the case of tracheal collapse, making it difficult to distinguish between both processes. In cases of redundant dorsal membrane, contraction or invagination of the membrane, the dorsal margin of the tracheal wall maintains a normal position (fig. 3.24), while in cases of collapse this margin appears displaced. However, in practice, it is not always possible to clearly establish this differentiation. Other causes of increased dorsal tracheal radiopacity include ventral displacement of the oesophagus plus tracheal rotation or overlapping of the oesophagus with the trachea.

Tracheal hypoplasia is a congenital disorder characterised by a uniform reduction in the diameter of the entire trachea, from the larynx to the carina, due to incomplete or abnormal development of the

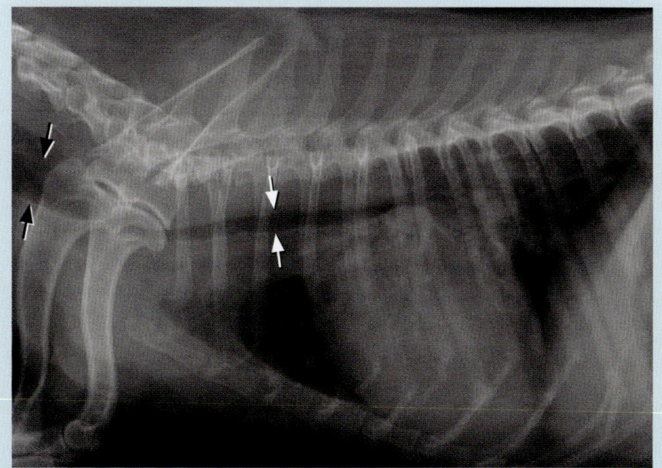

FIGURE 3.21. Lateral radiograph of the thorax and thoracic inlet of a dog with thoracic tracheal collapse. The reduction of the diameter exceeds 50 % (approximately 65 %). The diameter in the area of narrowing is shown with white arrows and the normal diameter of the cervical trachea with black arrows.

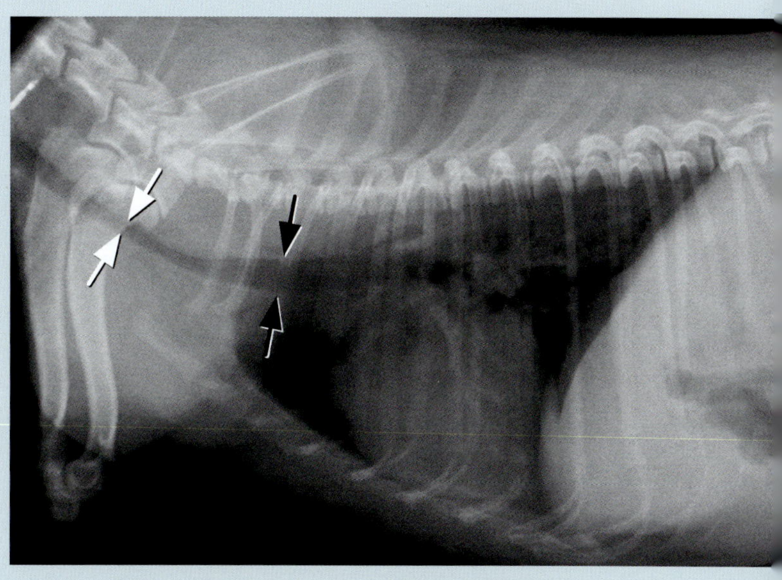

FIGURE 3.22. Lateral radiograph of the thorax and thoracic inlet of a dog with cervical tracheal collapse. The reduction of the diameter reaches 50 %. The diameter in the area of narrowing is indicated with white arrows and the normal diameter of the thoracic trachea is indicated with black arrows.

cartilaginous rings. Only very rarely does it affect a single segment of the trachea. Although more common in brachycephalic breeds (fig. 3.25), it can also appear in other breeds on an exceptional basis. It is important to calculate the tracheal diameter to thoracic inlet ratio to avoid subjective evaluations that may lead to misdiagnosis, especially in bulldog breeds (fig. 3.26). Patients with tracheal hypoplasia may also have other congenital abnormalities such as soft palate elongation, megaoesophagus or congenital heart defects.

Tracheal tears are caused by trauma or incorrect intubation. Following an anaesthetic procedure, a tracheal rupture should be suspected when progressive subcutaneous emphysema develops, which may affect the chest and abdomen. This emphysema will be evident on an X-ray, as well as signs of pneumomediastinum (fig. 3.27), which can spread to the abdomen and cause pneumoperitoneum or pneumoretroperitoneum. Pneumothorax may occur if it is accompanied by injury to the lung or pleura.

In cats, it may cause an **avulsion** of the trachea due to traumas involving a severe extension of the head and neck. Paradoxically, the animal may be taken to the veterinary practice several days or even weeks after the

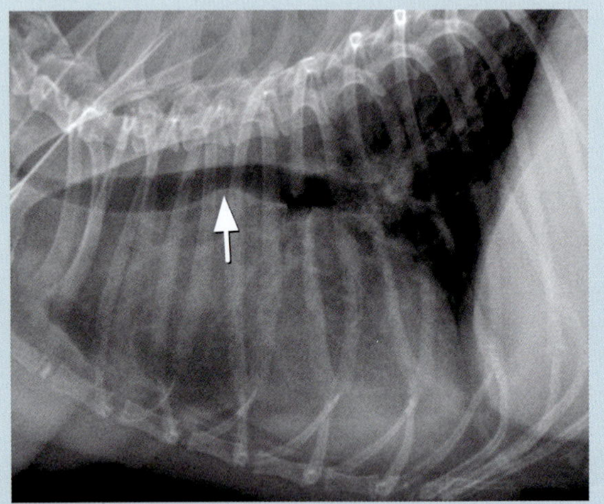

FIGURE 3.23. Lateral projection of the thorax of a dog with focal narrowing of the trachea (arrow) caused by external compression due to the presence of a chemodectoma at the heart base.

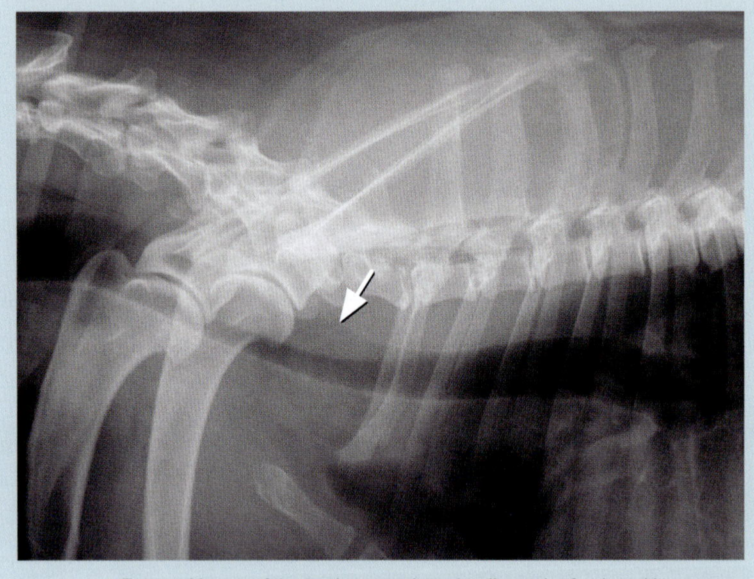

FIGURE 3.24. Enlarged image of the trachea on a lateral radiograph of a dog with clinical signs of respiratory abnormality. An apparent narrowing of the tracheal lumen is observed, extending from the central area of the cervical trachea to the central area of the thoracic trachea. However, a thin more radiopaque dorsal line compatible with the tracheal wall can be distinguished (arrow), which suggests that this finding is due to a redundancy of the dorsal tracheal membrane or to its contraction or invagination.

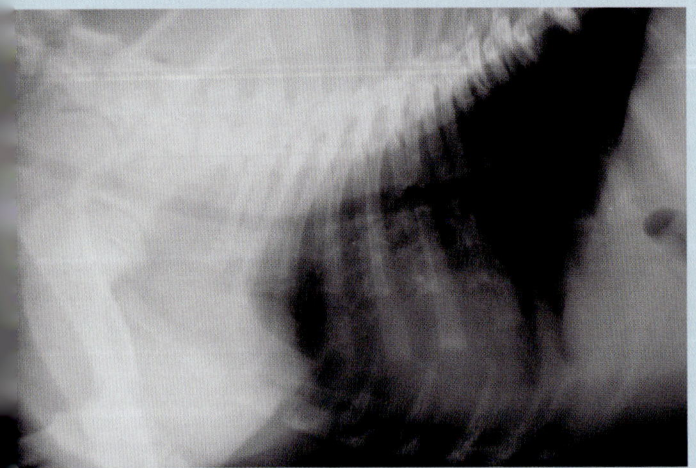

FIGURE 3.25. Lateral radiograph of the thorax of a Bulldog with tracheal hypoplasia. The ratio of the tracheal diameter to the height of the thoracic inlet is 0.07.

trauma occurred, when the subcutaneous emphysema or the pneumomediastinum may have disappeared. On radiographs, it is possible to observe severe focal dilatation of the trachea, which appears delimited by a thin wall formed by the intact adventitia or the surrounding mediastinal tissue.

Foreign bodies located in the trachea usually cause severe signs of respiratory obstruction. They may be

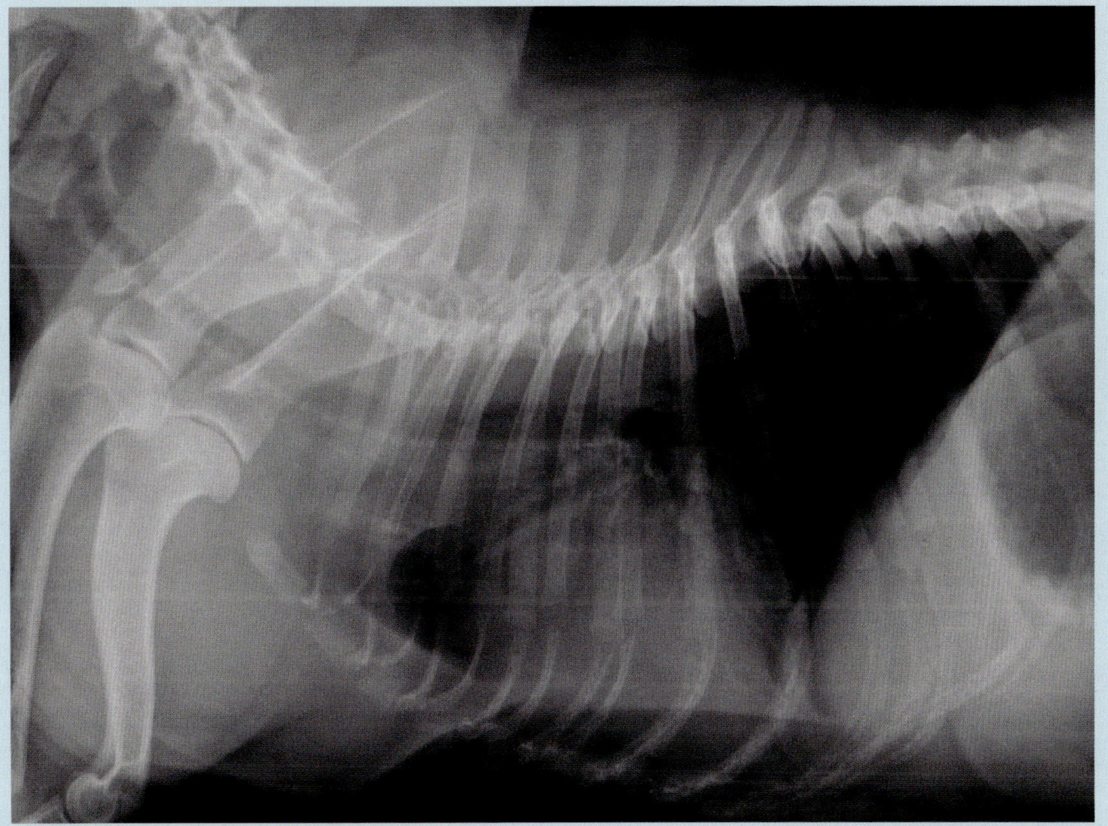

FIGURE 3.26. Lateral radiograph of the thorax of a Bulldog with no respiratory signs. The ratio of the diameter of the trachea to the height of the thoracic inlet is 0.11, which is considered to be within the limits of normality for this breed. The tracheal cartilages appear calcified (with no pathological significance).

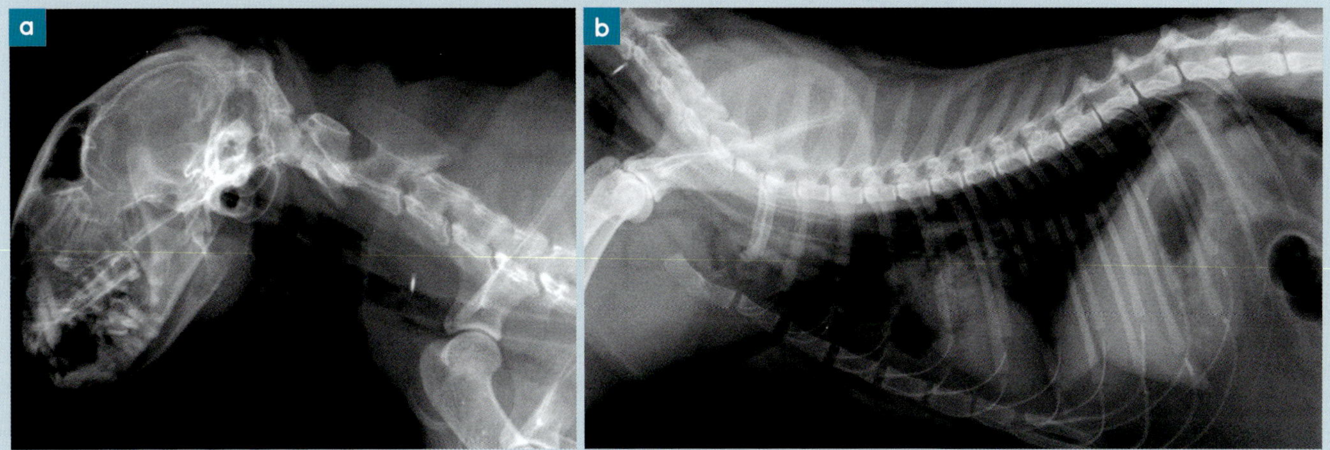

FIGURE 3.27. Lateral projections of the neck (a) and thorax (b) of a cat with subcutaneous cervical emphysema (bands of gas opacity dorsal and ventral to the pharynx and cervical trachea) and pneumomediastinum (band of gas opacity dorsal and ventral to the thoracic trachea) due to iatrogenic tracheal rupture following a tracheal intubation procedure.

identified or not on radiographs depending on their location, size and radiopacity. Radiopaque foreign bodies are easily identified, while radiolucent ones may or may not be identified depending on their shape. The accumulation of mucus around the foreign body creates focal areas of increased soft-tissue opacity at the site where it is located. These are usually found near the tracheal bifurcation.

Focal thickening of the tracheal wall may be due to neoplasms, granulomas (e.g. by *Oslerus osleri*), polyps or haematomas. More diffuse thickening may be due to tracheal haemorrhage caused by trauma or coagulopathy, or diffusely infiltrating neoplasms such as lymphoma, although rare. Inflammatory processes (tracheitis and tracheobronchitis) usually do not cause wall thickening that can be identified on an X-ray.

Computed tomography is an appropriate technique to evaluate and confirm cases of collapse, rupture, obstruction and mass in the trachea. Radiographs allow the follow-up of a tracheal stent in order to avoid any possible rupture, displacement or excessive formation of granulation tissue around it. However, computed tomography has the advantage of allowing the differentiation between excessive granulation tissue and accumulations of intraluminal fluid.

Oesophagus

Radiography is a valuable tool to diagnose diseases that affect the oesophagus. Lateral radiographs are usually used, since the oesophagus is superimposed with the spine and sternum on ventrodorsal and dorsoventral radiographs.

The normal oesophagus cannot usually be identified on plain radiographs, since it has the same radiographic density as most of the structures that surround it in the neck and mediastinum. Small accumulations of gas are sometimes visualised throughout its course (fig. 3.28), due to the swallowing of air in nervous patients or patients with respiratory difficulties. It is also common to observe, especially on left lateral projections, minimal fluid retention in the distal part of the oesophagus, just before its entry through the oesophageal hiatus of the diaphragm. This creates an elongated silhouette of soft-tissue density that appears centred between the course of the aorta and the course of the caudal vena cava on lateral radiographs (fig. 3.29). Non-significant, moderate oesophageal dilatation may be observed in anaesthetised patients (fig. 3.30) or in those in which an oesophageal catheter was placed.

Since the information provided by plain radiography is limited, contrast studies are often carried out to examine the oesophagus. Barium is usually used in the form of a paste or mixed with food, so as to slow down the passage of the contrast medium through the oesophagus, as it is very fast in normal conditions, especially when it is liquid. The administration of barium in the form of a paste is useful to examine the mucosa, because it adheres to it. It is usually used when oesophagitis or neoplasms are suspected, but it should not be used if the oesophageal study is going to be accompanied by a gastrointestinal study, as the paste does not fill the stomach or the intestine properly, and does not mix well with liquid barium if this is administered at the same time. Liquid suspensions of barium sulphate at a dose of 3 to 5 ml/kg do not adhere to the mucosa as well as the paste, but they easily surround obstructions. It is sometimes necessary to administer an additional amount to delimit the whole oesophagus when this is very dilated.

Barium should not be used when an oesophageal perforation or rupture is suspected, since it may lead to the formation of granulomas if it extravasates. In these cases, hyperosmotic, water-soluble iodinated contrast media may be used, such as meglumine amidotrizoate, or low-osmolarity organic iodinated contrast media, such as iohexol or iopamidol, at a dose of 7 ml/kg. Although the image of the oesophagus is more poorly defined with these contrast media than with barium, they would be absorbed if they extravasated, while barium would not. Despite their higher cost, it is recommended to use low-osmolarity contrast media. Hypertonic contrast media, due to their osmotic effects, may cause pulmonary oedema if they are aspirated or, if they are used in animals with hypovolaemia, the clinical status of the patient may worsen due to the loss of fluid through the gastrointestinal tract.

After administering barium, a temporary retention of the contrast medium may be observed between the folds of the oesophageal mucosa, which creates an image of parallel longitudinal bands in dogs. In addition to these longitudinal bands, transverse bands are also observed in the caudal third of the thoracic oesophagus in cats, which has been termed "herringbone" pattern. A minimal temporary retention of barium at the level of the pharynx or thoracic inlet may also be observed in normal conditions.

It is possible to examine functional anomalies of the oesophagus by means of fluoroscopy, as it allows real-time observation of the passage of the contrast medium from the oropharynx to the stomach (see video 3.5). It is recommended to first administer liquid barium and then solid food mixed with barium. This is particularly useful to diagnose stenosis or regional motility disorders.

Video 3.5.
Dynamic radiography of **normal transit through the oesophagus** of positive iodinated contrast mixed with food in a dog

The term **megaoesophagus** is used to describe an abnormal dilatation of the oesophagus, generally

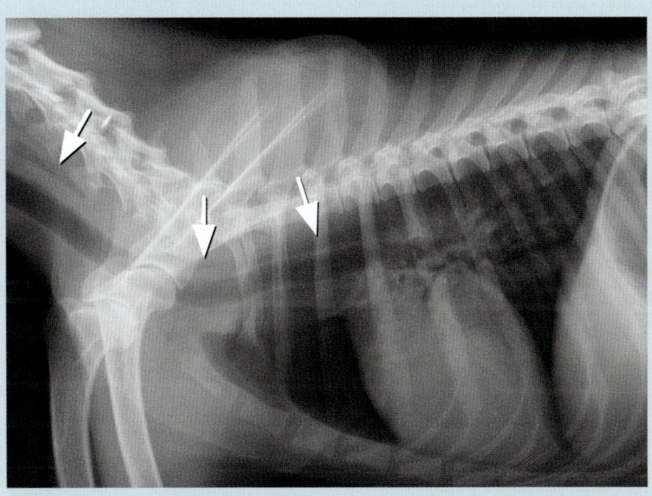

FIGURE 3.28. Lateral radiograph of the thorax and caudal area of the neck of a healthy dog. The normal oesophagus cannot be identified on plain radiographs, since it has the same radiographic density as most of the structures that surround it in the neck and mediastinum, but in this case, some small accumulations of gas in its lumen (arrows) allow the identification of its course. This finding is relatively usual in nervous patients or patients with respiratory difficulties because they swallow air. If the gas retention persists on consecutive radiographs, this may be indicative of a disease (for example, oesophagitis).

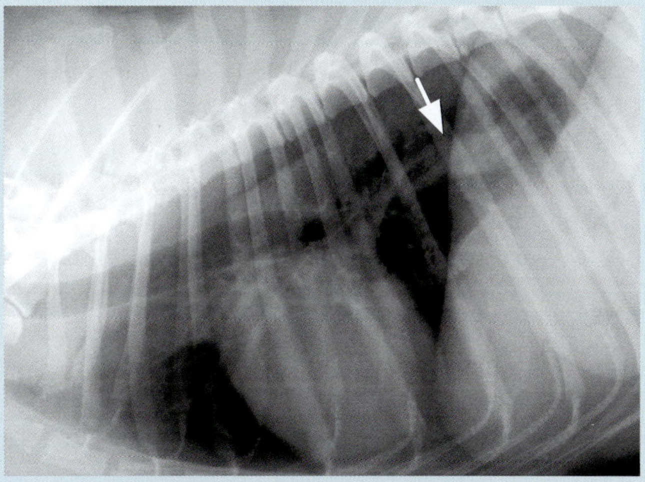

FIGURE 3.29. Lateral projection of the thorax of a healthy dog showing the silhouette of the caudal third of the thoracic oesophagus with minimal fluid retention of no pathological significance (arrow).

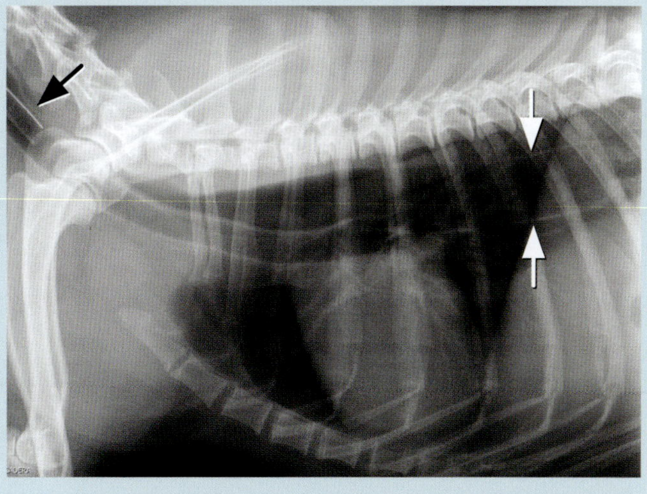

FIGURE 3.30. Lateral radiograph of the thorax of a dog with moderate dilatation of the oesophagus due to the anaesthesia. The dorsal and ventral walls of the oesophagus are indicated by white arrows and the endotracheal tube is shown with a black arrow.

associated with hypomotility of the wall. The dilatation is usually identified by means of plain radiography, although an oesophagogram may be indicated to confirm the diagnosis in case of doubt, to examine oesophageal motility (using fluoroscopy) or to detect the possible cause of the megaoesophagus. On both plain lateral and ventrodorsal or dorsoventral radiographs, it is possible to identify two thin lines of soft-tissue density in the area of the oesophagus. These lines converge in the diaphragm and correspond to the dilated oesophageal wall (fig. 3.31). These lines are clearly differentiated when the oesophagus is filled with gas but may also be identified when it contains fluid or food (fig. 3.32). The ventral line is sometimes masked by the superimposed caudal vena cava. When dilation is very pronounced, the trachea and cardiac silhouette may appear to be displaced ventrally (fig. 3.33). Ventral tracheal displacement is sometimes the only finding evident on the plain X-ray. On ventrodorsal or dorsoventral views, a moderately dilated oesophagus may be masked by the superimposed spine, although it is common to see a displacement of the trachea to the right. In patients with a megaoesophagus, special attention must be paid to the image of the lung fields, as aspiration pneumonia can often be detected (fig. 3.34).

Oesophagitis does not usually cause significant changes on plain radiographs, although a persistent retention of gas in the oesophageal lumen is sometimes observed. The oesophagogram may show an irregular retention of barium between the folds of the mucosa, which is accompanied by diffuse and non-uniform dilatation of the oesophagus.

Foreign bodies located in the lumen of the oesophagus are a common cause of oesophageal dysphagia. The most common sites where oesophageal foreign bodies are observed are:

- Upper oesophageal sphincter.
- Thoracic inlet.
- Base of the heart.
- Area cranial to the diaphragm.

It is easy to recognise radiopaque foreign bodies (fig. 3.35), but the diagnosis may be more complicated in cases of radiolucent ones. On the oesophago-gram, an accumulation of contrast medium is often observed cranial to the foreign body, although the contrast medium may also be absorbed if the object is porous. Foreign bodies may also cause a partial or complete

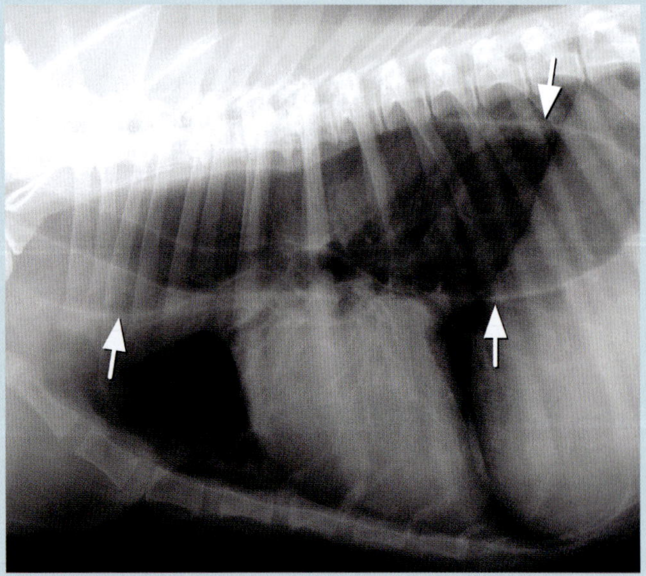

FIGURE 3.31. Lateral radiograph of the thorax a dog with a megaoesophagus. The walls of the oesophagus are shown with white arrows. The trachea appears slightly displaced in ventral direction.

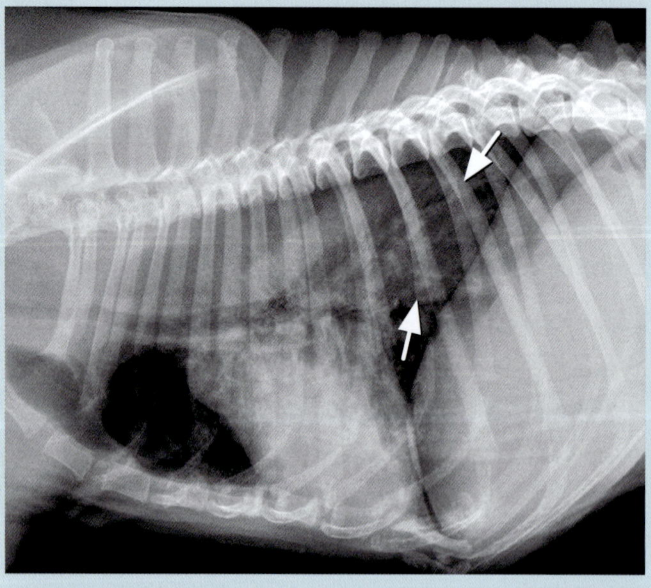

FIGURE 3.32. Lateral projection of the thorax of a dog with fluid-filled megaoesophagus. The arrows point to the dorsal and ventral margins of the dilated distal oesophagus.

obstruction or no obstruction at all. The complications associated with oesophageal foreign bodies are perforation and stenosis due to scarring**. Diverticula** are defined as localised dilatations of the oesophagus and are identified on radiographs by the focal accumulation of gas or granular material (food) in the oesophagus. By administrating a contrast medium, it is possible to determine the size and exact location of the lesion. When they are located in the cranial mediastinum, the diverticulum is usually seen ventral to the trachea (fig. 3.36).

An oesophageal image that may be confused with a diverticulum is sometimes referred to as a **redundant oesophagus**, which is characterised by the appearance of folds or kinks in the cranial portion of the thoracic oesophagus. In young dogs or short-necked brachycephalic breeds, this could just be a normal individual variation without clinical significance, but it could also be accompanied by altered motility in this segment, so fluoroscopy is recommended to determine the degree of significance of this finding (see video 3.6).

Stenoses are localised narrowings of the oesophageal lumen (fig. 3.37). They may appear as a result of the previous presence of a foreign body at the site where the stenosis is located, associated with anomalies of the vascular rings or with tumours, and in cases of oesophagitis due to reflux. An oesophagogram is necessary for their diagnosis. A normal peristaltic oesophageal contraction should not be mistaken for stenosis in static images. They can be differentiated by means of fluoroscopy or, if it is not available, by taking several radiographs at different times to observe whether the narrowing remains in the image.

Congenital anomalies of the vascular rings cause an external compression of the oesophagus. The most common is the persistence of the right aortic arch, which occurs more frequently in dogs than in cats. It is usually diagnosed in young animals with regurgitation. These anomalies usually cause localised oesophageal dilatation in the cranial mediastinum, cranial to the heart, which can be confirmed with a contrast study

Video 3.6. Videofluoroscopic examination of a dog with **redundant oesophagus**

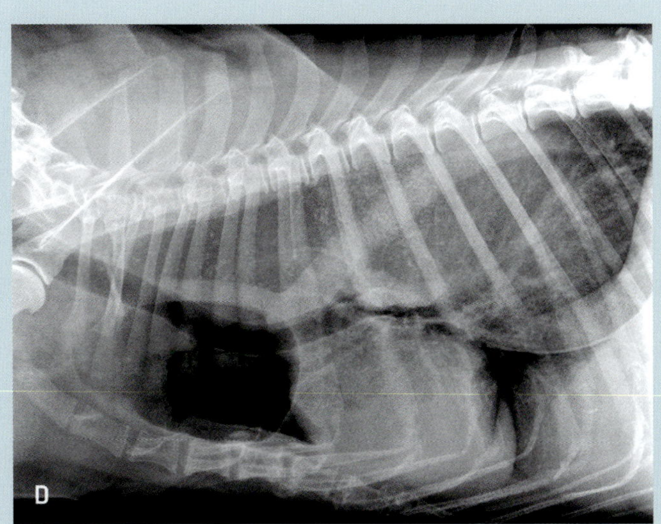

FIGURE 3.33. Lateral radiograph of the thorax a dog with a megaoesophagus. The degree of oesophageal dilation is very marked. There is a high gas and fluid content in the oesophagus, as well as radiopaque granular material. The trachea and heart appear slightly displaced in ventral direction.

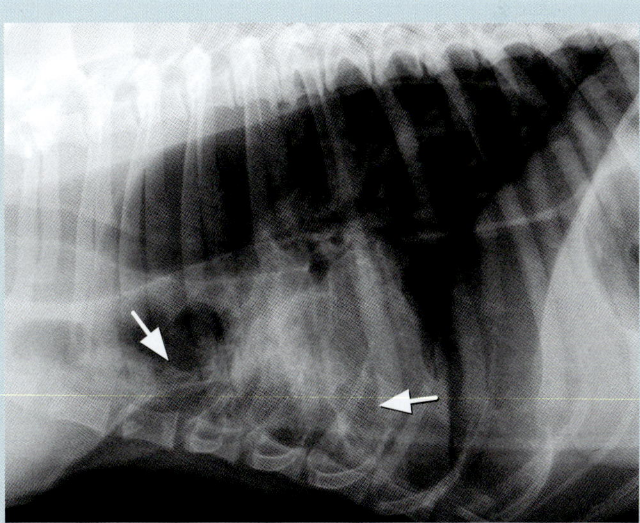

FIGURE 3.34. Lateral projection of the thorax of a dog with megaoesophagus and secondary aspiration pneumonia (arrows), located in the cranioventral portion of the lung.

(fig. 3.38) (see video 3.7). The image of the caudal oesophagus at the base of the heart is usually normal, although it may sometimes appear dilated. Persistent retention of food is often observed in the dilated area.

Oesophageal masses may correspond to benign or malignant neoplasms or to inflammatory masses. Oesophageal masses are rare in small animals.

Video 3.7.
Videofluoroscopic examination with focal dilation of the oesophagus due to **persistence of the fourth aortic arch**

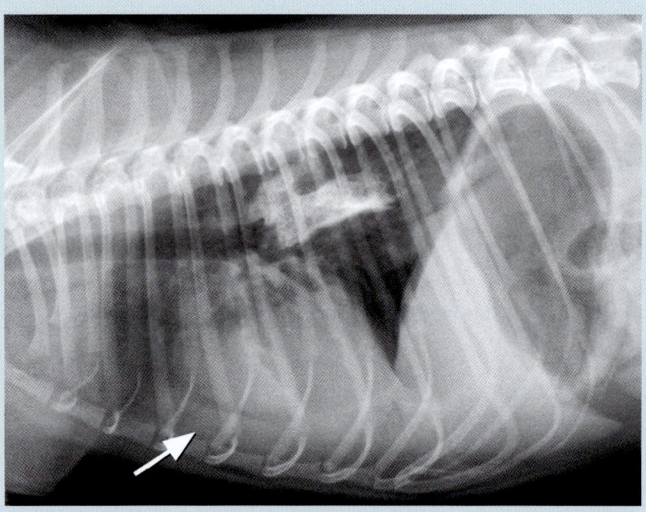

FIGURE 3.35. Lateral projection of the thorax of a dog with a mineral density foreign body (bone) in the oesophagus. The band of soft tissue/fluid density in the ventral portion of the chest (arrow) and masking part of the cranial margin and the apex of the heart is due to the presence of fluid in the mediastinum as a result of mediastinitis following perforation of the oesophageal wall by the foreign body.

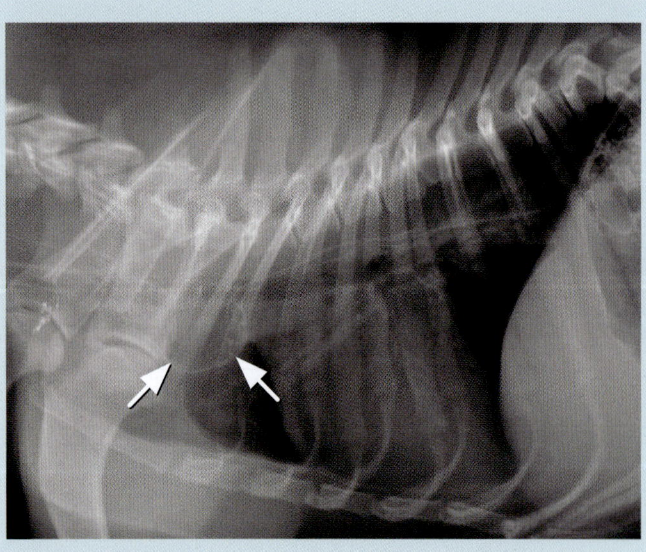

FIGURE 3.36. Lateral oesophagogram of a dog with an oesophageal diverticulum located in the cranial mediastinum, after the administration of barium.

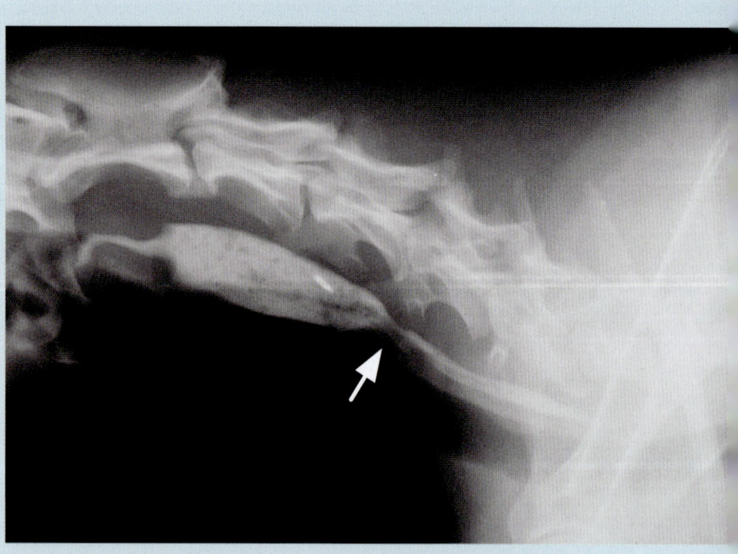

FIGURE 3.37. Lateral oesophagogram showing the neck of a dog with oesophageal stenosis (arrow), after the administration of barium. This image may be confused with that of a peristaltic wave and the persistence of the lesion must therefore be confirmed, either by means of fluoroscopy or by repeating the radiograph at different times.

On plain radiographs, it is possible to observe accumulations of food or associated diverticula, and soft-tissue opacity masses in some cases. A narrowed area is usually identified in contrast studies, with or without mucosal irregularity (fig. 3.39).

An oesophageal **perforation** may be suspected on a plain radiograph if there is subcutaneous emphysema of unknown origin in the neck, or signs of pneumomediastinum in the thorax. It may sometimes be accompanied by a pneumothorax, mediastinal effusion or pleural effusion. The diagnosis is confirmed by administering an iodinated contrast medium, which will be extravasated, although its identification may be difficult if the perforation is small. In case of doubt, fluoroscopy may facilitate the diagnosis.

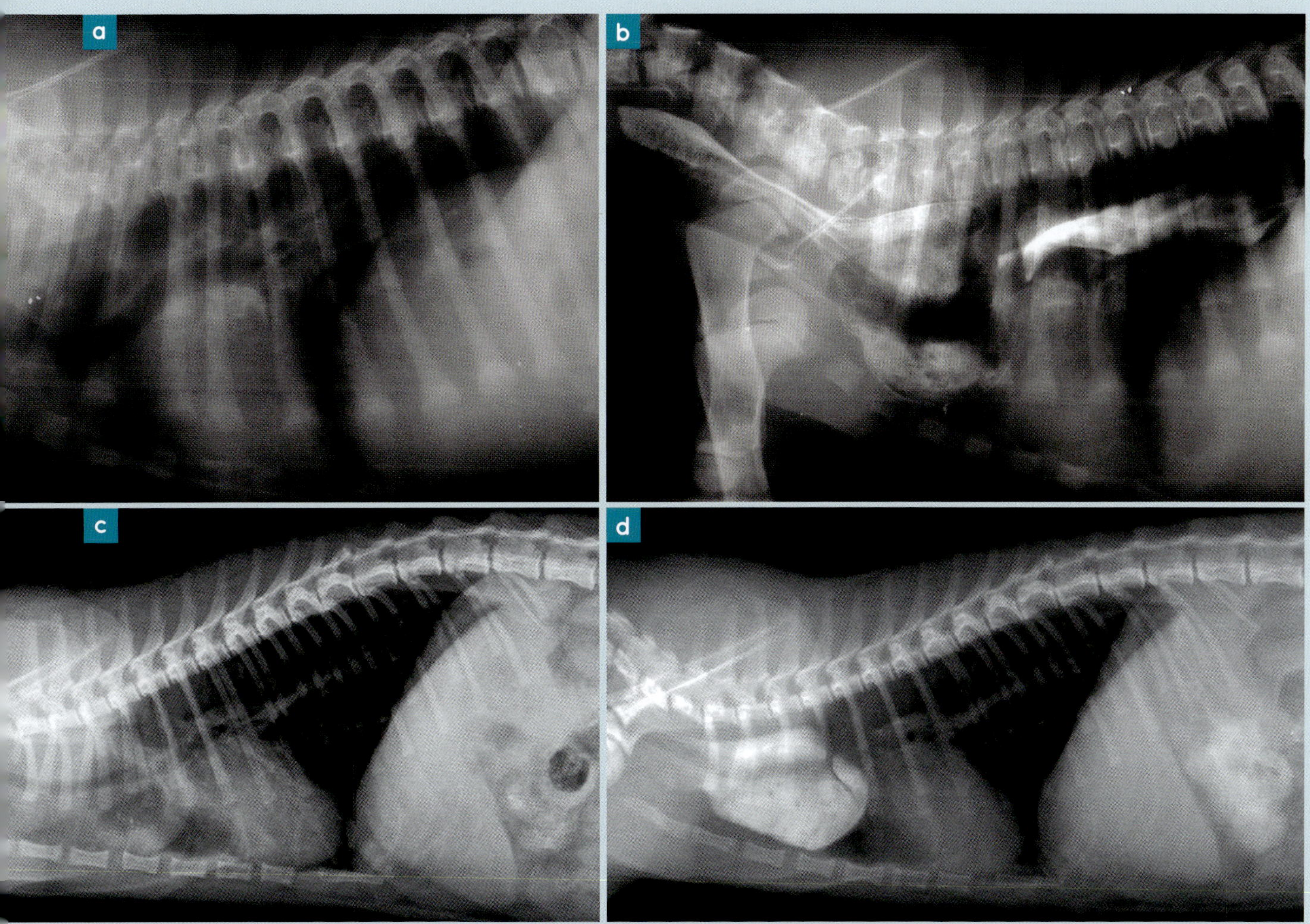

FIGURE 3.38. Lateral views of the chest of a 2-month-old dog before (a) and after (b) barium administration, and of a 5-month-old cat, before (c) and after (d) barium administration. There is marked focal dilation of the oesophagus cranial to the heart in both patients. This finding suggests the existence of a congenital anomaly of the vascular rings (the persistence of the right aortic arch is the most frequent anomaly), which causes external compression of the oesophagus at the level of the base of the heart. This condition is relatively common in dogs and very rare in cats. In image (a) the only radiographic sign indicative of oesophageal dilation is the marked ventral curvature of the trachea. In image (c), the dilated oesophagus with liquid, gaseous and granular contents could be confused with a non-oesophageal lung or mediastinal injury, given the central distribution of the gas and the peripheral distribution of the fluid.
Images (c) and (d) courtesy of María José Ruiz Fernández.

Fistulae may form between the oesophageal lumen and the respiratory system, although they are uncommon. The origin of the site of communication may be oesophagotracheal, oesophagobronchial or oesophagopulmonary. On oesophagograms, their image may be similar to that created when a contrast medium administrated by oral route is accidentally inhaled.

Hiatal hernias are usually transitory and may be associated with respiratory movements. They are difficult to diagnose on plain radiographs, in which case contrast and fluoroscopy studies are used. In the most evident cases, the stomach (with its characteristic folds) or part of it may be identified in the thorax (fig. 3.40). In other cases, a less defined soft-tissue density structure is visualised in the caudodorsal part of the thorax, and may disappear on subsequent radiographs. In contrast studies, part of the stomach is identified in the thorax (see video 3.8), although it may move in and out of the thoracic cavity with respiratory movements.

Gastrooesophageal invagination or intussusception is an uncommon alteration. The stomach or part of it moves into the lumen of the oesophagus, thus originating an anomalous shadow in the caudodorsal part of the thorax. If a contrast study is performed, the contrast medium may not reach the stomach and may delimit a large intraluminal oesophageal mass instead. In some cases, the intussuception appears intermittently.

Gastrooesophageal reflux occurs when stomach acids enter the oesophagus, which usually causes oesophagitis. Plain radiographs do not usually show any significant findings, although focal dilatation of the distal oesophagus with accumulation of gas or fluid is sometimes detected (fig. 3.41).

Video 3.8. Videofluoroscopic examination of a dog with **hiatal hernia**

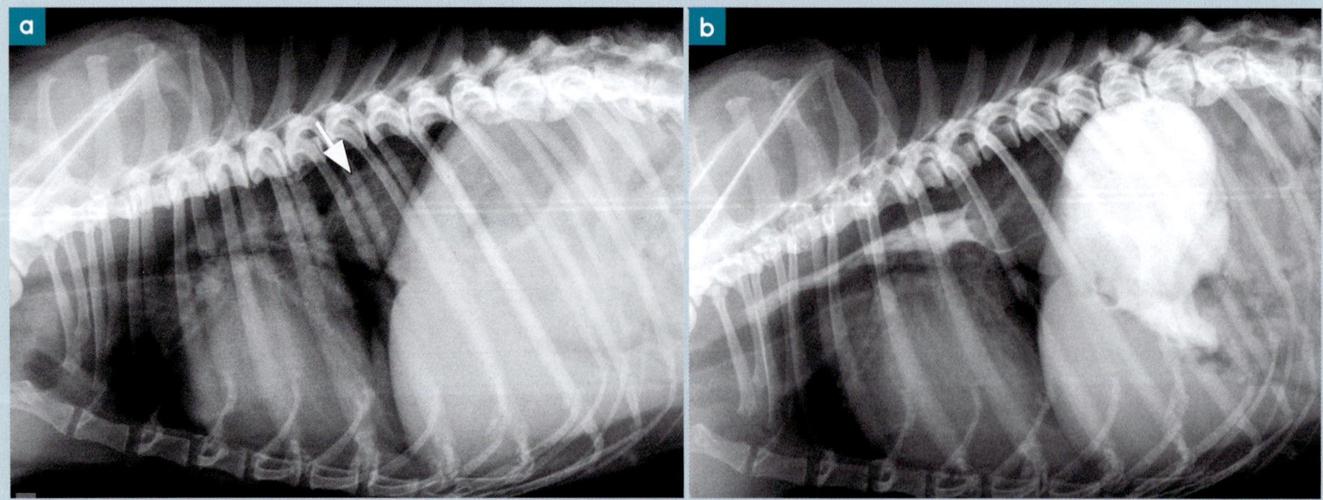

FIGURE 3.39. Lateral projection of the chest (a) and positive air oesophagogram in lateral projection (b) of a dog with an oesophageal neoplasm. On the plain X-ray, the mass (arrow) shows a rounded morphology, soft tissue opacity located in the dorsocaudal area of the chest, where it could be confused with a mass of pulmonary origin. After administration of contrast, moderate retention of the contrast immediately cranial to the mass is observed, as well as a marked deviation and reduction in the central portion of the oesophageal lumen diameter.

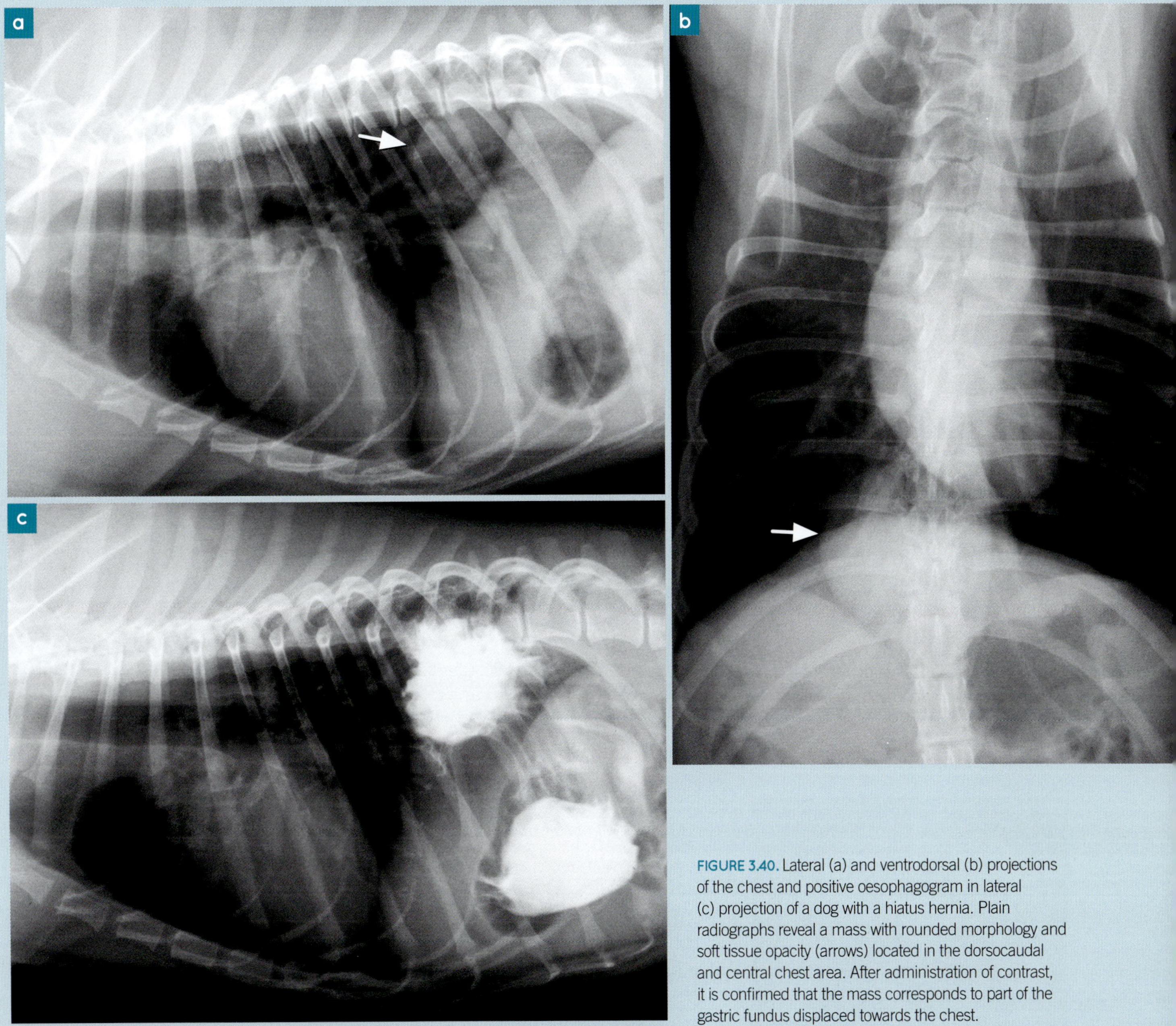

FIGURE 3.40. Lateral (a) and ventrodorsal (b) projections of the chest and positive oesophagogram in lateral (c) projection of a dog with a hiatus hernia. Plain radiographs reveal a mass with rounded morphology and soft tissue opacity (arrows) located in the dorsocaudal and central chest area. After administration of contrast, it is confirmed that the mass corresponds to part of the gastric fundus displaced towards the chest.

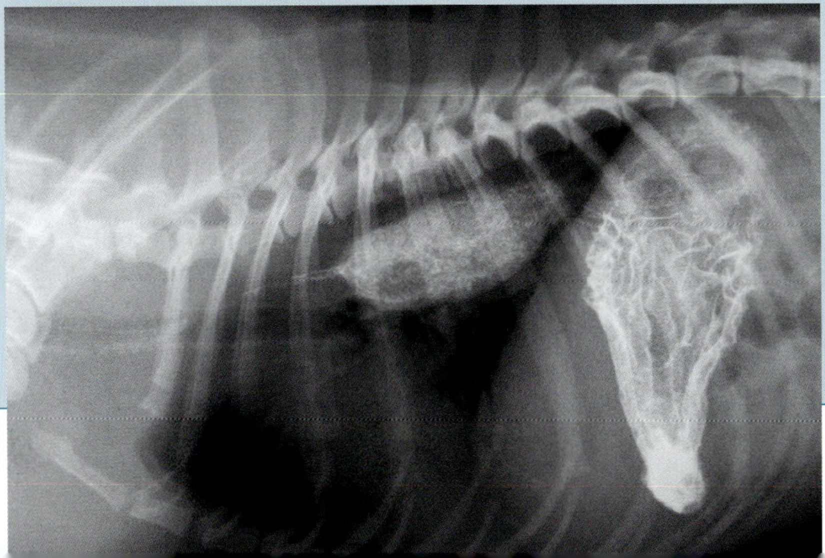

FIGURE 3.41. Positive oesophagogram in lateral projection of a dog with gastro-oesophageal reflux, which appears as a focal dilation of the distal thoracic oesophagus with accumulation of contrast (barium mixed with food).

Pleural space

The pleural space is the anatomical space included between the visceral and parietal layers of the pleura (fig. 3.42). The parietal pleura covers the internal aspect of the chest wall, the diaphragm and the mediastinum, and the visceral pleura covers the pulmonary surface and forms the interlobar fissures. It is a potential space, which, in normal conditions, contains a minimal amount of fluid that acts as a lubricant to minimise friction during breathing.

Plain radiography allows us to detect the presence of abnormal contents, which generally consist in fluid (pleural effusion) or gas (pneumothorax), in this anatomical space, as well as to identify masses of pleural origin. Calcifications and minimal pleural thickenings are usual findings in older animals and do not usually have any pathological significance.

Ultrasound examinations may provide diagnostic information of great interest in cases of effusion and pleural masses, but not in cases of pneumothorax, since the air contained in the pleural space is easily mistaken for that contained in the lungs. Moreover, this technique will facilitate sample collection for cytology or biopsy.

Computed tomography is also an excellent diagnostic alternative to assess the anomalies that affect this anatomical space.

Pleural effusion

In cases of severe pleural effusion, it is convenient to stabilise the patient first, before performing a radiographic study. Radiographs taken with the animal standing may be useful and, alternatively, the dorsoventral projection may be chosen in order not to worsen the state of the patient. If the respiratory involvement is not severe, a ventrodorsal is preferable to a dorsoventral radiograph, since there is greater fluid accumulation around the heart on the latter making visualisation of this organ more difficult (fig. 3.43 and 3.44), in addition to causing an enlargement of the mediastinum silhouette. On ventrodorsal radiographs, interlobar fissures will be better visualised in cases of mild or moderate effusion, since the fluid tends to enter in the fissures in dorsal recumbency, while it tends to accumulate dorsal to the sternum in sternal recumbency. If the respiratory

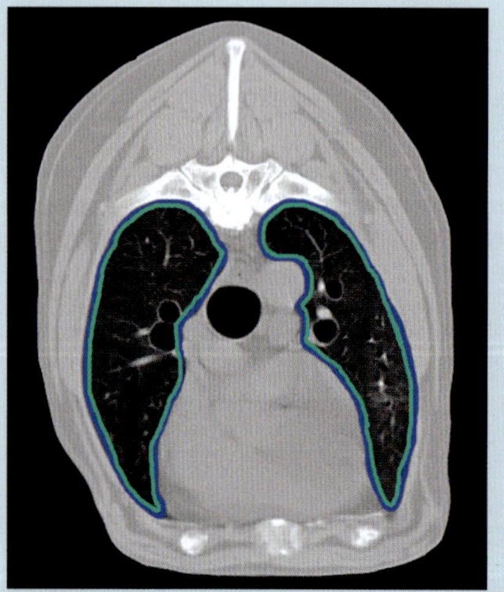

FIGURE 3.42. Representation of the parietal pleura (blue line) and visceral pleura (green line) on a computed tomography image of the thorax of a dog. In normal conditions, the pleural space is a potential anatomical space that only contains a minimal amount of fluid as a lubricant to minimise friction during breathing.

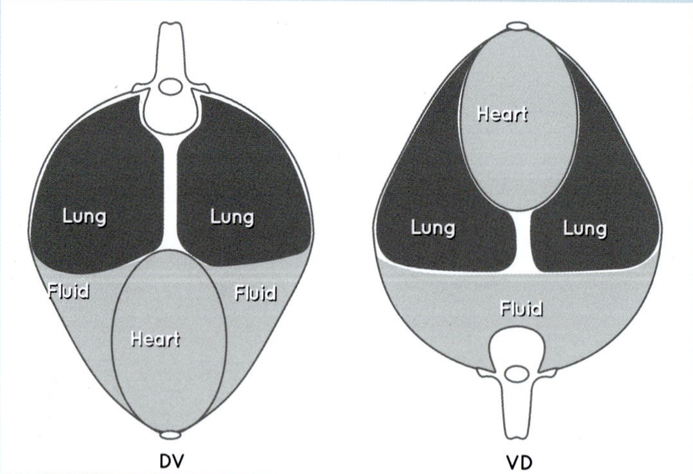

FIGURE 3.43. Schematic representation of the location of a moderate amount of pleural fluid when dorsoventral (DV) and ventrodorsal (VD) radiographs are taken. On the dorsoventral radiograph, the fluid is displaced to the ventral area of the thorax and surrounds the heart, so the cardiac silhouette is less defined. When a ventrodorsal radiograph is taken, the fluid moves to the roof of the thoracic cavity and is separated from the heart, so this latter will be better visualised in the image. In the case of a severe effusion, the cardiac silhouette is masked on both views.

involvement allows it, in these cases it is recommended to take, in addition, a lateral radiograph.

The radiological signs of a pleural effusion vary in function of the amount of fluid that accumulates. It could be transudate, exudate, blood or lymph, which are indistinguishable from each other on a radiograph. It starts to be detectable on radiographs from 50–100 ml. If the amount is very small, radiographs will only show thin bands of fluid density at the site of the interlobar fissures (fig. 3.45). As the amount of fluid increases, it is possible to observe retraction and rounding of the lung margins, which will appear separated from the thoracic wall by bands of fluid density. The cardiac silhouette and shadow of the diaphragm may appear partially or totally masked (fig. 3.46). If there is a very large amount of accumulated fluid, the

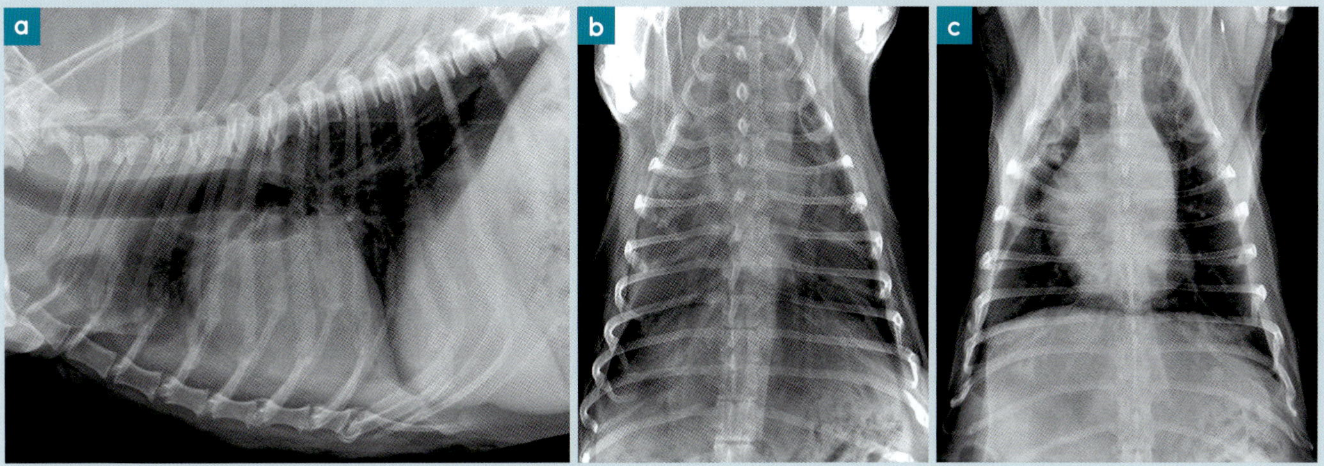

FIGURE 3.44. Lateral (a), dorsoventral (b) and ventrodorsal (c) projections of the chest of a dog with mild to moderate pleural effusion. If the patient's respiratory compromise is not severe, the ventrodorsal projection is preferred, as the signs of pleural effusion are better seen with this projection than with the dorsoventral projection. In dorsal recumbency, the fluid tends to enter the interlobular fissures, whereas in sternal recumbency it tends to accumulate dorsal to the sternum, somewhat masking the cardiac silhouette as occurs in image (b).

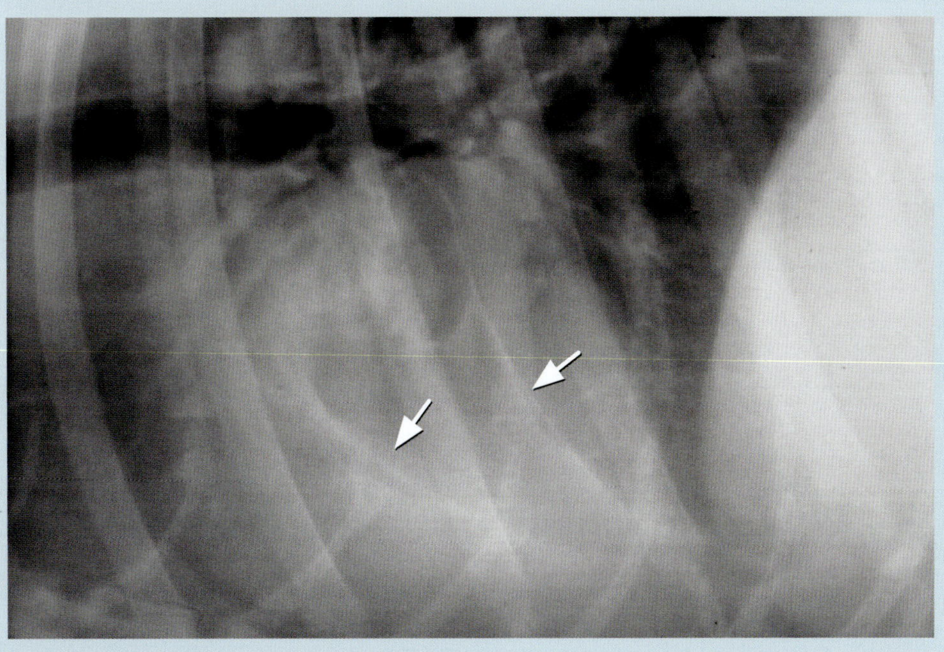

FIGURE 3.45. Enlarged image of the thorax on a lateral radiograph of a dog with mild pleural effusion. Thin bands of fluid/soft-tissue density that delimit the right middle lobe may be observed at the site of the interlobar fissures.

cardiac silhouette may be elevated and displace the trachea, which may give a false impression of cardiomegaly or mediastinal mass (fig. 3.47), although we must bear in mind that these conditions may coexist with a pleural effusion in some cases.

It is more common for the pleural effusion to be **bilateral** (fig. 3.48), as the fluid can pass from one hemithorax to another through the orifices in the mediastinum. However, if these orifices are no longer permeable, the effusion can be located in a single

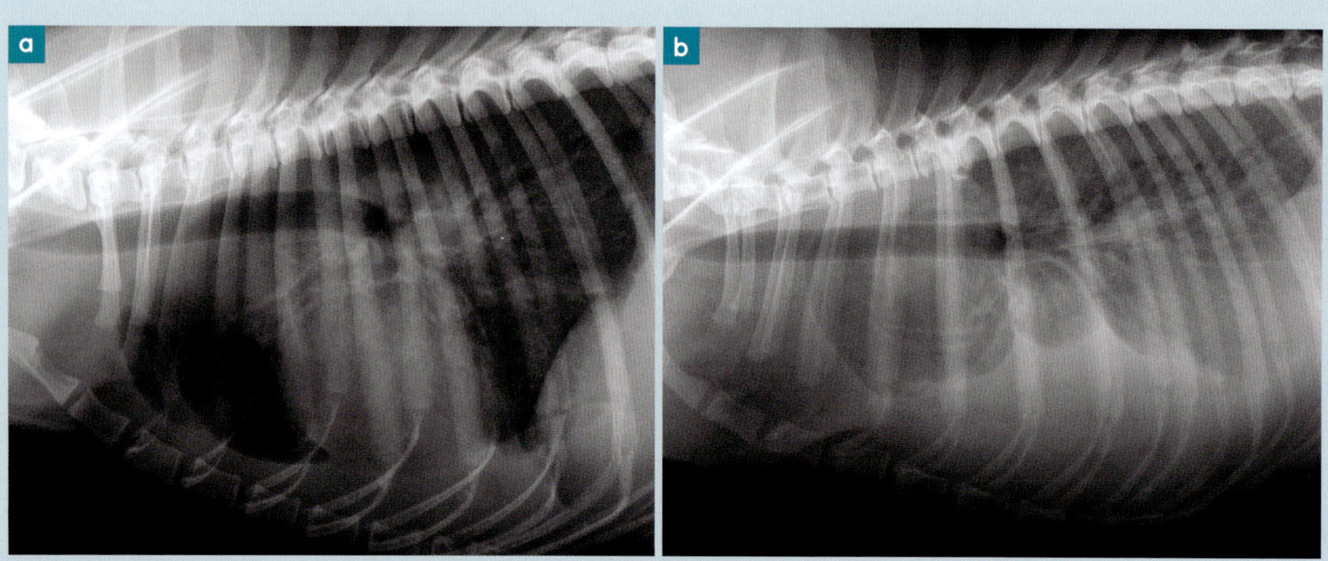

FIGURE 3.46. Lateral radiographs of the thorax of two dogs with pleural effusion, one moderate (a) and the other from moderate to severe (b). In both cases, the lung appears separated from the sternum by areas of fluid/soft-tissue density, but the degree of retraction and rounding of the lung margins is more marked in image (b). In image (a), only the ventral area of the cardiac silhouette and of the dome of the diaphragm is masked by the fluid, while in image (b), neither the cardiac silhouette nor most part of the shadow of the diaphragm can be visualised.

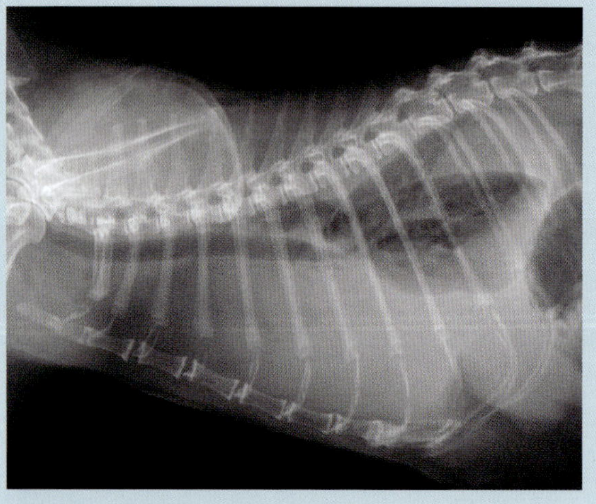

FIGURE 3.47. Lateral radiograph of a cat with a severe pleural effusion. The lungs are slightly distended and the trachea appears elevated. Most of the thoracic cavity has a practically homogeneous fluid/soft-tissue density and neither the cardiac silhouette nor the shadow of the diaphragm can be visualised in the image.

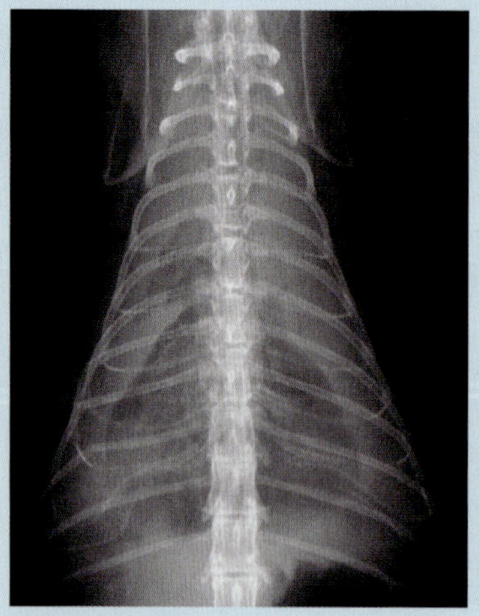

FIGURE 3.48. Dorsoventral radiograph of the thorax of a cat with severe bilateral pleural effusion. The fluid appears distributed in a more or less uniform manner between the two hemithoraces.

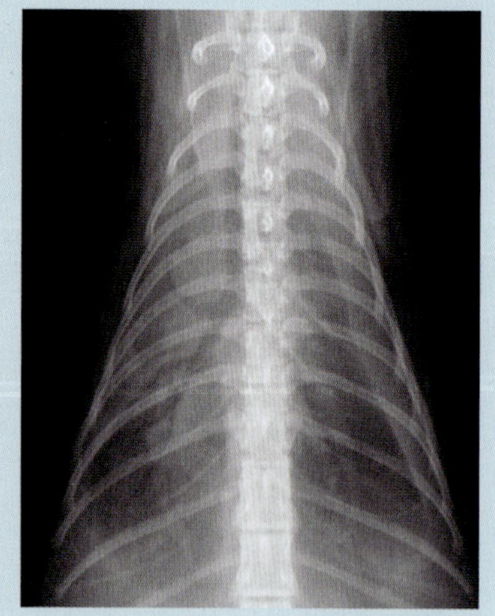

FIGURE 3.49. Dorsoventral radiograph of the thorax of a cat with unilateral left moderate pleural effusion. The right lung has an alveolar interstitial pattern that is mainly compatible with pneumonia, oedema or haemorrhage. The presence of a unilateral pleural effusion in cats suggests the presence of a pyothorax, although it may also appear due to other causes.

hemithorax. The causes of this loss of permeability may be:

- Inflammation or pathological processes that present with fibrin production (e.g. pyothorax, chylothorax, haemothorax or neoplasia). In cats, unilateral pleural effusion is common in cases of pyothorax.
- Congenital anatomical variations.
- Diaphragmatic hernia.
- Lung lobe torsion.

When the effusion is **unilateral**, the radiographic signs vary to some degree:

- On lateral radiographs, a more diffuse increase in intrathoracic density may be observed instead of lung retraction (this can even be mistaken for a pulmonary infiltrate).
- On ventrodorsal and dorsoventral radiographs, lung retraction is only observed on the affected side (fig. 3.49). In severe cases, the entire hemithorax may have a uniform soft-tissue density, whereas the contralateral one remains normal.
- There may be a displacement of the heart towards the healthy side.

A severe pleural effusion may mask a cardiomegaly, the presence of lung infiltrates, a pulmonary, pleural or mediastinal mass, a diaphragmatic hernia or a lung lobe torsion, so the patient should always be reassessed once the effusion has been drained, so as to rule out the presence of any of these conditions. When fluid rich in fibrin has been removed, the lungs may then not fully expand due to pleural thickening, and their margins may remain rounded until the process is resolved.

Ultrasonography is used to investigate the primary cause of an effusion, for example to assess cardiac function, identify masses and examine possible pleural thickenings, defects in the diaphragm or lung lobe torsion. It also allows the identification of areas of pulmonary atelectasis and the location of small accumulations of fluid in order to take samples and drain the thorax under ultrasound guidance in complicated cases.

In cases of pyothorax and chylothorax, computed tomography is particularly indicated to assess the extension and distribution of the fluid with more precision, as well as to determine the cause in some cases (e.g.: abscesses, fistulous tracts, thoracic duct leaks, etc.). It provides more complete diagnostic information than an ultrasound examination when the effusion is associated with masses, defects in the diaphragm or lung lobe torsion. In cases of chylothorax, a lymphangiogram is performed by administering an iodinated contrast medium through a mesenteric lymph vessel, or by injecting it in a mesenteric lymph node under ultrasound guidance. This way, leaks in the thoracic duct (or one of its branches) and lymphangiectases may be identified.

Pneumothorax

Pneumothorax is defined as the accumulation of gas in the pleural space, that is, between the parietal and visceral pleura. It usually occurs as a result of traumatic causes, although it can also occur spontaneously. The accumulation of air in the pleural space leads to pulmonary atelectasis, the degree of which is directly proportional to the severity of the pneumothorax. Atelectasis increases the opacity of the lung, visible on radiographs, as well as separating the lung margins from the normal anatomical borders, which can also be seen to some extent on the radiographs.

In the lateral projection, the radiological sign of the heart being elevated is very typical, where it appears separated from the sternum by a band of gas opacity. This image is actually due to the lateral displacement of the heart towards the hemithorax nearest the X-ray table, caused by the collapse of the lower lung (fig. 3.50). Elevation of the heart silhouette from the sternum in the lateral projection may also occur for other causes besides pneumothorax: in dogs with deep chest conformation, in animals with mediastinal deviation, in obese animals and in cases of hypovolaemia.

In ventrodorsal or dorsoventral projections, the lateral margins of the lung appear separated from the chest wall by bands of gas opacity (fig. 3.51). This image is best appreciated in the dorsoventral projection, since in the sternal recumbency position the gas ascends and lies between the lungs and the chest wall. Conversely, in the ventrodorsal projection, with animal in dorsal recumbency the gas rises to parasternal positions, more centred on the chest, where it overlaps with the mediastinal structures, and this makes identification difficult in the case of mild to moderate pneumothorax.

Taking an expiratory radiograph can also help to identify mild pneumothorax, as the lungs contain less air, which increases their opacity and therefore their contrast with the gas accumulated in the pleural space.

In the case of a tension pneumothorax, the pressure in the pleural space is greater than atmospheric pressure throughout inspiration and expiration. This is due to lesions in the lung that act as a one-way valve. The air passes from the lung to the pleural space during inspiration, but it is not returned to the lung during expiration. The chest wall remains intact, so the pressure in the pleural space increases with each breath. This, therefore, is considered an urgent need for immediate attention. Apart from the radiological signs already described, in tension pneumothorax, there could be signs of expansion of the chest cavity, the lungs are often markedly collapsed, and the heart and caudal vena may appear diminished in size. If it is unilateral, the mediastinal structures will appear displaced to the opposite side to that with the pneumothorax.

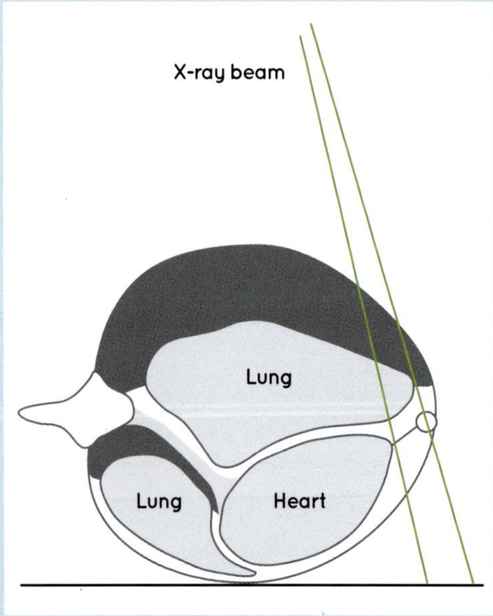

FIGURE 3.50. Schematic representation of the displacement of the heart, which creates an image of "elevation" of the cardiac silhouette on lateral radiographs in cases of pneumothorax. The heart is not supported as it would normally be by a healthy lung. The collapsed lung occupies a smaller volume and as a result, the heart is displaced to the centre of the thoracic cavity, which originates an image of elevation on lateral radiographs.

In pneumothorax that has evolved over several days, it is common to observe irregular-shaped bands of fluid/soft tissue densities due to the formation of pleural adhesions.

If the pneumothorax is unilateral, it will be possible to observe a displacement of the mediastinal structures to the contralateral hemithorax on dorsoventral and ventrodorsal radiographs. On lateral views, the cardiac silhouette may not appear elevated if the animal is placed with the affected side up.

A **hydropneumothorax** (presence of fluid and gas in the pleural space) due to trauma, pulmonary abscesses or oesophageal perforation may be detected. The radiographic findings will depend on the amount and proportion of accumulated fluid and gas.

On dorsoventral and ventrodorsal views, folds of skin may create an artefact that may be mistaken for the image of a pneumothorax, which is called **false pneumothorax** or **pseudopneumothorax**. The area medial to the fold has a higher opacity than the area lateral to it. If there is a high contrast, the lateral area may be mistaken for free gas in the pleural space (fig. 3.52). To differentiate it from a real pneumothorax, we must carefully examine the most radiolucent area and see if the pulmonary vessels can be identified in it. Their presence confirms that the image is due to an artefact. The small vessels are better visualised if we use a bright light source in the case of conventional images, or by significantly increasing image brightness on digital radiographs. An image similar to a pneumothorax may also be observed when lung radiopacity is reduced due to excessive inflation (for example, secondary to asthma or to chronic bronchial disease) or to cases of pulmonary emphysema, hypovascularisation of the lung or hypovolaemia.

It is difficult to distinguish the free gas located in the pleural space from the air contained in the normal lung in an ultrasound image, which is why ultrasonography is not routinely used for the assessment of a pneumothorax. A criterion of differentiation is that the gas contained in the pleural space remains static, while the air contained in the lungs is displaced with inspiration and expiration. An ultrasound examination may be useful to identify foreign bodies or fistulous tracts located in the thoracic wall when these are suspected to be the cause of the pneumothorax.

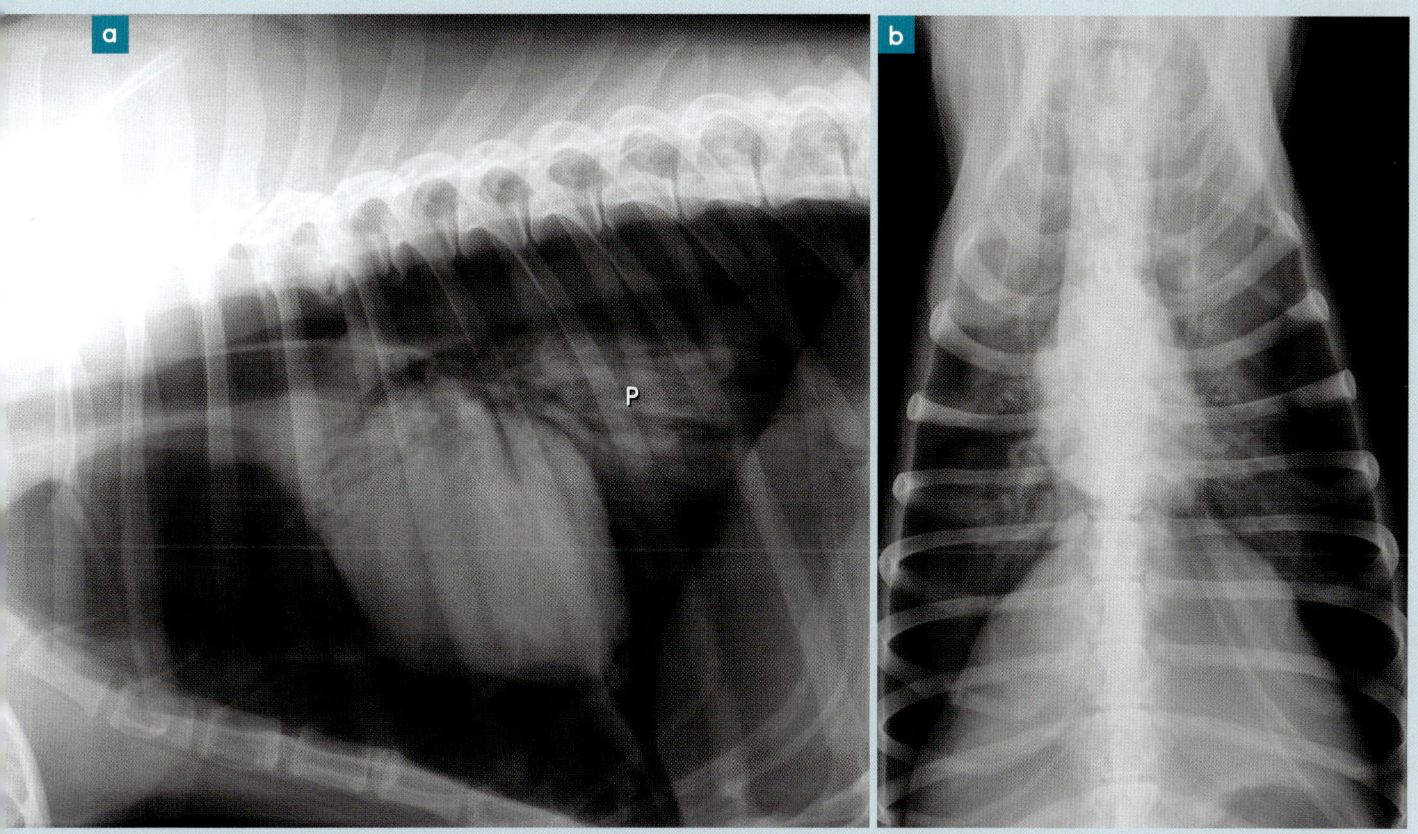

FIGURE 3.51. Lateral (a) and dorsoventral (b) radiographs of the thorax of a dog with a moderate to severe bilateral pneumothorax. In image (a), the cardiac silhouette appears separated from the sternum by a band of gas density and the lung (L) appears collapsed, which is why its radiopacity is increased. In image (b), both lungs are collapsed and separated from the costal wall by bands of gas density, although the degree of lung retraction is greater in the left hemithorax. The cardiac silhouette appears reduced in size, which is a common finding in cases of severe pneumothorax.

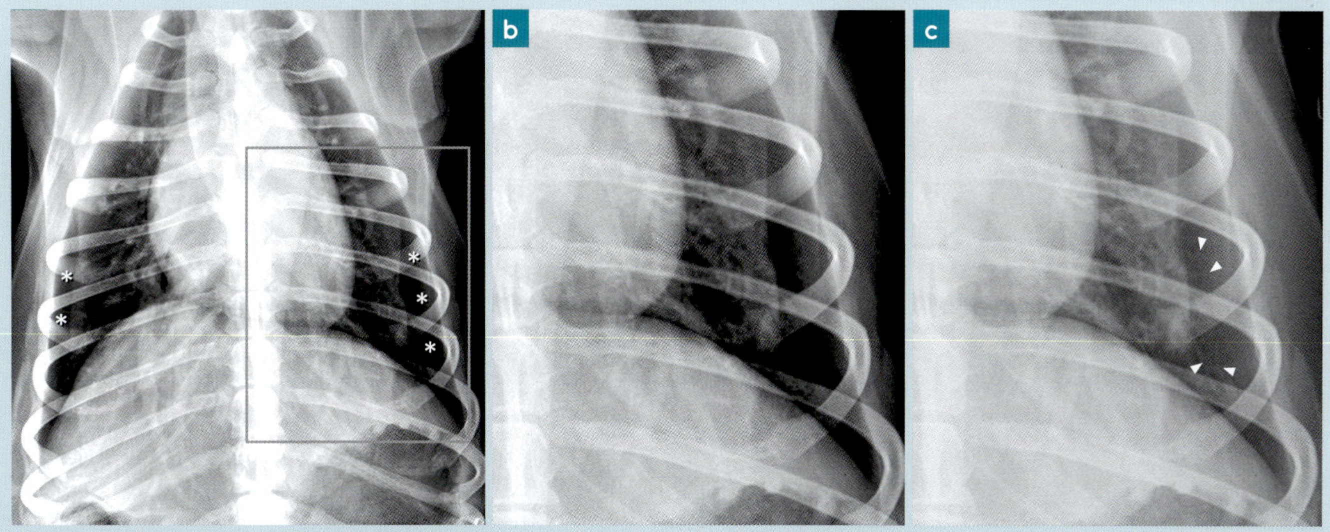

FIGURE 3.52. Dorsoventral projection of the thorax of a dog with image of pseudo-pneumothorax, marked with asterisks (a). Image (b) shows the affected area of the left hemithorax enlarged. Image (c) shows the same area after significantly increasing the brightness of the image, allowing identification of small peripheral pulmonary vessels (arrowheads), a finding that confirms that it does not correspond to a real pneumothorax.

Computed tomography will provide more complete diagnostic information in cases of recurrent or persistent pneumothorax with no known cause (fig. 3.53).

Pleural masses

The differential diagnosis of pleural masses includes neoplasia, abscesses/granulomas, haematomas or encapsulated pleural effusion. These lesions usually have relatively large areas of contact with the chest wall, but this criterion is not sufficient to differentiate them from lung masses on an X-ray.

Mesotheliomas is the only primary tumour that originates in the pleura. They often present a diffuse distribution, with the formation of very small, disseminated nodules, which may be undetectable on an X-ray. They usually cause pleural effusion, which may be the only radiological sign, or at least initially, identifiable on an X-ray (fig. 3.54). Occasionally, a larger focal pleural thickening may be detected which would usually be identified on an X-ray after chest drainage.

Metastatic infiltration of the pleura usually results in associated pleural effusion whose radiological signs, as in the case of mesotheliomas, may be the only detectable sign on an X-ray. The identification of lung lesions compatible with metastases in these patients may better guide the radiological diagnosis (fig. 3.55).

Ultrasonography allows the identification of pleural masses, whether there is a concomitant effusion or not, although it does not clearly differentiate a pleural origin from a possible pulmonary or mediastinal origin. In addition, it facilitates the collection of samples for cytology and biopsies.

Computed tomography will give a better definition of the margins of the mass, although in cases of mesotheliomas the pleural effusion may be the only recognisable finding. It is common to find associated pericardial masses or pericardial effusion in the study.

Pleural thickenings

In older animals, thin lines of soft-tissue or mineral density may be observed at the site of the interlobar fissures. These are normally due to thickenings of the pleura with no clinical significance. Pleural calcifications may also appear as small areas distributed throughout the lung fields on chest radiographs (fig. 3.56).

Pathological pleural thickenings appear as bands of soft-tissue opacity with an irregular morphology (fig. 3.57). They may be the sequela of any type of pleural effusion, although they are common and form more rapidly in cases of reactive effusion (pyothorax, haemothorax or chylothorax), in which fibrous adherences that capture and encapsulate small amounts of fluid may form. These focal accumulations of fluid may have a radiographic image similar to that of pleural masses.

Mediastinum

It corresponds to the anatomical space located between the right and left cavities (fig. 3.58). It communicates cranially with the soft tissues of the neck, through the thoracic inlet, and caudally with the retroperitoneum, through the aortic hiatus. The oesophagus, thoracic trachea, lymph nodes, thoracic lymph duct, thymus, some nerves, the heart and great vessels are located in the mediastinum. Of all these structures, only the trachea, cardiac silhouette, aorta and caudal vena cava may be identified on a normal chest radiograph of an adult animal. The lumen of the oesophagus can be visualised when it contains air or if fluid or mucus accumulates in its distal portion and the thymus is often identifiable in young animals (up to 6 months of age).

The mediastinum may be subdivided into three areas: the cranial portion (between the thoracic inlet and the heart), the middle portion (at the level of the heart) and the caudal portion (between the heart and the diaphragm). Cranioventral and caudoventral mediastinal reflections are sometimes identifiable on the X-rays of healthy patients, although they may be more evident in obese animals due to the accumulation of fat in them. The cranioventral reflection is located slightly left of midline because the right cranial pulmonary lobe extends in that direction, moving the mediastinum to the left. When identified, in dorsoventral and ventrodorsal projections, it appears as a slightly curved band of soft tissue density, extending from the T1–T2 vertebrae to the left margin of the cardiac silhouette, at the level of the main pulmonary artery. In the lateral projection, it appears as a band of soft tissue density between

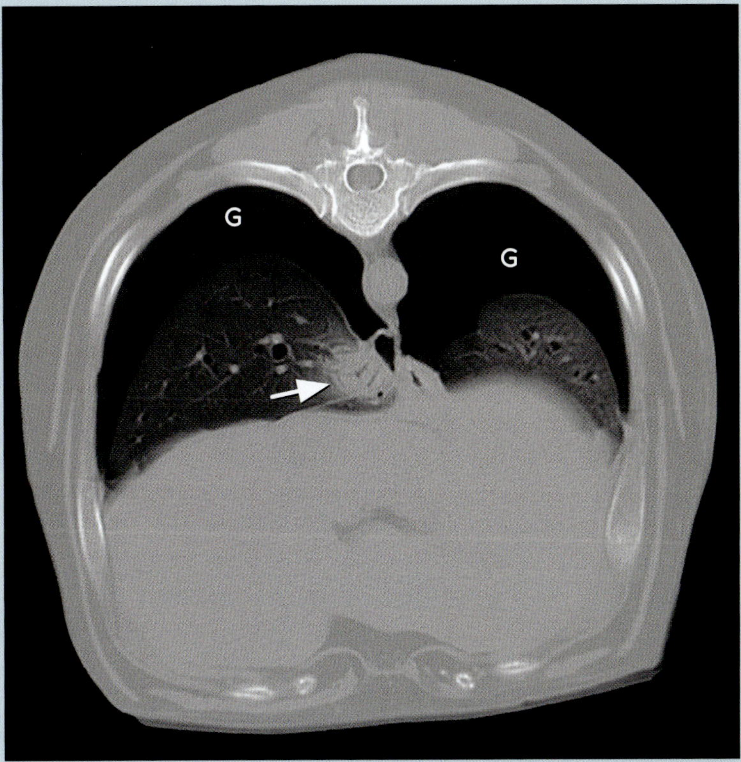

FIGURE 3.53. Computed tomography image of the thorax of a dog with a hydropneumothorax (accumulation of gas and fluid in the pleural space, although in this image it is only possible to observe the gas –G–) associated with a focal area of pulmonary infection (arrow), possible due to the penetration of a foreign body.

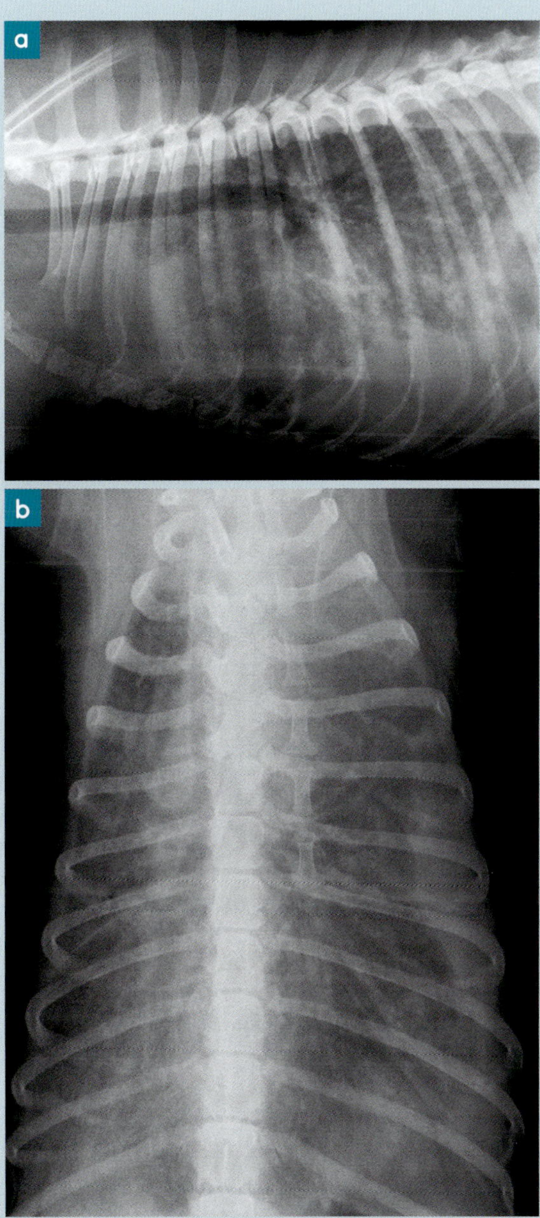

FIGURE 3.54. Lateral (a) and dorsoventral (b) projections of the thorax of a dog with mesothelioma. Signs of bilateral pleural effusion and a miliary pulmonary pattern are noted. The dorsoventral projection shows focal widening of the left pleural space at the level of the 6th, 7th and 8th intercostal spaces, which is suggestive of a pleural mass.

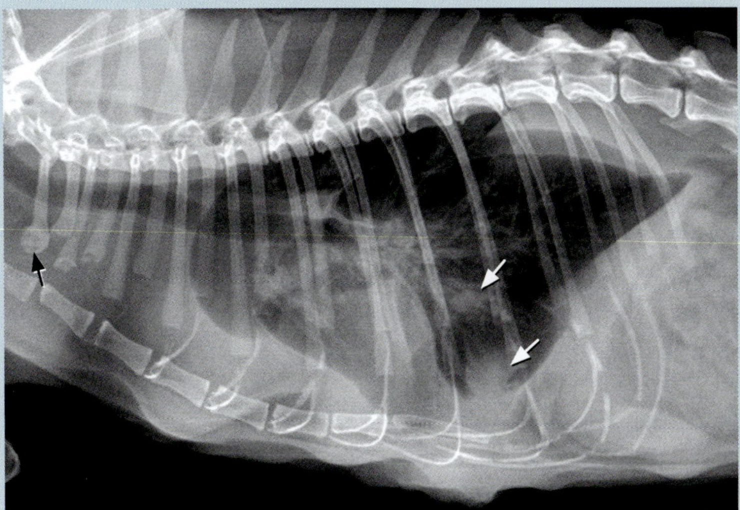

FIGURE 3.55. Lateral projection of the chest of a cat with mammary tumours (identifiable as superficial masses in the ventral chest wall), metastatic infiltration of the pleura causing pleural effusion, pulmonary metastases (white arrows) and bone metastasis in a rib (black arrow).

the right and left cranial lung lobe, located midway between the thoracic inlet and the heart (this may be mistaken for a gas-filled lung lesion in the cranial area of the lung) (fig. 3.59). The caudoventral mediastinal reflection can sometimes be identified on dorsoventral and ventrodorsal projections where it appears as a thin

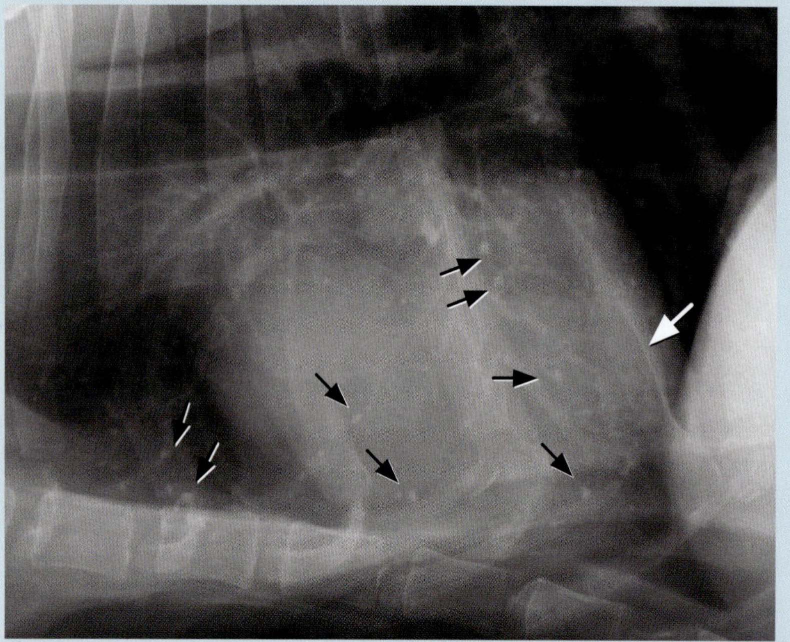

FIGURE 3.56. Enlarged imaged of the thorax on a lateral radiograph of an older dog. In older animals, it is often possible to visualise thin lines of soft-tissue or mineral density at the site of the interlobar fissures (white arrow). These are generally due to thickenings or calcifications of the pleura with no clinical significance. Pleural calcifications may also appear as small areas of mineral density distributed throughout the lung fields, which are visible in this image (some of them are shown with a black arrow).

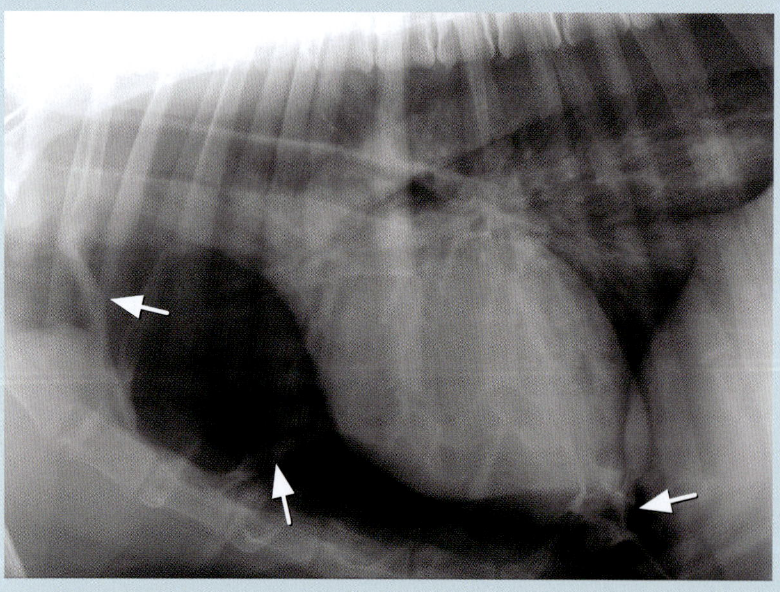

FIGURE 3.57. Lateral radiograph of the thorax of a dog with a hydropneumothorax possibly caused by the penetration of a foreign body, although this latter was not identified during surgery. The pneumothorax causes a displacement of the cardiac silhouette, which appears separated from the sternum by a gas density band. In various locations of the ventral area of the thorax, it is possible to observe soft-tissue density bands with an irregular morphology (arrows), which correspond to pleural thickenings and a focal accumulation of pleural fluid. The sternal lymph node also appears increased in size (dorsal to the manubrium and second sternebra).

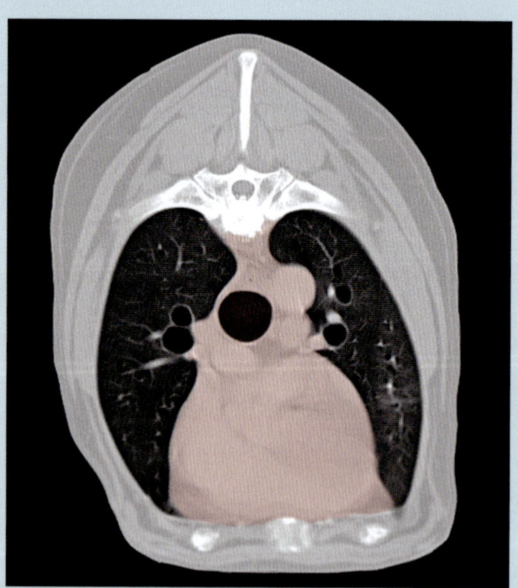

FIGURE 3.58. Representation of the mediastinum (coloured in red) on a computed tomography image of the thorax of a dog. The mediastinal space contains the oesophagus, the thoracic trachea, and lymph nodes, and thoracic lymphatic duct and thymus, some nerves, the heart and the great vessels of the thorax.

band of soft-tissue density located slightly left of midline between the apex of the heart and the diaphragm (fig. 3.60).

On dorsoventral and ventrodorsal radiographs, the shadow of the cranial mediastinum must have approximately the same width as the thoracic vertebrae in cats, while in dogs it should not exceed twice the width of these vertebrae in normal conditions. It should be taken into account that the mediastinum of brachycephalic dogs and obese cats and dogs may be wider, with a displacement of the trachea to the right on dorsoventral and ventrodorsal views, and a significant elevation of the cardiac silhouette due to an accumulation of fat ventral to it (fig. 3.61).

In young animals, it is often possible to identify the shadow of the thymus, which reaches its maximum size at approximately 4 months of age and is no longer visible at 6 months of age (fig. 3.62). On very rare occasions, a vestige of the thymus is observed in adults.

Most of the diseases that affect the mediastinum are secondary to pulmonary, oesophageal, pleural and lymphatic diseases.

Mediastinal effusion

It corresponds to the presence of free fluid (transudate, exudate, blood, lymph) in the mediastinal space. It may appear associated with mediastinitis, coagulopathies, trauma, feline infectious peritonitis, etc.

The radiographic image of a mediastinal effusion may be confused with that of a pleural effusion on lateral radiographs, but not on dorsoventral or ventrodorsal radiographs. On these views, there will be no retraction of the lateral margins of the lung, but an abnormal enlargement of the shadow of the mediastinum (fig. 3.63). In some cases, triangular or thorn-shaped shadows will appear with their wider base oriented towards the hilum (which differentiates them from interlobar fissures in a pleural effusion). These are called reverse fissure lines. A mediastinal effusion is often accompanied by pleural effusion.

The effusion, whether mediastinal, pleural or both, can mask the presence of localised masses in the mediastinal space, in which case an ultrasound examination will be particularly useful to assess the size and characteristics of the mass, as well as the amount of accumulated fluid. In these cases, ultrasound-guided sampling of the mass and fluid will be indicated. Computed tomography may provide complementary information about the possible origin of the effusion.

Pneumomediastinum

The presence of free gas in the mediastinal space may be indicative of a rupture of the trachea or oesophagus, or less likely of the bronchi or lung, but it may also be due to the presence of subcutaneous emphysema in the neck, since the gas may go from the spaces

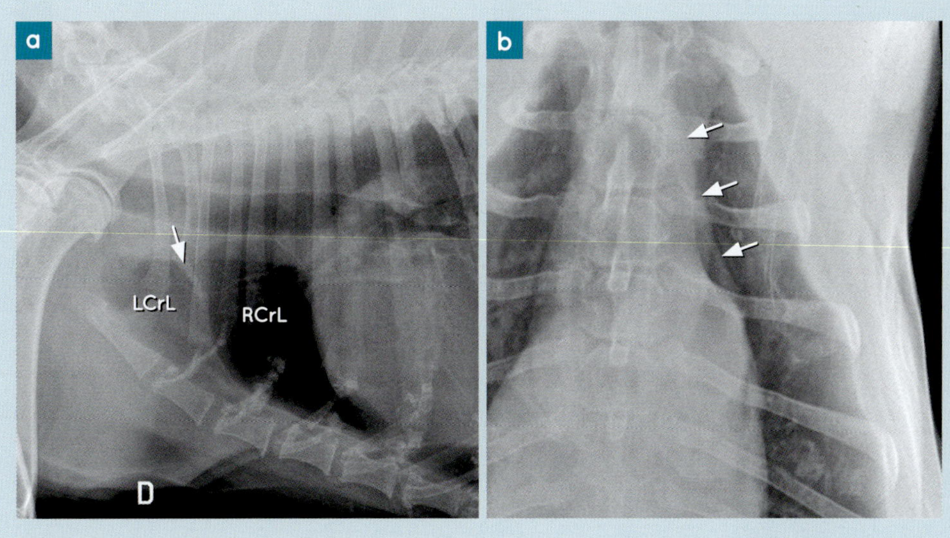

FIGURE 3.59. Enlarged images of the lateral (a) and ventrodorsal (b) projection of the chest of a healthy dog showing the cranioventral mediastinal reflection. In image (a) it appears as a band of soft tissue density (arrow) between the right cranial lobe (RCrL) and the left cranial lobe (LCrL), located midway between the thoracic inlet and the heart. In image (b) it appears as a band of soft tissue density (arrows), extending from the level of the T1-T2 vertebrae to the location of the left margin of the cardiac silhouette, at the level of the main pulmonary artery.

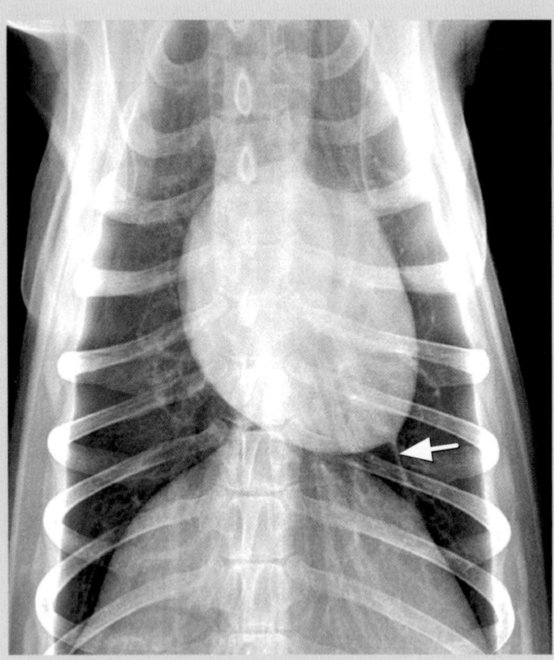

FIGURE 3.60. Enlarged image of the thorax in dorsoventral projection of a healthy dog identifying the caudoventral mediastinal reflection. It appears as a thin band of soft tissue density between the cardiac apex and the diaphragm (arrow).

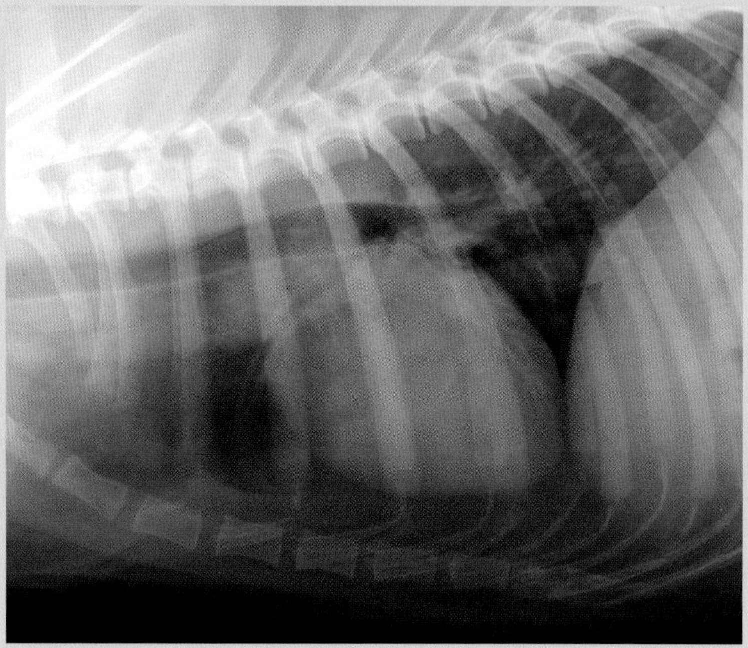

FIGURE 3.61. Lateral radiograph of the thorax of an obese dog. It is possible to observe a marked accumulation of mediastinal fat located ventral to the cardiac silhouette, which causes its elevation. This should not be mistaken for a pleural effusion. An effusion would mask the image of the cardiac apex, while in this case the definition of the whole ventral margin of the heart is improved due to the contrast between the radiographic density of soft tissue and that of fat.

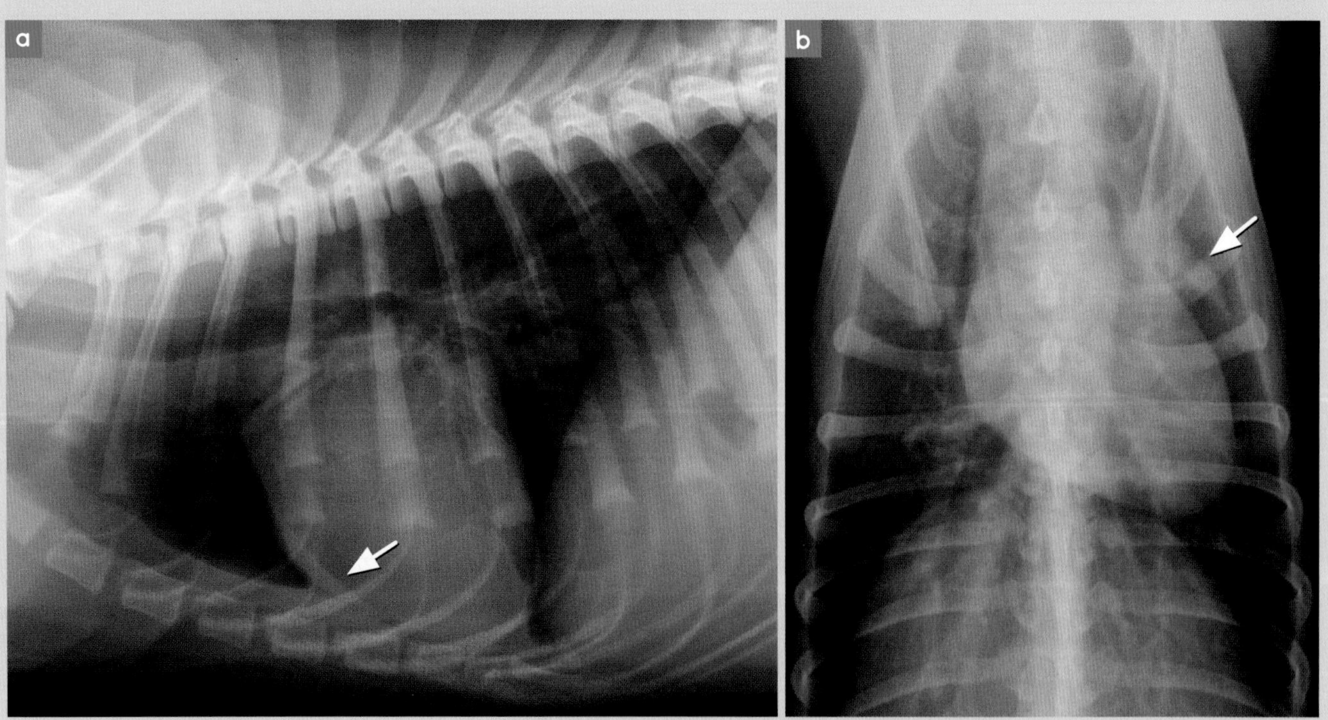

FIGURE 3.62. Lateral (a) and dorsoventral (b) radiographs of the thorax of a young dog, in which the normal shadow of the thymus may be observed. This organ reaches its maximum size at 4 months of age and is usually no longer visible on radiographs from 6 months of age.

between the fasciae of the neck to the mediastinal space through the thoracic inlet. If all the possible causes are ruled out, the possibility of an idiopathic pneumomediastimum should be considered.

In cases of pneumomediastinum, it will be possible to identify the shadows of some mediastinal structures, such as for example, the oesophagus or the blood vessels of the cranial mediastinum. It would not be possible to distinguish these structures from one another if no gas was located between them. When the amount of gas is relatively small, the most significant finding is the improved visualisation of the tracheal wall, which appears internally and externally limited by gas (fig. 3.64).

If air accumulates rapidly in the mediastinum, the mediastinal pleura may rupture and cause a pneumothorax. That is to say, a pneumomediastinum may progress to a pneumothorax. On the other hand, a pneumothorax is never the cause of a pneumomediastinum.

An ultrasound study is not indicated in cases of pneumomediastinum. However, contrast techniques or endoscopy are indicated to rule out a perforation or an oesophageal or tracheal rupture as the causes of the disease. Computed tomography is particularly useful to investigate the cause of a pneumomediastinum.

Mediastinal masses

These generally correspond to mediastinal lymphadenopathies (fig. 3.65) or tumours, although abscesses, granulomas, haematomas and cysts may also appear in this location.

The lymph nodes that can be found in the mediastinum are divided into:

- **Sternal** (there may be one or two in dogs and one in cats): when they increase significantly in size, they appear as a shadow of soft-tissue density dorsal to the second sternebra (fig. 3.66). They drain lymph

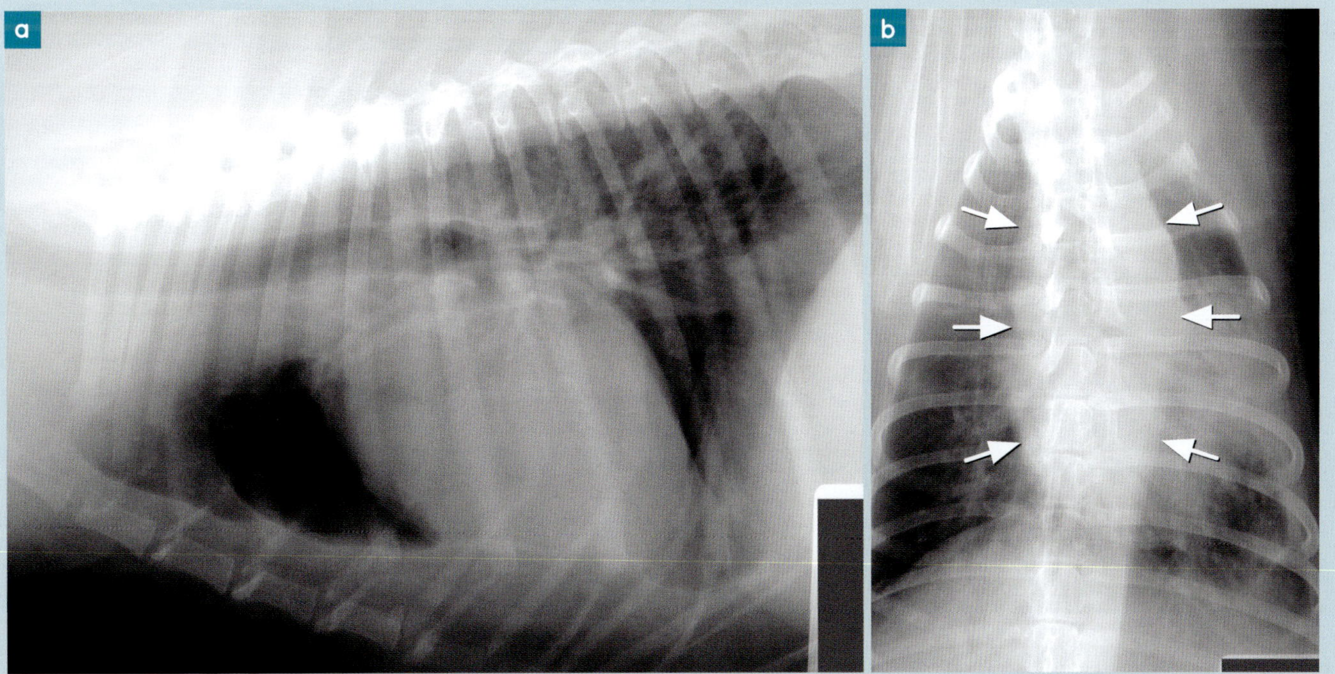

FIGURE 3.63. Lateral (a) and dorsoventral (b) radiographs of the thorax of a dog with a mediastinal effusion. On the lateral view, the findings are similar to those of a pleural effusion, but the dorsoventral view does not show a retraction of the lungs (except a minimal separation between the left caudal lobe and the chest wall, due to a mild pleural effusion) but an enlargement of the mediastinal shadow (arrows). It should be borne in mind that brachycephalic dogs have, in normal conditions, wider mediastinal shadows, as also occurs in obese cats and dogs. This patient has, in addition, a pulmonary infiltrate in the caudal area of the left cranial lobe.

from the thoracic wall and abdominal cavity. Therefore, if they are enlarged, the cause may be located in the thorax or in the abdomen.

- **Mediastinal lymph nodes:** they form a chain of lymph nodes that lies adjacent to the great vessels of the cranial mediastinum (cranial vena cava, brachiocephalic trunk and left subclavian artery). When they increase in size they originate an enlargement of the shadow of the cranial mediastinum, as well as a displacement of the trachea in dorsal direction on lateral radiographs, and to the right on dorsoventral and ventrodorsal radiographs.
- **Bronchial lymph nodes:** they are subdivided into pulmonary lymph nodes (often absent, but when present they are distributed throughout the main bronchi) and tracheobronchial lymph nodes (located around the carina). When the tracheobronchial lymph nodes become greatly enlarged, they originate a mass dorsal to the tracheal bifurcation, with a relatively oval morphology on lateral radiographs. The bifurcation of the trachea may be ventrally displaced. This image is similar to that produced by a significant enlargement of the left atrium, but in this case the bifurcation of the trachea appears displaced in the opposite direction –dorsally– and other signs of left cardiomegaly are usually observed. It is more difficult to visualise the mass on dorsoventral or ventrodorsal views, but it may cause a bronchial displacement that is identifiable in the image.

The most common location of mediastinal tumours is the cranial mediastinum. Heart base tumours are found in the middle mediastinum, and oesophageal tumours can occur in any part of the mediastinum, including the caudal portion.

Neoplastic lesions affecting the mediastinum include lymphomas, thymomas, neuroendocrine tumours, lymphomatoid granulomatosis, mastocytomas, melanomas and thyroid carcinomas. The radiological and ultrasound image of mediastinal granulomas, abscesses and haematomas may be identical to that of tumours. Idiopathic mediastinal cysts may appear in older cats, and can grow to a large size.

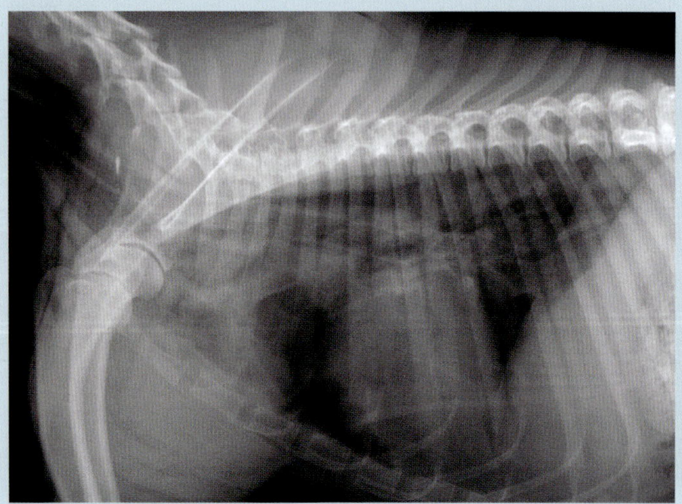

FIGURE 3.64. Lateral radiograph of the thorax of a dog with a pneumomediastinum caused by a bite in the neck. The gas that penetrates between the fasciae of the neck enters in the mediastinal space through the thoracic inlet. The same image may be observed in cases of tracheal or oesophageal perforation or rupture, since the free gas in the mediastinum may move towards the neck.

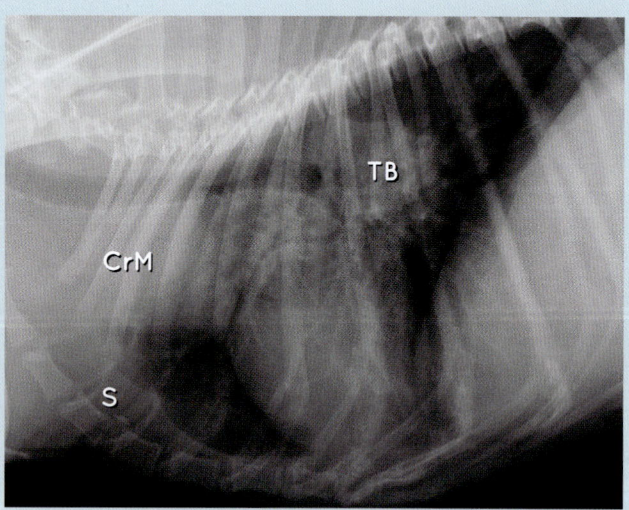

FIGURE 3.65. Lateral radiograph of the thorax of a dog with lymphoma. The enlargement of the sternal lymph node or lymph nodes (S) creates a shadow of soft-tissue density dorsal to the manubrium and most cranial sternebrae. The increase in size of the cranial mediastinal lymph nodes (CrM) causes an enlargement of the cranial mediastinal shadow and elevation of the trachea. Finally, the tracheobronchial lymph nodes (TB), which lie dorsal to the tracheal bifurcation, create an approximately oval shadow dorsal to the main bronchi, next to the carina.

In general, cranial mediastinal masses usually result in a somewhat marked increase in cranial mediastinal width in lateral, dorsoventral and ventrodorsal projections. They also usually cause dorsal displacement of the trachea in the lateral projection and lateral displacement in the dorsoventral and ventrodorsal projections (fig. 3.67). Depending on the size of the mass, the heart may also appear displaced, and with its border adjacent to the mass masked (fig. 3.68). Identifying tracheal displacement helps guide the radiological diagnosis of mediastinal masses when these are masked by pleural effusion, which is relatively common (fig. 3.69).

Thymomas usually present initially a more ventral position than masses of nodal origin, so they could be confused with lung masses on lateral projections, although their centred position on dorsoventral and ventrodorsal projections helps to differentiation them (fig. 3.70). They can grow quite large and extend beyond the lateral margin of the heart. Thymomas are sometimes associated with myasthenia gravis and megaoesophagus; the latter can be identified on X-rays (fig. 3.71).

Neoplasms in the middle mediastinum usually correspond to heart base tumours or lymphomas. Heart base tumours can be identified on X-rays as a mass of soft tissue opacity located immediately dorsal to the cardiac silhouette (fig. 3.72). In cases of tracheobronchial lymphoma, the "mass effect" usually occurs dorsally or around the carina. When visualising masses in this region of the mediastinum, other possible aetiologies should also be considered, including abscess, granuloma, oesophageal foreign body or reactive lymphadenomegaly.

Neoplasms located in the caudal mediastinum are rare and their origin is usually oesophageal. The radiological image could be confused with that of a pulmonary neoplasm, and may also be very similar to that of abscesses, granulomas, dorsal diaphragmatic or hiatus hernias (see figs. 3.39 and 3.40).

An ultrasound examination will allow the evaluation of the size and echogenicity of the mass and the presence of an associated effusion, in addition to allowing ultrasound-guided fine-needle aspiration or biopsy.

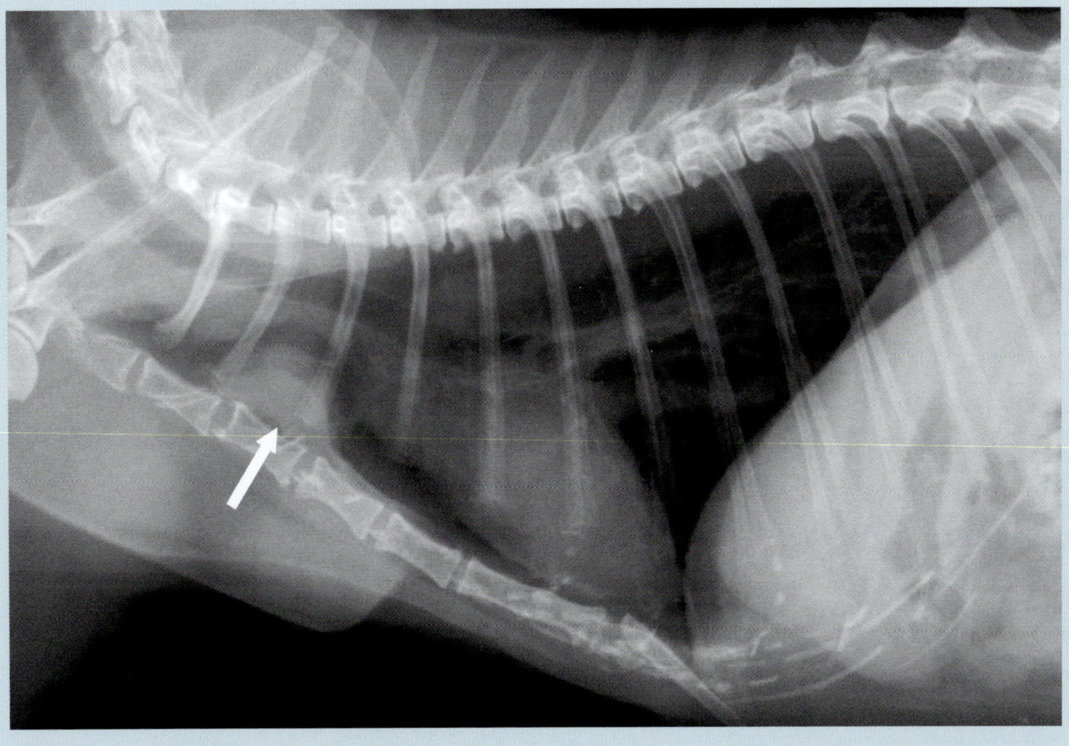

FIGURE 3.66. Lateral projection of the thorax of a cat with enlargement of sternal lymph nodes, appearing as a silhouette of soft tissue density dorsal to the second sternebra (arrow). Incomplete (partial) calcification of the costal cartilages is observed, giving a false impression of a rupture. This finding is common in cats.

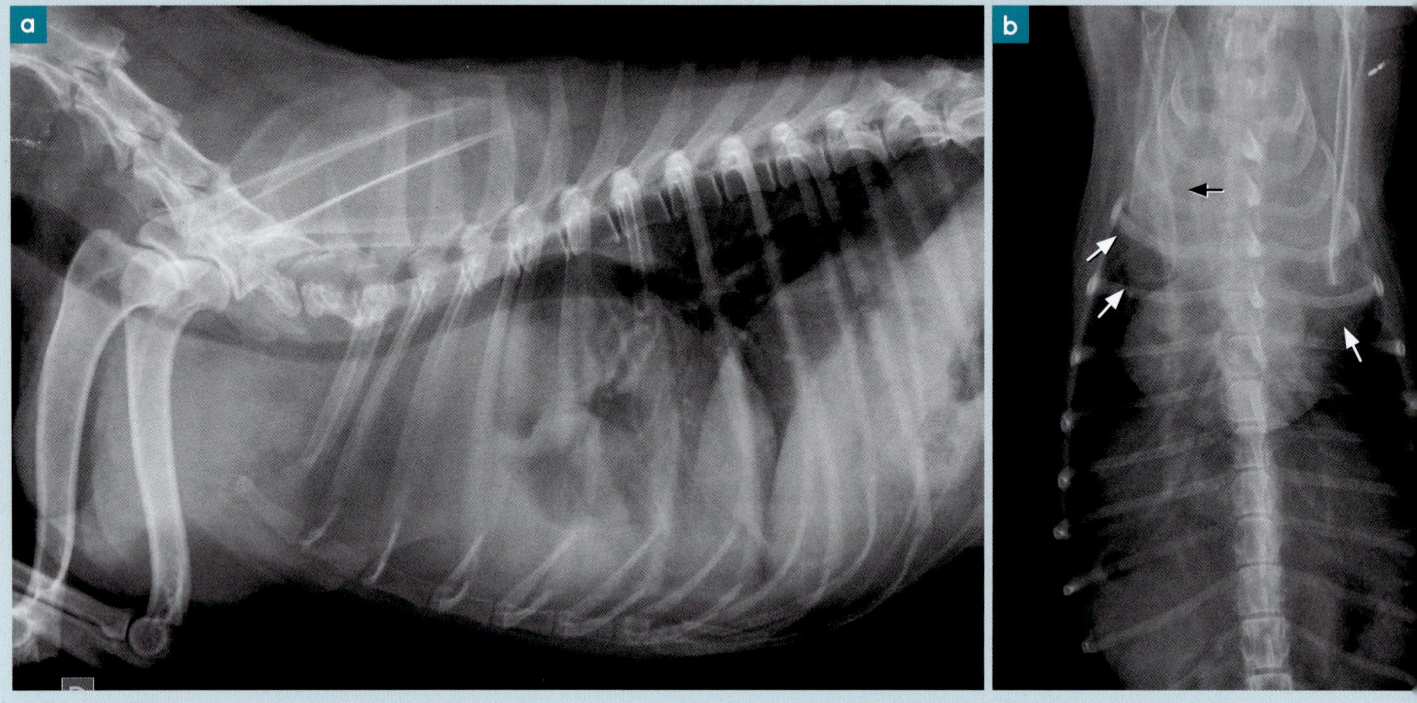

FIGURE 3.67. Lateral (a) and dorsoventral (b) projections of a dog with a large mediastinal mass causing marked displacement of the trachea dorsally and to the right (black arrow), also showing a reduction in its dorsoventral diameter in the proximal thoracic portion (this finding indicates compression of the tracheal lumen). The margins of the mass are better identified in image (b) (white arrows). The cardiac silhouette appears displaced caudally in both projections.

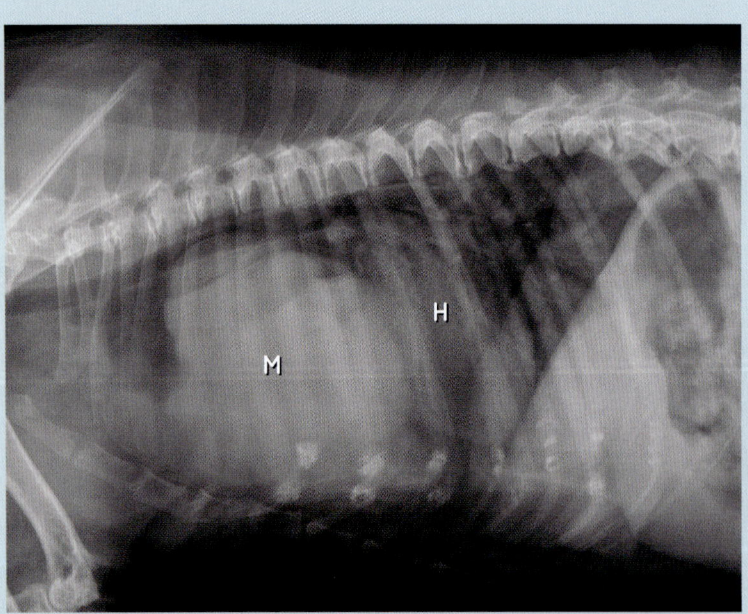

FIGURE 3.68. Lateral radiograph of the thorax of a dog with thymoma. A large mass (M) that causes a marked dorsal displacement of the trachea and a caudodorsal displacement of the heart (H) may be observed in the cranial area of the thorax.

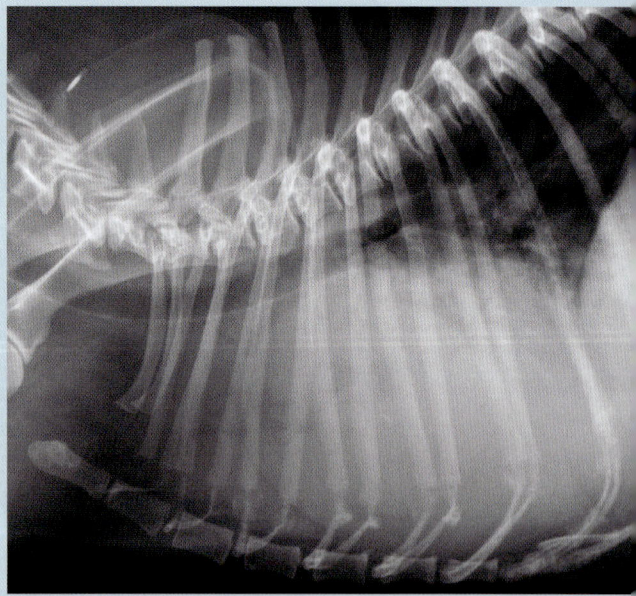

FIGURE 3.69. Lateral radiograph of the thorax of a dog with a cranial mediastinal mass, which is masked in the image due to the associated pleural/mediastinal effusion. The marked elevation of the trachea suggests the presence of a mass, although its outline cannot be visualised in the image. Ultrasonography allows the easy identification of the mass.

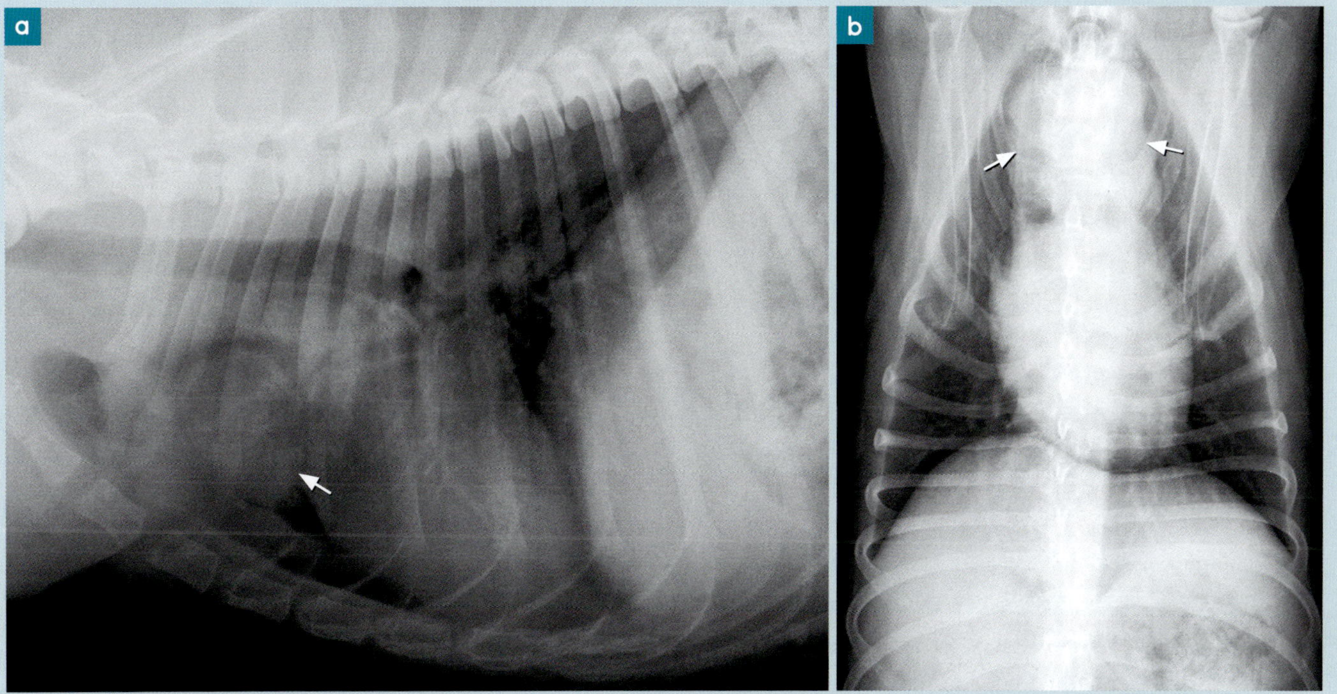

FIGURE 3.70. Lateral (a) and dorsoventral (b) projections of the thorax of a dog with a small thymoma (arrows). In the lateral projection, the lesion could be confused with a pulmonary mass, but its central location in the dorsoventral projection confirms the mediastinal origin as the most probable.

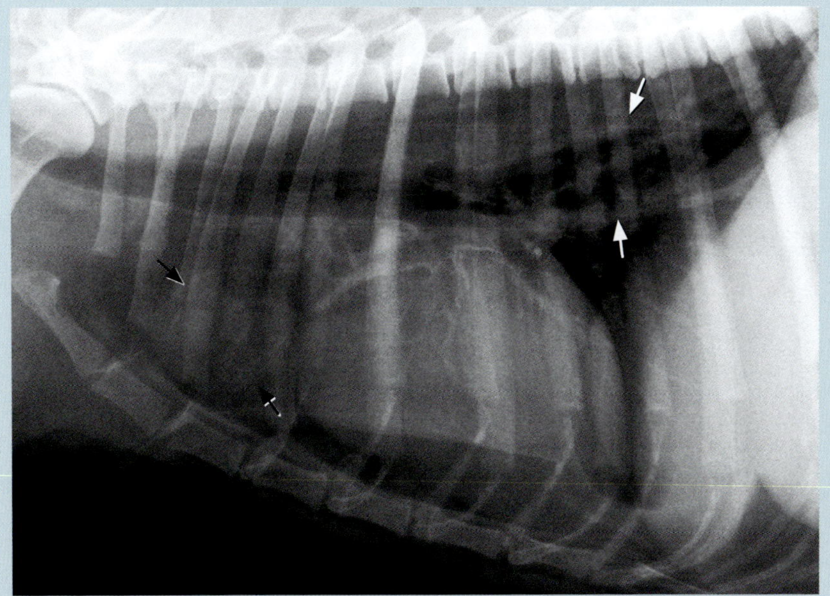

FIGURE 3.71. Lateral projection of the thorax of a dog with a thymoma (black arrows) and megaoesophagus (white arrows). Thymomas are sometimes associated with myasthenia gravis and megaoesophagus.

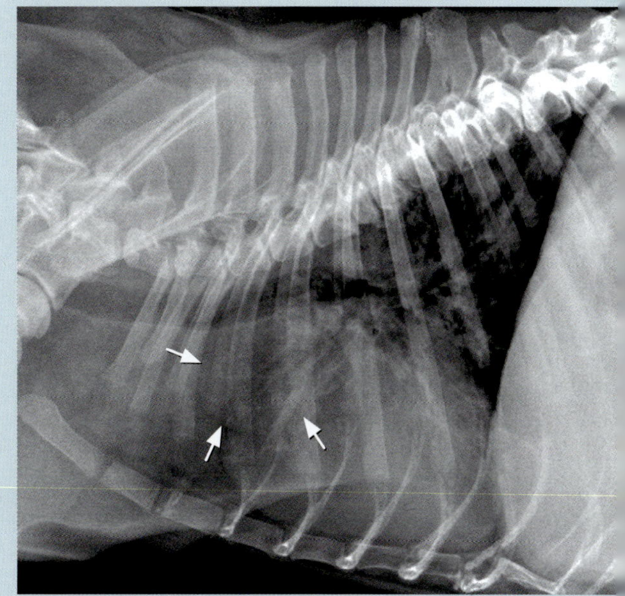

FIGURE 3.72. Lateral projection of the thorax of a dog with a chemodectoma (arrows), which appears as a soft-tissue dense mass located immediately dorsal to the cardiac silhouette.

Computed tomography is an excellent technique to identify mediastinal masses and establish their relationship with the other structures in the mediastinum (fig. 3.73).

Displacement of the mediastinum

The displacement of the structures that form the mediastinum indicates a change of volume in one of the hemithoraces. If the volume of a hemithorax increases, the mediastinum will be displaced to the opposite side, while if the volume of a hemithorax decreases, the mediastinal content will be displaced to the affected side. The most common cause is iatrogenic, due to a partial collapse of the lung, which has a lower position in patients that remain in lateral recumbency for a long period of time, especially if they are anaesthetised. On radiographs, it is possible to observe a displacement of the heart to the side on which the patient was lying and an increase in the density of the lung of the same side caused by temporary atelectasis.

A pathological displacement of the mediastinum may appear due to masses or accumulations located in one of the hemithoraces (unilateral pleural effusion, unilateral pneumothorax), in conditions causing an unequal expansion of the lungs (fig. 3.74), or when adherences that connect the mediastinum with the thoracic wall remain after a chronic pleural effusion.

Heart

Taking chest radiographs is an essential part of the assessment of patients with a suspected cardiovascular disease. Radiographs allow the assessment of the size and shape of the cardiac silhouette, as well as of the state of the lungs and circulation, thus showing the

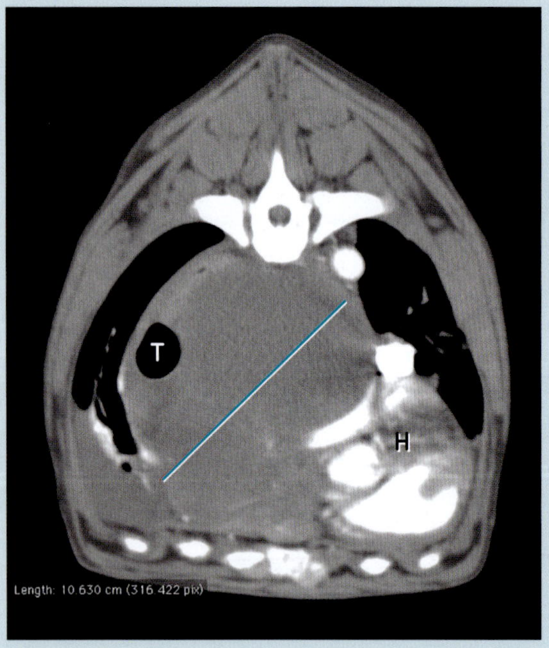

FIGURE 3.73. Computed tomography image of the thorax of a dog with a large mediastinal mass (its diameter is indicated by a blue line in the image), which causes an evident displacement of the trachea (T) to the right and of the heart (H) to the left. Tomography allows the assessment of the relationships of the mass with the adjacent anatomical structures and the detection of distant metastases.

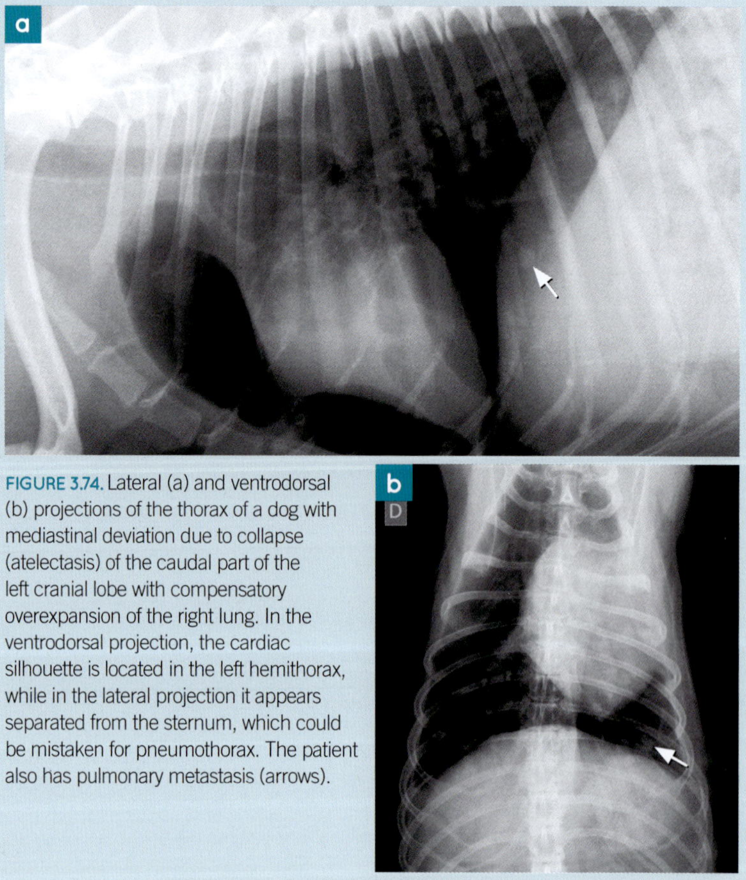

FIGURE 3.74. Lateral (a) and ventrodorsal (b) projections of the thorax of a dog with mediastinal deviation due to collapse (atelectasis) of the caudal part of the left cranial lobe with compensatory overexpansion of the right lung. In the ventrodorsal projection, the cardiac silhouette is located in the left hemithorax, while in the lateral projection it appears separated from the sternum, which could be mistaken for pneumothorax. The patient also has pulmonary metastasis (arrows).

degree of heart failure of the patient. Thoracic radiographs therefore help to determine the severity of the cardiac disease and allow the evaluation of the efficacy of the treatment.

Contrast studies (angiocardiography) have become less prevalent with the use of echocardiography, which is now an essential routine technique to establish a precise diagnosis of most of the diseases that affect the heart. The diagnostic information obtained by means of radio graphy and echocardiography is often enough for us not to need more advanced diagnostic imaging techniques. Computed tomography is useful for the diagnosis of heart tumours and some diseases of the pericardium.

Right lateral and dorsoventral radiographs are used for the radiological assessment of the cardiac silhouette. On left lateral radiographs, the silhouette appears falsely rounded, while on ventrodorsal radiographs it is more magnified than on dorsoventral ones. We should be particularly careful when positioning the animal before taking a radiograph. On lateral views, the rotation of the thorax causes a false increase of the cardiosternal contact and a false elevation of the trachea. On dorsoventral views, any degree of rotation of the thorax causes a deformation of the cardiac silhouette in the image, which does not allow its appropriate examination.

Size of the cardiac silhouette

The methods to assess the overall size of the cardiac silhouette are based on the measurement of its height and width on right lateral and dorsoventral radiographs. We will distinguish between the classic method and the Buchanan method.

According to the traditional method (fig. 3.75), the width of the cardiac silhouette (horizontal craniocaudal diameter) on lateral radiographs should be comprised between 2.5 and 3.5 intercostal spaces in the dog, although this interval varies depending on the conformation of the thorax:

- In dogs with a **narrow and deep thorax** (Greyhound type), the heart has a more vertical position in the thoracic cavity, so the limit of normal will be 2.5 intercostal spaces.
- In dogs with an **intermediate conformation** (German Shepherd type), the normal interval is from 2.5 to 3 intercostal spaces.
- In dogs with a **wide and shallow thorax** (Bulldog type), the normal range extends to 3.5 intercostal spaces, because the heart is anatomically more inclined on the sternum.
- In **cats**, the craniocaudal diameter is not measured horizontally, as in dogs, but perpendicularly to the longitudinal axis of the heart. However, the result obtained is compared to the width of the intercostal spaces horizontally. In normal conditions, its value is 2.

  This variation in the measurement system is due to fact that, with age, the feline heart tends to lie closer to the sternum because of a progressive elongation of the aorta (fig. 3.76). If the width is measured horizontally, as in dogs, it will therefore seem increased in older cats.

Both in dogs and cats, the height of the cardiac silhouette on lateral radiographs –measured from the centre of its base to its apex– corresponds approximately to two thirds of the height of the thoracic cavity at the same level. The width of the silhouette –measured at the level of the 5th intercostal space– should be approximately two thirds of the width of the thoracic cavity on dorsoventral radiographs.

The size of the heart in relation to the thoracic cavity is slightly greater in young animals than in adults. The cardiac silhouette also appears slightly larger during expiration when compared to inspiration, and during diastole when compared to systole. However, these changes are minimal and generally do not significantly affect the diagnosis.

When assessing the size of the cardiac silhouette, it must be taken into account that the exit of the aorta and pulmonary artery, the pericardium and the pericardial space are part of it. In addition, the abnormal presence of fluid or masses in the pericardial space or the enlargement of the great vessels will cause an increase in the size of the cardiac silhouette in the image. The presence of fat in the mediastinal space may also sometimes create a false impression of increased heart size in obese dogs.

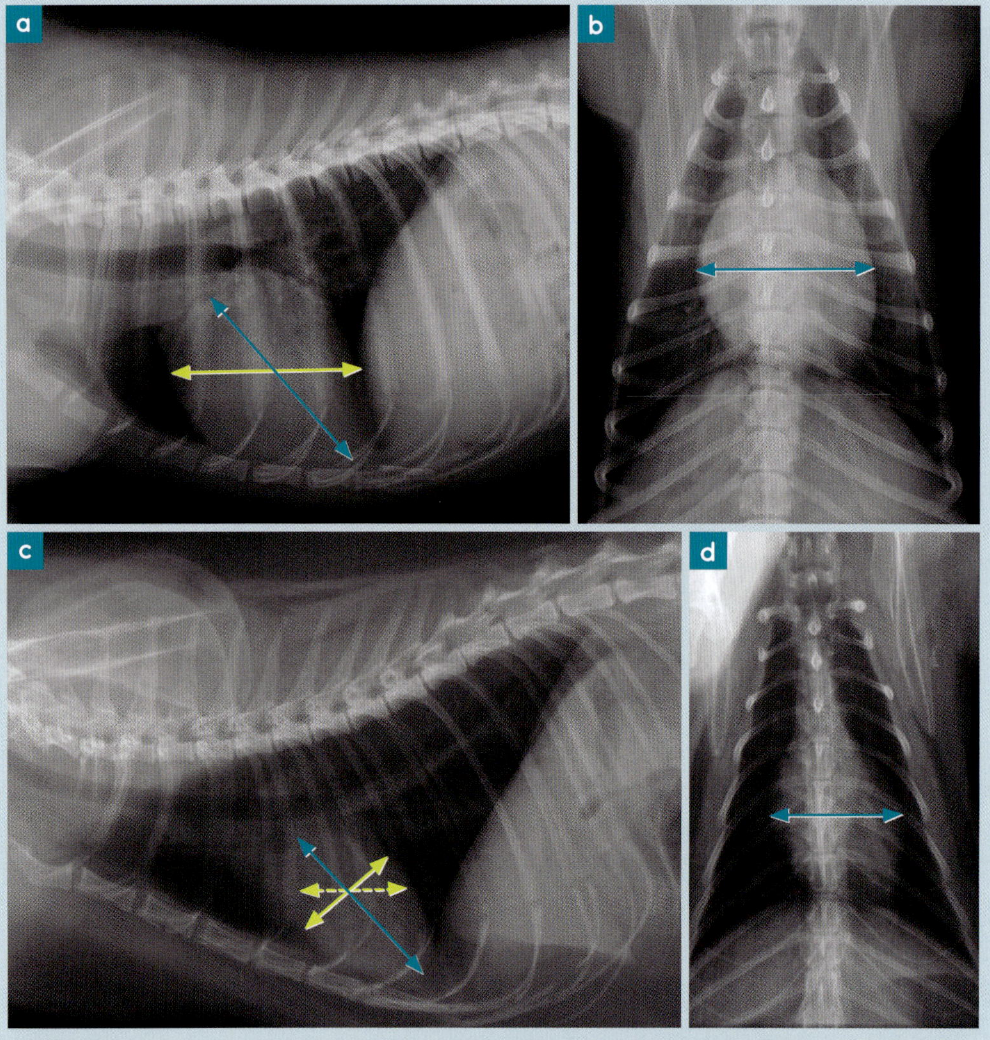

FIGURE 3.75. Normal images of the thorax of a dog in right lateral (a) and dorsoventral (b) projection and of a cat in right lateral (c) and dorsoventral (d) projection, in which the references for the measurement of the cardiac silhouette according to the traditional method are shown. The width of the cardiac silhouette (yellow line) on the lateral view should be between 2.5 and 3.5 intercostal spaces in the dog, although the normal range varies depending on the thoraci c conformation. In cats, the width is measured perpendicularly to the longitudinal axis of the heart (to avoid wrong diagnoses of cardiomegaly in old cats, as their heart may be very inclined on the sternum), and the result is then compared to the width of the intercostal spaces (broken yellow line) horizontally. The normal value is 2. Both in dogs and cats, the height of the cardiac silhouette on lateral radiographs –measured from the centre of its base to its apex– corresponds approximately to two thirds of the height of the thoracic cavity at the same level (blue line), while the width of the silhouette (blue line) –measured at the level of the 5th intercostal space– should be approximately two thirds of the width of the thoracic cavity on dorsoventral radiographs.

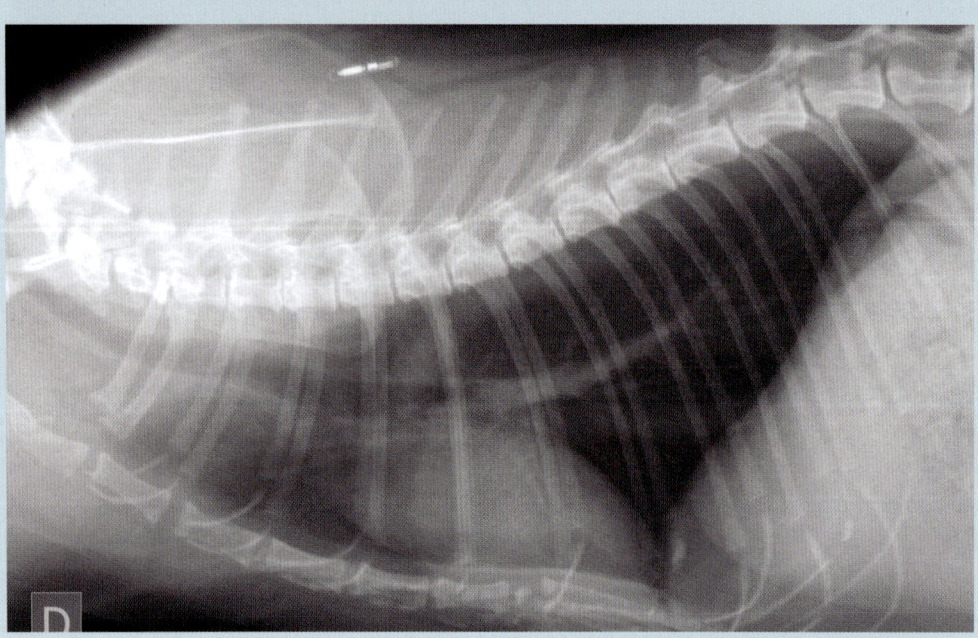

FIGURE 3.76. Lateral radiograph of the thorax of a healthy old cat. The cardiac silhouette appears very inclined on the sternum, which is due to a progressive elongation of the aorta with no clinical significance. This image should not be confused with that of cardiomegaly. The width of the cardiac silhouette, measured perpendicularly to the longitudinal axis of the heart, does not exceed 2 intercostal spaces. The identification microchip appears dorsal to the spinous process of T3.

THE BUCHANAN AND OTHER METHODS TO EVALUATE LEFT ATRIUM SIZE

The Buchanan method is also known as the vertebral scale system or the vertebral heart score (VHS). Two measurements are taken on the lateral radiograph: first, the distance between the ventral margin of the carina and the apex of the heart (the height), then, cranial to caudal, the widest portion of the silhouette perpendicular to the height axis. These two measurements are then aligned with the thoracic spine, counting the number of vertebral bodies that each one encompasses, starting at the cranial aspect of the 4th thoracic vertebrae. The sum of these two figures is the cardiovertebral index or VHS (fig. 3.77).

The general VHS value is 9.7 ± 0.5 vertebral bodies. By definition, 95 % of a normal population fall within the mean ±2 times the standard deviation of the mean, so the normal VHS range in dogs is 8.7 to 10.7. This value, however, varies with breed (see table 3.2) and it has been shown that it can also vary (by up to one vertebral body) with the respiratory and cardiac cycle in the same individual, hence the importance of always correlating it with the patient's clinical data. Nonetheless, it can prove extremely useful in the radiological follow-up of patients with heart disease.

Breeds with thoracic vertebral malformations (usually shortened) have higher VHS values, which would lead to misdiagnosis of cardiomegaly.

In cats, the generic VHS value is 7.5 ± 0.3 vertebral bodies. In a study of 67 cats with respiratory distress, it was concluded that heart disease is highly unlikely with values below 8.0, while values above 9.3 suggested a high probability of heart disease.

Table 3.2. Vertebral heart score (VHS) in different breeds published by various authors.

Breed	Vertebral Heart Size (VHS)
Yorkshire Terrier	9.9 ± 0.6
Pomeranian	10.5 ± 0.9
Chihuahua	10.0 ± 0.6
Shih Tzu	9.5 ± 0.6
Lhasa Apso	9.6 ± 0.8
Dachshund	9.7 ± 0.5
Pug (Carlino)	10.7 ± 0.9
Bulldog	12.7 ± 1.7
Boston Terrier	11.7 ± 1.4
Labrador	10.39 ± 0.19

Furthermore, in recent years, various methods to assess left atrium size in the lateral projection have been described. All of them, however, depend on the correct visualisation of the contour of this cardiac chamber on the X-ray, which is not always possible, especially in patients with increased pulmonary opacity. These methods are as follows:

- VLAS (vertebral left atrium score): The distance is measured from the centre of the ventral margin of the carina to the caudal margin of the left atrium at its intersection with the dorsal margin of the caudal vena cava. This measurement is then aligned with the thoracic spine, counting the number of vertebral bodies that it encompasses, starting at the cranial aspect of the 4th thoracic vertebrae (fig. 3.78). According to Malcom et al. (2018) a value greater than or equal to 2.3 is a good indicator of left atrial enlargement.
- RLAD (radiographic left atrial dimension): a line is drawn bisecting the 90-degree angle formed by the height and width axes of the cardiac silhouette (as per the Buchanan method) from the point of intersection of both axes to the dorsal edge of the left atrium. This measurement is then aligned with the thoracic spine, counting the number of vertebral bodies that it encompasses, starting at the cranial aspect of the 4th thoracic vertebrae (fig. 3.79). According to Sanchez Salguero et al. (2018) a value greater than or equal to 1.8 indicates an increase in the size of the left atrium.

- M-VLAS (modified-vertebral left atrium size): the distance between the centre of the ventral border of the carina to the caudal margin of the left atrium at the point where it intersects the dorsal border of the caudal vena cava silhouette, and then a second line is drawn perpendicular to the first line, starting from the most distal border of the left atrium. The two measurements are then aligned with the thoracic spine, counting the number of vertebrae that they encompass, starting from the cranial aspect of T4 (fig. 3.80). The sum of the vertebral bodies in these two lines is the M-VLAS index. According to Lam et al. (2021), the left atrium is enlarged with values greater than or equal to 3.4.

The consensus guidelines for the diagnosis and treatment of chronic myxomatous mitral valve disease in dogs, published by the American College of Veterinary Internal Medicine in 2019, include the radiographic evaluation of VHS and VLAS to identify increased cardiac size in patients with stage B2 of this disease when echocardiography is unavailable.

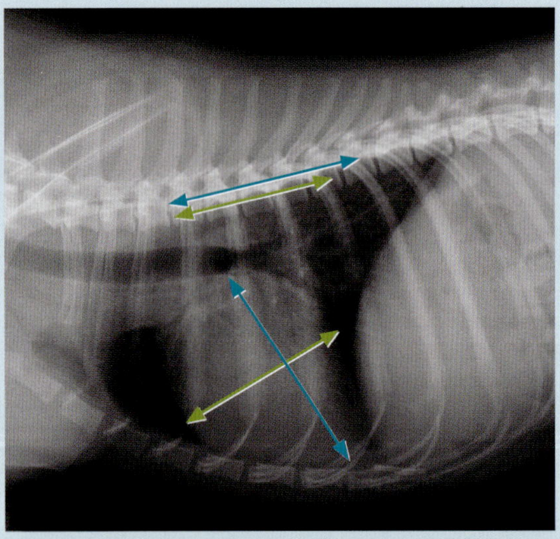

FIGURE 3.77. Normal lateral radiograph of the thorax of a dog, in which the references to measure the cardiac silhouette according to Buchanan's vertebral heart scale are shown. The distance between the ventral margin of the carina and the cardiac apex on lateral radiographs is used as a measure of height (blue line), and the craniocaudal diameter is then measured perpendicularly to the height axis (green line). This is done the same way in dogs and cats. The two measurements are then transferred to the thoracic spine to count the corresponding number of vertebrae, always starting from the cranial aspect of T4. The normal range is 9.7 ± 0.5 in dogs and 7.5 ± 0.3 in cats, although these may vary in some breeds. In this case the result is 10.2.

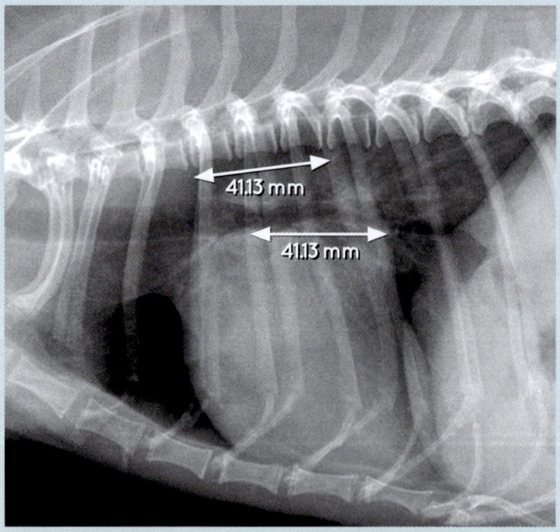

FIGURE 3.78. Lateral radiograph of the thorax of a dog with left atrium enlargement. The axes of measurement illustrate the left atrium size measurement system called VLAS: measuring the distance from the centre of the ventral margin of the carina to the caudal margin of the left atrium at its intersection with the dorsal margin of the caudal vena cava. This measurement is aligned with the thoracic spine and the number of vertebrae it encompasses counted, starting from the cranial aspect of T4. In this patient, the VLAS is 3 vertebral bodies.

Position of the cardiac chambers and great vessels

The position of the different cardiac chambers, the aortic arch and main pulmonary artery on right lateral and dorsoventral projections are shown in figure 3.81. On lateral views, the cranial border of the silhouette is formed by the outline of the right atrial appendage and right ventricle. The caudal border is formed by the outline of the left atrial appendage and left ventricle. The cardiac silhouette may be compared to that of a clock face (clock-face analogy) and time intervals may be used to locate the cardiac chambers and great vessels.

- **Lateral view** (fig. 3.82):
  - From 12 to 2 o'clock: left atrium.
  - From 2 to 5 o'clock: left ventricle.
  - From 5 to 9 o'clock: right ventricle.
  - From 9 to 10 o'clock: main pulmonary artery and right atrial appendage.
  - From 10 to 11 o'clock: aortic arch.
- **Dorsoventral view** (fig. 3.83):
  - From 11 to 1 o'clock: aortic arch.
  - From 1 to 2 o'clock: main pulmonary artery.
  - From 2 to 3 o'clock: left atrial appendage (the left atrial appendage is located between the two main bronchi, in the central area of the cardiac silhouette on this view).
  - From 2 to 5 o'clock: left ventricle.
  - From 5 to 9 o'clock: right ventricle.
  - From 9 to 11 o'clock: right atrium.

The identification of prominences of the silhouette in these locations helps to identify a possible enlargement of the different cardiac chambers, as well as of the exit of the aorta and pulmonary artery.

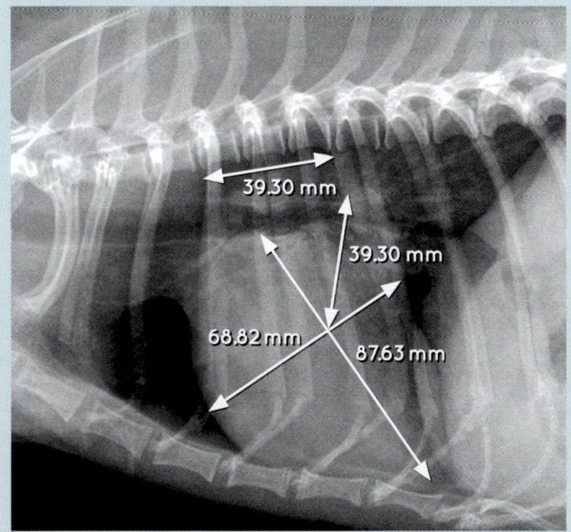

FIGURE 3.79. With the same X-ray as the previous figure using the RLAD method of measuring the left atrium size: a line is drawn bisecting the 90-degree angle formed by the height and width axes of the cardiac silhouette (as per the Buchanan method) from the point of intersection of both axes to the dorsal edge of the left atrium. This measurement is aligned with the thoracic spine and the number of vertebrae it encompasses counted, starting from the cranial aspect of T4. In this patient, the RLAD is 3 vertebral bodies.

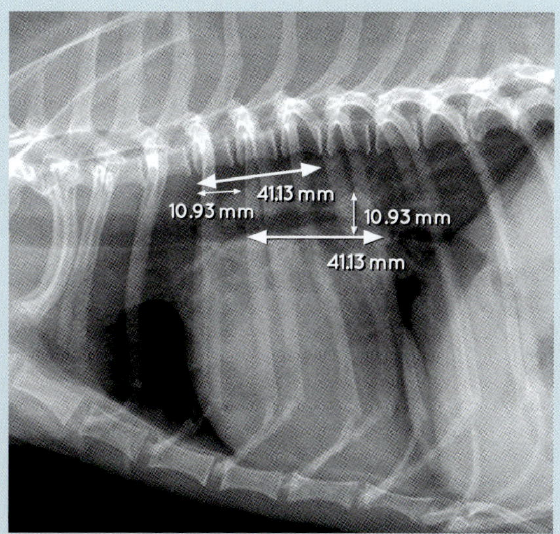

FIGURE 3.80. With the same X-ray as the previous figures but using the M-VLAS method to measure the left atrial size: the distance is measured from the centre of the ventral margin of the carina to the caudal margin of the left atrium where it intersects the dorsal margin of the caudal vena cava, and then a second line is drawn perpendicular to the first, starting from the most distal margin of the left atrium. These two measurements are then aligned with the thoracic spine, counting the number of vertebral bodies that they encompass, starting at the cranial aspect of the 4th thoracic vertebra. In this patient, the M-VLAS is 4 vertebral bodies.

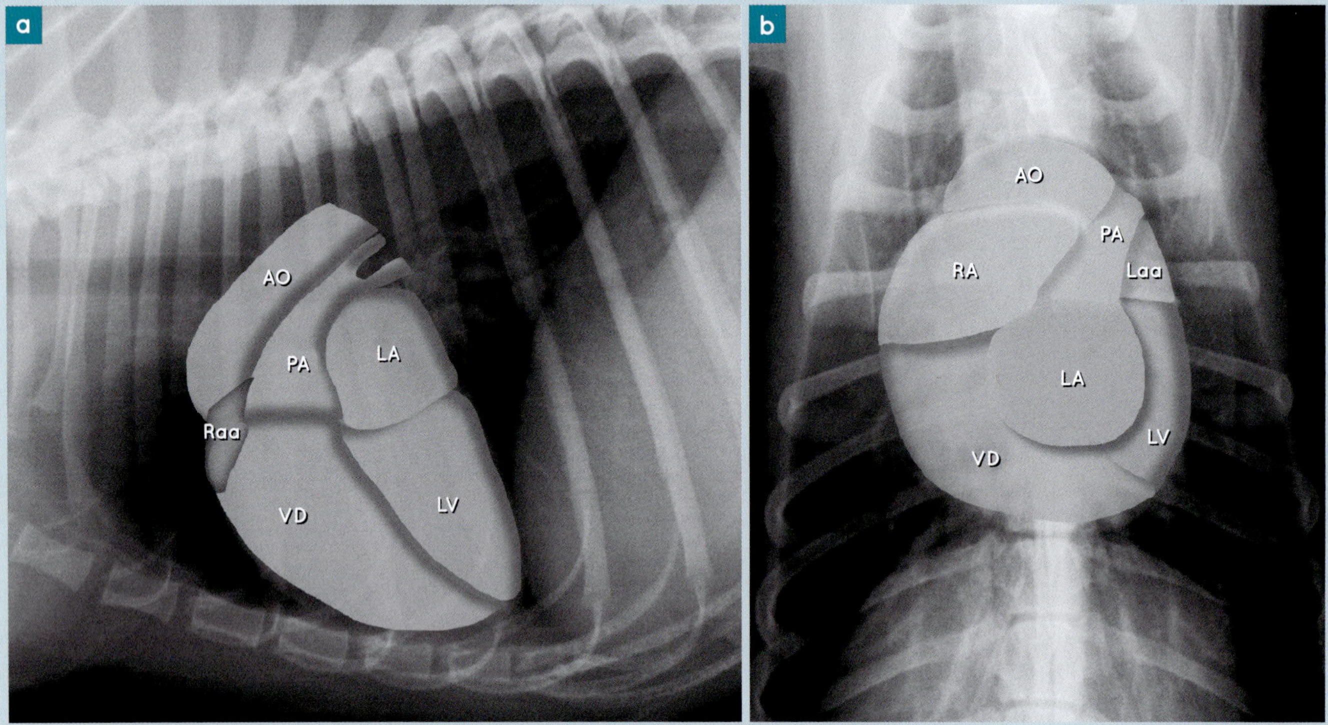

FIGURE 3.81. Normal lateral (a) and dorsoventral (b) radiographs of the thorax of a dog, in which the heart chambers, the aortic arch and the main pulmonary artery are shown in grey. RA, right atrium; LA, left atrium; RV, right ventricle; LV, left ventricle; Raa, right atrial appendage; Laa, left atrial appendage; AO, aortic arch; PA, main pulmonary artery.

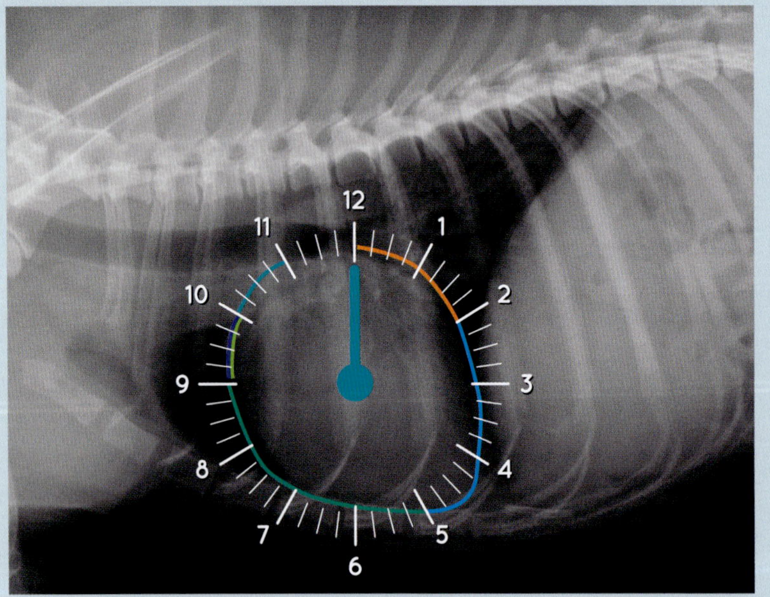

FIGURE 3.82. Normal lateral radiograph of the thorax of a dog, in which the position of the cardiac chambers and great vessels is shown according to the clock-face analogy. Left atrium: from 12 to 2 o'clock (orange line); left ventricle: from 2 to 5 o'clock (blue line); right ventricle: from 5 to 9 o'clock (dark green line); right atrial appendage (light green line) and pulmonary artery (purple line): from 9 to 10 o'clock; aortic arch: from 10 to 11 o'clock (red line).

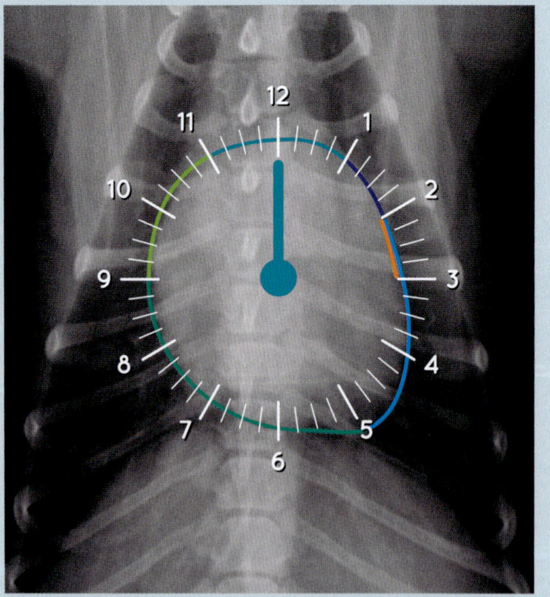

FIGURE 3.83. Normal dorsoventral radiograph of the thorax of a dog, in which the position of the cardiac chambers and great vessels is shown according to the clock-face analogy. Aortic arch: from 11 to 1 o'clock (red line); main pulmonary artery: from 1 to 2 o'clock (purple line); left atrial appendage: from 2 to 3 o'clock (orange line); left ventricle: from 2 to 5 o'clock (blue line); right ventricle: from 5 to 9 o'clock (dark green line); right atrium: from 9 to 11 o'clock (light green line).

Radiographic signs of enlargement of the heart chambers

From a didactic point of view, it is useful to describe the signs of enlargement of each of the cardiac chambers separately, although in practice it is rare to find a significant increase in the size of only one of them. It will be normal to detect signs of enlargement of the left heart (left atrium and ventricle), as well as global cardiomegaly (with or without predominance of the right or left side of the heart) at different degrees.

The radiographic signs of enlargement of each heart chamber are summarised in box 3.1 and are illustrated in figures 3.84–3.87.

In some cases, the enlargement of the left atrium may appear together with the narrowing of one or both of the main bronchi. This may be caused by the pressure exerted on the bronchi by the enlarged chamber, although it is more likely to be caused by bronchial chondromalacia and dynamic collapse of the bronchi which may be accentuated when the left atrium is significantly enlarged. This left atrium enlargement and bronchial collapse due to chondromalacia may cause the dog to cough, which the clinician should not confuse with a sign of heart failure.

The radiological signs of left atrial enlargement are less evident in cats. The most evident sign is usually the widening of the heart base silhouette in the dorsoventral projection (fig. 3.88). If the enlargement is very pronounced, it can produce what is known as the valentine-shaped cardiac silhouette, traditionally associated with biatrial enlargement in cases of hypertrophic cardiomyopathy. We now understand that visualisation of the valentine-shaped silhouette does not necessarily imply enlargement of the right atrium, in fact, it has been seen that most feline patients with this radiological sign present only a marked enlargement of the left atrium.

Radiographic signs of left cardiac failure may be observed when the left heart is enlarged: vascular congestion and pulmonary oedema. Dilatation of the pulmonary veins is the radiological sign that may be detected most early, although it is not always identified. Pulmonary oedema starts in the interstitial tissue, which makes the visualisation of the small pulmonary vessels more difficult. However, these remain visible until the oedema progresses and also affects the alveoli, which is when air bronchograms appear in the affected area. Cardiogenic pulmonary oedema in dogs is typically located in the perihilar area, although it extends to the median and peripheral area of the lung at advanced stages. It usually affects the right lung more than the left one. In cats, cardiogenic pulmonary oedema may appear in any part of the lung, often with a more patchy pattern. Pleural effusion is also common in cats as a sign of left heart failure (fig. 3.89).

When the right heart is enlarged, it is possible to detect signs of right cardiac failure, which include dilatation of the caudal vena cava, hepatosplenomegaly, ascites and pleural effusion. Pleural effusion due to right heart failure in cats differs from that caused by left failure: the patient does not also present associated hepatomegaly or ascites with left heart failure which do occur in cases of right failure.

If cardiomegaly is global, the silhouette will appear increased in width and height in the two projections (fig. 3.90). In many cases, the signs of an enlarged left heart predominate; in the other cases it is possible to observe signs of enlargement of the right heart, or a more or less uniform enlargement of both sides of the heart. Depending on which are the most affected chambers, the radiographs may show associated signs of left and/or right cardiac failure.

Moderate or marked cardiomegaly is a quite reliable indicator of cardiac disease, but mild cardiomegaly should be interpreted carefully, and always in correlation with the rest of the patient's clinical data.

On the other hand, a heart that appears normal on an X-ray may not be a healthy heart as some diseases do not have a significant impact on heart size or shape.

Recently, Huguet et al. (2021) published a study of 175 dogs and concluded that X-ray imaging is more accurate for diagnosing left heart enlargement than right heart enlargement, based on the correlation of radiographic findings in these patients with echocardiography. The authors found numerous false negatives in radiographic identification of right-sided cardiomegaly when it was mild, and false positives of right-sided cardiomegaly in cases of severe left-sided

BOX 3.1. SIGNS OF ENLARGEMENT OF THE CARDIAC CHAMBER

Left ventricle

It is located immediately ventral to the left main bronchus. The enlargement of the atrium leads to its dorsal displacement and to a prominence of the cardiac silhouette at this level, which are both visible on lateral radiographs. On dorsoventral radiographs, it is located between the two main bronchi, caudal to the tracheal bifurcation. An increase in the size of the atrium leads to a greater separation of these two bronchi, although this will only be visible on the radiograph if it is taken with a high kilovoltage so it is intentionally overexposed. In addition, the left atrial appendage is displaced, which originates an image of a prominent cardiac silhouette in the 2 to 3 o'clock position.

Right ventricle

When this chamber increases in size, it tends to do so in height, which therefore leads to an increase in the height of the cardiac silhouette and to a dorsal elevation of the trachea (along its whole length, from the thoracic inlet to the carina) on lateral radiographs. The caudal vena cava is also displaced dorsally. On dorsoventral radiographs, the left margin in the interval from 2 to 5 o'clock becomes rounded and lies closer to the thoracic wall.

Right atrium

On lateral radiographs, the increase in size of the atrium causes a dorsal displacement of the caudal part of the trachea (on the cranial part of the base of the heart), while the carina tends to maintain its normal position. It is difficult to assess on dorsoventral radiographs, although it may give rise to a prominence of the margin of the cardiac silhouette in the 9 to 11 o'clock position.

Left atrial appendage

When this chamber increases in size, it tends to do so in width, which therefore leads to an increase in the width of the cardiac silhouette and to a greater cardiosternal contact on lateral radiographs. On dorsoventral radiographs, the margin of the cardiac silhouette becomes rounded in the 5 to 9 o'clock position, and even acquires a "inverted D" shape when the enlargement is significant.

Left ventricle

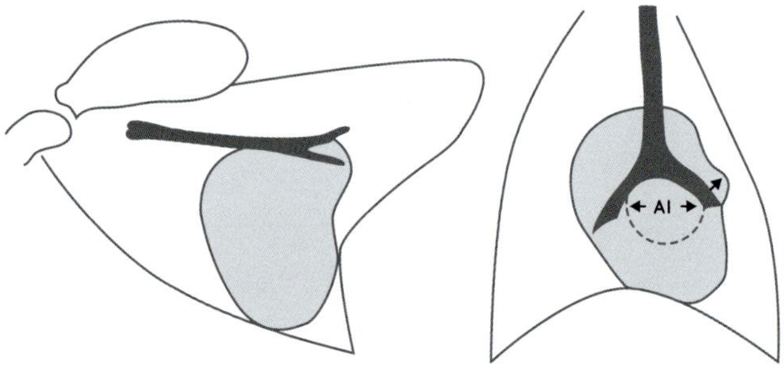

Right ventricle

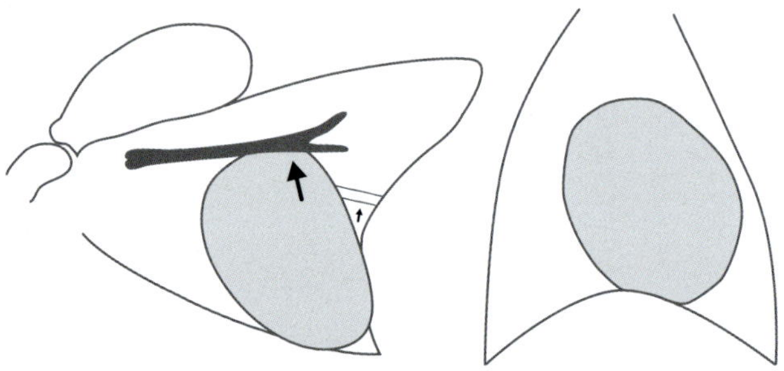

Right atrium

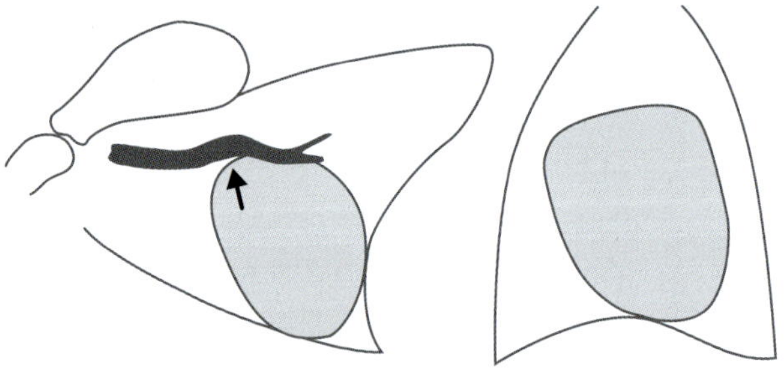

Left atrial appendage

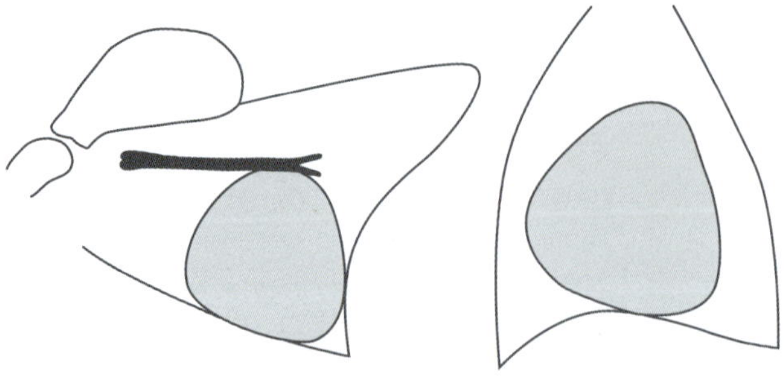

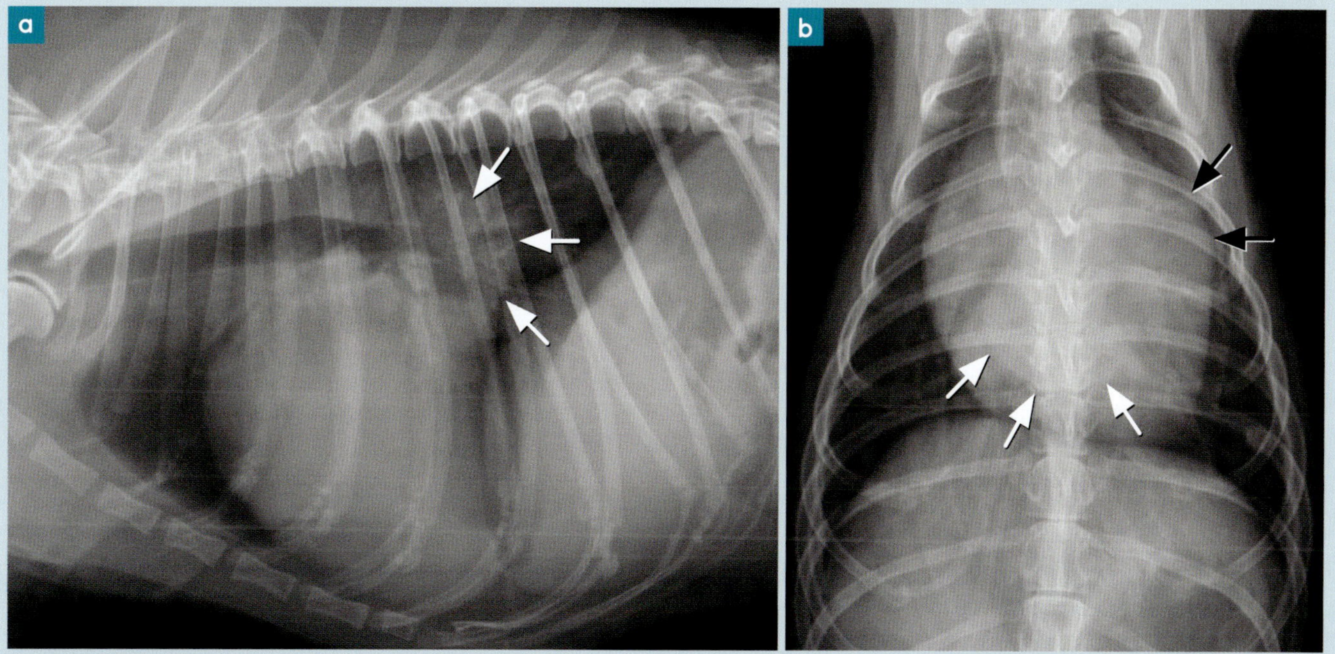

FIGURE 3.84. Lateral (a) and dorsoventral (b) radiographs of the thorax of a dog with signs of enlargement of the left atrium. In image (a), the left atrium is prominent in the caudodorsal margin of cardiac silhouette (white arrows). In image (b), the left atrium appears in the central area of the silhouette, where only part of its contour can be visualised (white arrows), and laterally displaces the left atrial appendage, thus causing a prominence in the 2 to 3 o'clock position (black arrows) according to the clock-face analogy.

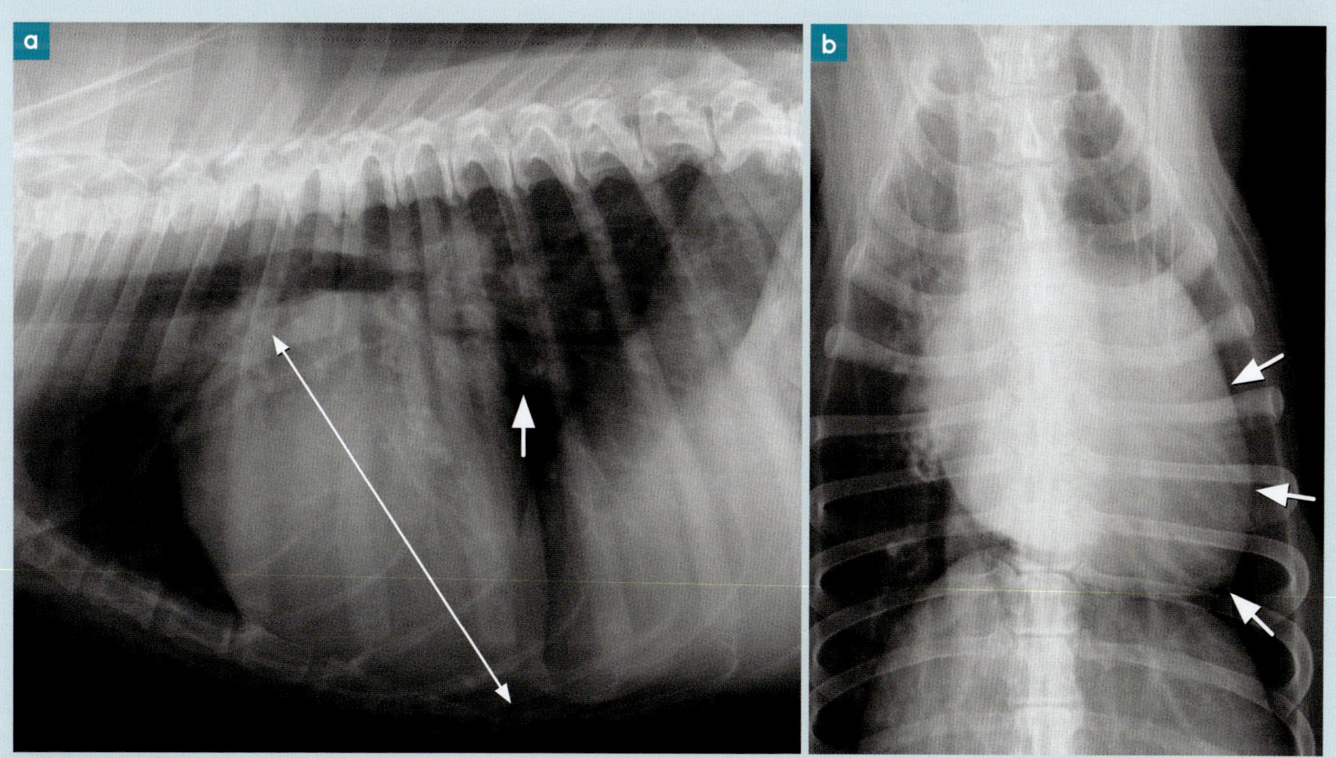

FIGURE 3.85. Lateral (a) and dorsoventral (b) radiographs of the thorax of a dog with signs of enlargement of the left ventricle. In image (a), the silhouette appears increased in height (white arrow), and the trachea and caudal vena cava (short white arrow) are displaced in dorsal direction. In image (b), the margin of the silhouette in the 2 to 5 o'clock position (white arrows) according to the clock-analogy lies closer to the thoracic wall. The left atrium is also moderately prominent on the lateral radiograph and venous congestion may be observed (initial sign of left cardiac failure).

cardiomegaly, which can cause significant alteration in the overall morphological appearance of the cardiac silhouette even in the absence of right-sided heart enlargement (fig. 3.91).

Great vessels

Changes in the image of the great vessels may provide additional information about possible alterations of the heart.

The diameter of the caudal vena cava (CVC), between the cardiac silhouette and the diaphragm, can be compared with the diameter of the descending aorta (Ao), measured at the same intercostal space and if possible, during inspiration (fig. 3.92). A CVC/Ao ratio > 1.5 is very indicative of right cardiac failure. A CVC diameter that exceeds T5 or T6 vertebral body length is another reference indicating enlargement, when measured on the lateral projection. Before reaching a definitive diagnosis of decreased size, we should bear in mind the diameter of this vessel varies slightly with both the respiratory and the cardiac cycles. If the decreased diameter size is maintained on serial radiography, hypovolaemia would be considered as the most likely cause.

The diameter of a normal aorta is similar to the height of the adjacent vertebral bodies. It may appear increased in cases of aortic valve stenosis, and occasionally, in patients with patent ductus arteriosus. On dorsoventral radiographs, an increase of the aortic diameter creates a prominence of the cardiac silhouette in the 11 to 1 o'clock position according to the clock-face analogy, while on lateral radiographs the aortic arch is more marked. In senior healthy cats, the aorta may be elongated, and its curvature may be more pronounced or it may even follow a more undulating course, which has been termed "redundant aorta" (see fig. 3.76). In these cases, the contour of the aortic arch may appear lateralised to the left in the dorsoventral and ventrodorsal projections, which can be mistaken for a pulmonary nodular lesion.

The main pulmonary artery (pulmonary trunk) may appear enlarged in cases of pulmonary stenosis, patent

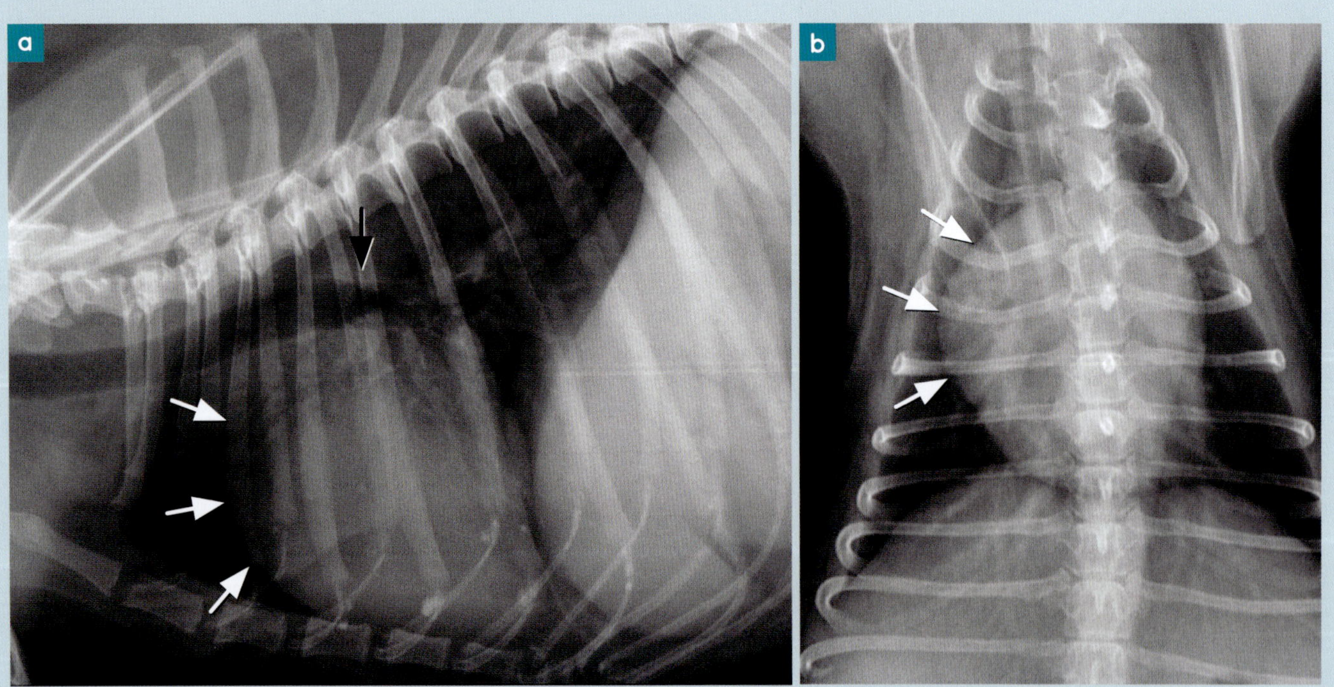

FIGURE 3.86. Lateral (a) and dorsoventral (b) radiographs of the thorax of a dog with signs of enlargement of the right atrium. In image (a), the craniodorsal margin of the silhouette is prominent (white arrows) and the trachea appears elevated on the base of the heart, while the carina (black arrow) tends to maintain a lower position. In image (b), the cardiac silhouette is prominent in the 9 to 11 o'clock position (white arrows) according to the clock-face analogy.

ductus ateriosus, pulmonary hypertension or dirofilariasis, essentially. On ventrodorsal radiographs, its enlargement gives rise to a prominence of the cardiac silhouette in the 1 to 2 o'clock position according to the clock-face analogy in dogs. In cats, its location is more medial. On lateral views, it is more difficult to identify its enlargement, although the superimposition with the trachea may facilitate its visualisation.

Acquired heart diseases

Acquired valvular disease

Primary acquired valvular disease in cats and dogs is usually degenerative (endocardiosis) or, on a less frequent basis, infectious (bacterial endocarditis).

Myxomatous mitral valve degeneration, also called mitral endocardiosis or chronic myxomatous mitral valve disease, is the most common heart disease in dogs. Clinical signs are generally observed in old animals, especially in small breeds. The incompetence of the mitral valve caused by valvular degeneration leads to the backflow of blood to the left atrium, which initially originates its dilatation, and will be followed by an enlargement of the left ventricle. As the process progresses, signs of left heart failure may appear.

Degeneration of the tricuspid valve is uncommon as an isolated lesion. It usually appears associated with degeneration of the mitral valve. It causes signs of enlargement of the right atrium and ventricle and may be accompanied by signs of right heart failure (dilatation of the caudal vena cava, hepatosplenomegaly, ascites and pleural effusion).

Bacterial endocarditis is rare in cats and dogs. Radiography does not provide any relevant information in most cases, at least in the early stages. The cardiac silhouette may appear normal, or show signs of enlargement of the left atrium and pulmonary oedema.

Cardiomyopathies

Dilated cardiomyopathy is one of the most frequent heart diseases in dogs. It usually produces signs of global cardiomegaly (fig. 3.93). In advanced stages, the silhouette may resemble that of pericardial effusion, and secondary signs of left and right heart failure may appear. In the Doberman, dilated cardiomyopathy may cause a very remarkable enlargement of the left atrium only.

Hypertrophic cardiomyopathy is the most common acquired heart disease in cats which usually presents with substantial left atrium enlargement (fig. 3.94). The valentine-shaped cardiac silhouette sign may appear, with widening of the cardiac base in the dorsoventral projection. As the disease progresses, signs of associated left and/or right heart failure may appear.

Dilated cardiomyopathy is much less frequent in cats, and usually causes global cardiomegaly with rounding of the apex. The cardiac silhouette is often masked by pleural effusion in these cases.

The diagnosis of cardiomyopathy is always confirmed by means of echocardiography.

Dirofilariasis

This is one of the main causes of pulmonary hypertension, which in turn causes right ventricular hypertrophy. Adult parasites inhabit the pulmonary arteries and sometimes the right ventricle and atrium. On chest X-rays, signs of right ventricle enlargement can be visualised, as well as the dilatation and tortuous course of the pulmonary arteries. When transverse silhouettes of these enlarged vessels are identified, their image may be confused with that of pulmonary nodules (see fig. 3.113c). The enlarged main pulmonary artery creates a prominence of the cardiac silhouette contour from the 1 to 2 o'clock position according to the clock-face analogy (fig. 3.95). A focal or multifocal alveolar lung pattern may appear in peripheral areas due to thromboembolism caused by the accumulation of parasite debris or secondary inflammation (pneumonitis). The latter may also cause an unstructured interstitial lung pattern.

Dirofilariasis is rare in cats. When present, enlargement of the main pulmonary artery is not usually evident, but enlargement of the peripheral pulmonary arteries can be identified. They may have a bronchointerstitial pattern similar to that of feline allergic or inflammatory lung diseases. This pattern may appear even in the absence of a vascular pattern, so this differential diagnosis should be taken into account in cats that present this radiological pattern, especially in geographical locations with the highest incidence of this disease.

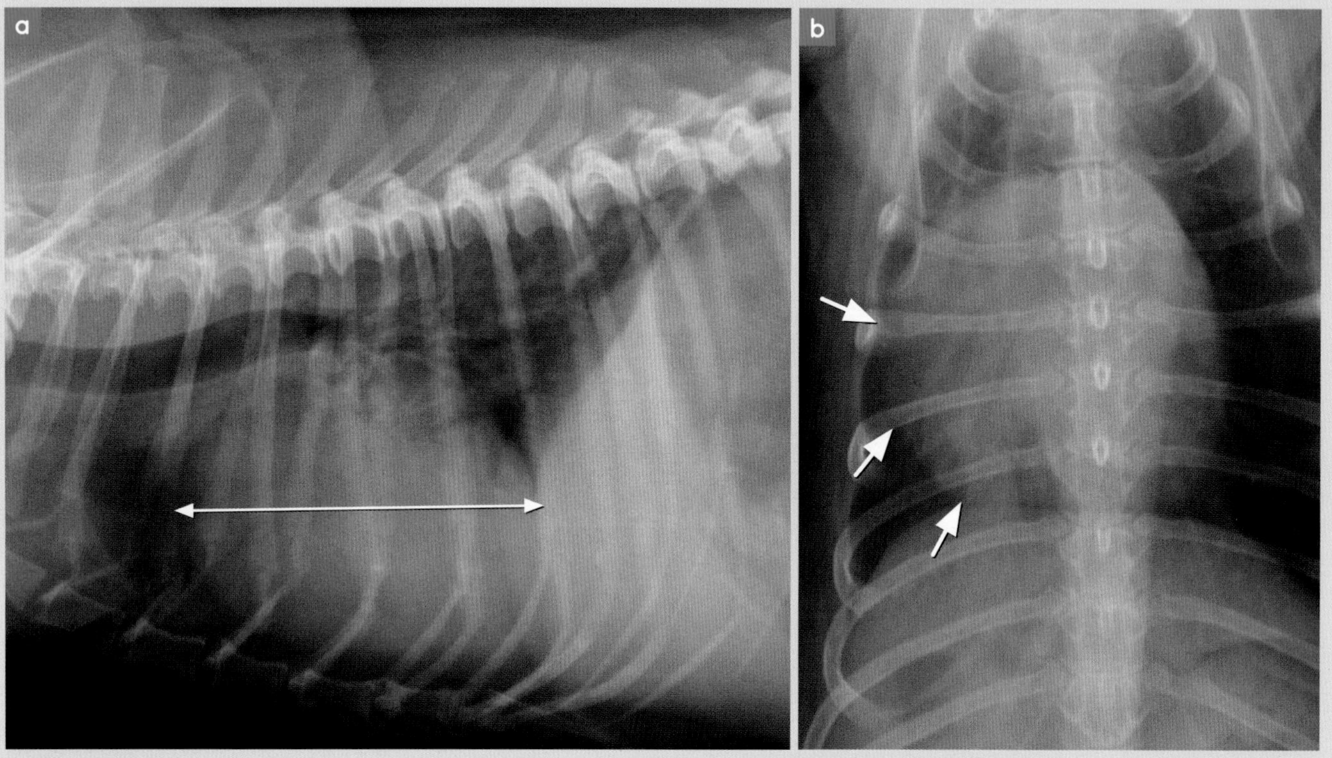

FIGURE 3.87. Lateral (a) and dorsoventral (b) radiographs of the thorax of a dog with signs of enlargement of the right ventricle. In image (a), the width of the cardiac silhouette appears enlarged (white line), thus leading to increased cardiosternal contact. In image (b), the cardiac silhouette is prominent in the 5 to 9 o'clock position (white arrows) according to the clock-face analogy, and the whole right margin of the cardiac silhouette has a more rounded shape ("inverted-D" shape).

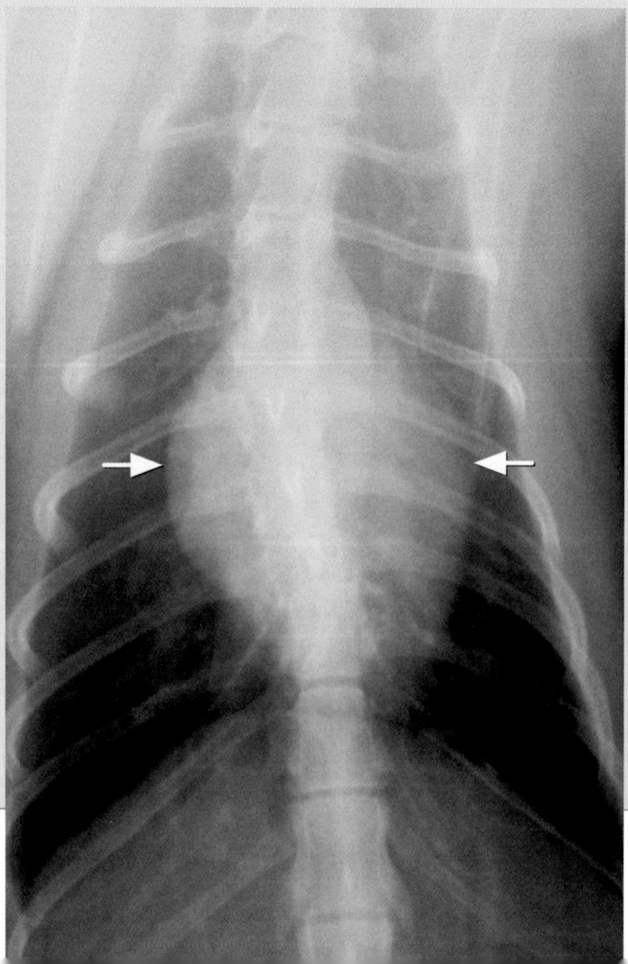

FIGURE 3.88. Dorsoventral projection of the chest of a cat with a valentine-shaped cardiac silhouette sign (term used to describe the widening of the heart base as indicated here by arrows) caused by left atrium enlargement. This sign had traditionally been associated with enlargement of both atria in cases of hypertrophic cardiomyopathy, but echocardiography has shown that most feline patients who show this radiological sign have only a marked increase in the size of the left atrium.

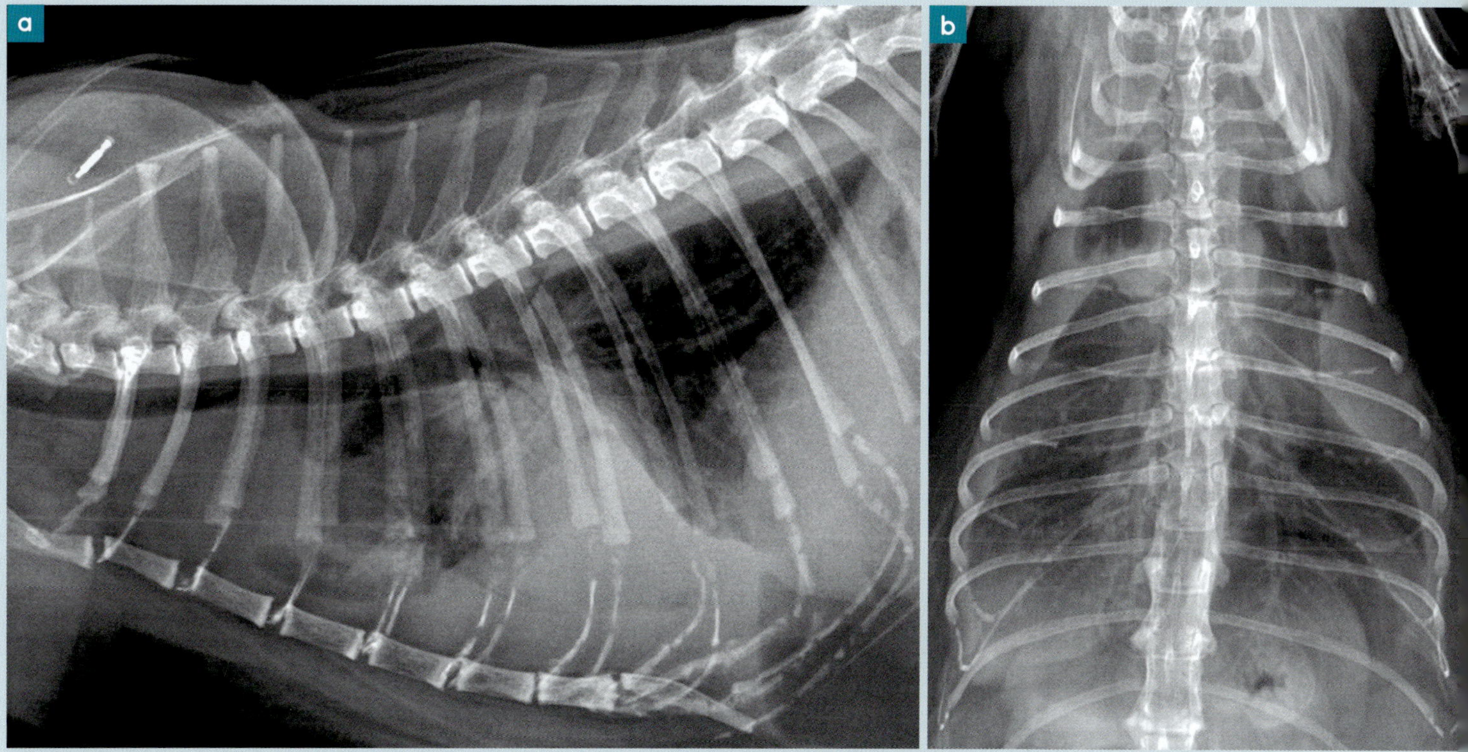

FIGURE 3.89. Lateral (a) and dorsoventral (b) projections of a cat presenting with pleural effusion due to left heart failure due to advanced hypertrophic cardiomyopathy.

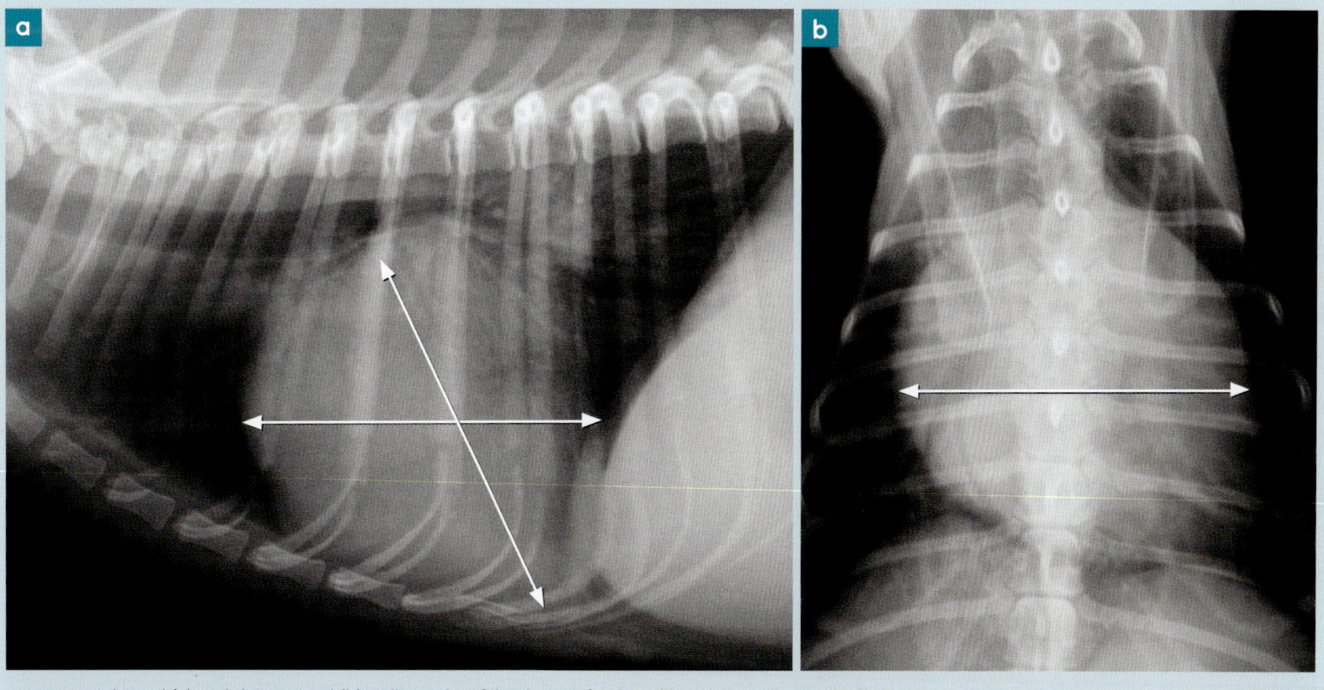

FIGURE 3.90. Lateral (a) and dorsoventral (b) radiographs of the thorax of a dog with global cardiomegaly. Signs of enlargement of all the heart chambers may be observed and the height and width of the cardiac silhouette are increased on the lateral view, as well as its width on the dorsoventral view.

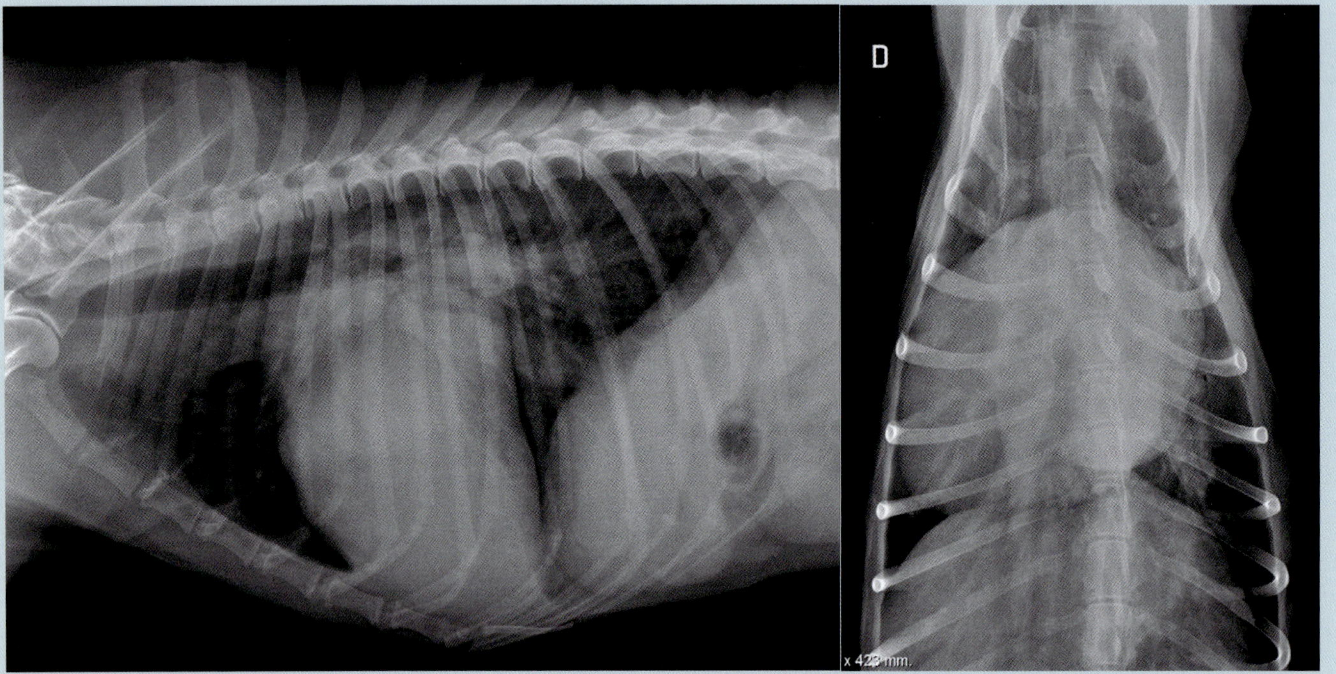

FIGURE 3.91. Lateral (a) and dorsoventral (b) projections of a dog with radiological signs suggestive of marked left and right heart enlargement. Echocardiography confirmed that the patient had no right heart enlargement. Radiography may result in false positives and false negatives in right-sided cardiomegaly, as published by Huguet et al. (2021). In this patient, a false identification of right-sided cardiomegaly was shown on the radiograph.

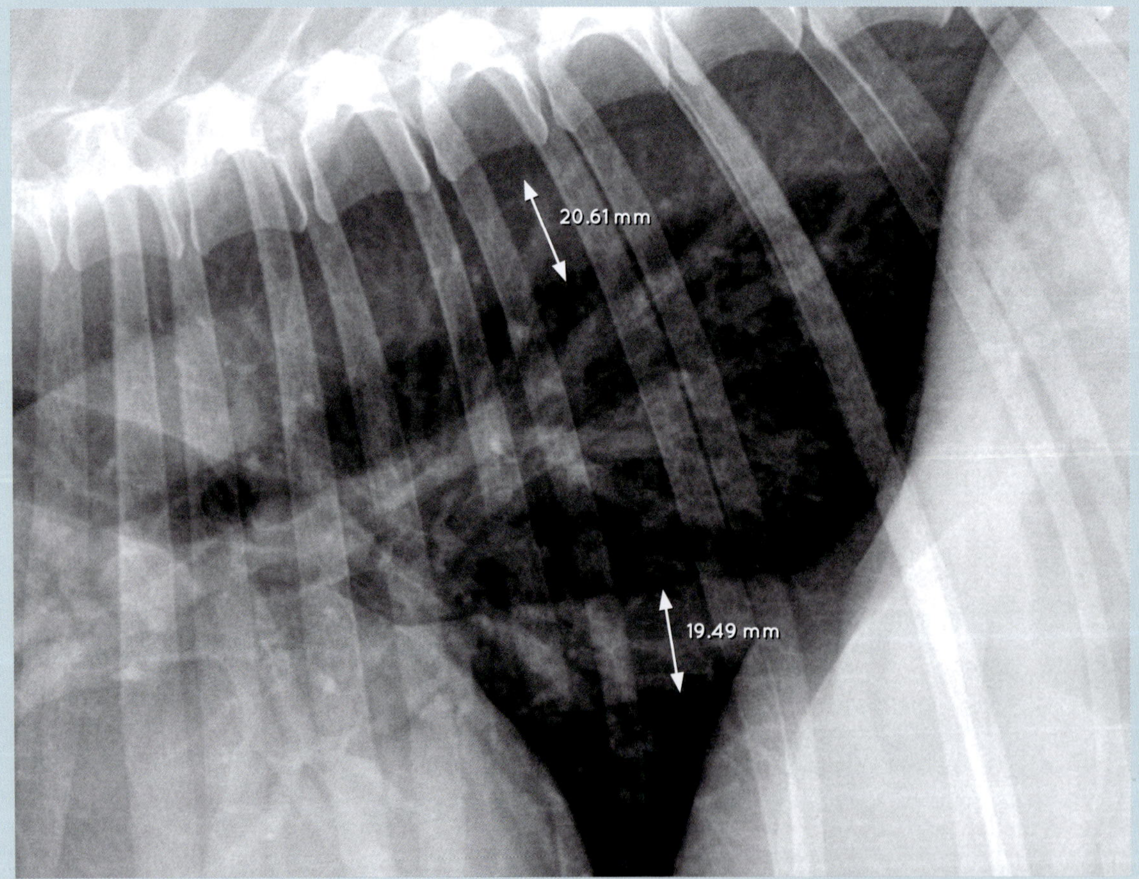

FIGURE 3.92. Enlargement of the lateral projection of the thorax of a healthy dog in which the measurements of the aorta (20.61 mm) and the caudal vena cava (19.49 mm) have been taken in the same intercostal space. The CVC/Ao ratio is 0.94 (within normal range).

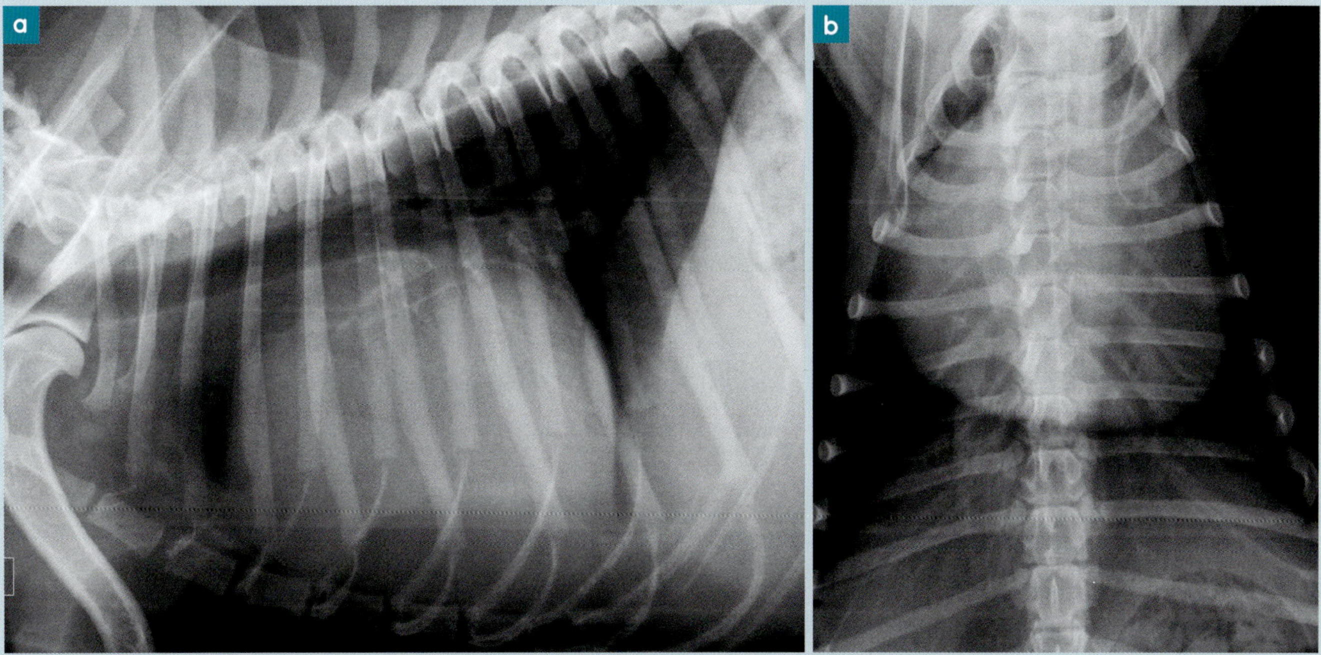

FIGURE 3.93. Lateral (a) and dorsoventral (b) projections of a dog with severe dilated cardiomyopathy.

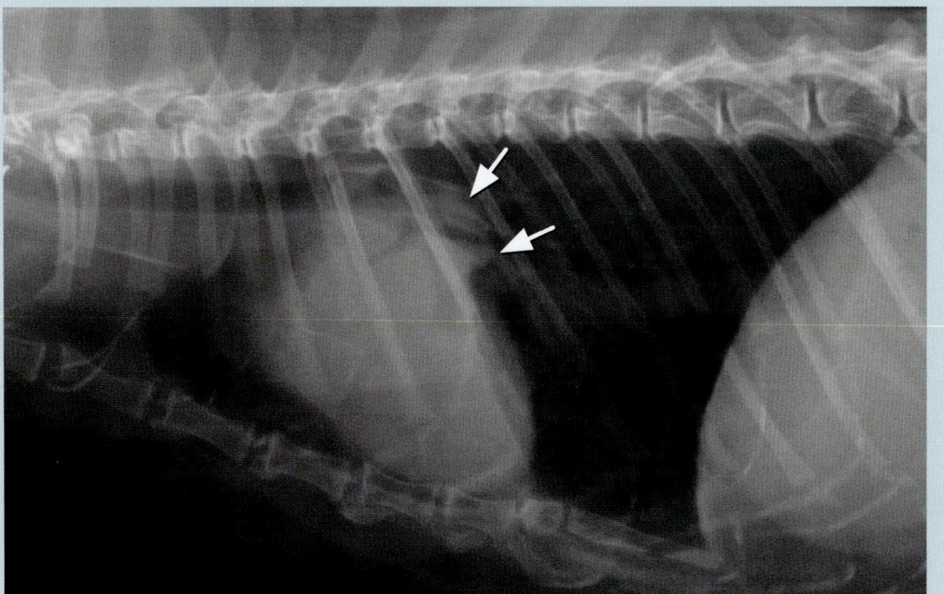

FIGURE 3.94. Lateral radiograph of the thorax of a cat with hypertrophic cardiomyopathy. It is possible to observe an increase in the height of the cardiac silhouette, an elevation of the trachea and caudal vena cava and a marked prominence of the left atrium (arrows).

Congenital cardiac diseases

The value of plain radiography in the diagnosis of congenital diseases of the heart and great vessels is limited. Contrast techniques have been almost totally replaced by echocardiography, which is the method of choice for the diagnosis and assessment of these diseases.

The most common congenital heart defects in dogs are patent ductus arteriosus, pulmonary stenosis, aortic stenosis, ventricular septal defect and tetralogy of Fallot. *Mitral valve dysplasia, atrial septal defect, tricuspid valve dysplasia,* cor triatatum dexter and mitral valve stenosis are diagnosed on a less frequent basis. Persistent truncus arteriosus, tricuspid valve stenosis, right ventricular hypoplasia, double outlet right ventricle and transposition of the great vessels are rarer. In cats, the most frequent defects are mitral valve or tricuspid valve dysplasia, patent ductus arteriosus, tetralogy of Fallot, ventricular septal defect, aortic valve stenosis, tetralogy of Fallot, persistent common atrioventricular canal or endocardial fibroelastosis.

In some cases, plain radiography provides data that may help or guide us in case of a clinical suspicion of a congenital heart or vascular disease.

Patent ductus arteriosus

In the foetal circulation, the ductus arteriosus shunts the oxygenated maternal blood to the aorta. The permanent closure of this duct occurs soon after birth, thus forming the ligamentum arteriosum. A failure in the closure of the duct maintains a communication between the aorta and the main pulmonary artery, and is called patent ductus arteriosus. The consequences of this failure to close will depend on the diameter of the duct and on the pulmonary vascular resistance. When the pulmonary vascular resistance is normal, there is a continuous shunt flow from the aorta (high resistance) to the pulmonary circulation (low resistance). This type of flow (systemic to pulmonary) is termed left-to-right shunt and is the most common pattern. Reverse or right-to-left patent ductus arteriosus refers to those

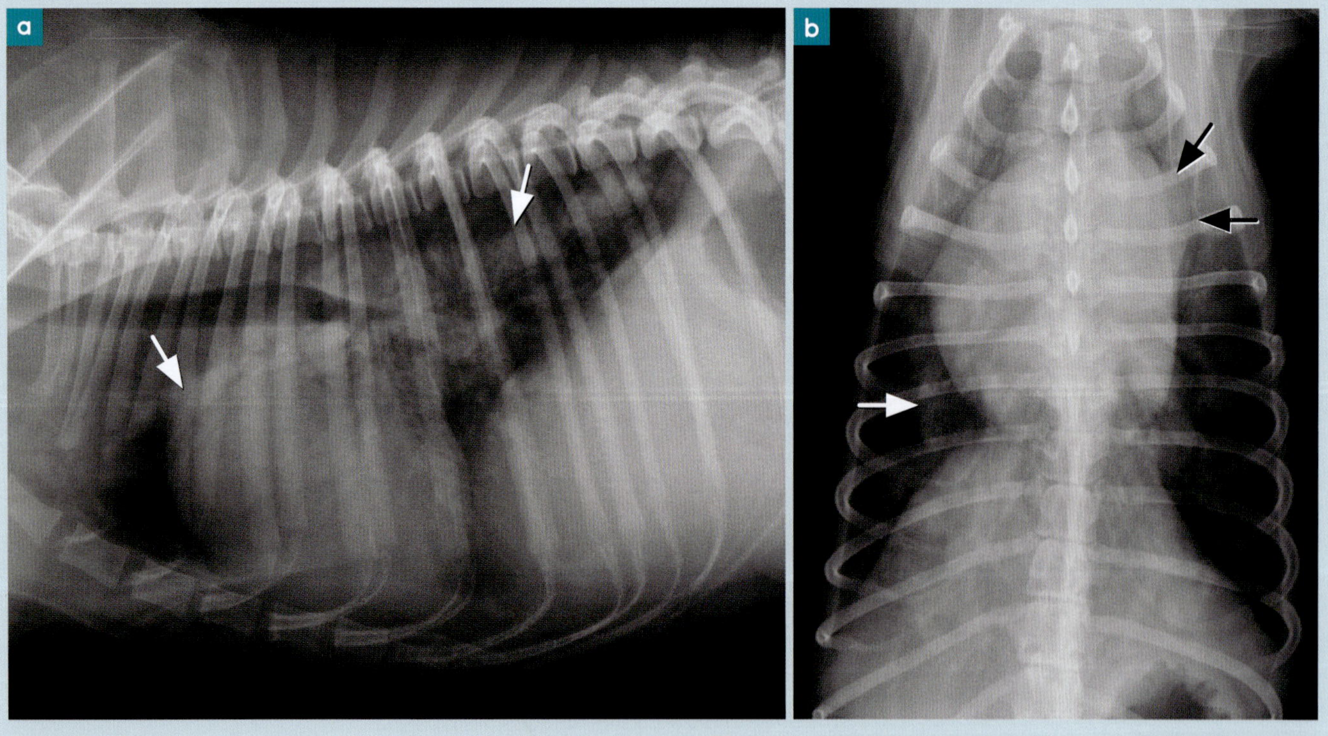

FIGURE 3.95. Lateral (a) and ventrodorsal (b) radiographs of the thorax of a dog with dirofilariosis. It is possible to observe signs of enlargement of the right ventricle and dilatation and tortuous course of the pulmonary arteries (indicated by white arrows). In image (b), the enlarged main pulmonary artery creates a prominence of the cardiac silhouette in the 1 to 2 o'clock position (black arrows) according to the clock-face analogy.

cases in which blood flows back from the pulmonary artery to the aorta (pulmonary to systemic), and occurs because the pulmonary vascular resistance is higher than the systemic vascular resistance.

The radiographic signs of a patent ductus arteriosus considerably vary depending on the volume of blood being shunted, the age of the animal and the degree of cardiac decompensation. In left-to-right shunts, it is possible to observe a mild to moderate enlargement of the left atrium and ventricle due to volume overload and vascular congestion. It is common to observe three prominences in the margin of the cardiac silhouette on dorsoventral radiographs: in the 11 to 1 o'clock position due to aortic arch enlargement; in the 1 to 2 o'clock position due to enlargement of the outflow tract of the pulmonary artery; and in the 2 to 3 o'clock position, due to lateral displacement of the left atrial appendage. Pulmonary oedema occurs with the development of left heart failure. In animals with severe pulmonary hypertension, caused by a right-to-left patent ductus arteriosus, an enlargement of the right ventricle and tortuous pulmonary arteries (fig. 3.96) are observed.

Pulmonary stenosis

It is a narrowing of the outflow tract of the right ventricle at the valvular (pulmonary valve dysplasia), subvalvular or supravalvular level. The most common type is the first one. When blood passes through the area of narrowing, the flow accelerates and poststenotic turbulences that cause dilatation of the main pulmonary artery appear. The pressure overload in the right ventricle leads to its enlargement.

The radiographic signs of this condition depend on the degree of narrowing, although it is often possible to see signs of enlargement of the right heart and main pulmonary artery in the two projections. It is easier to see the prominence of the pulmonary artery on dorsoventral radiographs, in the 1 to 2 o'clock position according to the clock-face analogy (fig. 3.97), although its shadow may be seen superimposed with

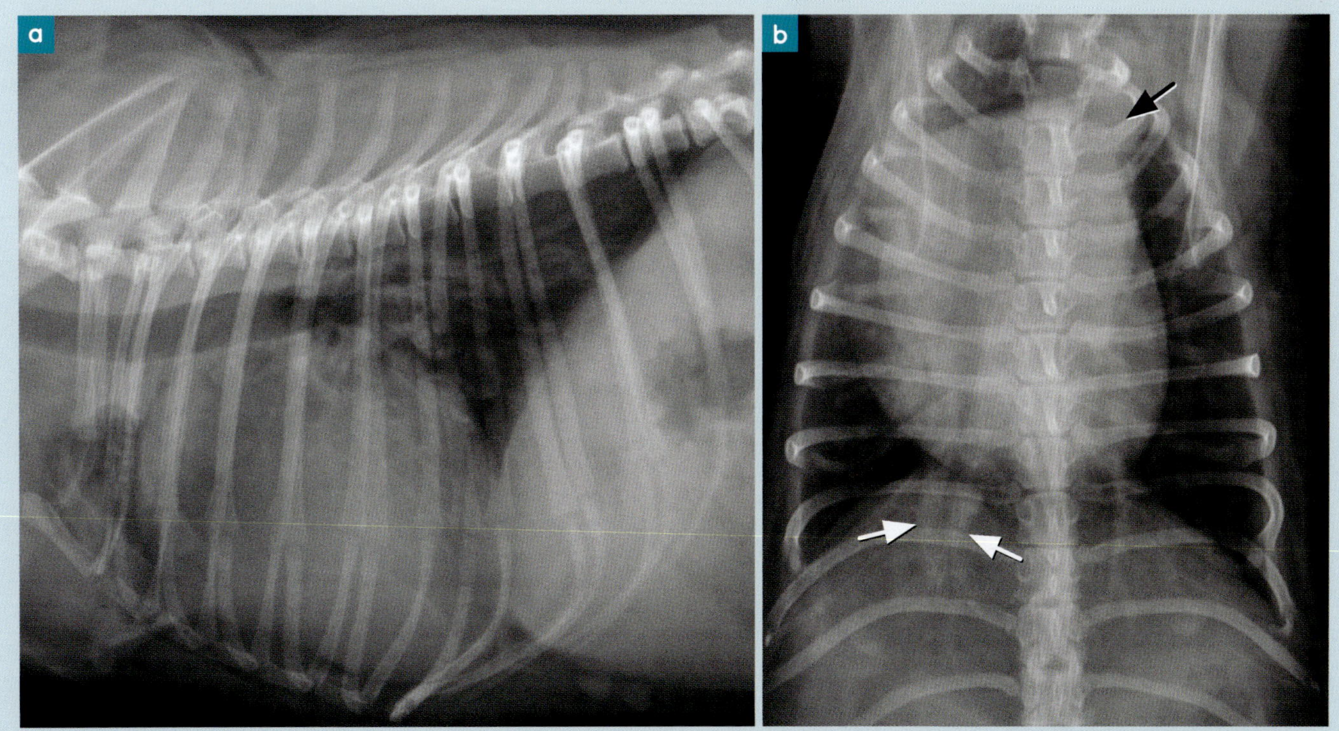

FIGURE 3.96. Lateral (a) and ventrodorsal (b) radiographs of the thorax of a dog with patent ductus arteriosus. These images show marked global cardiomegaly with a prominence of the cardiac silhouette in the 12 to 2 o'clock position (black arrow) according to the clock-face analogy, which indicates an enlargement of the main pulmonary artery, and, to a lesser extent, of the aortic arch. Dilatation of the pulmonary arteries and veins may also be observed (white arrows).

the trachea on lateral radiographs (as a kind of "hat"). The pulmonary arteries may appear normal or have a reduced diameter.

Aortic stenosis

It is a narrowing of the outflow tract of the left ventricle at the subvalvular (fibrous or muscular ring), valvular or supravalvular level. The subvalvular type is the most common type in dogs (subaortic stenosis). When blood passes through the area of narrowing, the flow accelerates and poststenotic turbulences that cause dilatation of the aortic arch appear. Secondarily, the left ventricle dilates due to pressure overload.

The radiographic signs of this disease depend on the degree of the narrowing. An enlargement of the aortic arch and signs of increased height of the left ventricle may be observed on lateral radiographs (fig. 3.98), as well as a prominence of the cardiac silhouette in the 1 to 1 o'clock position, and in the 2 to 5 o'clock position on dorsoventral radiographs. Signs of enlargement of the left atrium will appear at advanced stages.

Ventricular septal defect

Interventricular septal defects may occur in any area of the septum, but they are more frequent in its membranous part, in its most dorsal area. They may be isolated defects or be associated with other congenital anomalies, such as atrial septal defects or patent ductus arteriosus. If the right and left ventricular pressures are normal, the blood flow will be shunted from left to right because the left ventricular systolic pressure is higher than the right one. However, if the defect is very dorsal, the blood will flow directly into the pulmonary artery, which causes almost no effects on the right ventricle. The blood that is shunted to the pulmonary circulation returns to the left atrium and ventricle, which causes pulmonary (arteries and veins) congestion and enlargement of the left heart. If the defect has a more ventral location, a large volume of blood may enter the right ventricle, so this latter may also appear enlarged in these cases.

Small defects do not usually cause any alterations on chest radiographs. If the defect is large, there will

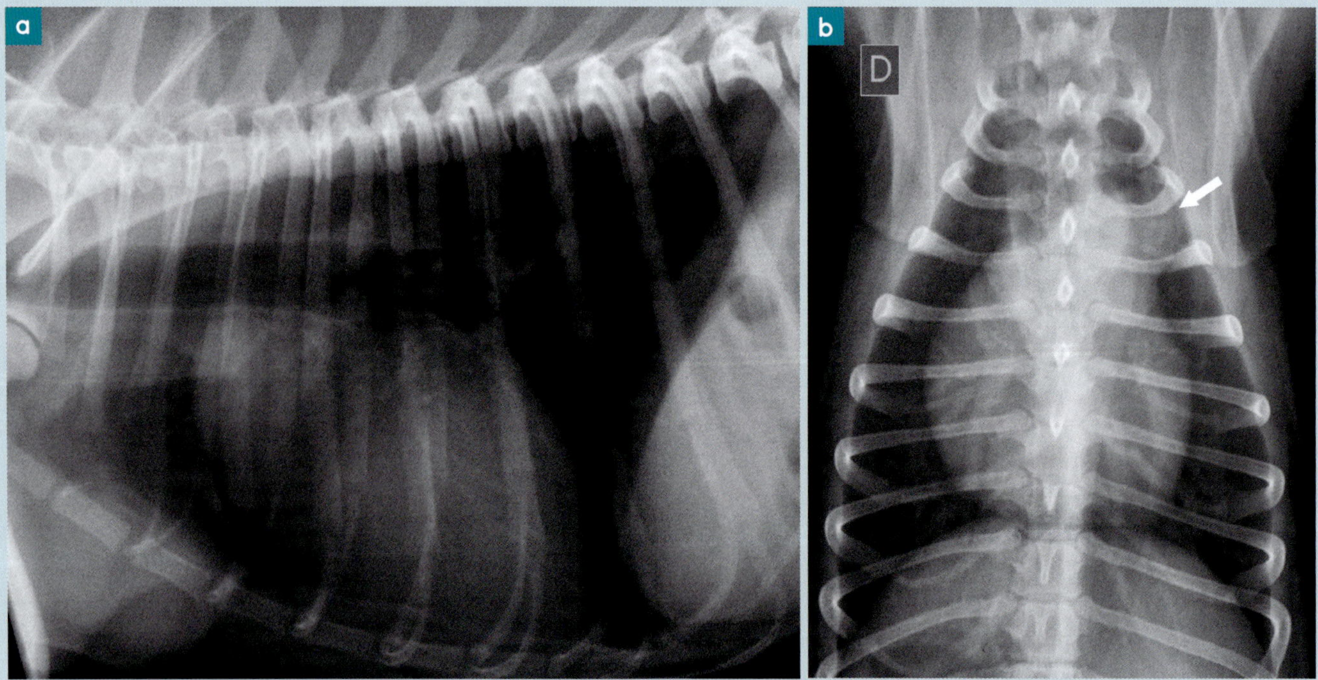

FIGURE 3.97. Lateral (a) and dorsoventral (b) radiographs of the thorax of a dog with pulmonary stenosis. Image (a) shows a prominence of the cranioventral margin of the silhouette and image (b) its right margin appears rounded, with marked prominence at 1 to 2 o'clock position (arrow), according to clock-face analogy, due to the enlargement of the main pulmonary artery.

be signs of enlargement of the left ventricle and atrium, although this will be less marked in the later, as well as signs of enlargement of the right ventricle on some occasions (if the defect is ventral) and pulmonary congestion.

Tetralogy of Fallot

Tetralogy of Fallot is the congenital defect that most often causes cyanosis. It is the result of the combination of pulmonary stenosis, ventricular septal defects, secondary hypertrophy of the right ventricle and several degrees of dextroposition and overload of the aorta.

The radiographic signs of this disease may greatly vary depending on the severity of the pulmonary stenosis and size of the ventricular septal defect. An enlarged right heart and reduced pulmonary vessels are usually observed.

Diseases of the pericardium

The disease that most frequently affects the pericardium is pericardial effusion. It causes a generalised enlargement of the cardiac silhouette, which acquires the aspect of a water bottle when the volume of fluid that has accumulated in the pericardial sac is very large (fig. 3.99). When the amount of fluid is minimal or moderate, the cardiac silhouette does not necessarily acquire a characteristic water-bottle shape and its enlargement is variable. On radiographs, the globally rounded shape of the cardiac silhouette in the two projections and the fact that the heart chambers cannot be identified help us to differentiate this image from that of global cardiomegaly. Even so, it is necessary to perform an echocardiogram to establish a differential diagnosis between both conditions. In many cases, this technique will also allow detection of tumours as the cause of the effusion.

Peritoneopericardial hernias may have a congenital origin and are characterised by a communication between the peritoneal space and the pericardial space through a defect in the diaphragm. The identification of clumped abdominal structures that mask the image of the normal cardiac silhouette in the centre of the thorax is a typical radiological finding in this anomaly (fig. 3.100). The liver is the most frequently herniated organ, followed by the gallbladder, the stomach, the intestine and the omentum. If there is communication but passage of abdominal contents to the pericardial sac is minimal, the cardiac silhouette may appear enlarged with an asymmetric morphology (fig. 3.101). In such cases, the communication and abnormal content in the pericardial space can be confirmed via echocardiography. The oral administration of barium may confirm the anomalous position of the stomach and intestine if these are herniated.

Cardiac tumours

Most cardiac tumours are associated with a pericardial effusion. Haemangiosarcoma is the most frequent tumour in dogs, while lymphoma is the most frequent type in cats. Haemangiosarcomas originate in endothelial cells and may appear in any part of the heart, although their most common location is the wall of the right atrium. Chemodectomas originate in neuroepithelial cells and are typically located at the base of the heart, where they create a more or less defined "mass effect" on radiographs depending on their size (fig. 3.72). Other tumours (myxomas, ectopic thyroid carcinomas, fibrosarcomas, etc.) are less frequent.

Microcardia

The term microcardia is used to describe the reduction of the size of the heart. The decrease in the size of the cardiac silhouette may be real or apparent on radiographs. An increase in the amount of air in the lungs (emphysema) or in the pleural space (pneumothorax) may create an image suggestive of microcardia. Real decreases in size are always the result of conditions that cause hypovolaemia, mainly haemorrhage, severe dehydration or Addison's disease. In the latter, the image may be particularly remarkable because hypovolaemia is accompanied by atrophy of the muscular mass of the heart. The size of the pulmonary vessels is usually reduced (hypovascularisation) as an associated finding in cases of microcardia (fig. 3.102). Microcardia and pulmonary hypovascularisation can sometimes be encompassed with the identification of signs of megaoesophagus in patients with Addison's disease.

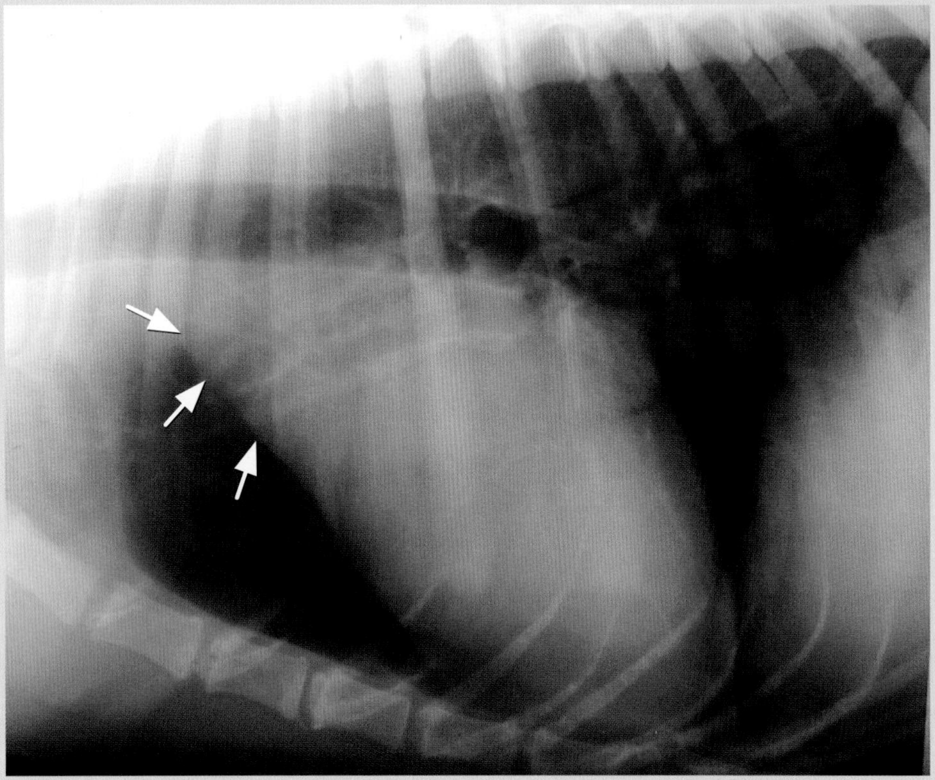

FIGURE 3.98. Lateral radiograph of the thorax of a dog with aortic valve stenosis. The shadow of the aortic arch appears enlarged.

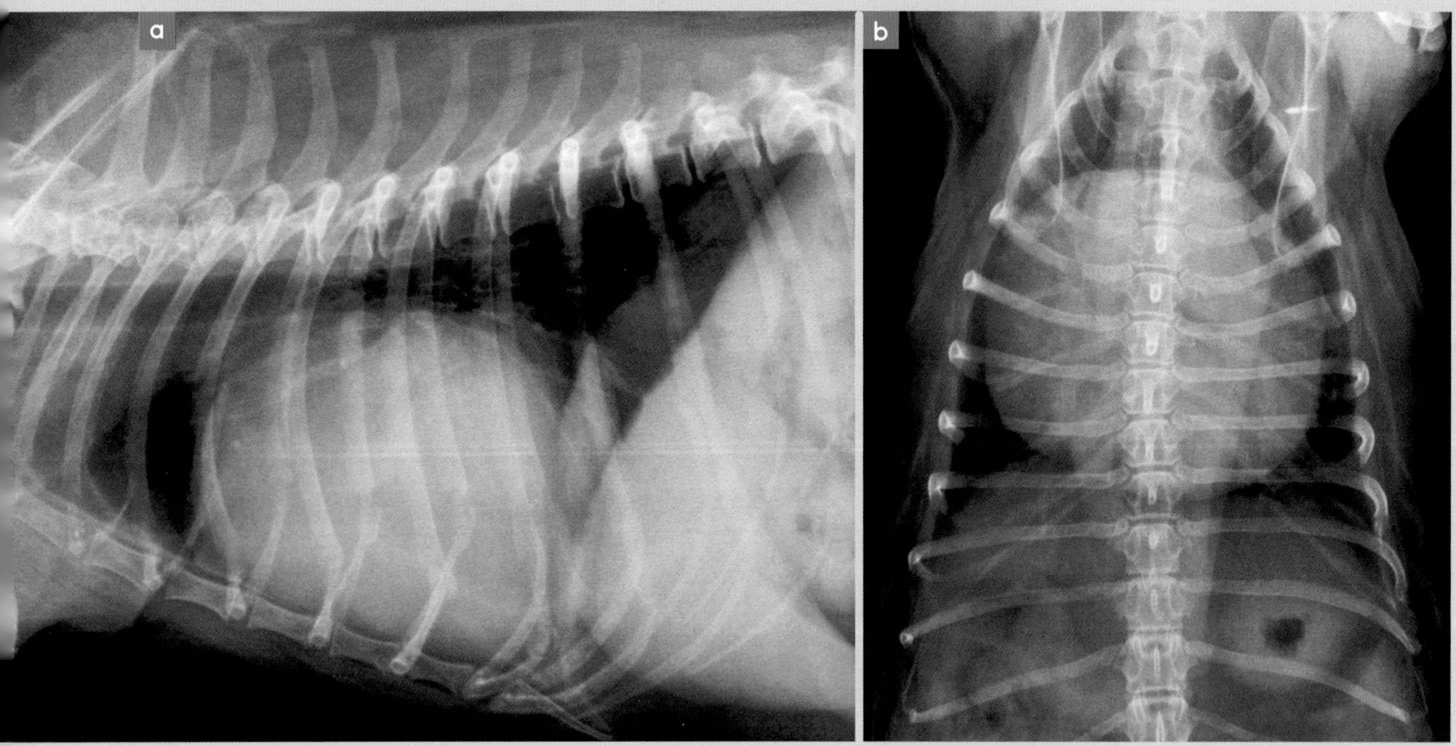

FIGURE 3.99. Lateral (a) and dorsoventral (b) radiographs of the thorax of a dog with a pericardial effusion. The cardiac silhouette appears enlarged and with a "water-bottle" shape. A dilated cardiomyopathy may give rise to a similar image, although it is usually possible to distinguish the cardiac chambers to some extent, while in the image of a pericardial effusion it is not. However, an echocardiogram is necessary to confirm the diagnosis with certainty.

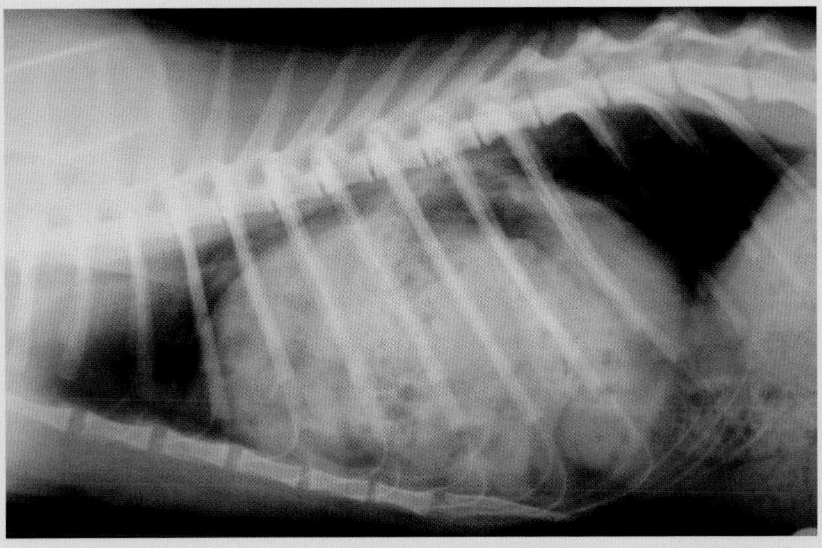

FIGURE 3.100. Lateral radiograph of a cat with a peritoneopericardial hernia. It is possible to identify the presence of the small and large intestines in the pericardial sac, which probably contains other abdominal organs, such as the liver or stomach. Their presence may be confirmed by means of echocardiography.

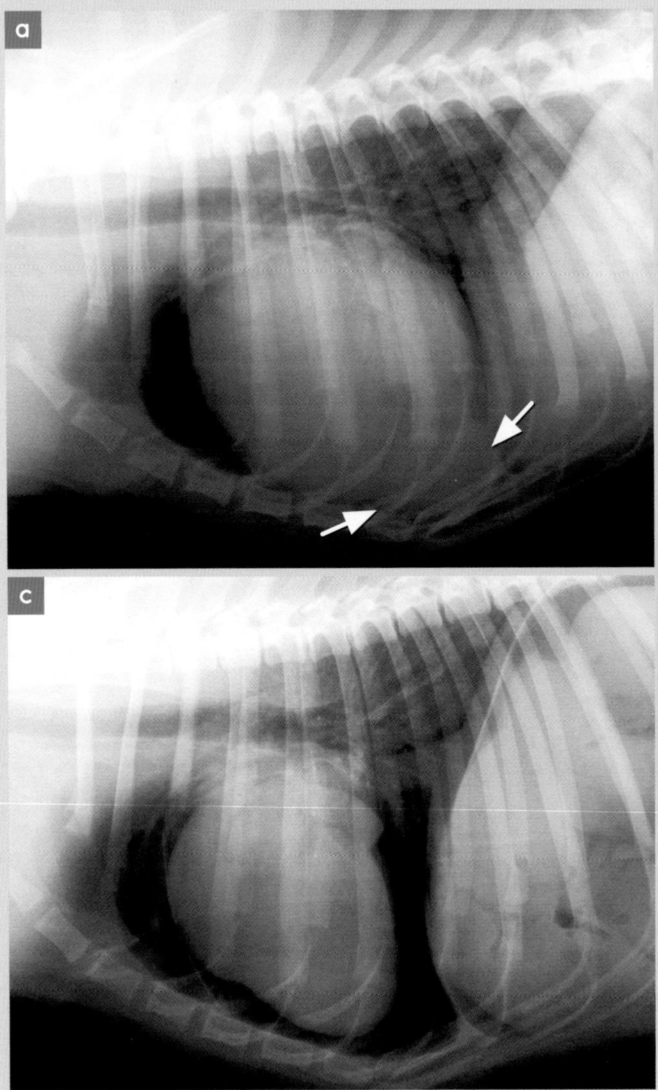

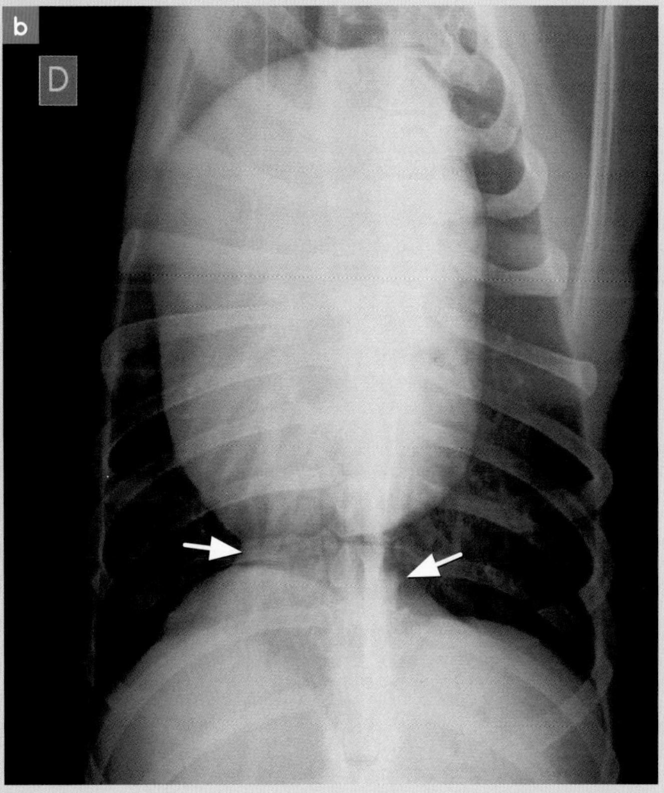

FIGURE 3.101. Lateral (a and c) and dorsoventral (b) projections of the thorax of a dog with a peritoneopericardial hernia before (a and b) and after surgery (c). Image (a) shows an enlarged cardiac silhouette with loss of normal cardiac apex visualisation. A soft tissue density silhouette appears in its place, blending in the image the caudoventral area of the cardiac silhouette with the ventral area of the diaphragmatic dome (arrows). In image (b) the cardiac silhouette appears enlarged and deformed; the arrows indicate the soft tissue opacity silhouette that blends the caudal zone of the cardiac silhouette and the central zone of the diaphragm. Image (c) shows signs of iatrogenic pneumopericardium and pneumoperitoneum due to surgical procedure for the hernia.

Cor pulmonale

The radiological identification of an enlargement of the right ventricle in a patient with a pulmonary or vascular disease is very indicative of cor pulmonale, which is defined as a right heart failure caused by a pulmonary or thoracic disease. By definition, there must be pulmonary hypertension in cor pulmonale for right heart failure to happen. In dogs, the most common cause of cor pulmonale is dirofilariasis, although any obstruction of the pulmonary vessels may cause hypertension and, therefore, cor pulmonale. The obstruction of the pulmonary arteries may occur as a result of the presence of blood clots (pulmonary thromboembolism) or by embolisation of fat, septic material, neoplastic cells or nematodes of the genus Dirofilaria.

Lung

In cats and dogs, the right lung is divided into four (cranial, middle, caudal and accessory) lobes and the left lung is divided into two (cranial and caudal) lobes. The approximate areas occupied by each lung lobe are shown in figure 3.103.

The lungs contain air in the alveoli and in the lumen of the bronchi and bronchioles, and are formed by structures of soft-tissue density, which include the alveolar walls, the interstitial tissue, the blood vessels and the walls of the bronchi and bronchioles. Of these latter, only the blood vessels and walls of the bronchi with a larger diameter can be identified on a radiograph of a normal thorax.

If we divided the radiograph in three concentric areas –perihilar area, middle area and peripheral area of the lung–, in normal conditions it would only be possible to visualise the walls of the bronchi in the area most proximal to the pulmonary hilum, since these are usually too thin to be identified in the image in the middle and peripheral areas. The blood vessels, however, are visible in the three areas as they have soft-tissue density walls and content. They appear as structures with a linear morphology that branch out and become narrower as they run from the hilum to the periphery of the lung. Following this criterion, the concept of normal lung pattern refers to the lung that appears basically radiolucent, due to its air content, and in which the pulmonary vessels–with a normal size and morphology–and the walls of bronchi with a larger diameter are identified (fig. 3.104). The pulmonary vessels and bronchi follow a parallel path. In lateral projections, the arteries are dorsal to the veins, while in dorsoventral and ventrodorsal projections, the arteries are lateral to the veins. The path of the main bronchi can be identified among the silhouettes of the larger arteries and veins (fig. 3.105).

Cranial lobar pulmonary vessels are better appreciated on lateral projections. There is generally less overlapping between them in the left lateral projection, which improves their assessment in this projection compared to the right lateral projection. Caudal lobar pulmonary vessels are better evaluated in dorsoventral and ventrodorsal projections. However, dorsoventral are preferred as these vessels appear more magnified, their path is more perpendicular to the X-ray beam and there is less pulmonary atelectasis in adjacent areas compared with ventrodorsal projections.

In healthy patients, the arteries and veins should be equal in size. In the lateral projection, the width of the cranial lobar vessels where they cross the 4th intercostal space should not exceed the width of the proximal third of the 4th rib. The caudal lobar vessels are evaluated in the dorsoventral and ventrodorsal projections, the width of which under normal conditions should not exceed the width of the 9th rib at the point where they overlap. In cats, it is easier to visualise the cranial lobar arteries and veins than the caudal ones.

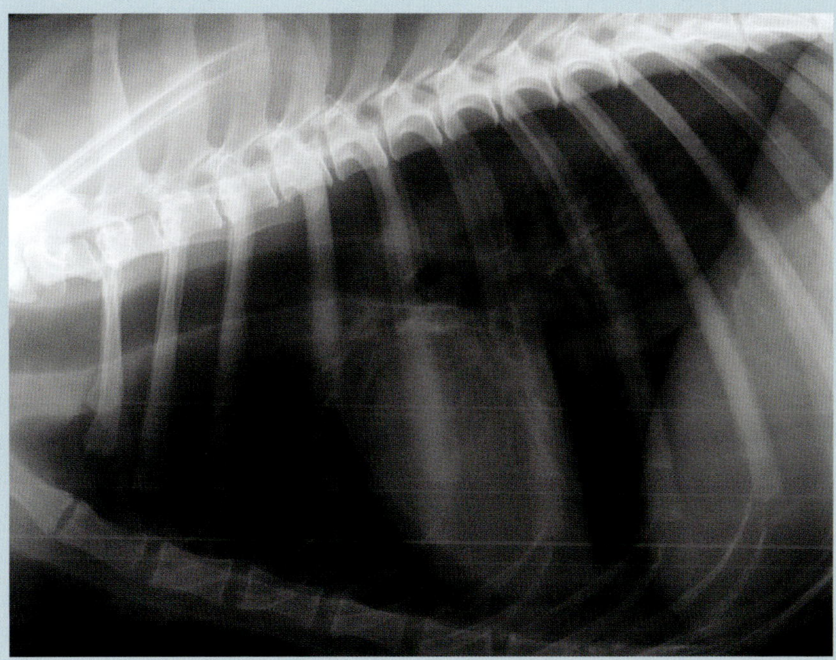

FIGURE 3.102. Lateral radiograph of the thorax of a dog with microcardia and hypovascularisation. The cardiac silhouette and pulmonary lungs appear smaller, which leads to the lung fields appearing wider and more radiolucent. This may be mistaken for pulmonary emphysema.

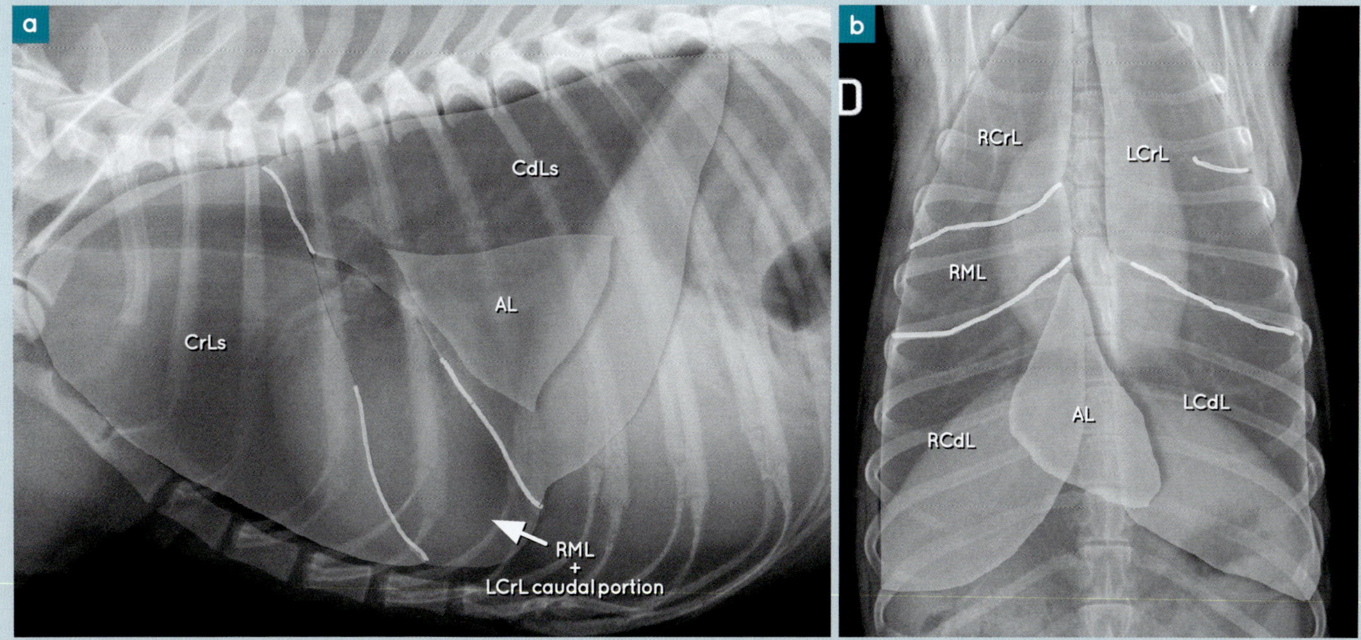

FIGURE 3.103. Normal lateral (a) and ventrodorsal (b) radiographs of the thorax of a dog, in which the location of the different lung lobes is indicated by the grey areas. RCrL refers to right cranial lobe; LCrL, left cranial lobe. RML: Right middle lobe. RCdL, right caudal lobe; LCdL, left caudal lobe; AL, accessory lobe; CrLs, cranial lobe overlap area; CdLs, caudal lobe overlap area. The white lines between lobes represent the location of interlobular fissures, including the incomplete fissure located between the cranial and caudal portions of the left cranial lobe.

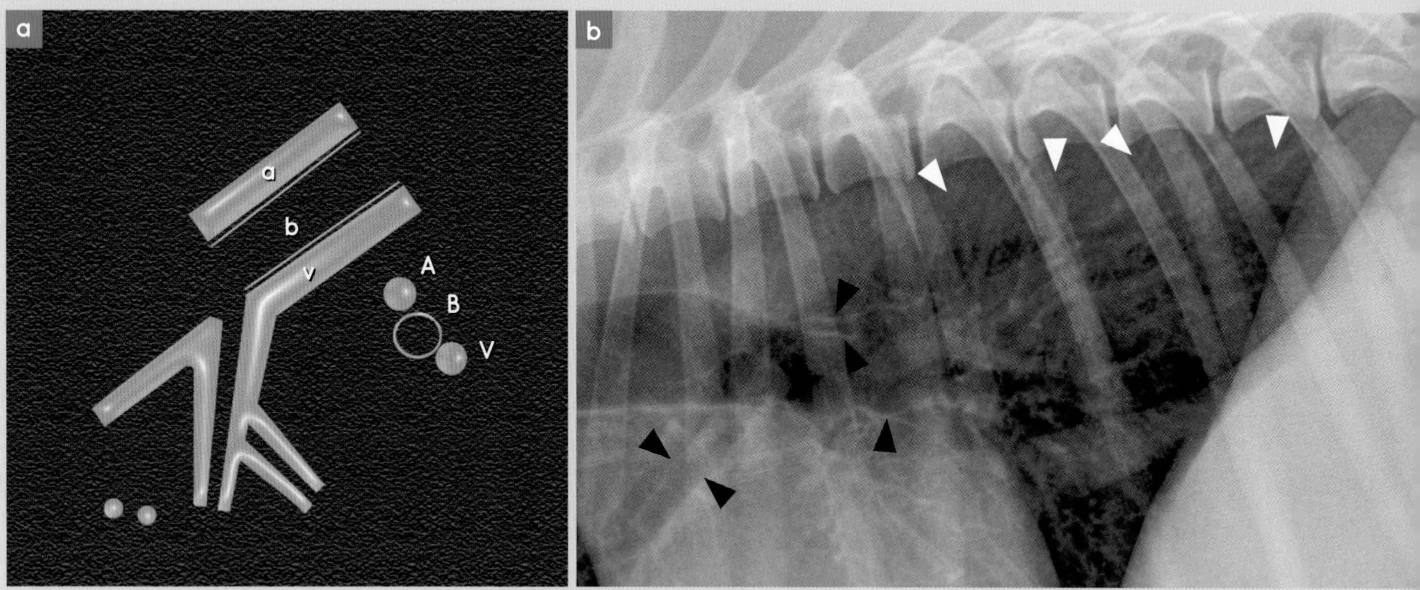

FIGURE 3.104. Schematic representation of the normal (a) pulmonary pattern and enlarged image of the caudodorsal area on a lateral radiograph of the thorax of a healthy dog. Image (a) represents the normal lung parenchyma, which is mainly radiolucent (dark grey background), with parallel pulmonary vessels (arteries and veins with a similar diameter) that branch out as they run towards the peripheral area, and bronchial walls that are only visible in the area where the diameter is larger; the vessels and bronchi are represented longitudinally (a: artery, b: bronchus, v: vein) and transversally (A: artery, B: bronchus, V: vein). In image (b) the walls of the larger bronchi (black arrowheads) and the pulmonary vessels can be identified. White arrowheads point to small normal pulmonary vessels located in the peripheral area of the lung.

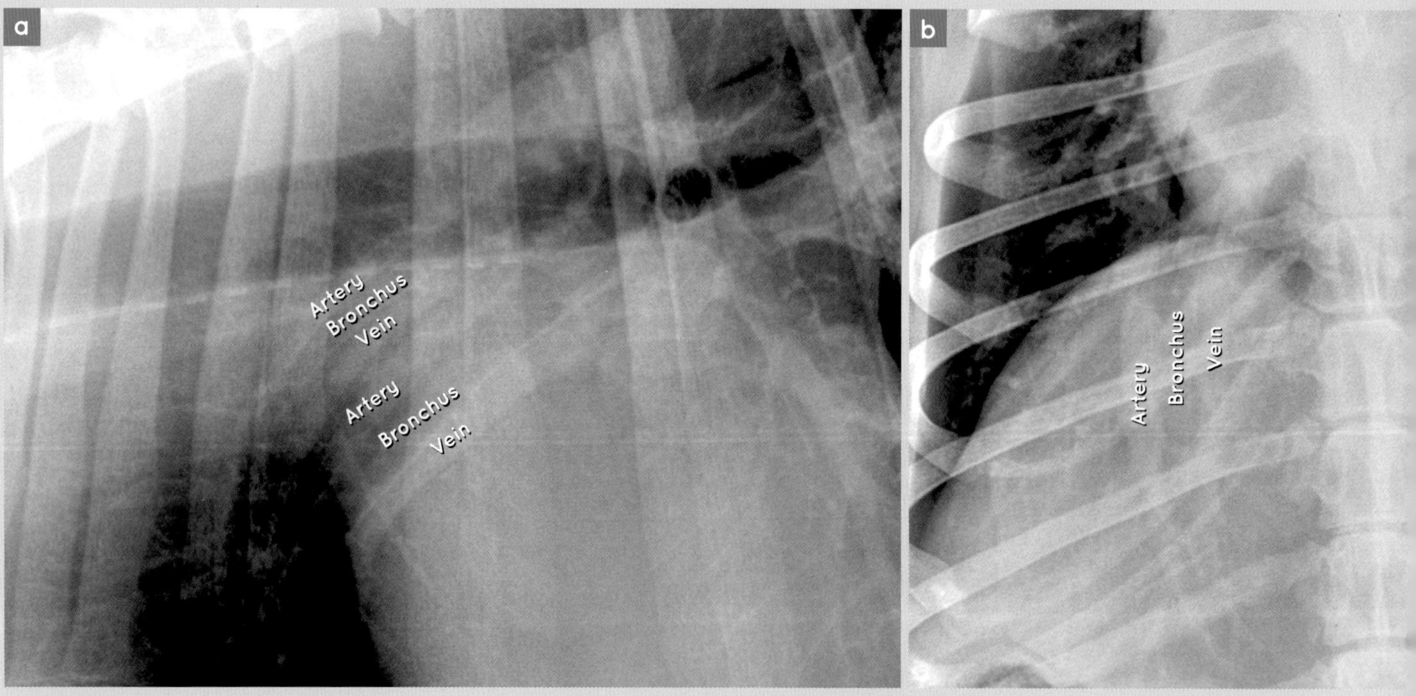

FIGURE 3.105. X-ray of cranial lobar vessels identified in the lateral projection (a) and caudal lobar vessels identified in the dorsoventral projection (b) in the dog. The arteries are situated dorsal to the veins in the lateral projection, while in the dorsoventral projection the arteries are located laterally, and the veins are medial. The bronchi lie between the arteries and the veins.

As discussed above, the factors that have the greatest impact on lung radiography are:

- **Exposure values:** on underexposed conventional radiographs, the lung has a higher radiopacity, which may be mistaken for an interstitial infiltrate of the parenchyma, while on overexposed conventional radiographs, all the structures in the image appear darker, which may be confused with emphysema, and on overexposed digital radiographs, only the lung areas with less thickness would appear as black areas which cannot be corrected with post-processing tools.
- **Moment of the respiratory cycle:** if the radiograph is taken during expiration, the lungs contain a lesser amount of air, which slightly increases their radiopacity.
- **Obesity:** an excess amount of subcutaneous fat leads to a slight increase in pulmonary radiopacity, as the density of fat is added to that of the lungs. In addition, the accumulation of intrathoracic fat somewhat limits lung expansion, which also contributes to the increase in pulmonary radiopacity.
- **Age:** the lungs of young animals may be more radiopaque than those of adults because they contain more water. The lungs of old animals may be slightly more radiopaque due to interstitial fibrosis, as well as to calcification or fibrosis of the bronchial walls, which make these more visible on radiographs (it will also be possible to visualise them in the middle area of the lungs).
- **Prolonged lateral recumbency:** the animals that remain in a recumbent position for a relatively long period of time, especially if they are anaesthetised, will have a partial collapse of the lung that corresponds to the side on which they had been lying. In the ventrodorsal and dorsoventral view, a deviation of the mediastinum towards the affected side is observed, which helps to differentiate atelectasis caused by a recumbent position from a true pulmonary pathological alteration.
- **Digital radiographs:** digital radiographs have a much higher contrast resolution than conventional radiographs and make the lungs appear less radiolucent. They also improve the visualisation of soft-tissue density structures, such as the pulmonary vessels and walls of the bronchi, which will sometimes be identified in the middle area of the lungs despite having no anomalies.

Lateral and ventrodorsal radiographs are recommended for a general assessment of the lungs. If ventrodorsal and dorsoventral views are compared, the capacity of the lungs to expand is greater with the first one, which improves the definition of the lung in the image. On a lateral radiograph, the lung that is higher will be better visualised, since its capacity of expansion is at its maximum, while the lung that is lower will always have some degree of partial collapse, which may limit its radiological examination. The right lateral projection is usually used as the standard view. However, in the specific case of an assessment of pulmonary metastases, the combination of the two lateral projections, right and left, is used, since if there are small lesions, these will be better viewed in the most distended lung (higher position). In case of doubt, a ventrodorsal radiograph is added in order to obtain complementary information, although small lesions that are visible on one or the two lateral views often cannot be identified on the ventrodorsal view.

Ultrasound examinations of the lungs have important limitations. It will only be possible to visualise areas of the lungs that do not contain air and are in contact with the thoracic wall, since the presence of air will hinder the examination in other locations. In cases of pleural effusion, the fluid facilitates the visualisation of the pulmonary content. Ultrasonography is indicated in the study of pulmonary masses and consolidation, since it provides information about the internal structure of the lesion, its vascularisation may be examined with Doppler ultrasound and it allows the collection of samples for cytology or biopsies under ultrasound guidance.

As opposed to magnetic resonance imaging, which provides low-quality lung images with conventional equipment, computed tomography will be indicated whenever the findings on the radiographs are suspicious, when a torsion is suspected, in cases of bronchial foreign body or pulmonary thromboembolism, for a thorough examination of metastases and for the assessment of masses (it allows the determination of its exact location and examination of the rest of the lung to rule out any associated lesions), as well as for guided punctures or biopsies of lesions that are not identifiable by means of ultrasonography.

Abnormal lung patterns

The radiological assessment of the lungs is based on the identification of abnormal lung patterns, which have been classified in function of the affected components of the lung:

- Bronchial.
- Vascular.
- Alveolar.
- Interstitial.
- Mixed (combination of two or more of the previous patterns).

The identification of the pattern may be more or less difficult depending on the location and extension of the lesions. Once it is identified, a differential diagnosis is made for each abnormal lung pattern. The length of the list of diseases may vary depending on the correlation of the radiological findings with the rest of the patient's clinical data (anamnesis, examination, laboratory tests, etc.). The main limitation in the interpretation of lung radiographs lies in this fact: very different diseases may have a similar radiographic image.

Bronchial pattern

A bronchial pattern is identified when bronchial walls that could not be observed become visible in normal conditions, in general in the middle or peripheral area of the lung, although we must remember that digital radiography can allow the visualisation of walls of normal bronchi in the middle area.

The typical radiological sign is the visualisation of "ring-" or "donut-"shaped images, which correspond to transverse shadows of bronchial walls (of those bronchial branches with a course that is parallel to the X-ray beam), and "train track" images, which correspond to the longitudinal shadows of these branches (bronchial branches with a course that is perpendicular to the X-ray beam).

The bronchial pattern may be due to the thickening of the bronchial walls, the presence of peribronchial infiltrates (indistinguishable from wall thickening on an X-ray) (fig. 3.106) or increased radiopacity caused by bronchial wall calcification (fig. 3.107). The latter is usually due to a degenerative process associated with the advanced age of the patient, although in some cases it may appear secondary to primary pathological alterations such as Cushing's disease. A radiographic finding of bronchial wall calcification is not considered significant. It is, however, not always easy to differentiate on an X-ray a bronchial pattern caused by some disease from that caused by bronchial wall calcification.

It is important to keep in mind that the absence of any identifiable bronchial pattern on the X-ray does not rule out bronchial pathology, especially in acute processes.

Identification of bronchial lung patterns should always be correlated with the patient's clinical data. Patient's age and whether or not they have clinical signs consistent with bronchial pathology at the time the X-rays are taken should be taken into account. In a young patient, a radiographic finding of a bronchial pattern is usually due to pathological causes that is either occurring at the time of the X-ray or the after-effects of previous bronchial pathologic processes. In a senior animal with no clinical signs consistent with bronchial pathology, this pulmonary pattern is usually associated with an age-related degenerative process. Finally, when an adult patient, senior or not, presents clinical signs consistent with a bronchial process, the radiographic visualisation of a bronchial pattern should be considered *a priori* as significant, although, as in a young patient, it may also be a sequela of previous pathological processes. If in doubt, a transtracheal wash will allow a more precise diagnosis to be established.

The typical lung pattern of feline asthma is bronchial (fig. 3.108), although it may be associated with other lung patterns. The severity of the clinical signs often does not directly correlate with the magnitude of the radiological findings. In patients with feline asthma, it is common to observe secondary atelectasis of the right middle lobe and emphysema.

In chronic or severe bronchial diseases, the bronchi may have irreversible sac-like dilatations, a condition known as bronchiectasis (fig. 3.109). These may also be caused by obstructions of the airway or smoke inhalation.

Bronchial neoplasms rarely produce an evident bronchial pattern but tend to cause pulmonary consolidation and nodular lesions.

Computed tomography is of great interest in the study of the diseases of the bronchi. It allows the visualisation of bronchi and bronchioles with a small diameter, bronchiectases that are not detectable by means of radiography or bronchial ruptures, and the differentiation between foreign bodies, presence of intraluminal mucus and bronchial masses (fig 3.110). In the case of bronchial neoplasms, it also facilitates the identification of pulmonary metastases and lymphadenopathies. With CT virtual bronchoscopy, it is possible to follow the course of the trachea and large bronchi (fig. 3.111).

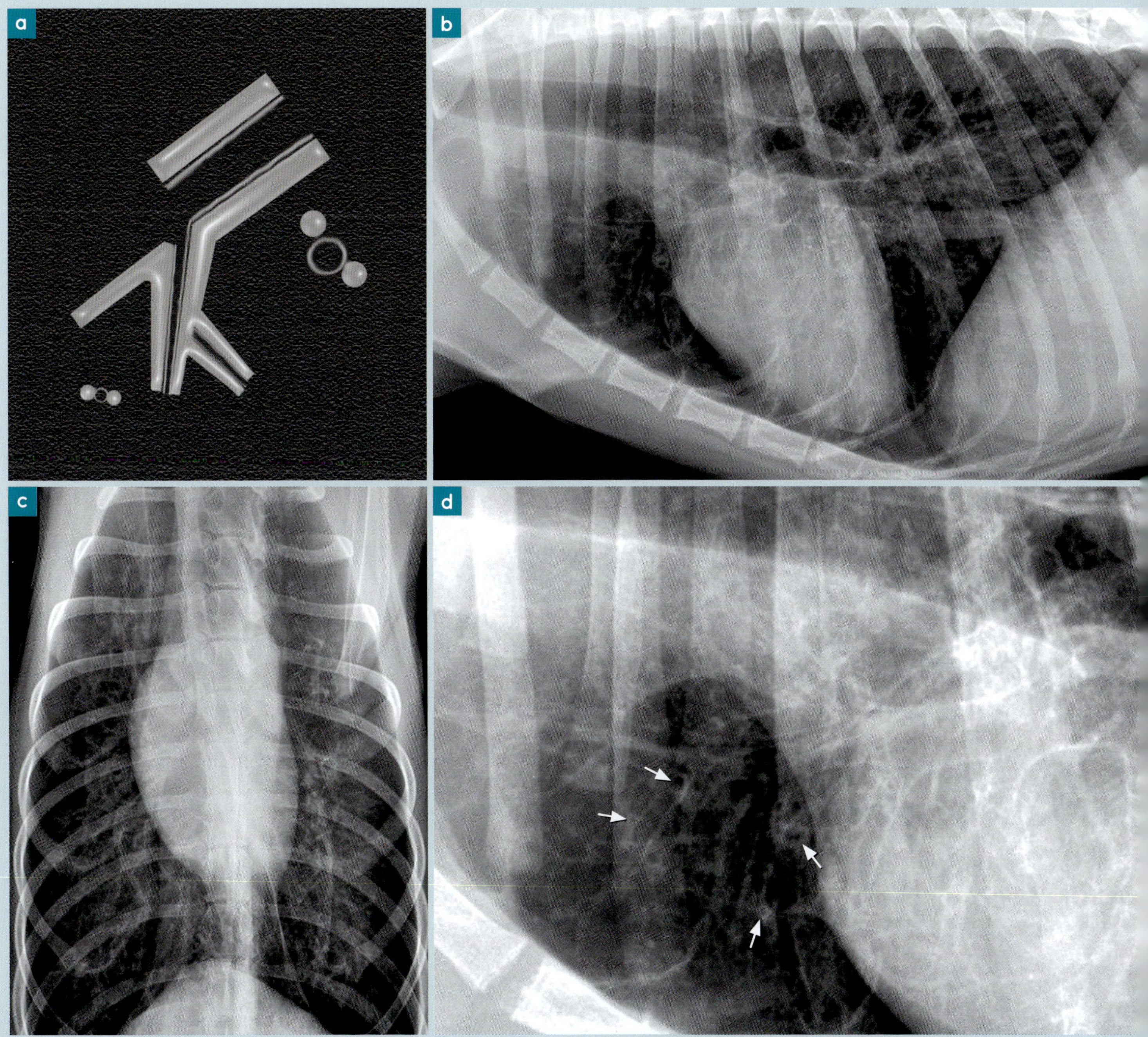

FIGURE 3.106. Schematic diagram of the bronchial lung pattern caused by thickening of walls or peribronchial infiltrates (a) and lateral (b) and ventrodorsal (c) projections, as well as the enlarged image of the cranioventral area of the lung in lateral projection (d) of the thorax of a dog with marked bronchial pattern due to allergic bronchitis. White arrows (d) point to "ring-like" shadows of varying sizes.

Vascular pattern

The pulmonary vascular pattern is characterised by changes in pulmonary blood vessel size and/or morphology. It is inadvisable to evaluate the size and shape of the vessels subjectively. The image of the cranial lobar vessels in the lateral projection and the caudal lobar vessels in the ventrodorsal or dorsoventral projections should be taken as reference. Vascular patterns may be arterial, venous, or mixed. In a venous vascular pattern, the width of the veins exceeds that of the arteries (fig. 3.112); in an arterial vascular pattern, the width of the arteries exceeds that of the veins (fig. 3.113);

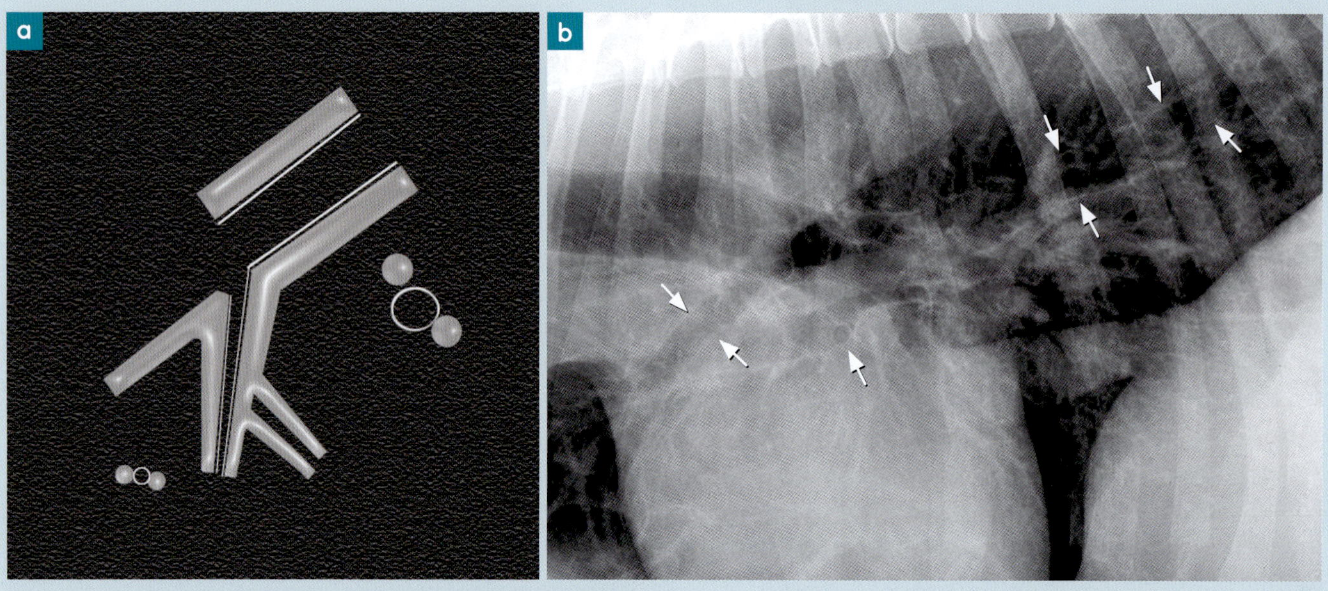

FIGURE 3.107. Schematic diagram of the bronchial lung pattern due to calcification (a) and enlarged image of the dorsocaudal zone of the thorax in lateral projection (b) of a dog with calcified bronchial walls (arrows) of no clinical significance.

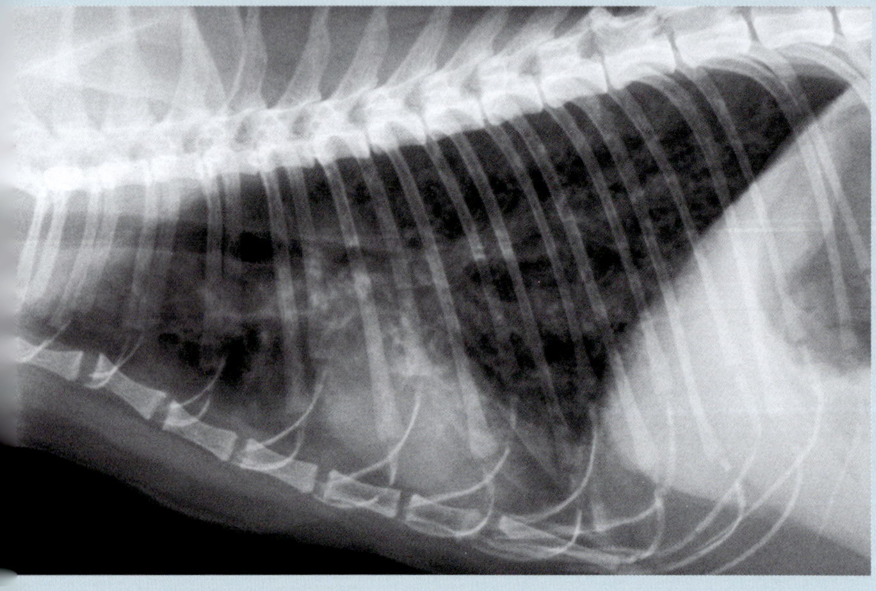

FIGURE 3.108. Lateral radiograph of the thorax of a cat with a bronchial pattern due to feline asthma.

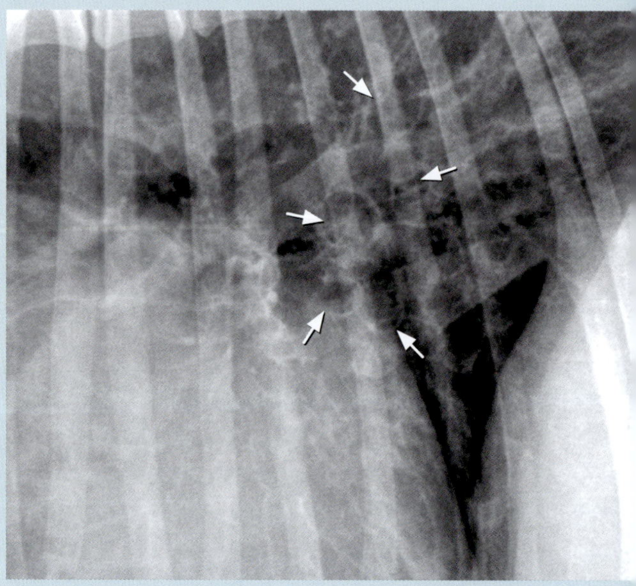

FIGURE 3.109. Enlarged image of the dorsocaudal area of the thorax in lateral projection of a dog with bronchiectasis (arrows).

and in a mixed vascular pattern, both the arteries and the veins appear enlarged (fig. 3.114). In the latter case, it is important to use reference landmarks comparing vessels against rib diameter (as explained earlier), rather than relying on subjective assessments which could lead to misdiagnoses.

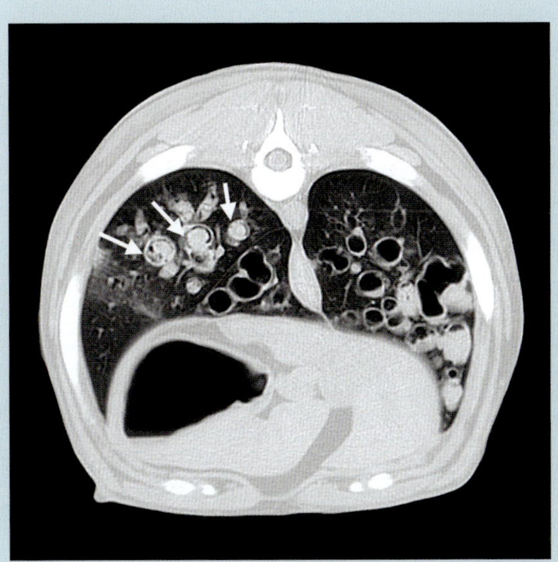

FIGURE 3.110. Computed tomography image of the thorax of a dog with bronchiectases and presence of multiple masses in the lumen of numerous bronchial branches (arrows), which may correspond to parasite granulomas or neoplastic nodules.

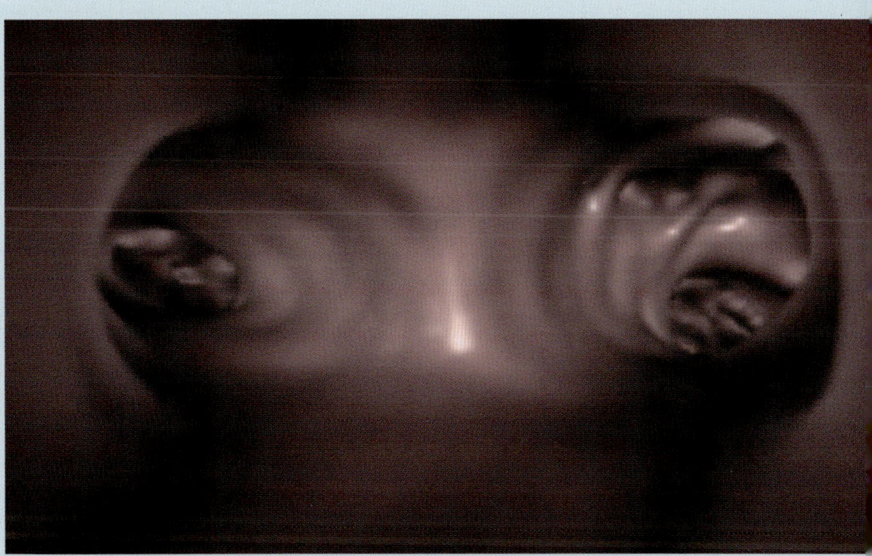

FIGURE 3.111. Image of a CT virtual bronchoscopy of a healthy dog, in which the bifurcation of the trachea in the two main bronchi may be observed. Subdivisions into smaller branches may be identified in the lumen of these latter.

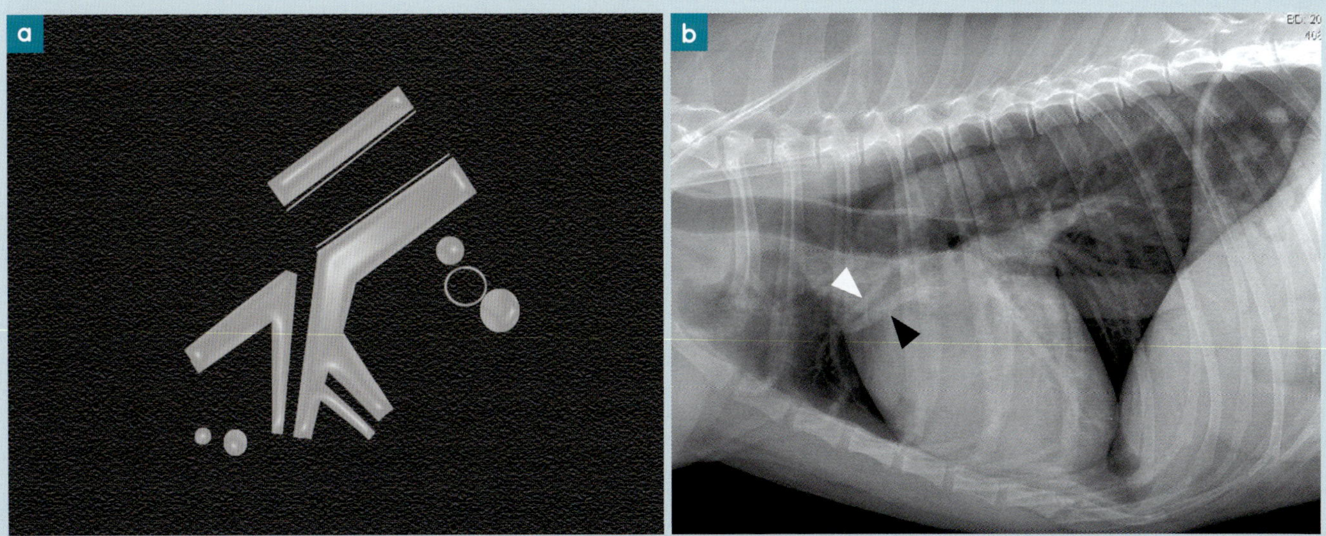

FIGURE 3.112. Schematic diagram of the vascular lung pattern caused by an enlargement of the pulmonary veins (a) and left lateral projection radiograph of the thorax of a dog with venous congestion (b). The right cranial lobar artery (white arrowhead) and vein (black arrowhead) appear more magnified, which facilitates their evaluation. The vein is wider than the artery.

The most common causes of venous vascular lung pattern are:

- Left heart failure.
- Fluid overload (iatrogenic).
- Left atrial obstruction (thrombus, neoplasm).
- Intracardiac communication with right-to-left flow (e.g.: Tetralogy of Fallot).
- On rare occasions, intracardiac communication with left-to-right flow.

An arterial vascular lung pattern may appear in patients with:

- Dirofilariasis, *Angiostrongylus vasorum* infection or *Aelurostrongylus* infection (cats).
- Large left-to-right intracardiac communication (e.g. septal defects).
- Pulmonary thromboembolism.
- Pulmonary hypertension.
- Chronic lung disease.
- Peripheral arteriovenous fistula.

A mixed vascular pattern, with enlargement of both arteries and veins, may be observed in patients with:

- Fluid overload (iatrogenic).
- Intracardiac communication with left-to-right flow (e.g. patent ductus arteriosus, inter-ventricular or atrial septal defects).
- Feline cardiomyopathy.

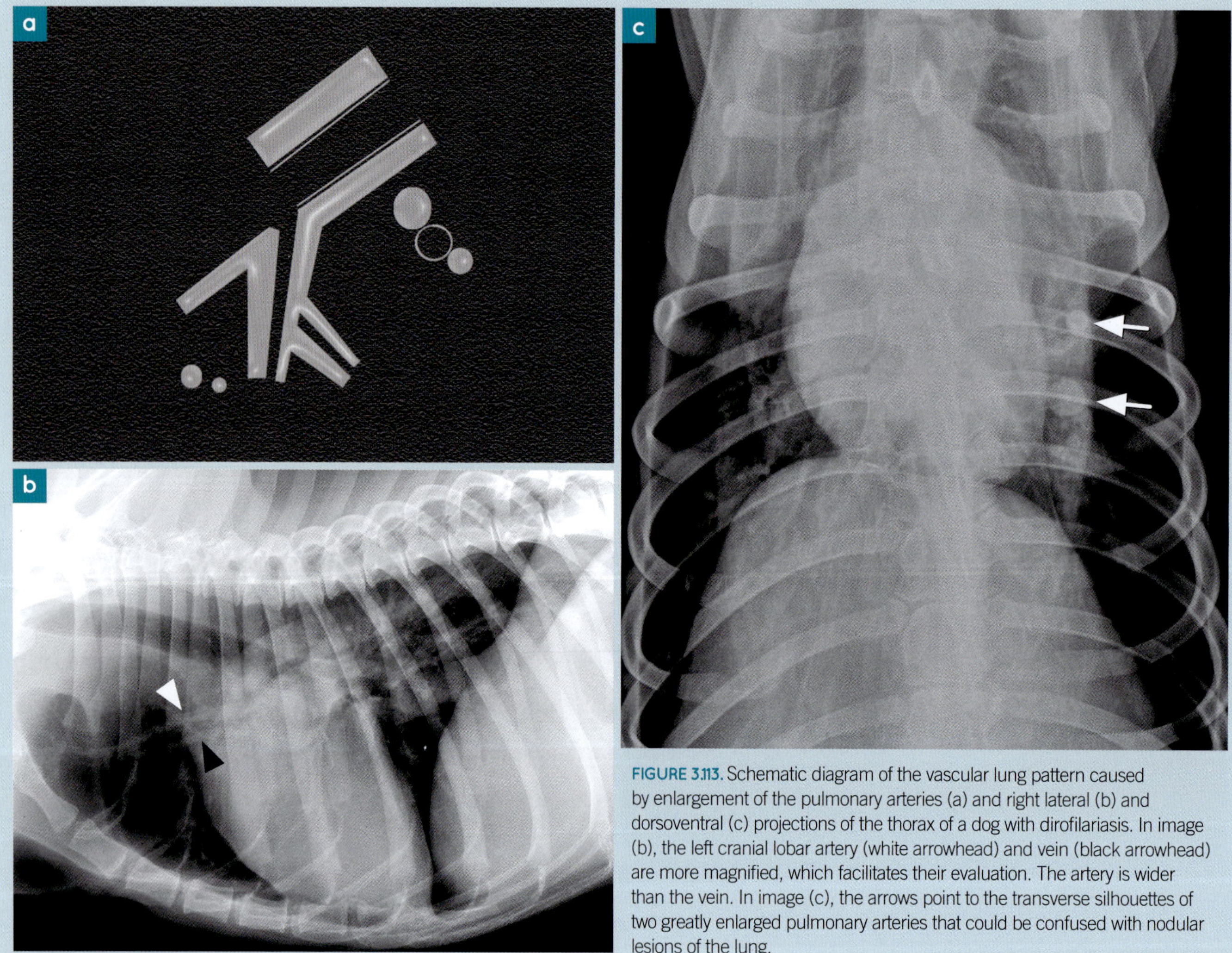

FIGURE 3.113. Schematic diagram of the vascular lung pattern caused by enlargement of the pulmonary arteries (a) and right lateral (b) and dorsoventral (c) projections of the thorax of a dog with dirofilariasis. In image (b), the left cranial lobar artery (white arrowhead) and vein (black arrowhead) are more magnified, which facilitates their evaluation. The artery is wider than the vein. In image (c), the arrows point to the transverse silhouettes of two greatly enlarged pulmonary arteries that could be confused with nodular lesions of the lung.

- Pulmonary congestion prior to pneumonia.
- Left heart failure.
- Chronic anaemia.
- Hyperthyroidism.
- Arteriovenous malformations.
- Upper airway obstruction.

Visualisation of tortuous (wavy) pulmonary vessels is also considered to be an abnormal vascular pattern (fig. 3.115). It is common to observe this type of image in pathologies that cause pulmonary hypertension, such as dirofilariasis.

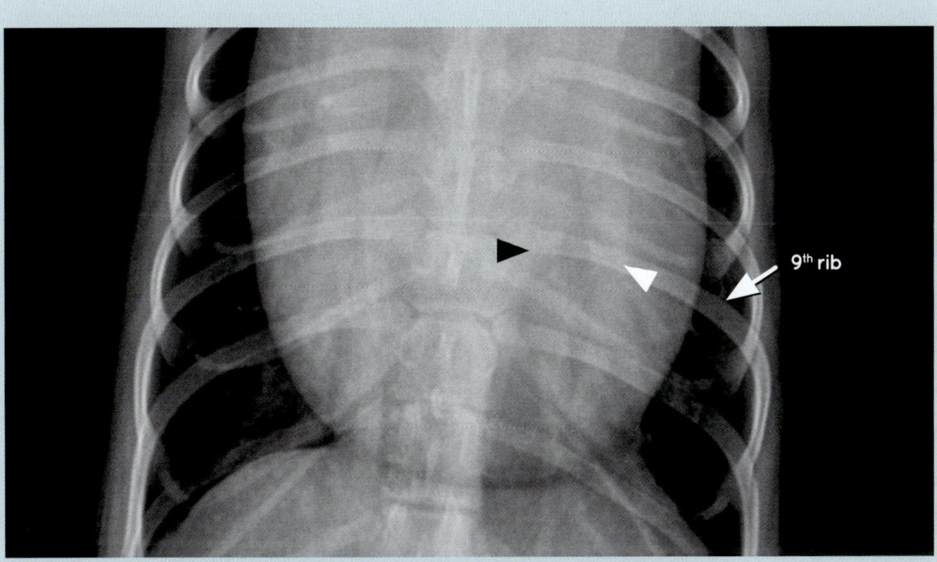

FIGURE 3.114. Enlarged image of the dorsoventral projection of the thorax of a dog with mixed vascular congestion. The width of the caudal lobar arteries and veins exceeds the width of the 9th rib at the point where they overlap. The white arrowhead points to the left caudal (lateral) lobar artery and the black arrowhead points to the left caudal (medial) lobar vein.

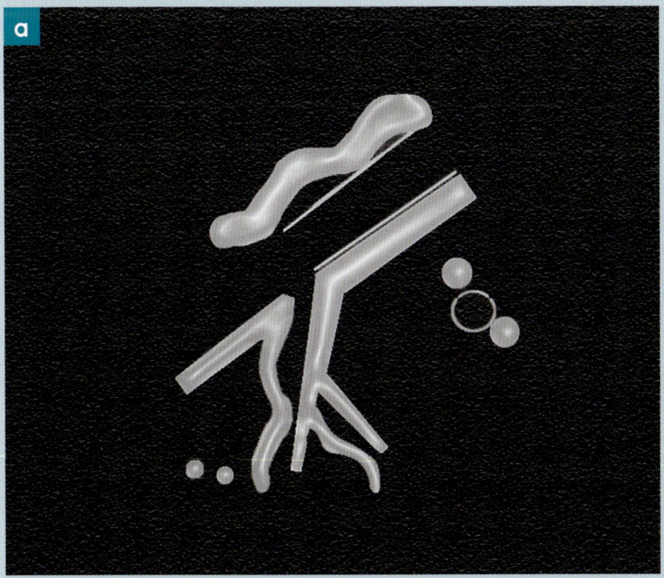

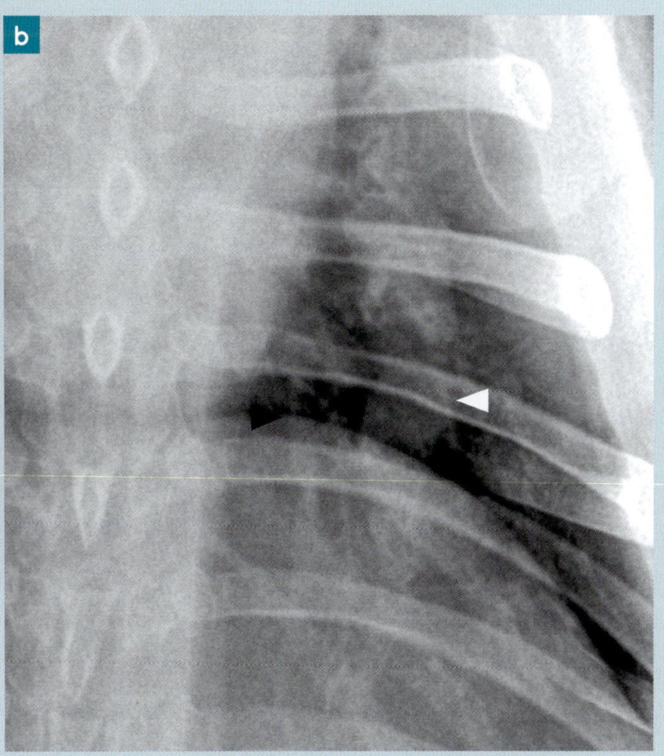

FIGURE 3.115. Schematic diagram of the vascular lung pattern caused by tortuosity of the pulmonary arteries (a) and enlarged image of the left caudal hemithorax (b) of a dog with dirofilariasis. The white arrowhead points to the left caudal lobar artery, which is extremely enlarged and following a slightly wavy path, and the black arrowhead points to the left caudal lobar vein, which is normal in size, but also slightly wavy.

A reduction in the size of the pulmonary vessels is also considered a pathological vascular pattern, which is called **pulmonary hypovascularisation** (fig. 3.116), which appears in processes that cause hypovolaemia, such as haemhorrage, severe dehydration or Addison's disease. It can also occur in some congenital conditions with right-to-left flow and in severe cases of pulmonary stenosis. As the size and number of vessels visible on the X-ray decrease, the lung fields appear darker, and it may be difficult to identify vessel silhouettes in peripheral areas.

Alveolar pattern

This occurs when the pulmonary alveoli fill with fluid (oedema, pneumonia, haemorrhage) or when they become deflated (atelectasis). Alveolar pattern due to the proliferation of neoplastic cells, at least in isolation, is much less common. Figure 3.117 shows the different phases in the evolution of an alveolar lung pattern.

When a small number of alveoli are affected by one of these processes, the increased opacity of the affected areas may be negligible or very difficult to identify on an X-ray. This means that, at very early stages, oedema, pneumonia, haemorrhage or pulmonary atelectasis may not be detected on an X-ray examination. As the affected areas in the lung expand, the possibilities for radiographic identification also increase. They appear on the image as areas of soft tissue/fluid opacity with irregular morphology and poorly defined borders (fig. 3.118), distinguishing them from nodular lung lesions which have regular morphology and usually well-defined borders.

When the areas of increased alveolar opacity become larger and surround the bronchial branches, the air content of the latter will be highlighted on the radiographic image, a sign known as **air bronchogram**. An air bronchogram occurs when the normal lumen of the bronchi is made visible on the X-ray by the opacification of the surrounding pulmonary parenchyma. In other words, the lumen of the bronchi is normal and what is altered is the parenchyma surrounding them. Air bronchograms on the lung image are considered the hallmark sign of an alveolar pattern. But air bronchograms are not always identified in an alveolar pattern. If the affected areas are small and close to a relatively large diameter bronchial branch, the lumen of the bronchi will not be highlighted and therefore the bronchograms will not be noted. Air **alveolograms** are the areas of lung parenchyma that retain some air but appear surrounded by parenchyma zones with alveoli filled with fluid or without any air (fig. 3.119).

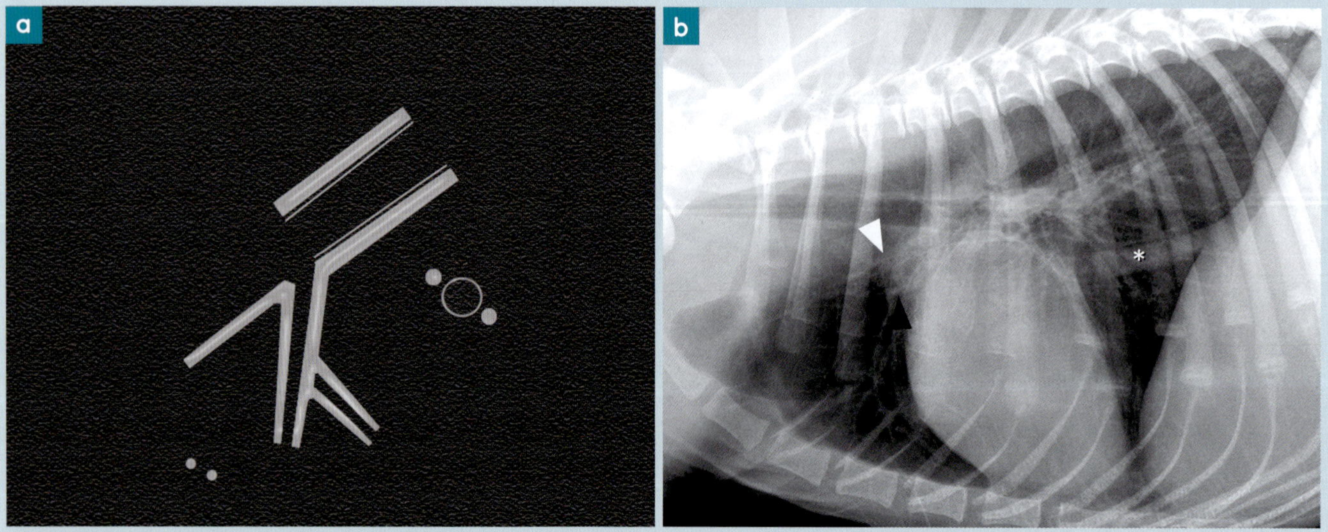

FIGURE 3.116. Schematic diagram of the vascular lung pattern caused by a decrease in the size of the pulmonary vessels (a) and lateral projection of the thorax of a dog with pulmonary hypovascularisation (b). The left cranial lobar artery (white arrowhead) and vein (black arrowhead) are indicated, both reduced in size; other radiographic findings suggestive of hypovolaemia are also noted, such as microcardia and decrease in the size of the caudal vena cava (asterisk).

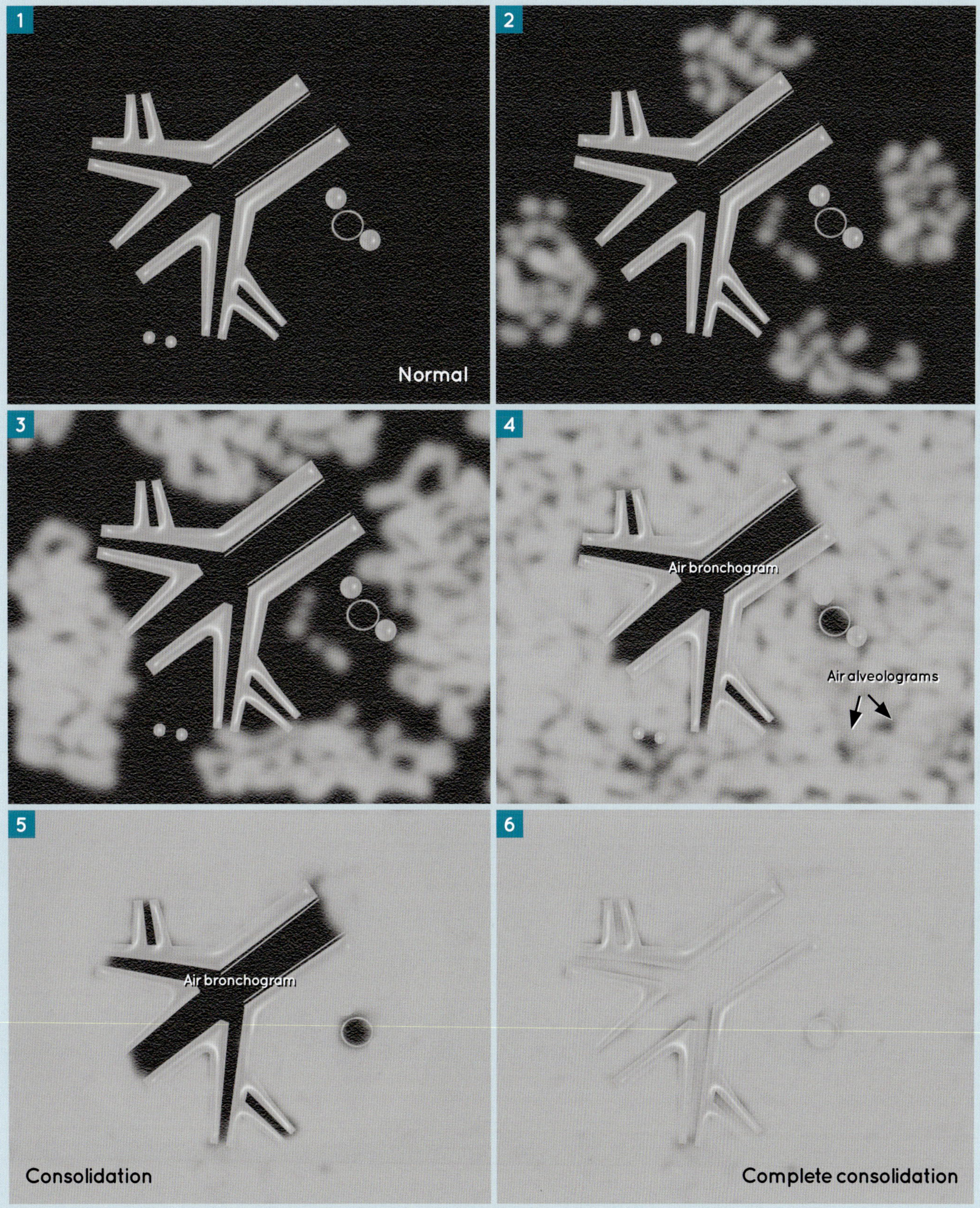

FIGURE 3.117. Schematic representation of the different phases (1-6) in the evolution of an alveolar pattern.

When all the alveoli are fluid-filled or deflated in a large area of pulmonary parenchyma, this area acquires a homogeneous fluid/soft tissue opacity, without alveolograms, which is called **pulmonary consolidation**. Air bronchograms may be observed in an area of pulmonary consolidation (fig. 3.120), but if they collapse or become filled with fluid, they will no longer be visible in the affected area. This is what is known as complete consolidation and would represent the most advanced phase of an alveolar pattern (fig. 3.121).

When a consolidated area coincides with the margin of a pulmonary lobe and the contiguous lobe is not affected, we get what is known as a **lobar sign**, so called because the lobe margin can be seen which is not possible on an X-ray of a healthy lung. The alveolar pattern may also cause a **silhouette sign** (also termed loss of silhouette sign or loss of outline sign) in areas where the affected lung parenchyma abuts other soft tissue opaque anatomical structures, such as the heart, pulmonary vessels or diaphragm. As they are in contact and are of the same opacity, it is not possible to distinguish the margins of one structure from the other on the X-ray (fig. 3.122).

The most common causes of an alveolar lung pattern are pulmonary oedema, pneumonia and pulmonary haemorrhage. As all these pathologies produce the same pulmonary pattern, they cannot be differentiated by radiological study alone. However, the rest of the patient's clinical data, other radiographic findings identifiable on the image (fig. 3.123), the location of the area of pulmonary involvement and, in some cases, treatment response and progression may adequately guide the differential diagnosis. For example, oedema may develop and disappear in a few hours if the appropriate treatment is administered (fig. 3.124). However, a haemorrhage or aspiration pneumonia may appear in a few minutes, but it may take days before they disappear. On the other hand, bacterial pneumonia develops within a few hours or days, but takes several days or weeks to resolve when treated.

Oedema of cardiogenic origin (due to left heart failure) appear in patients with heart disease which can generally be identified on an X-ray as cardiomegaly, with some exceptions, such as endocarditis. In dogs, its location is typically perihilar in the early stage,

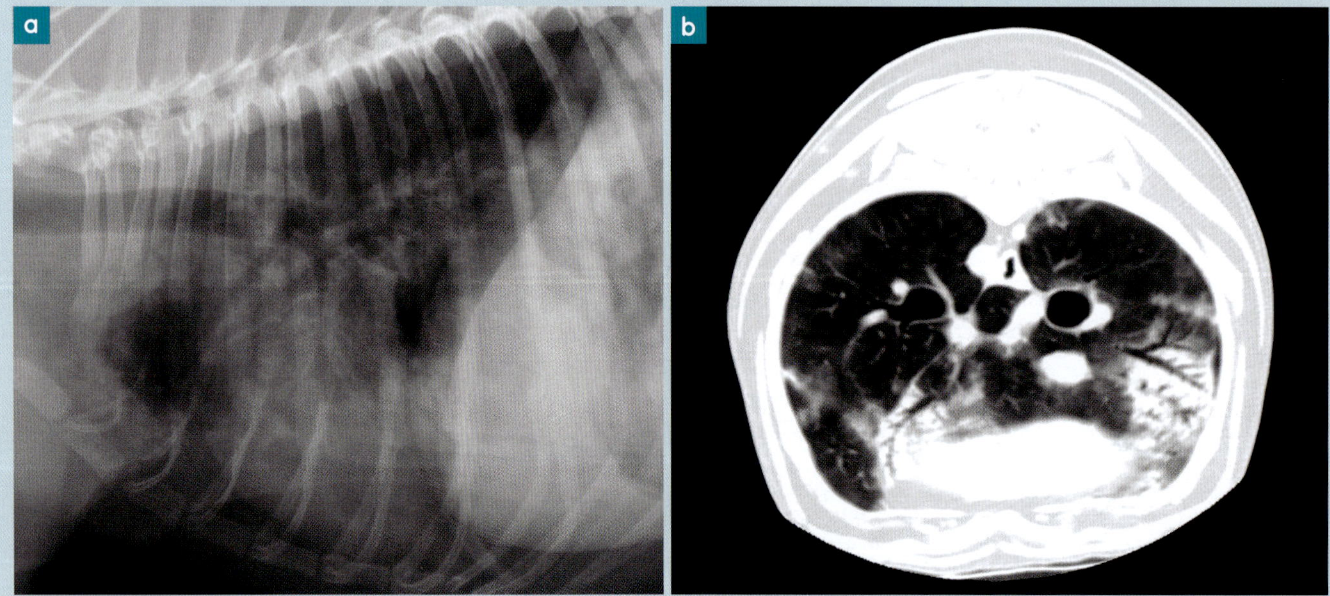

FIGURE 3.118. Lateral radiograph (a) and computed tomography image (b) of the thorax of a dog with an alveolar pattern due to pneumonia. In image (a), areas of soft-tissue density with an irregular morphology may be observed in the peripheral areas of the lung, where some air bronchograms can be identified, though with difficulty. The affected areas and air bronchograms are much more evident in the computed tomography image.

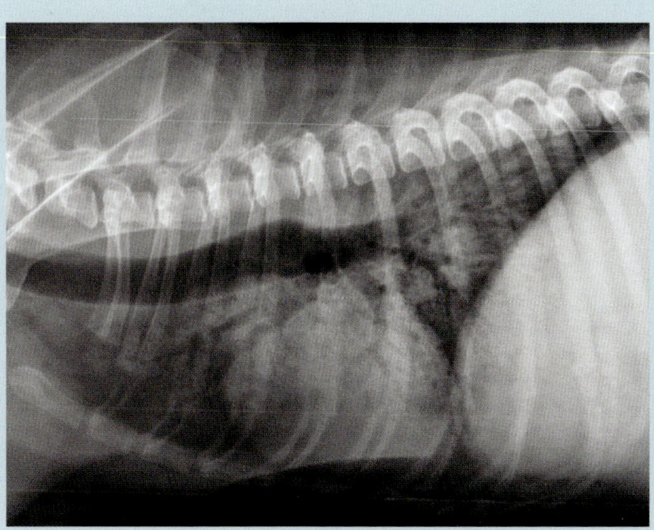

FIGURE 3.119. Lateral radiograph of the thorax of a dog with an alveolar pattern due to bronchopneumonia, which affects all the lung lobes. Large air bronchograms and numerous small air alveolograms, which give the lung the appearance of a "sponge", can be observed.

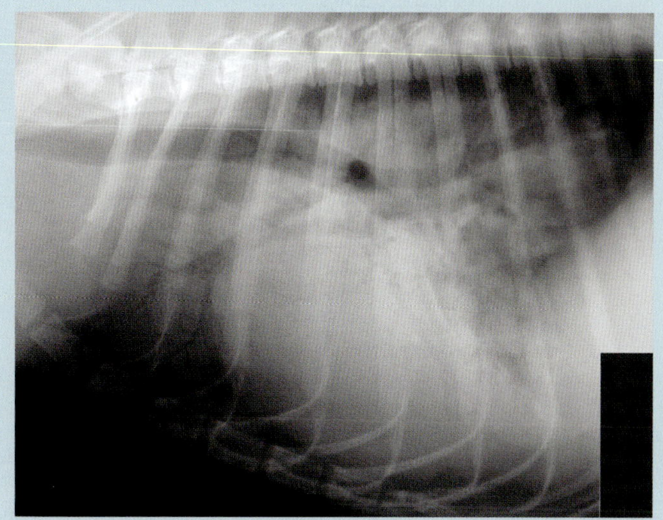

FIGURE 3.120. Lateral radiograph of the thorax of a dog with an alveolar pattern due to a bronchopneumonia, which affects all the lung lobes, but particularly the cranial and right middle lobes, where air bronchograms surrounded by consolidated lung parenchyma can be identified (with homogeneous soft-tissue density).

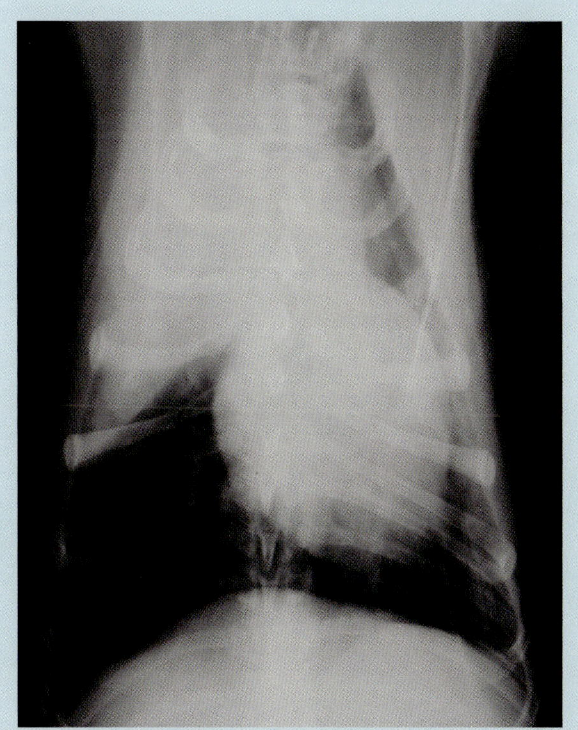

FIGURE 3.121. Ventrodorsal radiograph of the thorax of a dog with complete consolidation of the right cranial lobe, which has homogeneous soft-tissue density with no air bronchograms. This indicates that the lumen of the bronchi is filled with fluid or no longer contains air. A severe pneumonia or haemorrhage may cause the complete opacification of the lobe, but its volume would not change. Atelectasis of the lobe would cause the displacement of the mediastinum towards the affected side. However, in this case the mediastinum appears displaced to the left. In these cases, a lung ultrasound or computed tomography is indicated.

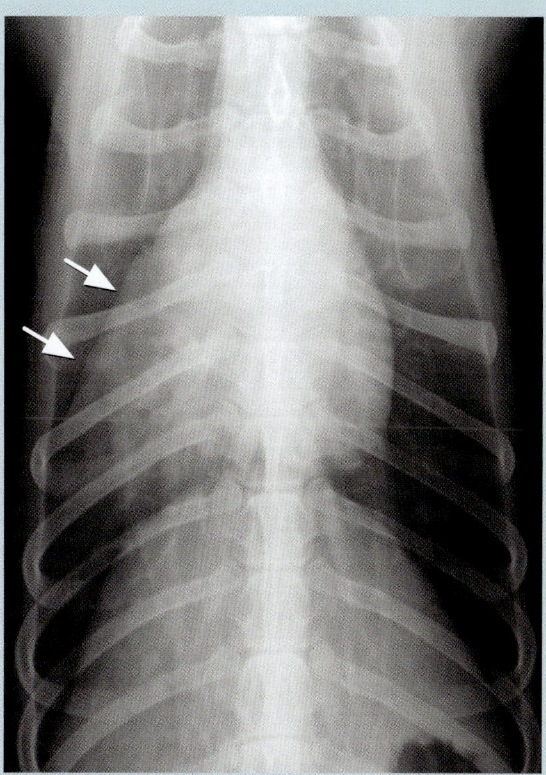

FIGURE 3.122. Dorsoventral radiograph of the thorax of a dog with localised pneumonia in the right middle lobe. The opacification of the lobe allows the clear identification of the margin of the cranial lobe (arrows). This is termed lobar sign and causes a loss of the cardiac border that is adjacent to the lesion, which is referred to as silhouette sign.

spreading first to the middle and then to the periphery (fig. 3.125). In cats, however, cardiogenic oedema can occur in any location and its pattern is often multi-focal ("patchy"). If cardiogenic pulmonary oedema is suspected, the radiological image of the lung should be reassessed after appropriate treatment.

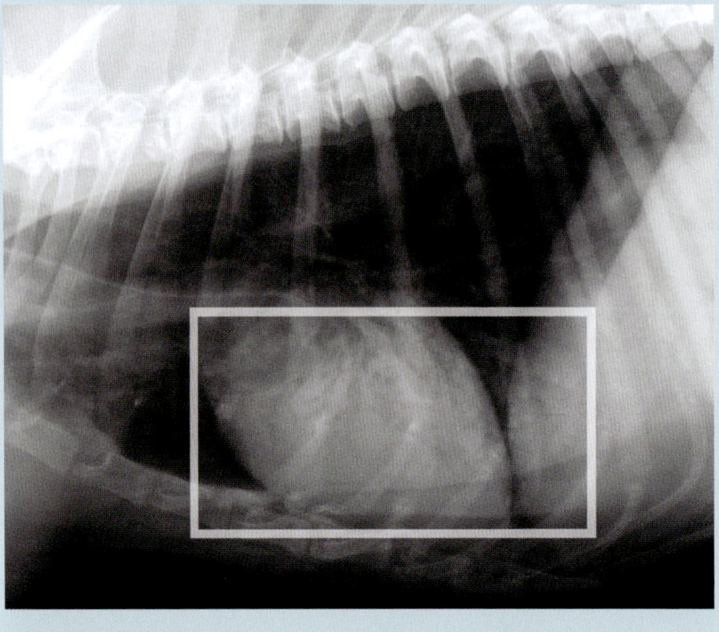

FIGURE 3.123. Lateral radiograph of the thorax of a dog with an alveolar pattern in the area of the right middle lobe and ventral area of the caudal lobes (shown in the rectangle) due to aspiration pneumonia. The additional findings in the image may be of help to establish a differential diagnosis. In this case, it is possible to identify the dilated walls of the oesophagus and a slight ventral displacement of the trachea and cardiac silhouette caused by the megaoesophagus.

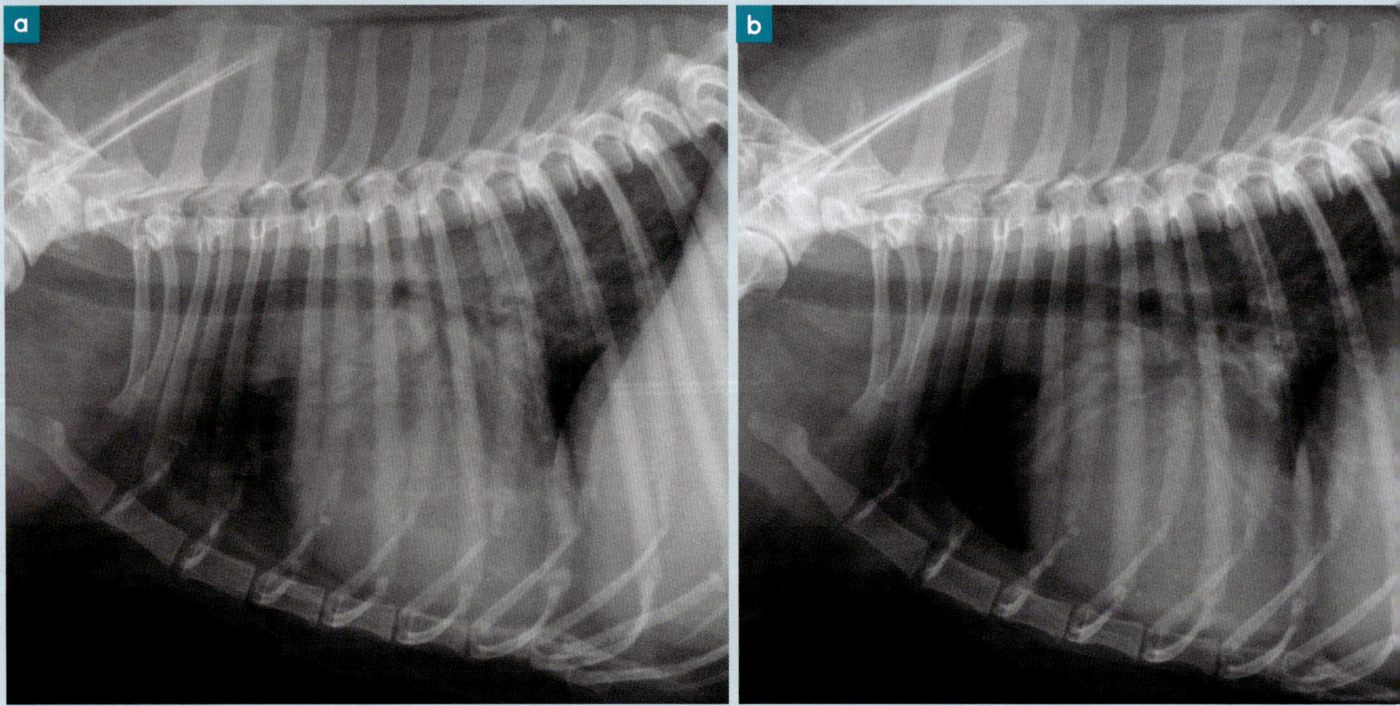

FIGURE 3.124. Lateral radiographs of the thorax of a dog with an alveolar pattern in the caudodorsal area of the lung due to cardiogenic oedema, before (a) and a few hours after (b) the treatment. The time an alveolar pattern takes to appear and disappear may be of help to establish a differential diagnosis. An oedema takes several hours to disappear or reduce with the appropriate treatment, while a haemorrhage or pneumonia will take days to do so.

Non-cardiogenic oedema is uncommon. While it can occur in any part of the lung, dorsocaudal lung involvement is more common, and especially the right caudal lobe. Medical history and examination findings can help guide the radiological diagnosis in these patients who present with an episode of acute dyspnoea. The most common causes are upper airway obstruction, neurogenic (e.g. secondary to seizures), electrocution and near-drowning.

Pneumonia may present at any location in the lung, with involvement of one or more lobes. Bacterial pneumonia is often found in the cranioventral area (fig. 3.126). Ventral location is also common for aspiration pneumonia, although it may appear in other locations depending on the patient's position at the time of aspiration. If aspiration occurs as a result of an alteration of the oesophagus, the X-ray may also provide some information about this. Foreign body penetration of the lung (e.g. grass awns) usually causes focal pneumonia, sometimes difficult to identify on X-rays, especially when the affected area overlaps with other chest structures, such as the heart (fig. 3.127). Peripheral involvement may suggest *Angiostrongylus* infection. The absence of cardiomegaly and venous congestion on the image may help distinguish pneumonia from cardiogenic oedema.

Pulmonary haemorrhages usually occur as a result of trauma to the chest but can also be due to coagulation disorders. In the event of trauma, the most affected area is usually closest to the impact (fig. 3.128). They may present a more diffuse pattern of distribution or cause more focal haematomas (fig. 3.129), usually adjacent to the chest wall.

The accumulation of cells in the alveoli is uncommon, although it may occur in some types of neoplasia (e.g. bronchoalveolar carcinoma).

In the case of pulmonary atelectasis, the alveolar pattern is accompanied by radiographic signs of decreased volume of the lung or the affected area of the lung. This is usually identified on dorsoventral and ventrodorsal radiographs by the displacement of mediastinal structures toward the affected lobe or lobes (fig. 3.130), unless the atelectasis affects both lungs to a similar extent, as may occur in pneumothorax or bilateral pleural effusion. It is more difficult to appreciate the signs of decreased volume in a lung or

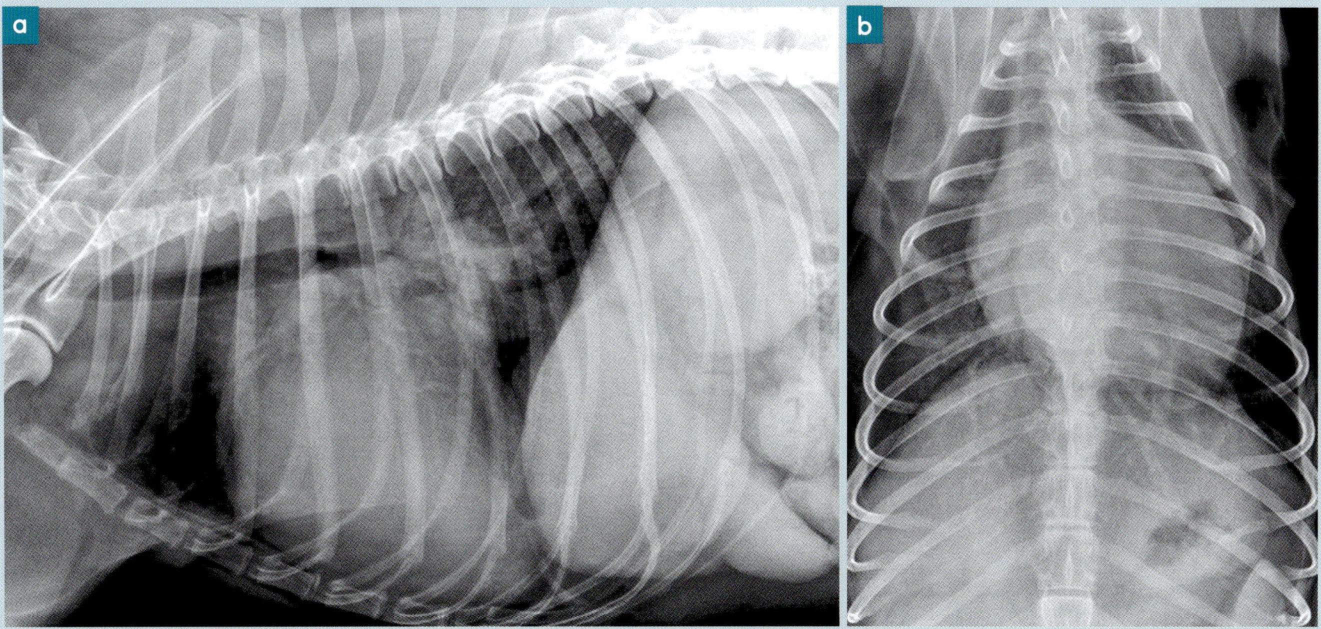

FIGURE 3.125. Right lateral (a) and dorsoventral (b) projections of a dog with cardiogenic pulmonary oedema. In the lateral projection, the perihiliar and dorscaudal areas of the lung appear more affected. The right lung is more affected than the left lung.

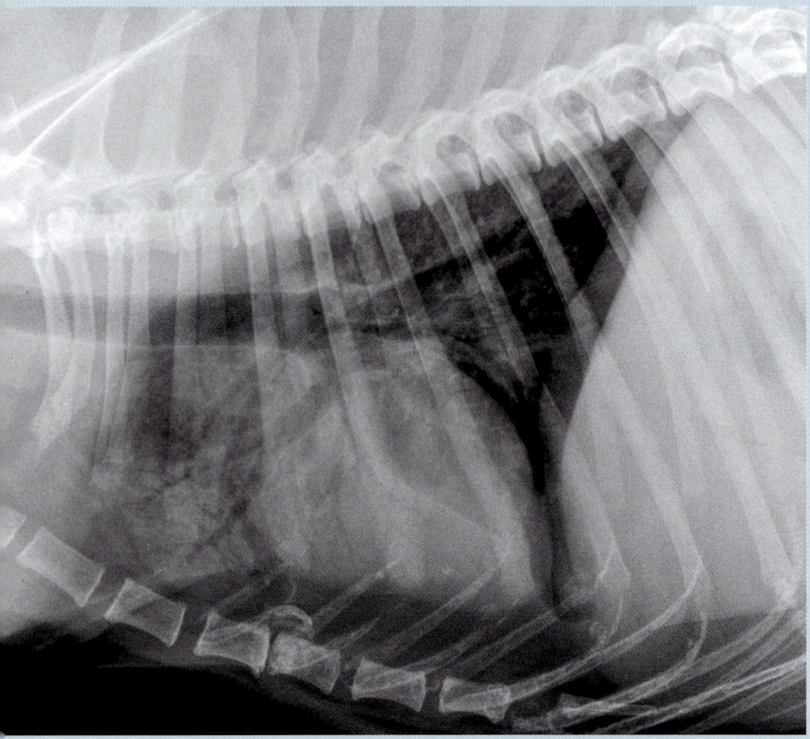

FIGURE 3.126. Lateral projection of the thorax of a dog with pneumonia of bacterial origin, mainly affecting the cranioventral area of the lung.

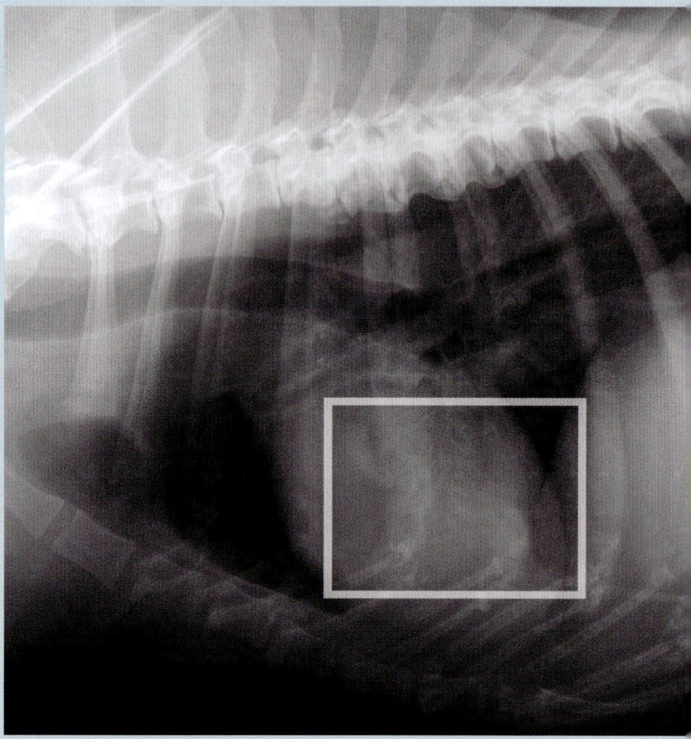

FIGURE 3.127. Lateral radiograph of the thorax of a dog with an alveolar pattern in the area of the right middle lobe (shown in the rectangle) due to focal pneumonia caused by the penetration of a plant awn in the lung. The affected area is very small, but the identification of an air bronchogram in it confirms the diagnosis of alveolar pattern.

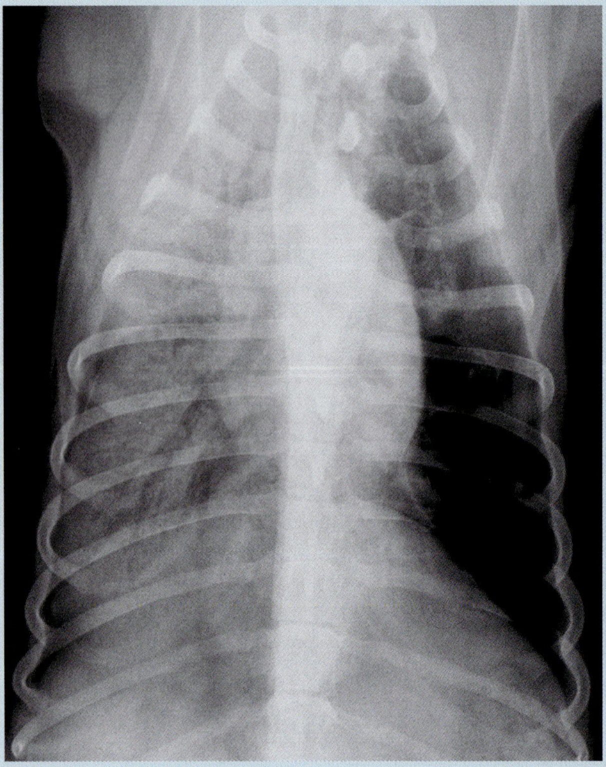

FIGURE 3.128. Dorsoventral projection of the thorax of a dog with pulmonary haemorrhage located in the right lung and cranial area of the left. The X-ray was performed one hour after the patient was hit by a car, with impact on the right chest wall.

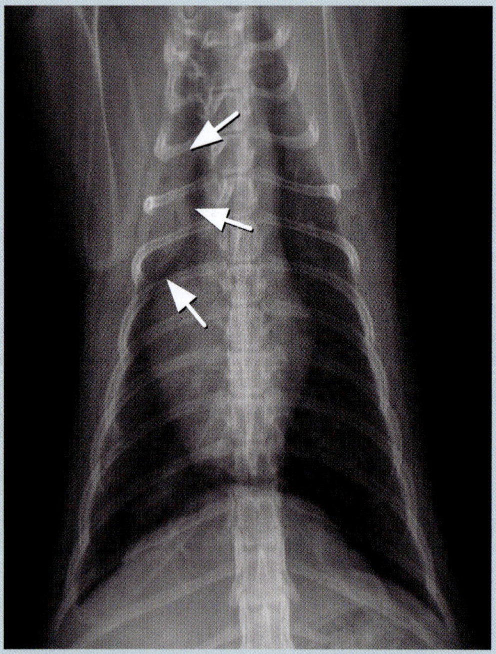

FIGURE 3.129. Ventrodorsal radiograph of the thorax of a cat with a pulmonary contusion, which appears as an area of focal consolidation (arrows) in the same side as that of the trauma that caused it.

lung area in lateral projections. In cases of more pronounced atelectasis, the cardiac silhouette can appear elevated over the sternum by the displacement of the heart towards the affected hemithorax (fig. 3.131) or towards the most affected in the case of atelectasis of both lungs.

Interstitial pattern

The lung interstitial pattern is characterised by abnormalities affecting the pulmonary interstitium. Two types of patterns are clearly distinguished: nodular interstitial, due to the focal proliferation of cells in the interstitium that leads to the formation of nodular lesions, and unstructured interstitial pattern, when involvement of the pulmonary interstitium occurs diffusely.

Nodular interstitial pattern

The differential diagnosis of a nodular pattern varies in function of the number and size of the lesions. A nodular lesion may be distinguished from an area of alveolar infiltration because a nodule has a regular shape (typically round or oval) and well-defined borders, while an area of alveolar infiltration has an irregular morphology and poorly defined limits (fig. 3.132). Nodular lesions may be identified on radiographs when they reach a diameter of 5 mm or more. With smaller diameters, they may be confused with transverse images of the pulmonary blood vessels. However, if the lung has an elevated number of nodular lesions smaller than 5 mm (referred to as a **miliary nodular interstitial pattern**), these will no longer be mistaken for vessels.

The differential diagnosis of a nodular interstitial pattern with lesions larger than 5 mm (fig. 3.133) includes: pulmonary metastases (the most common diagnosis), primary lung neoplasms, abscesses and pulmonary granulomas (not frequent). A miliary nodular interstitial pattern (fig. 3.134) may be due to metastases or mycotic pneumonia as the most probable diagnoses, followed by mycobacterial or haematogenous bacterial pneumonia, pulmonary lymphoma or disseminated intravascular coagulation.

Pulmonary bone metaplasia (fig. 3.135), which is a benign process characterised by the appearance of numerous very small, calcified nodules in the lung parenchyma, should not be confused with a miliary pattern caused by metastases, mycosis, lymphoma, etc.

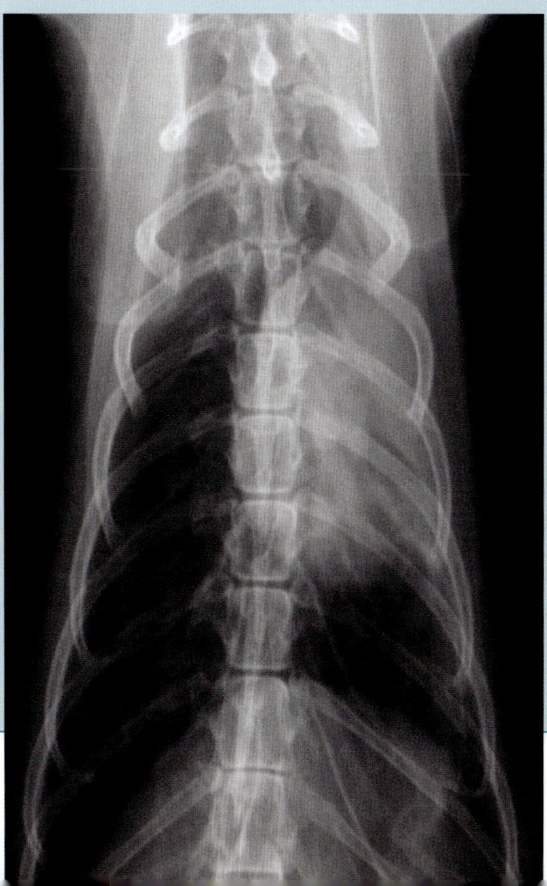

FIGURE 3.130. Dorsoventral radiograph of the thorax of a cat with atelectasis of the caudal segment of the left cranial lung lobe. The displacement of the cardiac silhouette (displacement of the mediastinum) to the left hemithorax indicates a loss of volume in the affected lung lobe. A mass was detected by means of bronchoscopy in the bronchus of the caudal segment of the left cranial lobe.

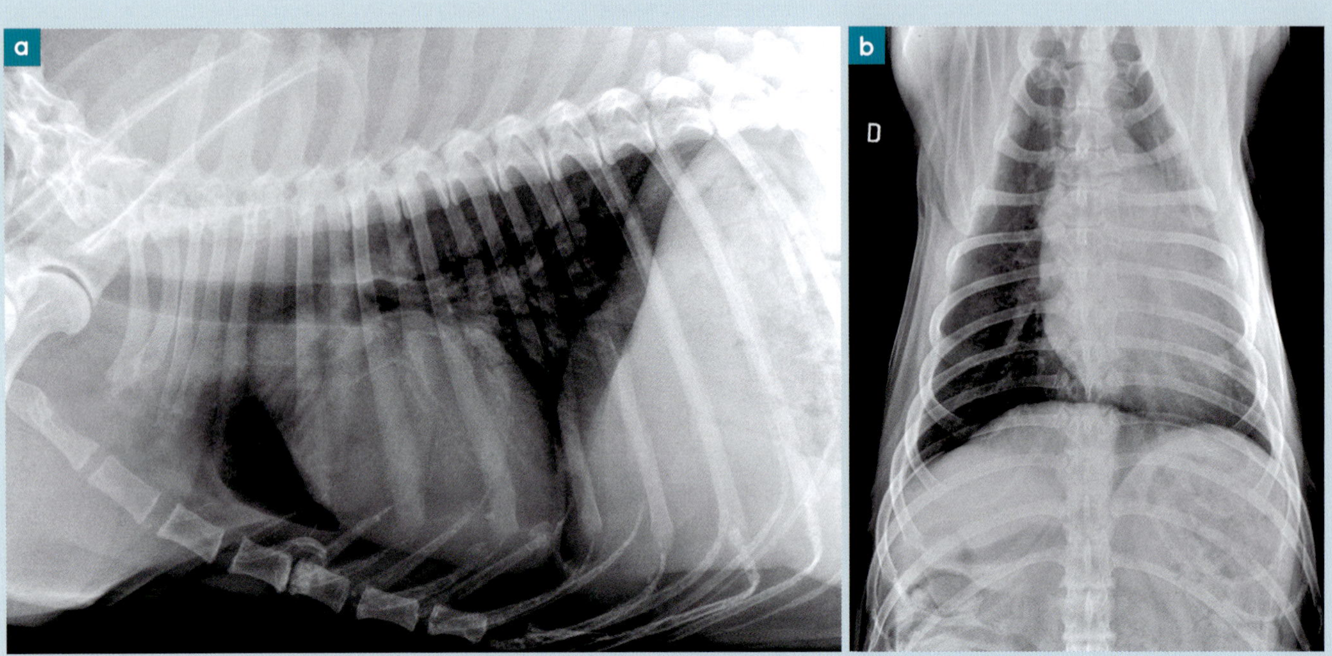

FIGURE 3.131. Lateral (a) and ventrodorsal (b) projection of the thorax of a dog with partial atelectasis of the left lung. In the lateral projection, elevation of the cardiac silhouette and a slight retraction of the ventral pulmonary border can be observed. The ventrodorsal projection shows mediastinal displacement towards the atelectatic lung, that is, to the left.

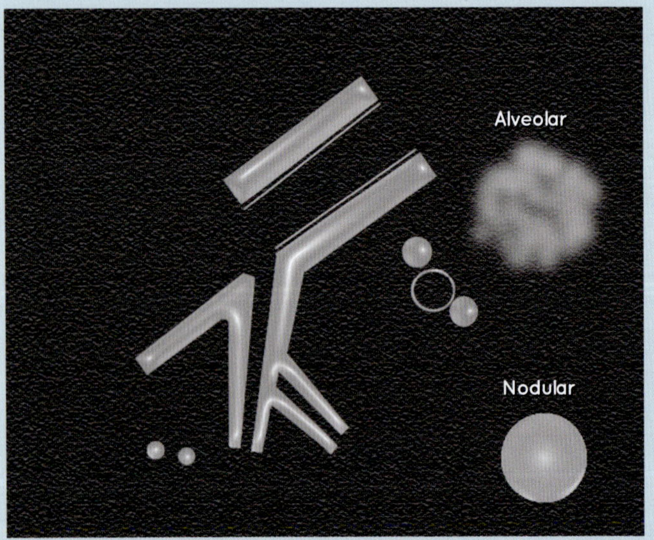

FIGURE 3.132. Schematic representation of a nodular interstitial pattern in comparison with an area of alveolar infiltration. A nodular lesion has a regular shape (generally round or oval) and well-defined limits, while the area of infiltration has an irregular morphology and ill-defined borders.

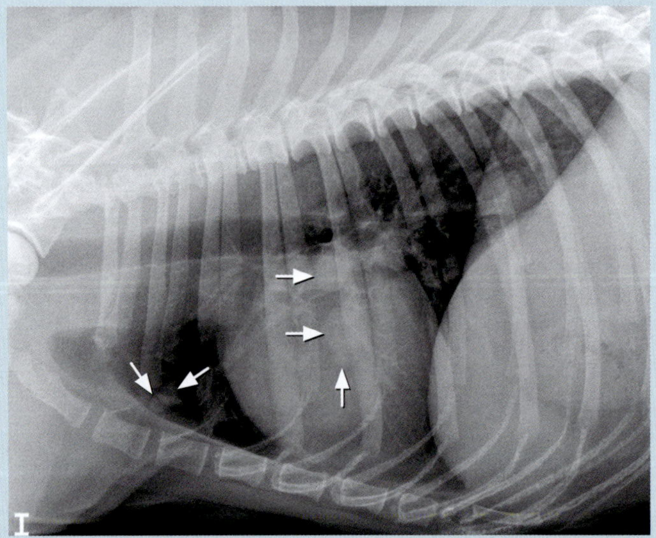

FIGURE 3.133. Lateral projection of the thorax of a dog with pulmonary metastases. The arrows point to several of the pulmonary nodular lesions, measuring over 5 mm in size (nodular interstitial lung pattern) presented by the patient.

The calcification of nodular lesions caused by metastases, even from osteogenic tumours such as osteosarcoma, is very rare.

The use of the terms pulmonary "nodule" or "mass" depends on the size of the lesion: if its diameter is less than 3 cm, it is called nodule, and if it exceeds this value, the term "mass" is used. It is important not to confuse nodules with transverse images of pulmonary vessels, images created by the superimposition of ribs and other structures, or with calcified pulmonary or pleural plaques.

The most probable cause of a single pulmonary mass (fig. 3.136) is primary lung neoplasm, although abscess, granuloma, haematoma or fluid-filled bulla should also be included in the list of possible differential diagnoses. Pulmonary masses may occasionally be calcified in the centre due to dystrophic calcification, or have a more or less irregular central area with gas density (**cavitary mass**). The most likely diagnoses of a cavitary pulmonary mass are a tumor with necrotic center and an abscess (fig. 3.137).

It is important not to confuse a cavitary mass with a pulmonary bulla (also called pneumatocele), which often appears as an incidental finding. A pulmonary bulla is due to a focal accumulation of gas in the lung caused by loss or rupture of the alveolar walls, which may be of congenital, traumatic or idiopathic origin. The wall of the bulla is usually thin and is formed by pulmonary connective tissue and the visceral pleura (fig. 3.138).

When a large lung mass is observed next to others with a smaller diameter, these latter usually correspond to metastases of the first mass. In dogs, lung metastases usually appear as well-defined, round lesions, while in cats they often have a more irregular shape and a more poorly defined outline. The metastases of haemangiosarcomas may also appear less defined because they are usually accompanied by haemorrhage.

A large lung mass may mimic the image of lung lobe consolidation due to other causes, such as lobar pneumonia (fig. 3.139). One criterion that facilitates their differentiation is that masses generally have convex margins, not consistent with the normal morphology of interlobular fissures. It is uncommon to identify air bronchograms in a lung mass, but when visualised they are usually narrow or distorted.

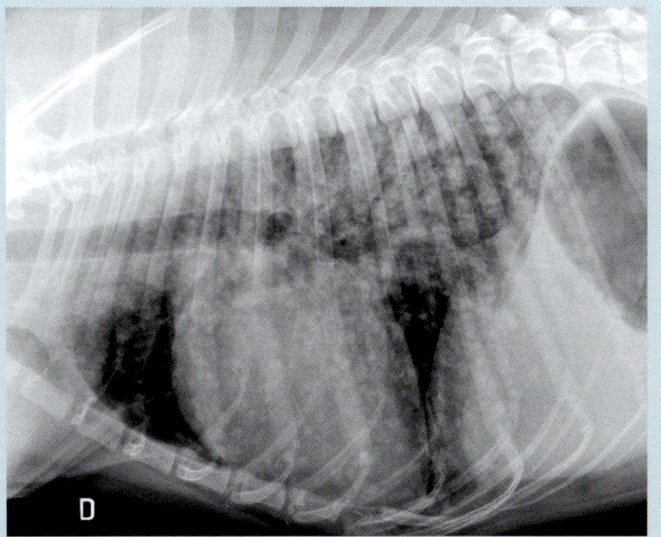

FIGURE 3.134. Lateral projection of the thorax of a dog with pulmonary metastases. There are very numerous pulmonary nodular lesions measuring less than 5 mm (miliary nodular interstitial lung pattern).

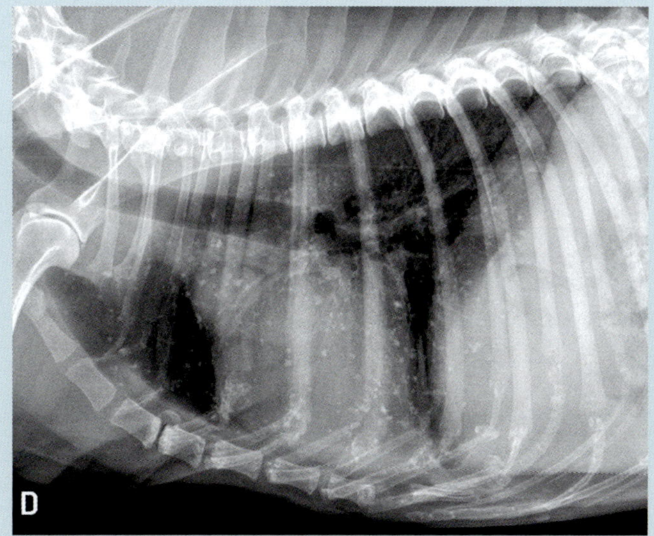

FIGURE 3.135. Lateral projection of the thorax of a dog with pulmonary osseous metaplasia, a benign process characterised by the appearance of numerous tiny, calcified nodules in the lung parenchyma.

When a mass is located adjacent to the thoracic wall, it is possible to assess it by means of an ultrasound examination, and thus to determine whether it is solid or cystic, to examine its vascularisation and to perform an ultrasound-guided fine-needle aspiration or biopsy.

Computed tomography is particularly indicated to look for metastases (nodules smaller than 2 mm can be detected) and for the study of lung masses, since it allows us to determine their exact location for a possible surgical treatment, assess their extension to adjacent structures (fig. 3.140) and perform a guided biopsy if this cannot be done by means of ultrasonography.

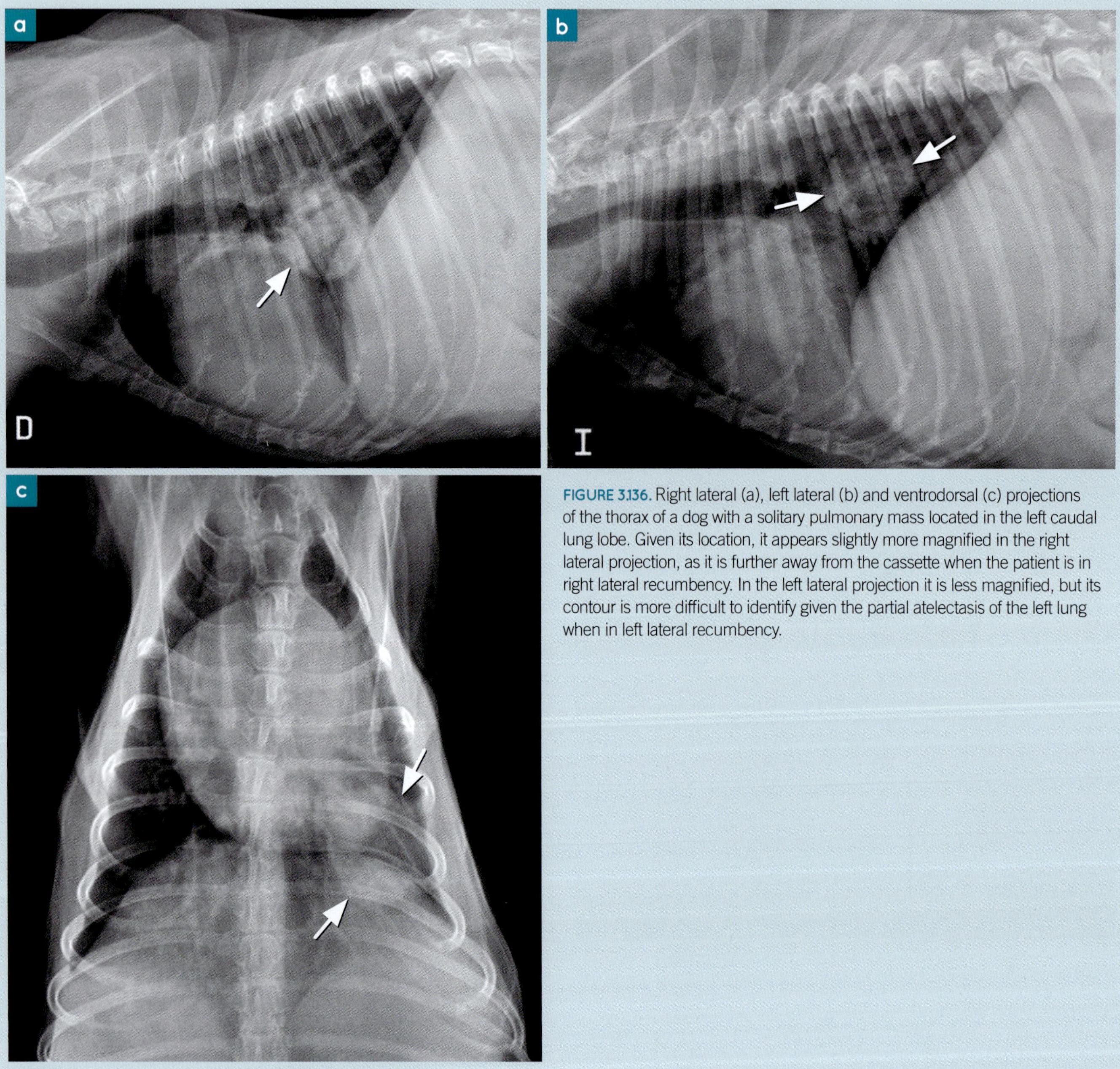

FIGURE 3.136. Right lateral (a), left lateral (b) and ventrodorsal (c) projections of the thorax of a dog with a solitary pulmonary mass located in the left caudal lung lobe. Given its location, it appears slightly more magnified in the right lateral projection, as it is further away from the cassette when the patient is in right lateral recumbency. In the left lateral projection it is less magnified, but its contour is more difficult to identify given the partial atelectasis of the left lung when in left lateral recumbency.

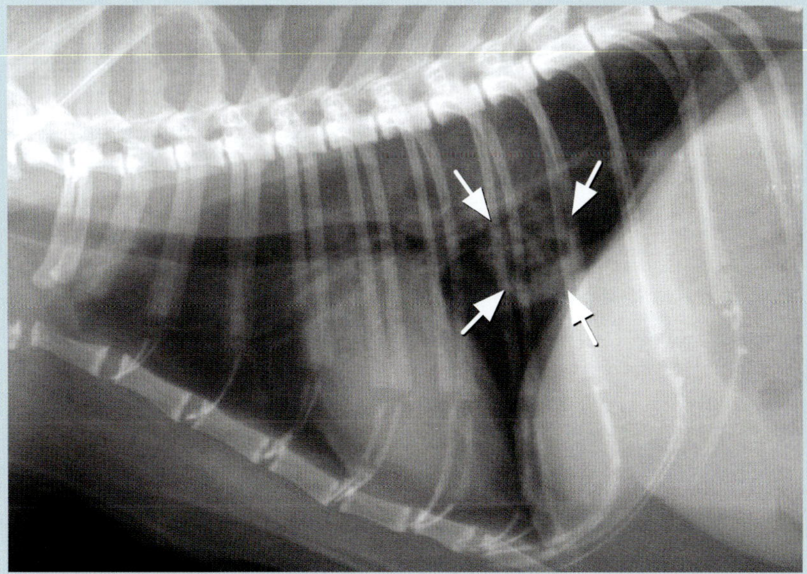

FIGURE 3.137. Lateral projection of the thorax of a cat with a solitary lung mass. The most likely cause is a primary but cavitary lung neoplasm (arrows). It is possible to observe areas of gas density with an irregular morphology in the central area of the mass. The list of possible differential diagnoses should include abscess, granuloma, haematoma or pulmonary cysts.

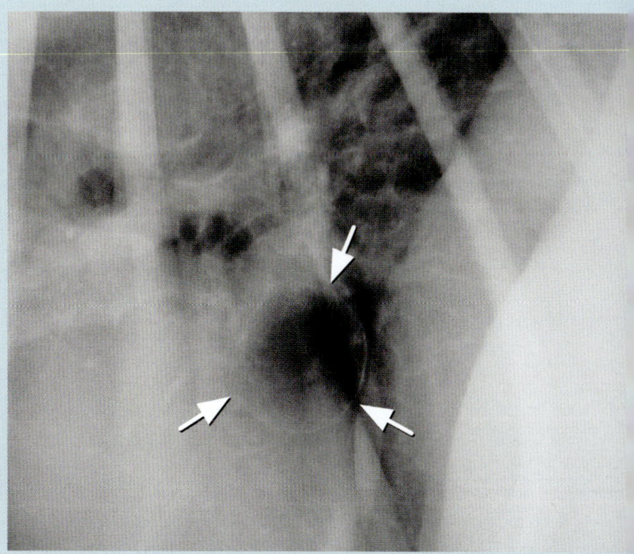

FIGURE 3.138. Enlarged image of the perihilar region on a lateral radiograph of the thorax of a dog with a pulmonary bulla (arrows). As opposed to cavitary lung masses, bullae usually have a very thin wall and are incidental findings.

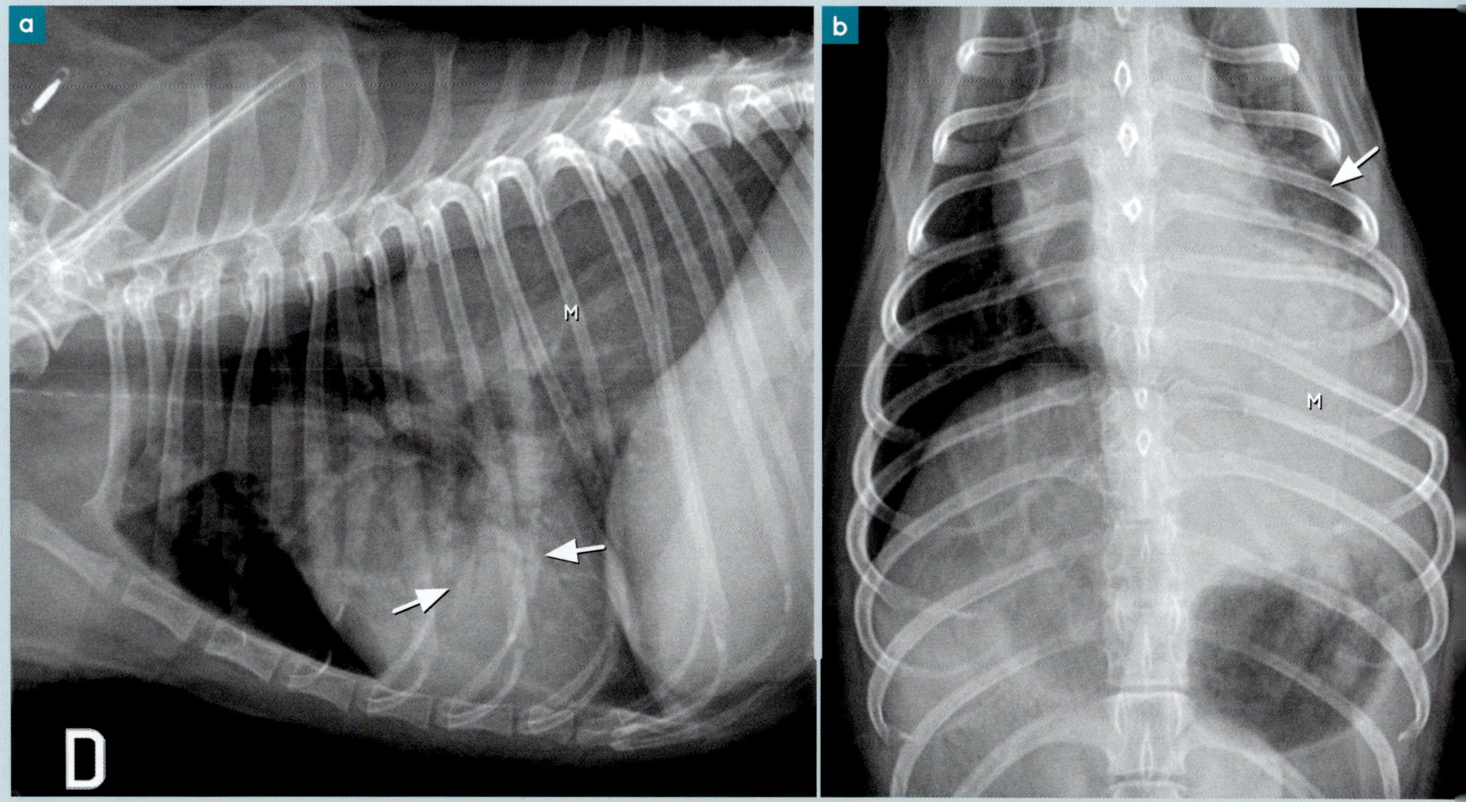

FIGURE 3.139. Right lateral (a) and dorsoventral (b) projections of the thorax of a dog with a large mass (M) located in the left caudal lung lobe. The mass has a morphology similar to that of the lobe, but its borders are convex, and this help guide the radiological diagnosis. The white arrows point to lung areas with an alveolar pattern, possibly due to atelectasis caused by adjacent mass.

Unstructured interstitial pattern

The unstructured interstitial pattern (also called diffuse interstitial) is the most difficult to identify on X-rays. It causes a discrete diffuse increase in pulmonary opacity in the affected areas, which makes it difficult to differentiate the pulmonary vessels, although these are still visible in the image (fig. 3.141). It differs from the alveolar pattern in that the latter causes a more marked increase in opacity, which completely obscures the image of the pulmonary vessels in the affected areas. In fact, if a pathological process affects the interstitium and alveoli, the unstructured interstitial pattern will be masked by the alveolar component, which is common in the case of oedema, pneumonia or haemorrhage that affects both pulmonary components. Cardiogenic oedema is only interstitial in the earliest phase (often difficult to identify on radiographs due to the typical perihilar location in dogs). Afterwards it evolves towards greater alveolar interstitial involvement at which point the alveolar radiological pattern predominates and masks the interstitial pattern.

The increased pulmonary opacity caused by the unstructured interstitial pattern is usually homogeneous in appearance, although it can sometimes acquire a reticular or linear appearance (fig. 3.142).

The most common causes of pure unstructured interstitial pattern (not associated with an alveolar component) are interstitial oedema (initial or resolution phase), viral or protozoan pneumonia, pulmonary fibrosis, diffuse neoplastic infiltration (lymphoma or metastasis of mammary carcinoma), herbicide poisoning and haemorrhage (initial or resolution phase).

Pulmonary fibrosis may appear as a degenerative sign associated with ageing in older animals and causes a slight increase in interstitial radiopacity. It may also appear as the final consequence of a great variety of lung diseases leading to an irreversible alteration of the support tissue of the interstitium. The initial cause may be inflammatory, infectious or idiopathic. Idiopathic pulmonary fibrosis mainly affects senior dogs of the Terrier breeds, especially the West Highland White Terrier and Cairn Terrier (fig. 3.143).

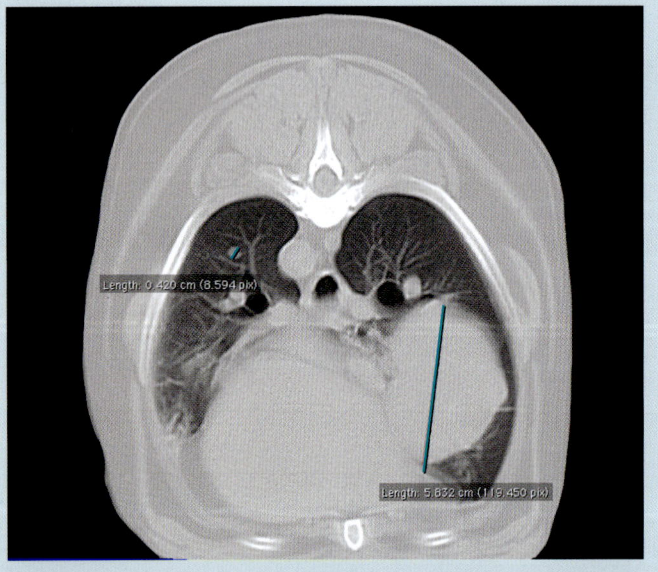

FIGURE 3.140. Computed tomography image of the thorax of a dog with a 6-cm mass in the left lung (long red line), previously diagnosed by means of radiography. Computed tomography allowed the determination of the exact location of the mass and the detection of small metastases (short red line) that had not been identified in the right lung.

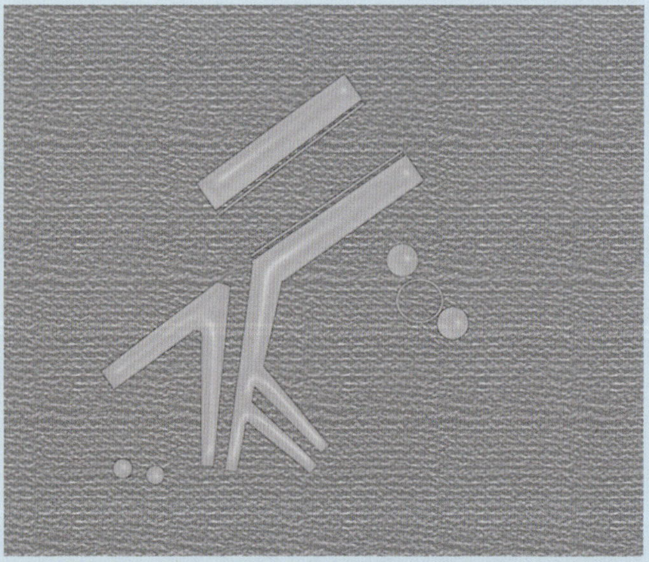

FIGURE 3.141. Schematic representation of the unstructured interstitial pattern, which is characterised by a diffuse increase of lung radiopacity, which reduces the visibility of the pulmonary vessels.

Mediastinal lymphadenopathies are also often found in patients with pulmonary lymphoma, especially in dogs. It may also be accompanied by pleural effusion and/or pulmonary oedema. Ultrasound examination of the abdomen usually reveals organomegaly and intra-abdominal lymphadenopathies in these patients.

Computed tomography is very sensitive to detect or confirm this type of lung pattern (fig. 3.144).

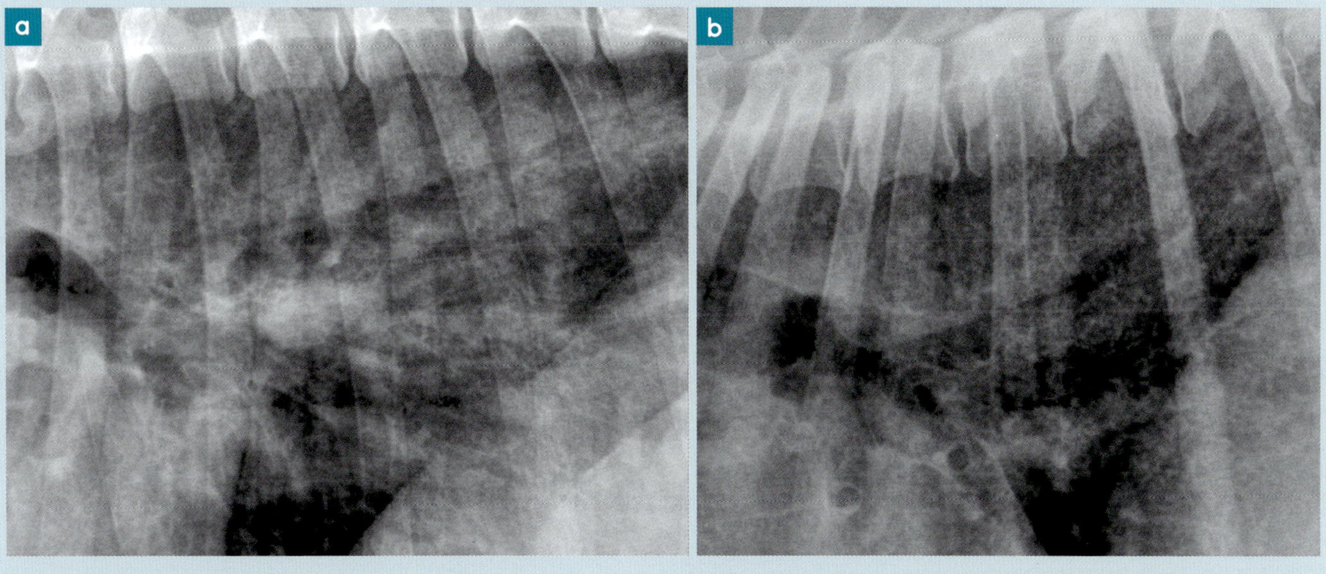

FIGURE 3.142. Enlarged images of the dorsocaudal area of the thorax in lateral projection of two dogs with an unstructured interstitial lung pattern due to lymphoma. In image (a) the increased opacity is more homogeneous, while image (b) has a more reticular appearance. The pattern obstructs proper visualisation of smaller diameter pulmonary vessels.

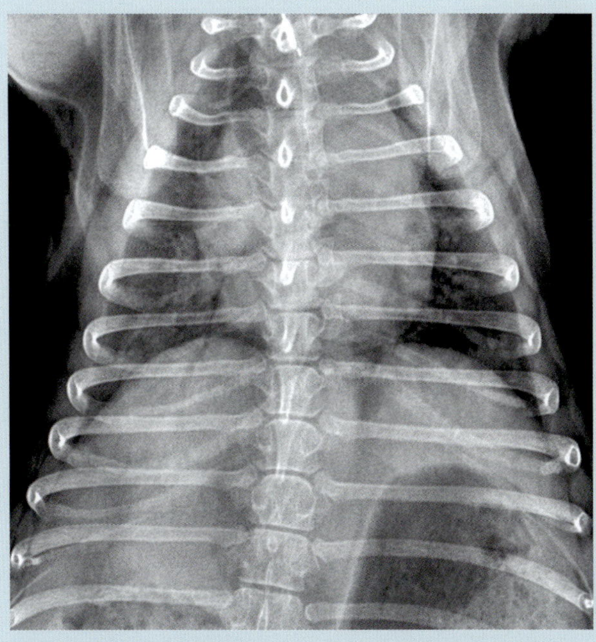

FIGURE 3.143. Dorsoventral projection of the thorax of a West Highland White Terrier with a generalised unstructured interstitial lung pattern caused by pulmonary fibrosis. Involvement is more marked in the right lung.

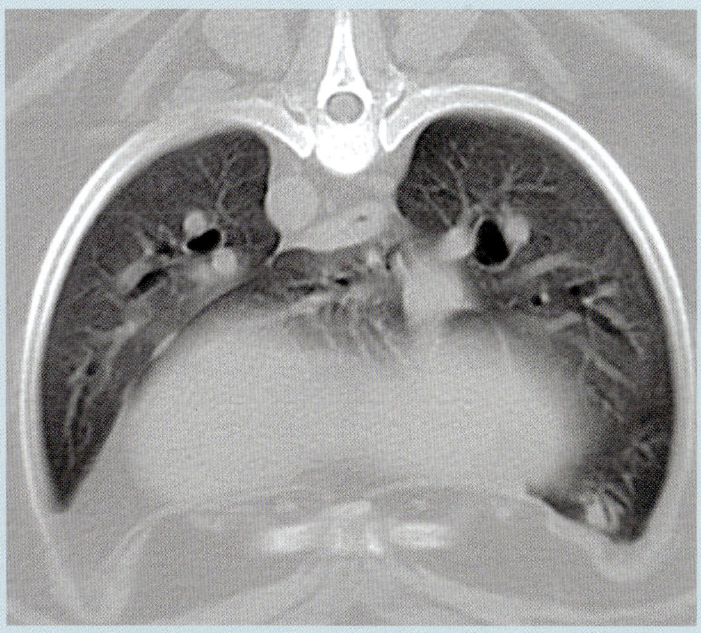

FIGURE 3.144. Computed tomography image of the thorax of a dog with a generalised unstructured interstitial pattern.

Mixed pattern

Pathological processes affecting the lung often cause abnormalities in more than one pulmonary component, so it is very common to identify mixed lung patterns on the X-ray (fig. 3.145). Bacterial bronchopneumonia, for example, usually elicits a mixed pattern with bronchial, alveolar and interstitial components, although the latter is usually masked by the alveolar. In pulmonary fibrosis, the co-appearance of an unstructured interstitial and a bronchial pattern is also common. Whereas with primary pulmonary neoplasms, an interstitial component (nodular and/or unstructured), a bronchial component and in some cases an alveolar component (secondary atelectasis or alveolar infiltration) are common.

The predominant pattern is usually taken into account when establishing the order of probability of the possible differential diagnoses.

Lung hypertranslucency

Generalised hypertranslucency may appear due to an increase in the volume of air contained in the lungs (due to an obstruction of the intrathoracic airways or emphysema) or as a result of a reduction in the size of the pulmonary vessels. Real hypertranslucency should not be confused with an overexposed radiograph.

Pulmonary emphysema is characterised by an excessive, focal or diffuse, accumulation of air in the lung parenchyma, and may be congenital or acquired. Acquired emphysema usually occurs secondary to chronic obstructive pulmonary disease, which causes irreversible expansion of the alveoli or destruction of their walls. One or more lung lobes may be affected showing up as hyperlucent (less opacity than normal) and this does not vary with the inspiration and expiration cycle. The chest cavity may appear expanded, with the ribs more perpendicular to the spine and the diaphragm flattened and displaced caudally, with little variation in its position with inspiration and expiration. The cardiac silhouette may appear diminished in size and more distant from the diaphragm (fig. 3.146). If only one lung is affected, the mediastinal structures tend to lean toward the unaffected lung, and if only a single lobe is affected, it can partially collapse the adjacent lobe, causing a sharp contrast in the opacity between the affected and the adjacent lobe. Pulmonary bullae can also be identified in these patients.

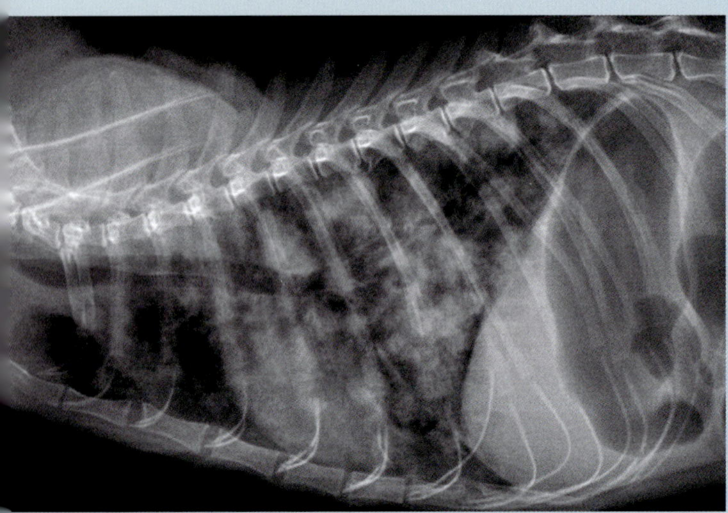

FIGURE 3.145. Lateral projection of the thorax of a cat with a mixed pulmonary pattern (nodular interstitial, alveolar and bronchial) caused by a lymphoma.

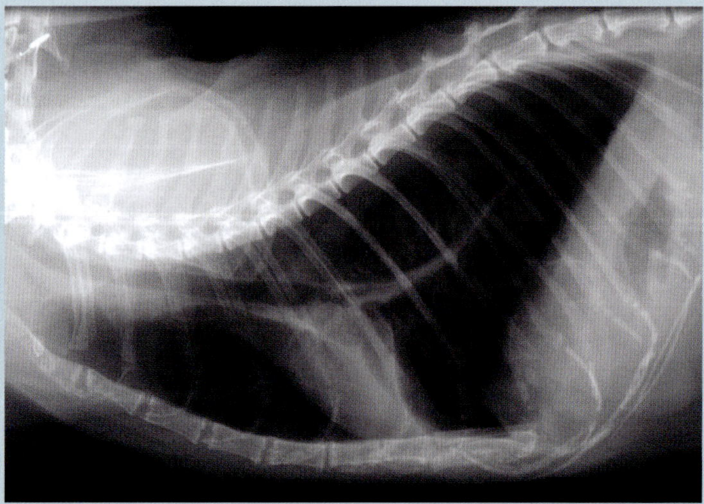

FIGURE 3.146. Lateral radiograph of the thorax of a cat with hyperlucency and increase of the lung volume due to emphysema. The cardiac silhouette appears reduced in size and the diaphragm is flattened and caudally displaced. Emphysema is a common complication of feline asthma.

Pulmonary neoplasia

The most common radiological image of primary lung neoplasms is characterised by the appearance of a solitary mass with a regular and clearly defined contour. Multiple nodules, homogeneous lobar consolidation, a diffuse reticulonodular pattern or an interstitial-alveolar pattern may also be observed. Bronchioloalveolar carcinoma may produce a mixed pattern with nodules of irregular morphology and peribronchial infiltrates.

Areas of consolidation, that appear associated with a primary lung neoplasia, may correspond to the tumour itself but could also be caused by pulmonary atelectasis due to secondary inflammatory changes or tumour invasion of the airways.

In dogs, pulmonary histiocytic sarcomas are most commonly found in the right middle lobe (predominantly in the ventral area) and the left cranial lobe, and usually involve the peripheral area of one lobe or the whole lobe. The appearance of air bronchograms in the lesion is more common in histiocytic sarcomas than in other primary tumour types.

Identifying chest lymphadenopathies associated with primary lung neoplasms on X-rays is not common. However, studies have been published indicating that they are more common in dogs with histiocytic sarcomas, in which greater sternal and tracheobronchial node involvement was observed compared with cranial mediastinal nodes.

The radiological pattern that can be identified on X-rays of patients with pulmonary lymphoma varies greatly in both dogs and cats. In dogs, the most common radiological pattern is unstructured interstitial, followed by nodular interstitial (single or multiple lesions), alveolar infiltration and bronchial infiltration. In cats, pulmonary masses and/or nodules and bronchial infiltration are the most common findings. In some cases, the pulmonary infiltration pattern appears together with images of sternal, cranial mediastinal and/or tracheobronchial lymphadenopathies, and less frequently pleural effusion.

Pleural effusion associated with a primary lung neoplasm is more common in cats than in dogs. In these patients, ultrasound may facilitate more accurate identification of lung lesions, provided that they extend to the peripheral area of the lung. To properly assess the lung image, the X-ray should be repeated after thoracentesis.

In addition to the increased frequency of associated pleural effusion, other common radiographic findings in cats with primary lung neoplasia are:

- The radiological pattern is usually that of a well-defined mass, although the margins can often be irregular.
- The most common location is in the caudal lobes, with a predominance of the right.
- Bronchioloalveolar carcinoma may generate a mixed bronchial pattern that is more alveolar, with no evident nodular component, a focal alveolar pattern or one or more cavitary masses (fig. 3.147).
- Gas-filled cavities are more common in tumours of bronchial origin, although they can also appear with other types of lung tumours. If calcification appears in association with these lesions, this further increases the suspicion of neoplasia.
- Adenocarcinomas, squamous cell carcinomas and bronchogenic carcinomas can metastasise to the distal phalanges, and can affect various digits and phalanges. If lysis is identified in one or more distal phalanges in the cat, which may spread to the middle phalanges, metastasis of a lung carcinoma should be considered as a differential diagnosis. Cases of monoparesis as a result of arterial thromboembolism have also been described in patients with primary lung carcinoma, hence a chest X-ray is recommended in senior cats without heart disease presenting this clinical sign.

Lung lobe torsion

Lung lobe torsion can occur spontaneously, especially in deep-chest dogs, or it can be secondary to pathologies that cause lobar collapse and the presence of air or fluid around it, which facilitates lobe mobility. The most affected lobe is the right middle, followed by the cranial part of the left cranial lobe (especially in Pugs) and the right cranial lobe; caudal lobe involvement is unlikely.

Initially, signs of increased volume of the affected lobe can be observed, but when secondary necrosis develops, the volume of the lobe tends to decrease, and its margins may appear concave. Consolidation can be observed, sometimes with small identifiable air bronchograms. The appearance of a "vesicular pattern", with numerous small "sponge-like" areas of trapped gas is relatively typical; a finding that is highly indicative of lobe torsion. The lobar bronchi may present a sudden interruption of their path or an abnormal direction. The development of a secondary pleural effusion is common, which can be located in both hemithoraces, only in the affected lobe or only around the affected lobe. Pneumothorax or pneumomediastinum may also appear if there is a rupture of the bronchi.

Doppler ultrasonography may be of great help in the diagnosis as it allows the detection of the absence of venous flow and of the reduction or absence of arterial flow in the affected lobe. However, in practice, good quality images may not be obtained due to the breathing difficulties of patients with torsion.

The most appropriate diagnostic technique is computed tomography, as it provides accurate data on the abnormal bronchial and vascular structure positioning as well as an evaluation of their permeability. The administration of an intravenous contrast medium allows the differentiation between the vascularised collapsed lung and the necrotic lobe with torsion.

Pulmonary thromboembolism

This is caused by blockage of an artery by a blood clot or migration of an embolus, which may be composed of small blood clots as well as other components such as bacteria, parasites, fat, air or foreign bodies (e.g. an intravenous catheter). The patient presents with lethargy, weakness and tachypnoea and poorly response to oxygen and other support measures. Computed tomography or pulmonary angiography are usually required to confirm the diagnosis. X-rays may show no obvious abnormalities, even in patients with severe clinical signs. Up to 27 % of dogs and cats with a necropsy-confirmed pulmonary thromboembolism do not show any anomalies on chest radiographs. In an animal with tachypnoea that does not respond to oxygen administration, a normal chest radiograph will strongly suggest the presence of thromboembolism.

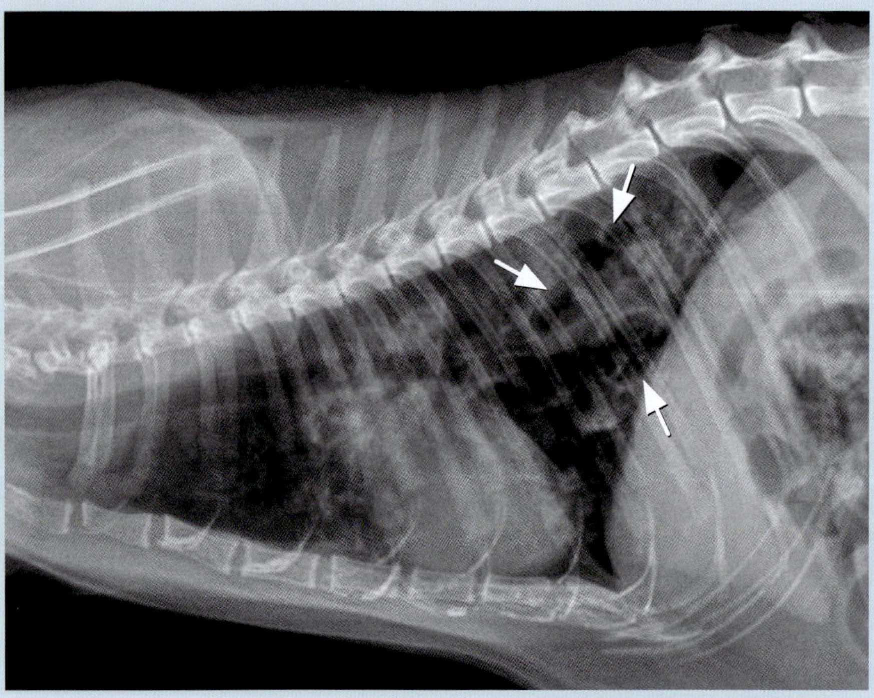

FIGURE 3.147. Lateral projection of the thorax of a cat with a mixed bronchoalveolar pattern together with several cavitary masses (arrows), caused by a bronchoalveolar carcinoma.

Peripheral hypovascularisation may sometimes be observed, with images of smaller or absent vessels. The affected vessel is rarely identified; it may appear dilated in the segment prior to the obstruction point and appear sharply reduced in size in the segment after it. Sometimes mild pleural effusion appears. Computed tomography may be very useful to identify grade 1 and 2 thrombi in arteries, although very small thrombi may not be detectable in the images.

Cases for **self-assessment**

Case 3.1.

Presentation Explanation

Case 3.2.

Presentation Explanation

Appendicular skeleton 4

Normal radiographic anatomy of the appendicular skeleton
https://goo.by/oKtDO

Principles of interpretation

Radiography is an excellent technique for skeleton assessment. As with other anatomical regions, the main difficulty in the radiological diagnosis of some appendicular diseases is that the same radiological findings are shared by different diseases. In such cases, it is essential to correlate findings with other clinical data (history, examination, laboratory data, etc.) from the patient. Useful information for the diagnosis can be obtained in some cases by assessing the evolution in time of the radiographic image of a lesion. This is why serial radiographs are often performed.

When studying the appendicular skeleton, a comparison of the obtained images with those from radiographic atlases is of special interest, especially when examining complex anatomical joints, such as the tarsus or the carpus. When an animal has a lesion only in one limb, we can obtain a better reference of normality by radiographing the contralateral limb.

A few technical tips to optimise appendicular skeleton images are summarised below:

- **Projections:** in general, two radiographic projections should be always taken at a 90° angle, although in some cases it may also be useful to obtain oblique radiographs or radiographs taken in forced flexion, extension or lateralisation of a joint. When radiographing a large bone, the corresponding proximal and distal joints should be included.
- **Positioning:** in order to avoid image distortions caused by obliquity, it is important to correctly centre the anatomical region that is to be radiographed. In addition, the median plane of the bone structures should be parallel to the cassette, if possible.
- **Collimation:** it is very important to correctly collimate the anatomical region that is to be radiographed. Thus, the image quality will be optimised, unnecessary radiation to other anatomical regions of the animal can be avoided, and the amount of diffuse radiation that can affect the operator who holds the patient can be reduced.
- **Anti-scatter grid use:** only needed when radiographing anatomical regions over 10-cm thick, which generally correspond to the scapula, the scapulohumeral joint and the humerus in the forelimb, and the hip and femur in the hind limb. The rest of limbs are radiographed without the grid.
- **Image observation:** on a conventional radiograph, small-sized lesions can be better observed using an intense focal source of light (e.g.: placing the film next to a halogen lamp). On a digital radiograph, the same effect can be achieved using image post-processing tools.

A good appendicular skeleton radiograph should provide good detail of the trabeculae of bone and the cortex. At the same time, it should offer sufficient contrast of soft parts, so soft tissues and fat (e.g.: the infrapatellar fat pad) can be differentiated.

Ossification and closure of growth plates

Calcification of bone structures begins during gestation. At birth, only the diaphyses of long bones and the cranial bones are calcified, whereas the epiphyses are still cartilaginous, thus having the density of soft tissue, and cannot be distinguished from the soft tissues surrounding the bone. Subsequently, progressive calcification of the ossification centres located in the epiphyses, the apophyses and smaller-sized bones occurs. Table 4.1 shows the ages of onset and fusion of the different ossification centres in dogs and cats.

The metaphysis, located between the epiphysis and the diaphysis of long bones (fig. 4.1), can present slightly irregular margins in growing animals, especially in large breeds. It should not be mistaken for a periosteal reaction or for pathological osteolysis.

It is important not to mistake growth plates for fracture lines in young animals. In case of doubt, radiographic atlases can be consulted, although the best reference of normality is obtained by radiographing the contralateral limb of the same animal (provided the disease is not bilateral). In adult animals, the closed growth line can appear as a sclerotic band that binds the epiphysis with the metaphysis.

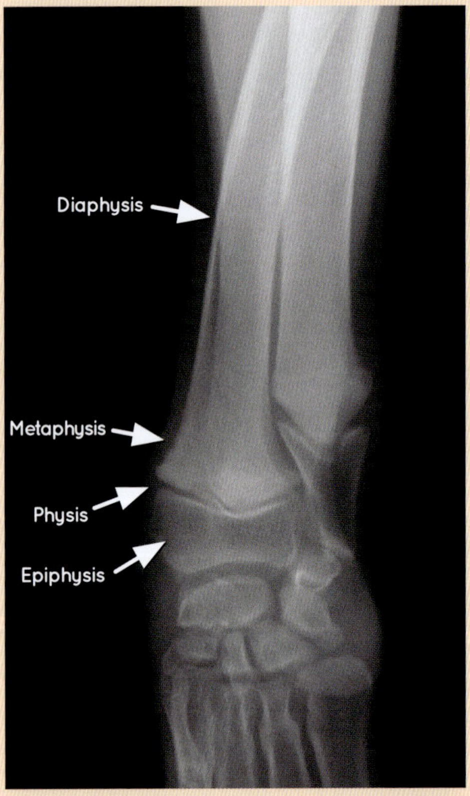

FIGURE 4.1. Dorsopalmar radiograph of the carpus of a healthy 10-week-old dog. The growth line (physis) appears as a soft tissue density band that separates the epiphysis from the metaphysis. The latter can present slightly irregular edges during growth, especially in large breed dogs. The metaphysis is joined to the bone diaphysis.

Osteolysis and osteogenesis

Bone lesions basically present in two forms: with bone destruction (osteolysis) and with new bone production (osteogenesis). The terms osteolysis and osteogenesis should not be mistaken for osteopaenia and sclerosis, although they are related. In osteopaenia, general reduction in radiopacity of a bone is observed, and the term sclerosis is used to describe increased bone radiopacity.

Several patterns in osteolysis and osteogenesis are described, and correct identification of the pattern leads to a more precise radiological diagnosis.

Patterns of osteolysis (fig. 4.2)

Geographical pattern

One or more areas of osteolysis appear, generally more than 1 cm in diameter and with well-defined edges, with a narrow zone of transition between the lesion and normal bone. Geographical lesions may or not have a sclerotic margin and are usually found in the bone marrow. The adjacent cortical zone can appear interrupted, thinned or displaced (expansile lesion). This pattern usually appears in benign or low-grade malignant lesions.

Moth-eaten pattern

Multiple osteolytic areas appear in different sizes, usually 3–10 mm in diameter, and may coalesce in the central area to form a bigger lesion. Margins are not well-defined and show a relatively wide area of transition to normal bone. They can be localised both in the bone marrow and cortex. The affected cortical zone usually appears irregularly eroded. This pattern usually appears in more aggressive processes, such as malignant tumours, osteomyelitis and multiple myeloma.

Permeative pattern

Many small-sized osteolysis zones appear, 1–2 mm, with pinpoint shapes. The margins of the lesion are ill-defined and show a relatively wide area of transition to normal bone. The cortical zone usually appears irregularly eroded. It is characteristic of more aggressive bone lesions, such as highly malignant tumours or severe osteomyelitis.

TABLE 4.1. Age at appearance and fusion of ossification centres in the dog and cat (taken from F.J. Barr, 2006; R. Dennis et al., 2001; J.P. Morgan, 1981; R.N. Smith, 1968, 1969 and G. Summer-Smith, 1966).

	Dog		Cat	
	Ossification centre appearance	Fusion	Ossification centre appearance	Fusion
Supraglenoid tubercle	6–9 weeks	3–7 months	7–9 weeks	4 Months
Humerus-proximal	1–2 weeks	10–13 months	1–2 weeks	18–24 months
Humerus-distal and medial parts of the condyle	2–4 weeks	6–9 weeks	2–5 weeks	3.5 months
Humerus-medial epicondyle	–	6 months	6–8 weeks	4 Months
Humerus-condyle to remainder of the bone	–	5–8 months	–	4–4.5 months
Radius-proximal	3–5 weeks	5–11 months	3–4 weeks	5–7 months
Radius-distal	2–4 weeks	6–12 months	2–4 weeks	14–22 months
Ulna-olecranon	7–9 weeks	5–10 months	4–5 weeks	9–12 months
Ulna-anconeal process	–	3–5 months	–	–
Ulna-distal	7–9 weeks	6–12 months	3–4 weeks	14–24 months
Carpal bones	2–6 weeks	–	3–8 weeks	–
Metacarpals/metatarsals-proximal (finger 1)	3–5 weeks	6 months	–	–
Metacarpals/metatarsals-distal (fingers 2–5)	3–4 weeks	5–7 months	3–4 weeks	7–10 months
First phalanx-proximal	4–6 weeks	4–6 months	3–4 weeks	4–5 months
Second phalanx-proximal	5–7 weeks	4–6 months	3–4 weeks	4–5 months
Femur-greater trochanter	4–10 weeks	6–10 months	5–6 weeks	7–9 months
Femur-lesser trochanter	3–4 weeks	8–13 months	–	–
Femur-proximal	2–3 weeks	6–11 months	2 weeks	7–10 months
Femur-distal	3–4 weeks	6–11 months	1–2 weeks	13–19 months
Patella	8–9 weeks	–	8–9 weeks	–
Tibia-tibial tuberosity	7–9 weeks	6–8 months (to the epiphysis)	6–7 weeks	9–10 months (to the epiphysis)
Tibia-proximal	2–5 weeks	6–12 months	2–3 weeks	12–19 months
Tibia-distal	3 week	5–11 months	2–3 weeks	10–12 months
Tibia-medial malleolus	12 week	5 months	–	–
Fibula-proximal	9–10 weeks	6–12 months	6–7 weeks	13–18 months
Fibula-distal	2–6 weeks	6–11 months	3–4 weeks	10–14 months
Calcaneus and astragalus	Birth– 1 week	–	Birth– 1 week	–
Other tarsal bones	2–6 weeks	–	2–7 weeks	–

Mixed pattern

A combination of the above-mentioned patterns can be found in a lesion, usually indicating evolution to the most aggressive type. This can be observed when a benign process becomes more active, becomes fractured or when it progresses to malignancy.

Osteopaenia

It is defined as a general reduction in bone radiopacity. It is usually accompanied by thinning of the cortices and apparent sclerosis of the subchondral bone. The most frequent causes of osteopaenia are:

- **Osteoporosis:** decreased bone calcification with reduced bone mass. A frequent cause for osteoporosis is secondary hyperparathyroidism of nutritional or renal origin. It can also appear after immobilisation of a limb (disuse osteoporosis) or as a sequela of distal fractures (post-traumatic osteoporosis).
- **Osteomalacia:** decreased bone calcification maintaining bone mass. It is caused by vitamin D deficiency and it is rare in small animals.

Patterns of osteogenesis (fig. 4.3)

A common characteristic of many skeletal lesions is new bone formation. This happens as a direct or indirect result of a lesion, infection, tumour or other local or systemic diseases. Most of the new bone is formed in the periosteum (periosteal reaction), although it can also be formed in the endosteum or bone trabeculae. It therefore corresponds to the bone response after an abnormal stimulus that can be short, repeated or maintained over time.

Several classifications of periosteal reactions have been made. The classification below has been sorted from moderate to high aggressiveness.

Solid periosteal reaction

Cortical thickening occurs, and may have smooth (chronic mild trauma, subperiosteal haematoma, panosteitis) or rough margins (trauma, inflammation of tissue adjacent to the bone).

Lamellated periosteal reaction

It is also known as “onion skin”. New bone forms in layers due to repeated periosteum elevation periods. This reaction type is observed in many pathological processes, from focal trauma to bone infections and tumours.

Palisading periosteal reaction

It presents as a series of small bone columns perpendicular to the cortex. This type of reaction is usually observed in bacterial osteomyelitis and hypertrophic pulmonary osteoarthropathy.

Brush border periosteal reaction

Thin and short bone spicules are formed very close together and perpendicular to the cortex, occupying a wide cortical area. It can appear due to inflammation of tissue adjacent to the bone, in acute osteomyelitis or in early stages of bone neoplasms.

Spiculated periosteal reaction

Bone spicules are formed roughly set apart and perpendicular to the cortex. It is considered suggestive of malignancy.

Sunburst periosteal reaction

Bone spicules that irradiate from the lesion in various directions are formed. It is suggestive of lesion expansion through the cortex into adjacent soft tissue.

Amorphous periosteal reaction

Different sized, shaped and oriented new bone deposits appear in the soft tissues surrounding the damaged area of the bone. It is considered highly suggestive of malignancy.

Aggressive bone lesions versus non-aggressive

In order to classify a bone lesion as aggressive or non-aggressive several factors should be considered:

- Degree of lesion margin definition.
- Width of the zone of transition between damaged and healthy bone.
- Pattern of osteolysis.
- Pattern of osteogenesis.
- Cortex involvement.
- Occurrence of sclerotic margins.
- Progress of the lesion over time.

Findings suggestive of aggressive and non-aggressive lesion are summarised in Table 4.2. When a lesion presents a combination of signs of both columns of the table, those which are more suggestive of aggressiveness should be considered.

Soft tissues

Soft tissues can show alterations associated to the presence of lesions in the appendicular skeleton. They often appear thicker due to inflammation or because of the presence of masses, although a reduction in size due to muscular atrophy can also be appreciated (fig. 4.4).

Presence of gas in soft tissues (subcutaneous emphysema) is usually due to air penetration from the outside, in case of penetrating wounds (fig. 4.5) or after surgery in the area, although it can also be caused by anaerobic infections.

In soft tissue, radiopaque foreign bodies or areas of calcification can also be identified on radiographs (fig. 4.6). The latter can be mistaken for small bone fragments or overgrowths when localised next to the bone.

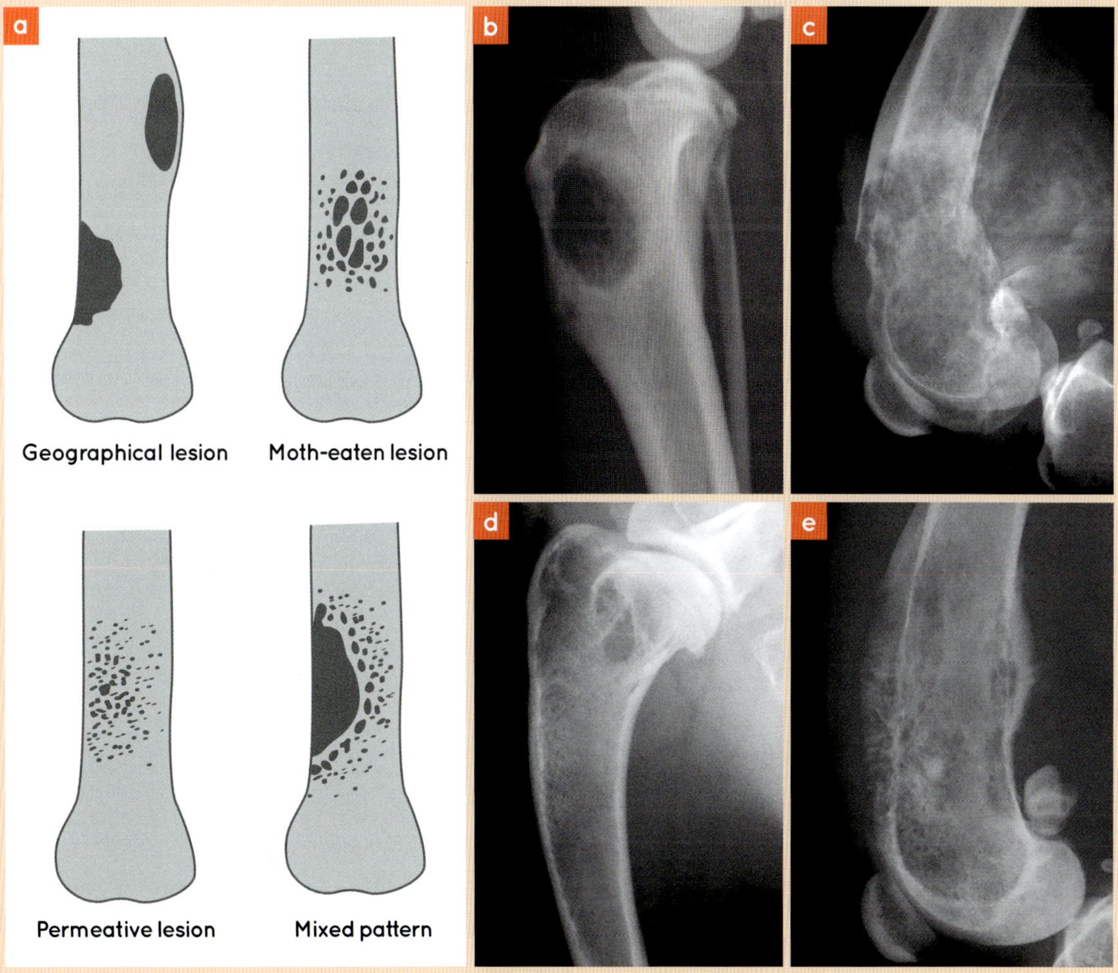

FIGURE 4.2. Schematic diagram (a) and radiographs of the different osteolysis patterns: geographic (b), moth-eaten (c), permeative (d) and mixed (e) pattern.

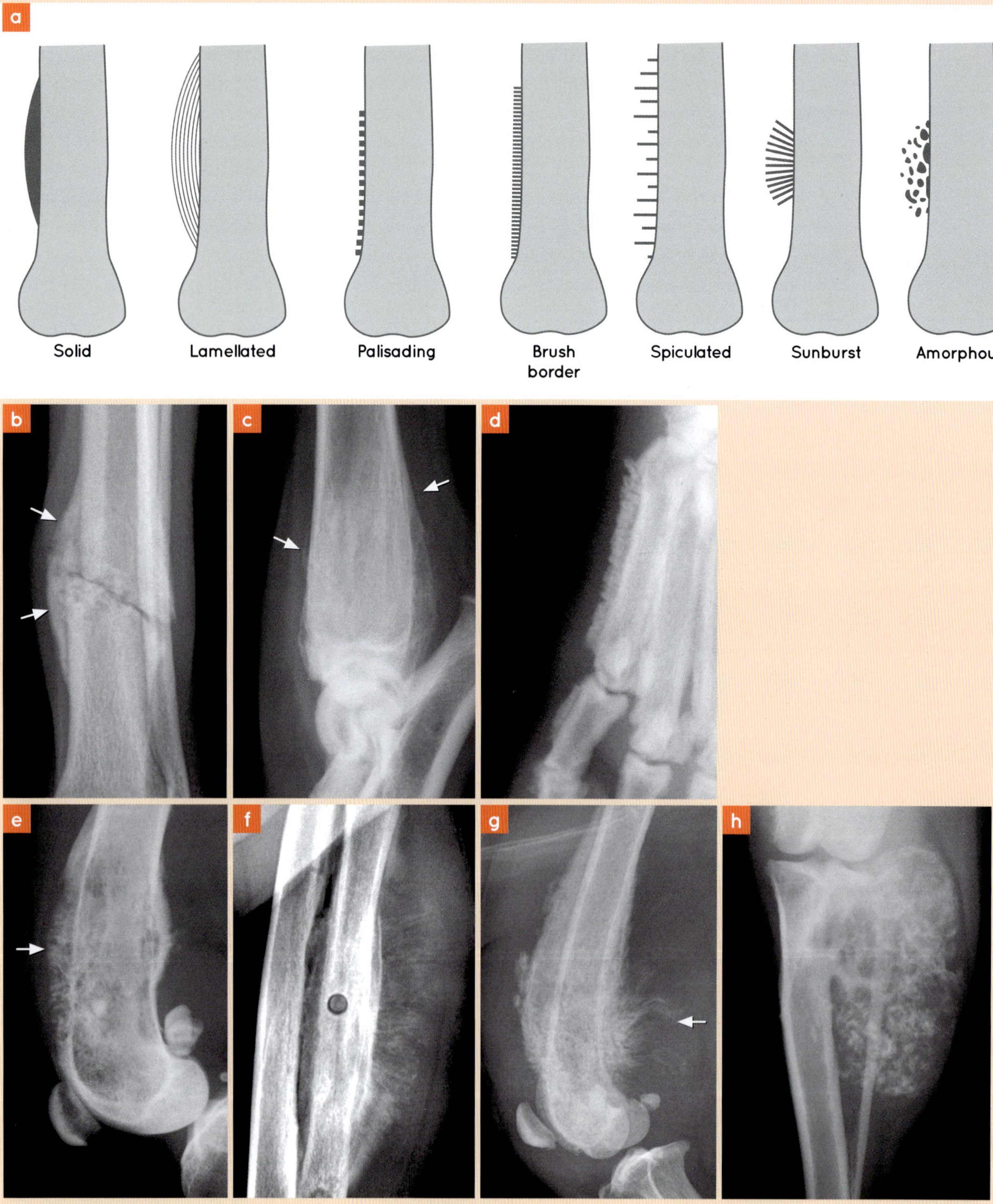

FIGURE 4.3. Schematic diagram (a) and radiographs of the different types of periosteal reaction: solid periosteal reaction (b), lamellated periosteal reaction (c), palisading periosteal reaction (d), brush border periosteal reaction (e), spiculated periosteal reaction (f), sunburst periosteal reaction (g) and amorphous periosteal reaction (h).

Other imaging diagnostic techniques

In recent years, the use of ultrasonography has spread as a supplementary diagnostic technique to radiography for the evaluation of the musculoskeletal system. It is usually used to examine soft tissues and is of special interest in the study of muscular and tendon lesions. The associated joints and ligaments can also be examined, although very high resolution transducers and wide experience are required to correctly interpret the images for small animals.

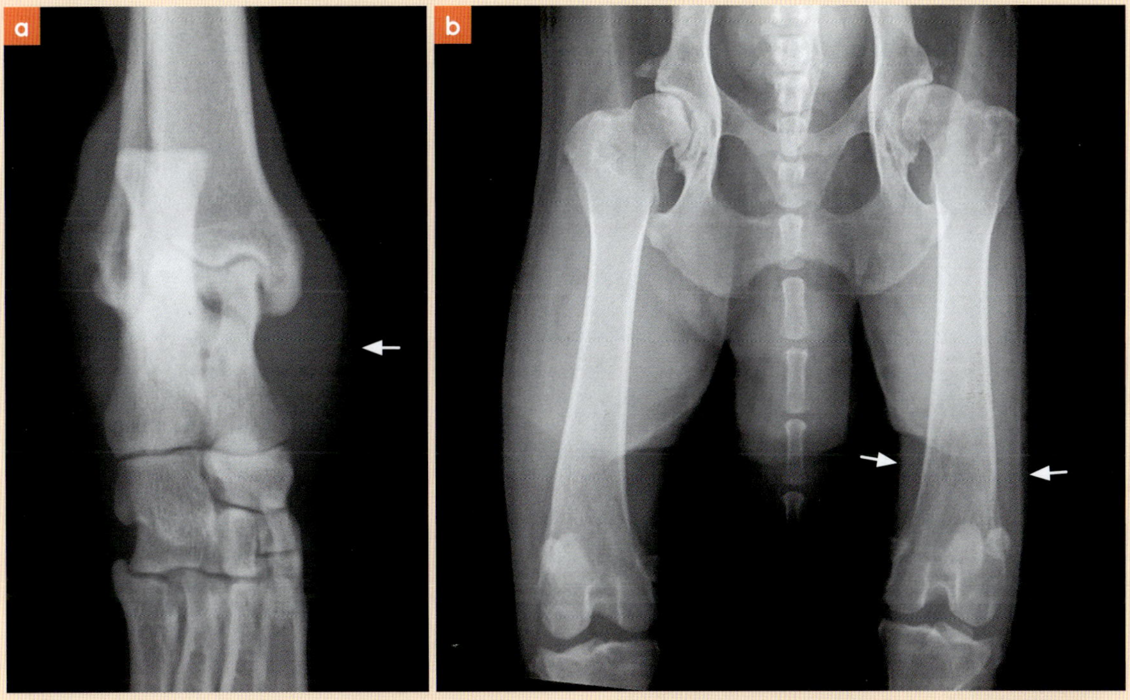

FIGURE 4.4. Dorsoplantar projection of the tarsus of a dog with increased soft tissue thickness at the medial aspect of the joint (a) and enlarged view of the ventrodorsal projection of the hip and femurs of a dog with severe bilateral coxarthrosis, causing muscle atrophy in both limbs, more marked on the left (arrows).

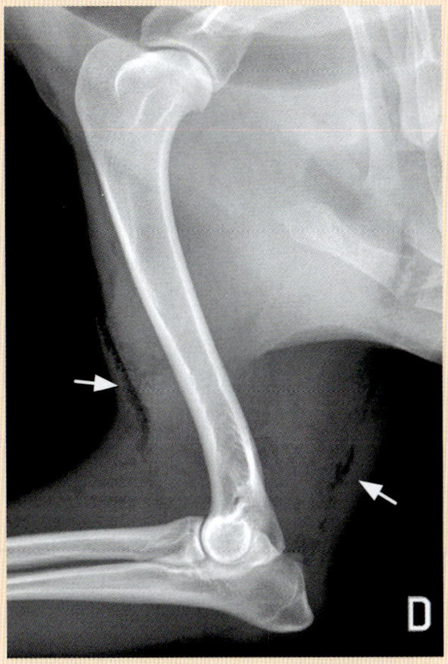

FIGURE 4.5. Mediolateral projection of the humerus of a dog with gas in soft tissues (arrows) from injuries sustained in car accident.

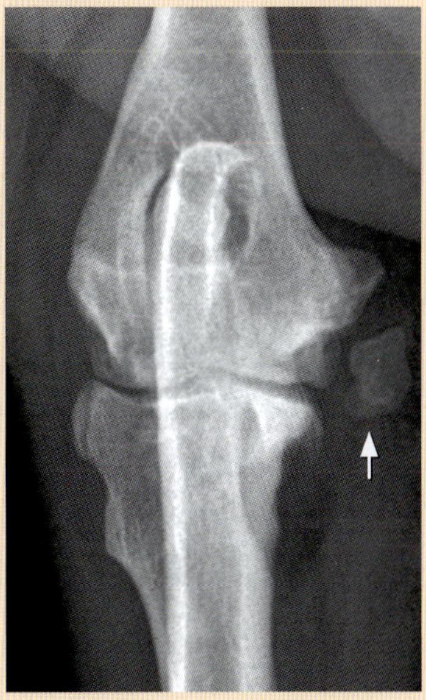

FIGURE 4.6. Craniocaudal projection of the elbow of a dog showing large soft tissue mineralisation (arrow) on the medial aspect of the joint.

TABLE 4.2. Radiological findings suggestive of aggressive versus non-aggressive bone lesions. When a lesion shows a combination of signs of both table columns, those which are more suggestive of aggressiveness should be considered.

NON-AGGRESSIVE BONE LESION Lesions due to trauma, degenerative, bone cysts, benign neoplasms.	AGGRESSIVE BONE LESION Malignancies, severe osteomyelitis
Well-defined edges.	Poorly-defined edges
Narrow zone of transition.	Wide zone of transition.
With or without geographical osteolysis.	Moth-eaten or permeative osteolysis.
The cortex can appear displaced or thinner, but does not usually present discontinuation.	Cortex discontinuation.
Solid or laminated periosteal reaction	Palisading, spiculated, sunburst or amorphous periosteal reaction.
With and without sclerotic margins.	Without sclerotic margins.
Slow progress or no changes.	Rapid progress.

Computed tomography offers excellent images of bone structures. It is specially indicated to evaluate less-evident bone lesions or those difficult to detect by radiography, or to examine anatomically complex joints such as the carpus or tarsus. It is also indicated for the preoperative assessment of bone deformations and complex fractures because three-dimensional image reconstruction at different angles enables the surgeon to know the exact location and morphology of the deformed bone or fragments in order to decide the most appropriate surgical approach.

In human medicine, magnetic resonance is the imaging technique of choice for the diagnosis of diseases of joints and soft tissues of the limbs. It is, however, limited for assessing bone structures, especially in those lesions that can mostly affect the bone cortex, given that it produces no signal. Despite this, it is most useful to evaluate bone tumours, osteomyelitis, haematomas and processes which cause bone necrosis. Due to the smaller size of the joints, its use in small animals is limited by the patient size and the resolution offered by the equipment.

Congenital, hereditary and developmental abnormalities

Chondrodysplasia

The term chondrodysplasia is applied to a wide group of diseases, all of them due to abnormal cartilage growth. It can affect long bone epiphyses, vertebral body epiphyses, long bone epiphyses and metaphyses, or a combination of the above.

One or several of the following radiological signs can be observed:

- Slower growth of long bones, which may appear shorter and thicker than normal.
- The physes can appear wider.
- Retained growth cartilage can be observed in the metaphyseal region.
- Calcification of the epiphyseal ossification centres can be delayed.
- Punctated or distorted epiphyses may be observed.
- Vertebral epiphyses can be partially or irregularly ossified.

Chondrodysplasia is classified based on the bone region that is mostly affected, as described below.

Epiphyseal chondrodysplasia

In dogs, it has been described in Beagles and Poodles. It is characterised by a delay in the calcification of the epiphyseal ossification centres. The epiphyses can have a punctate appearance and although ossification may be completed, they are often deformed, thus causing early onset of osteoarthritis. It has also been described in some cat breeds.

Physeal chondrodysplasia

It has been described for the Pointer breed and causes a disproportionate dwarfism. Marked widening of the physis is radiologically observed, especially in the radius, ulna and tibia. Long bones are shortened and curved. It is accompanied by articular cartilage erosion, thus causing early onset of osteoarthritis. The same process occurs in the Alaskan Malamute, although without articular cartilage erosion. It has also been described in cats.

Metaphyseal chondrodysplasia

It has been described in the Pyrenean Mountain Dogs. It basically affects long bone metaphyses and vertebrae. All long bone metaphyses appear wider, especially in the radius, ulna, tibia, metacarpals and metatarsals. Vertebral body epiphyses are irregularly or incompletely ossified. In the Labrador Retriever and the Samoyed, a form of oculoskeletal dysplasia has been described. It causes shortening and deformation of the limbs, associated with ocular defects

Retained core of growth cartilage

In growing large and giant breed dogs, a retained core of growth cartilage can be observed, generally affecting the distal physis of the ulna, although it has also been described at other sites, such as the distal physis of the radius or the femur. It appears as a radiolucent triangular area that spreads from the physis to the metaphysis, with a sclerotic margin (fig. 4.7). It may cause limb deformity.

Retained core of growth cartilage can be observed associated with other pathological alterations of the physis, but in those cases the lesion usually has non sclerotic, ill-defined margins.

Polymelia

It indicates a higher number of limbs or parts of a limb than normal. Supernumerary fingers (polydactyly) are most frequent, especially observed in cats and other dog breeds such as the Pyrenean Mountain Dogs. Supernumerary fingers often start at the medial part of the limb and can include full or partial metacarpals or metatarsals and a variable number of phalanges. This abnormality is not usually clinically significant.

Ectrodactyly

The distal part of the limb appears split, with split phalanges, metacarpals, and carpal bones and associated abnormally to the radius and ulna (fig. 4.8). Aplasia, hypoplasia or fusion of distal bones in the limbs can occur. It is a rare alteration in cats and dogs, and considered hereditary in the latter.

Hemimelia

Absence or hypoplasia of one of the bones forming a pair (most frequently affecting the ulna–radius, but also can affect the tibia–fibula) (fig. 4.9).

Osteochondrosis and osteochondritis dissecans

Osteochondrosis is defined as a failure of endochondral ossification, resulting in thickening of the cartilage. The thickest areas do not receive enough quantity of nutrients, which results in necrosis and fissure formation in the affected area. When a chondral flap or an osteochondral fragment is separated from the adjacent subchondral bone, the process is called osteochondritis dissecans. The cartilage flap or even the osteochondral fragment cannot be radiologically identified in many patients, thus generally receiving the name osteochondrosis.

This developmental disease appears in young dogs of large and rapid growth breeds. Clinical signs usually appear between 6–9 months of age. It is usually bilateral, even though the animal may only present with lameness in one limb. It usually appears at specific anatomical locations and affects weight-bearing joint surfaces:

- Caudal or caudolateral surface of the humeral head (fig. 4.10).

- Distal and medial surface of the humeral condyle (fig. 4.11).
- Distal surface of the lateral femoral condyle (fig. 4.12) and less frequently, in the same area of the medial condyle.
- Medial or lateral trochlear edge of astragalus.

Flattening or concavity of the affected subchondral bone surface is radiologically observed, as well as sclerosis of the subchondral bone surrounding it. The cartilage flap is usually not observed, unless it is calcified. If osteochondral fragments are identified inside the joint, the clinical signs are usually more evident.

At times, a subchondral defect can be identified on the joint surface opposite the lesioned joint, which is known as a "kissing lesion". Although rare, the appearance of intra-articular gas has also been described in dogs with shoulder osteochondrosis, known as "vacuum phenomenon", which is attributed to an accumulation of nitrogen gas due to the negative pressure exerted during the traction of the joint for X-ray positioning.

When the lesion is located in the lateral margin of the astragalus, overlapping of the calcaneus in the dorsoplantar projection may impede its identification. A dorsolateral–plantaromedial oblique or a flexed dorsoplantar view may be useful in these cases.

Sacral osteochondrosis, which affects its craniodorsal edge, has also been described. It basically affects the German Shepherd and, less frequently, the Boxer and Rottweiler. Irregularity of the dorsal edge of the cranial vertebral endplate of the sacrum is observed. As in other sites, the osteochondral fragment is occasionally identified; in this example, on the vertebral canal floor.

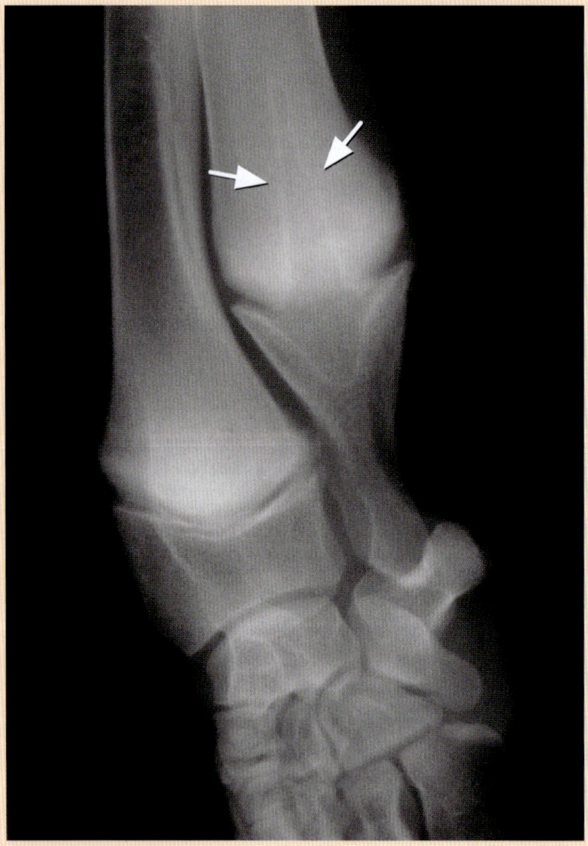

FIGURE 4.7. Enlarged image in mediolateral projection of the radius and distal ulna of a dog with retained core of growth cartilage of the ulna that appears as a radiolucent triangular area spreading from the physis to the metaphysis, with a thin sclerotic margin (arrows).

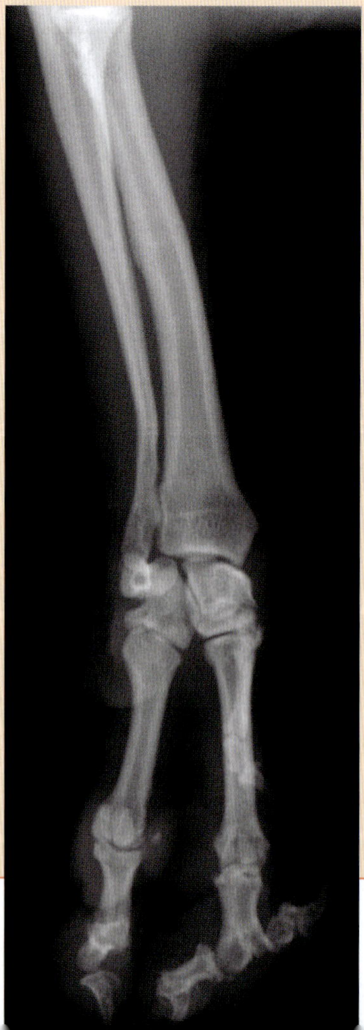

FIGURE 4.8. Dorsopalmar radiograph of the carpus, metacarpals and phalanges in a dog with ectrodactyly. The distal part of the limb appears split, with split phalanges, metacarpals, and carpal bones. In this case aplasia of some carpal bones is observed, as well as of metacarpals and phalanges in two fingers. Finger 2 shows duplicity of the medial and distal phalanges.

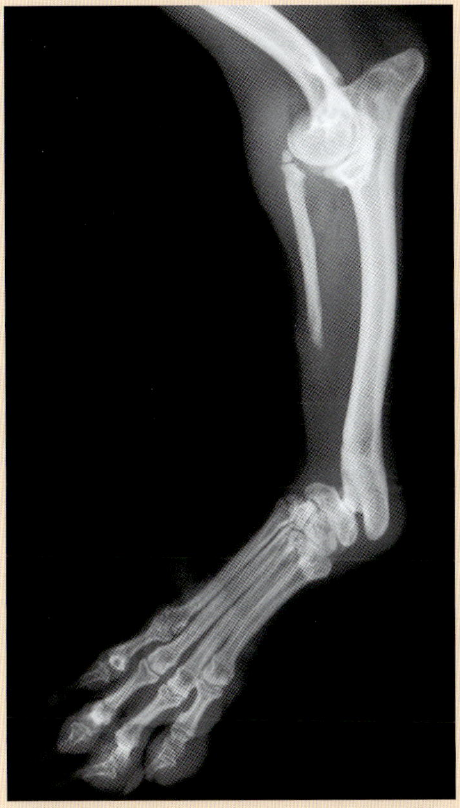

FIGURE 4.9. Mediolateral radiograph of the radius and the ulna of a dog with radial hemimelia due to hypoplasia. Image courtesy of María José Ruiz Fernández.

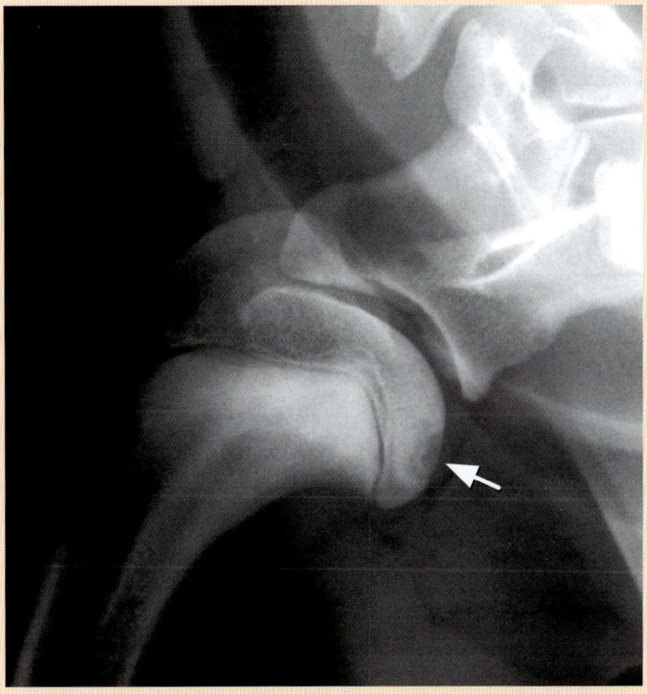

FIGURE 4.10. Mediolateral radiograph of the scapulohumeral joint of a dog with osteochondritis dissecans of the humeral head. A radiolucent area delimited by a thin sclerotic margin is observed at the caudal surface of the humeral head (arrow).

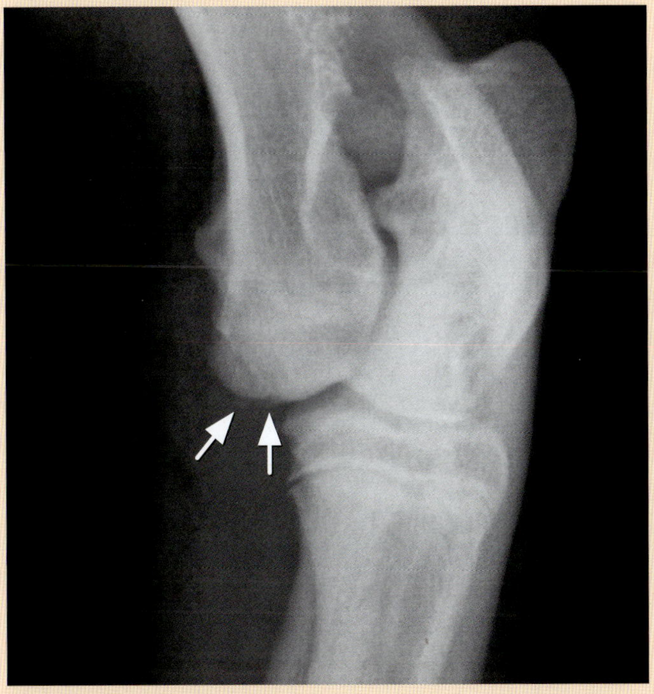

FIGURE 4.11. Craniocaudal oblique radiograph of the elbow of a dog with osteochondritis dissecans in the humeral medial condyle. A small concavity is observed in the distal and medial margins of the humeral condyle and beside it, two small osteochondral fragments (arrow).

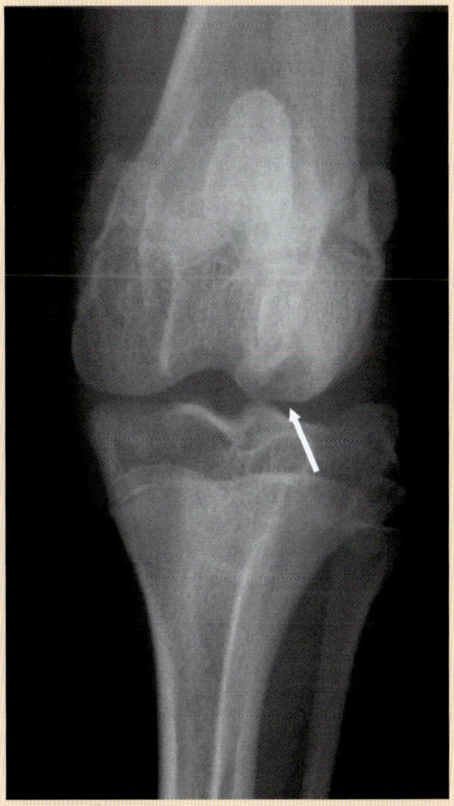

FIGURE 4.12. Craniocaudal projection of the knee of a dog with osteochondrosis of the lateral condyle of the femur. A radiolucent area of concave morphology and flattening of the distal margin is observed in this condyle (arrow).

Elbow dysplasia

Elbow dysplasia is a non-specific term that refers to a triad of developmental lesions which include:

- Osteochondrosis of the humerus.
- Failure of anconeal process to fuse with the ulna.
- Fragmentation of the medial coronoid process of the ulna.

One, two or all three lesions can be observed in one animal, and most frequently there is affectation of both limbs. Elbow joint incongruity, due to non-uniform contact of the joint surfaces that form the elbow, can lead to ununited or fragmented anconeal process and hyperostosis or fragmented medial coronoid process of the ulna. X-ray can identify severe elbow joint incongruity, but CT is much more accurate in diagnosing this abnormality, especially if the severity of the lesion is mild or moderate.

The anconeal process should fuse with the ulna at 5 months of age. Lack of fusion at this age is considered pathological. It affects large dog breeds, especially the German Shepherd. To adequately observe the lesion, the elbow radiograph should be taken in lateral projection, forcing flexion of the joint (fig. 4.13).

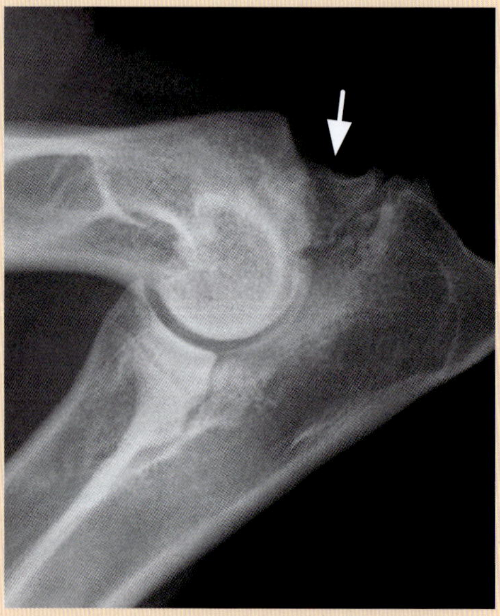

FIGURE 4.13. Mediolateral radiograph with hyperflexion of the elbow of a dog with an ununited anconeal process of the ulna (arrow). The hyperflexion makes it easier to identify the lesion.

Fragmentation of the medial coronoid process of the ulna affects large or medium breed dogs, more males than females, and clinical signs usually appear between 4–6 months of age. It is the primary cause of elbow dysplasia in dogs. The radiological study of these patients should include the two standard orthogonal projections, mediolateral and craniocaudal elbow, plus the craniolateral-caudomedial oblique view with limb pronated 15 to 25°, which reduces the overlapping of the medial coronoid process of the ulna with the radius, thus improving its evaluation. In many cases, the fragment is not identified on the radiograph due to superimposition with the radius, because it is partially adhered to the ulna or when it is basically made of cartilage. Thus, the radiological diagnosis is very frequently based on the observation of degenerative signs secondary to the primary lesion.

The radiographic signs that indicate fragmentation of the medial coronoid process of the ulna (fig. 4.14) are:

- Visualisation of the bone fragment at the area where the medial coronoid process is located (uncommon).
- Loss of definition or irregularity of the cranial edge of the medial coronoid process in mediolateral projection.
- Rounding of the medial edge of the medial coronoid process in the craniocaudal projection.
- Incongruence or subluxation of the elbow joint. Computed tomography is much more precise than radiography to evaluate joint incongruency (nonuniform contact of joint surfaces).
- Degenerative secondary signs: osteophyte formation at the proximal edge of the anconeal process, distal humerus, proximal radius, trochlear notch, and in the medial coronoid process itself; also, trochlear plate sclerosis.

Computed tomography is an excellent alternative to accurately diagnose this anomaly (fig. 4.15).

Hip dysplasia

The term hip dysplasia refers to an abnormal development of coxofemoral joints. It is a hereditary disease that can appear in any dog breed, but especially in large breeds, although also in medium and small breeds, as well as in cats. It is usually bilateral although it can also be unilateral (in approximately 11% of cases). At birth, the coxofemoral joint is normal but, due to the increase in joint laxity experienced by these animals, they develop a greater or lesser degree of subluxation/luxation and signs of degenerative joint disease (coxarthrosis).

The standard projection that is normally used when assessing hip dysplasia is ventrodorsal. In order to avoid diagnostic errors, a correct positioning is essential (fig. 4.16):

- Symmetric pelvis (it can be checked by comparing the two obturator foramina, which should be of the same size in the image, and the width of the wings of the ilium, which should also be the same).
- The femurs should appear in parallel.
- The patellas should appear aligned with the trochlear groove (to achieve this, internal rotation of the knees should be forced).
- The full pelvis and both knees should appear on the radiograph.

This projection is used to assess dysplasia when issuing official certificates, usually from 1 year of age.

Radiographic signs for dysplasia include:

- Femoral head subluxation or luxation: usually the acetabular coverage of the femoral head is at least 50 %. When there is coxofemoral subluxation, widening of the medial joint space will be observed (fig. 4.17). The degree of luxation is also measured by the Norberg angle, that requires specific templates or angle-measuring devices. In digital radiography, the angle can be measured using specific post-processing tools (fig. 4.18).
- Signs of joint degeneration (fig. 4.19):
    - Acetabular remodelling (usually flattening), with rounding of the cranial acetabular edge.
    - Femoral head and neck remodelling.
    - Periarticular osteophyte formation on the edges of the femoral head and the acetabulum.
    - A sclerotic line appearing on the femoral neck called Morgan's line. It is due to osteophyte formation at the caudal surface of the femoral neck and is considered an early sign of coxarthrosis.
    - Subchondral sclerosis of the acetabular edge.

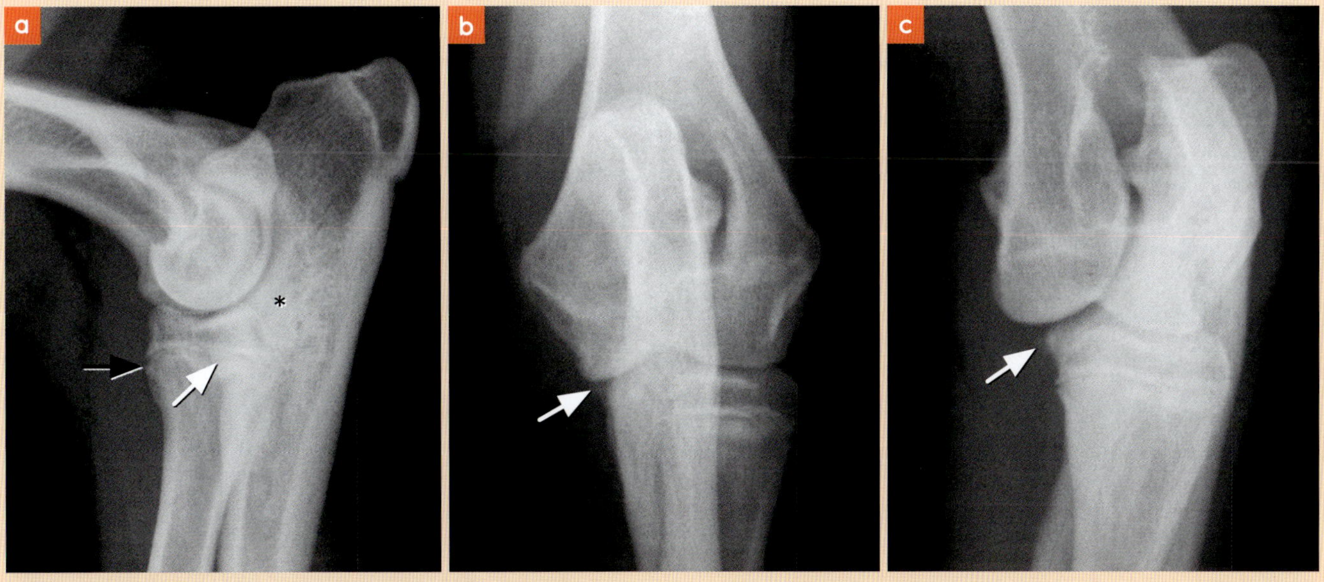

FIGURE 4.14. Mediolateral (a), craniocaudal (b) and oblique caniolateral-caudomedial radiographs of a dog with fragmentation of the medial coronoid process of the ulna. Image (a) showing flattening of the cranial margin of the medial coronoid process of the ulna (white arrow), remodelling of the cranial margin of the radial head (black arrow) and sclerosis in the trochlear notch of the ulna (asterisk). Image (b) shows a slight rounding of the margin of the medial coronoid process of the ulna (arrow), while image (c) identifies a small bone fragment adjacent to the medial coronoid process of the ulna (arrow) thanks to the oblique projection.

Dysplasia is less prevalent in cats than in dogs. In the cat, most degenerative changes appear at the craniodorsal edge of the acetabulum, whereas remodelling of the femoral head and neck is less frequent.

The Norberg angle is measured at the intersection of two lines: one drawn between the centres of both femoral heads, and another one starting at the centre of each femoral head and moving tangentially to the craniolateral acetabular edge. The Norberg angle measures 105° or more in most healthy dogs, and at least 95° in healthy cats. Inferior measurements are suggestive of dysplasia. The smaller the angle value is, the higher the subluxation degree, and therefore the severity of the dysplasia. Nevertheless, it is important

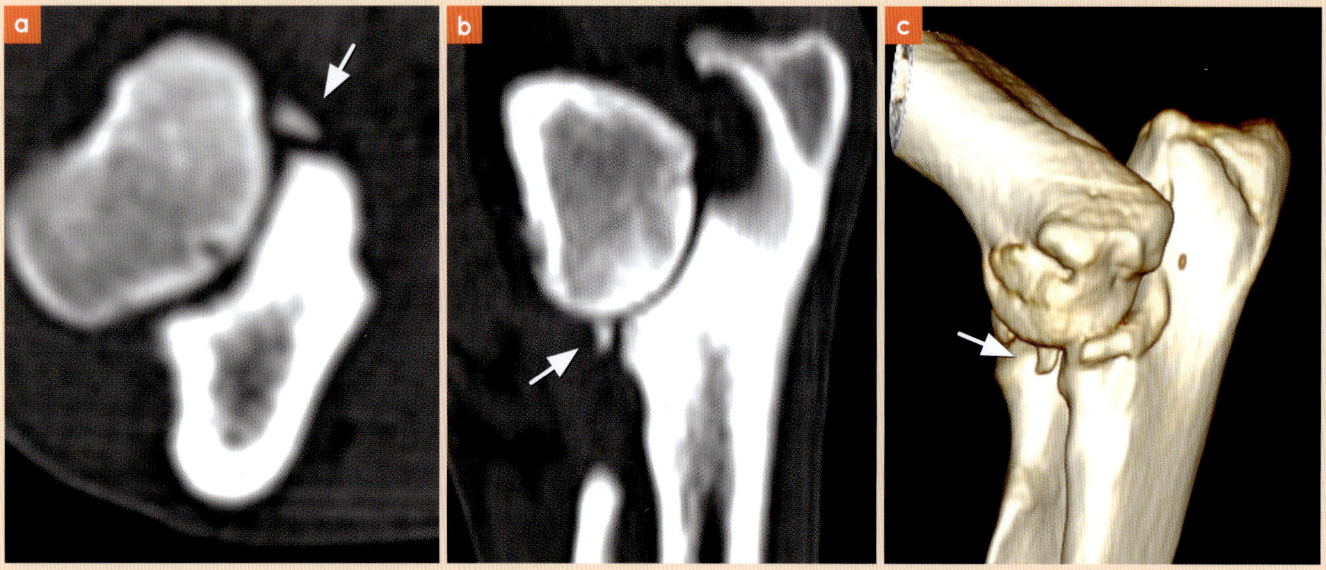

FIGURE 4.15. Computed tomography images in transverse plane (a), sagittal reconstruction (b) and volumetric reconstruction (c) of the elbow of a dog with fragmentation of the medial coronoid process of the ulna. In the three images the arrows are pointing at the fragment. The fragment is easily identified in the image (a) because there is no structural superimposition in these types of images. By means of post-processing computer programmes, multiplanar reconstructions can be performed (in any plane of space), as well as volumetric reconstructions (three-dimensional) that may more or less contribute to the diagnosis.

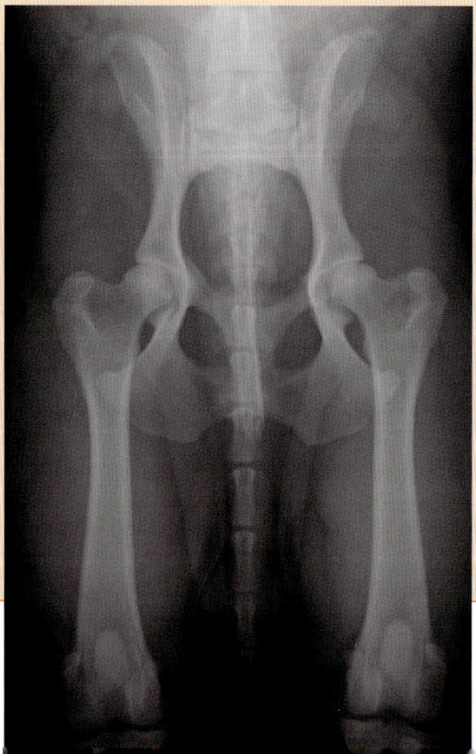

FIGURE 4.16. Ventrodorsal radiograph of a healthy dog's hip. To correctly assess coxofemoral joints, the pelvis should appear symmetric, the femurs in parallel and the patellas aligned with the trochlear channel.

to remark that there are many factors influencing the correct measurement of this angle, such as the positioning of the femurs and pelvis and changes in the acetabular edge.

The PennHIP method is a way to assess the degree of laxity of the coxofemoral joint at an earlier stage, from 16 weeks of age. Three radiographic projections are used: the standard ventrodorsal with the femurs pulled

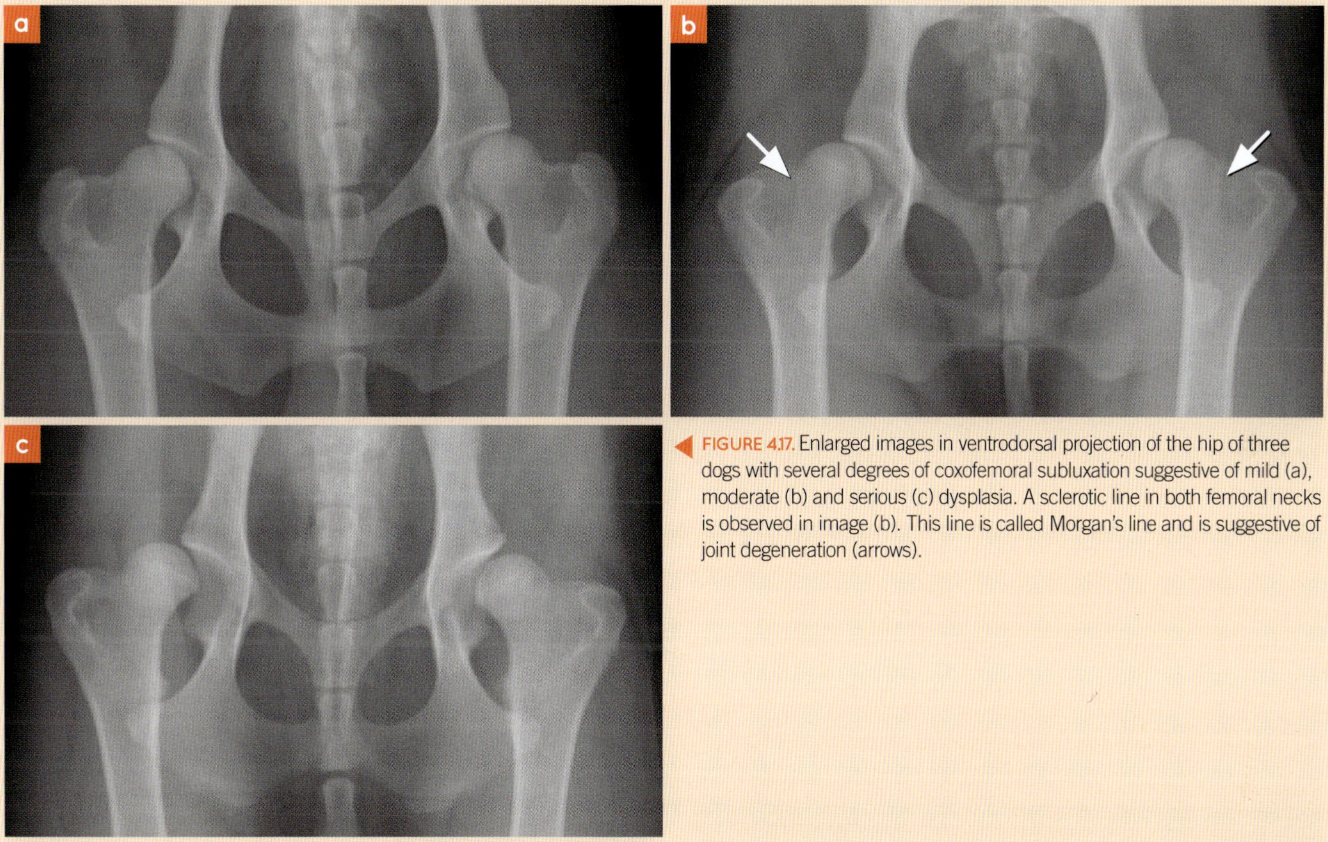

FIGURE 4.17. Enlarged images in ventrodorsal projection of the hip of three dogs with several degrees of coxofemoral subluxation suggestive of mild (a), moderate (b) and serious (c) dysplasia. A sclerotic line in both femoral necks is observed in image (b). This line is called Morgan's line and is suggestive of joint degeneration (arrows).

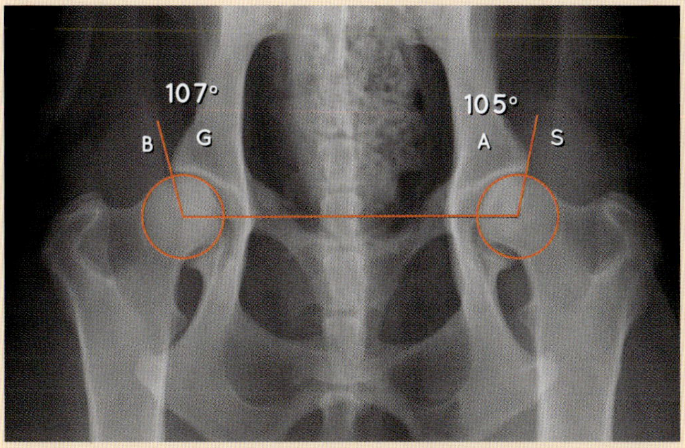

FIGURE 4.18. Enlarged image in ventrodorsal projection of the hip of a healthy dog, on which the Norberg angle has been measured using digital image post-processing tools. The value of this angle is 105º or higher in healthy animals.

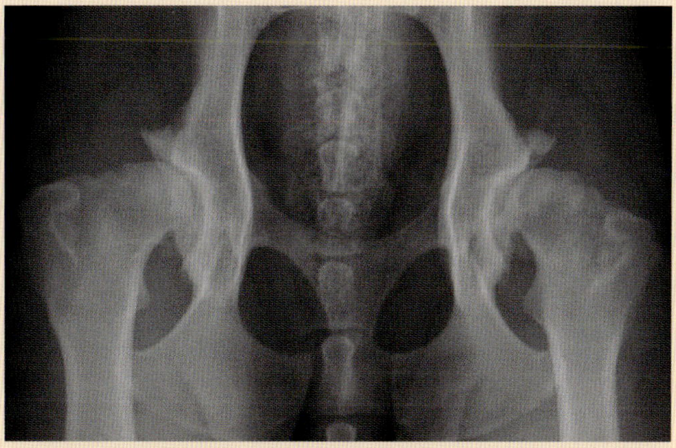

FIGURE 4.19. Enlarged image in ventrodorsal projection of the hip of a dog with severe coxoarthrosis caused by dysplasia. Marked remodelling of the acetabula, and femoral heads and necks is observed, with periarticular osteophyte formation at the edges of the femoral and acetabular heads, as well as subchondral sclerosis of the acetabular edge.

into extension; a ventrodorsal projection with compression of both coxofemoral joints; and a ventrodorsal with distraction of both joints. A specific device is used to cause the distraction. The distraction index is calculated by dividing the distance from the femoral head centre to the centre of the acetabulum, between the radius of the femoral head. The value of this index can vary from 0 to 1. A value of 0 indicates perfect joint congruity and a value of 1 indicates complete luxation. This method was developed by researchers from the University of Pennsylvania, where an international database is elaborated and there are specific courses to obtain official certification as a PennHIP certified technician.

Hypertrophic osteodystrophy

Also called metaphyseal osteopathy or metaphyseal osteodystrophy. It affects young dogs between 2 and 7 months of age, generally large and giant breeds. It is uncertain how this disease is originated, but in some cases it has been related to distemper and nutritional alterations (an excessive administration of vitamin complexes is thought to cause onset, but this is not clear). Great Danes and Weimaraners could be somewhat predisposed. Clinically, the animal can develop fever and the metaphysis area of long bones appears swollen, warm and painful. It is generally self-limiting and is usually resolved in a few weeks, although most severe cases can cause premature or abnormal closure of growth lines as a sequela.

Radiological signs (fig. 4.20):

- Lesions are usually bilateral and symmetrical.
- A radiolucent band usually appears at the metaphysis, parallel to the epiphyseal line. This sign is more evident in the distal metaphysis of the radius, ulna and tibia, although it may affect the metaphyses of all long bones.
- A sclerotic band usually appears at the metaphysis, parallel to the radiolucent band.
- Inflammation of the soft tissues adjacent to the affected metaphysis.
- In advanced stages, calcified areas are formed around the metaphysis, apparently separated from the bone cortex by a radiolucent band. These areas can extend to the diaphysis.

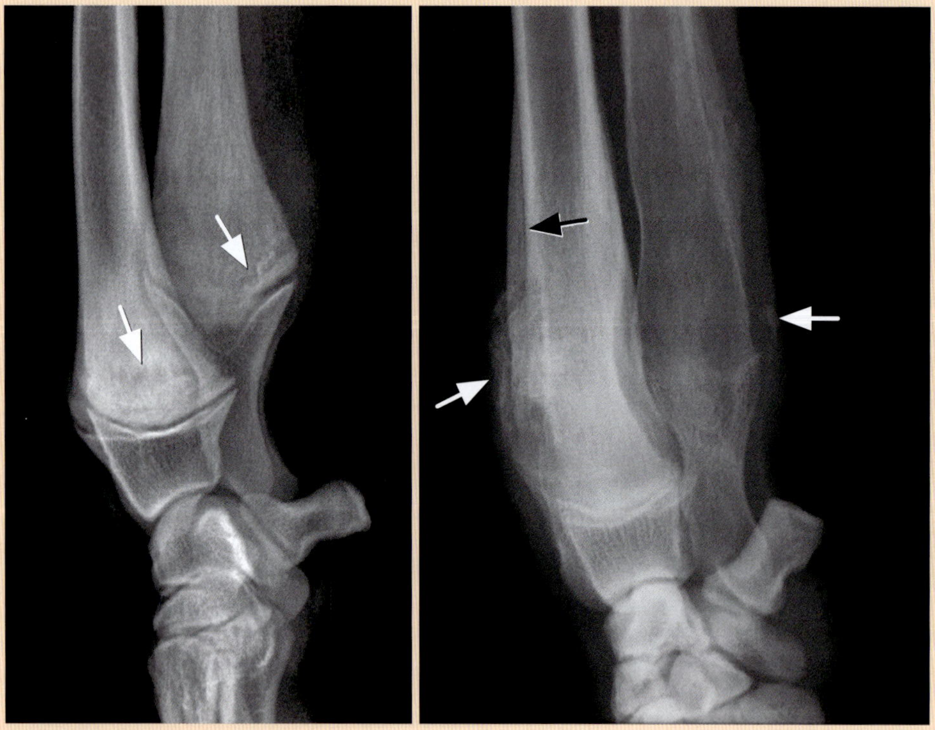

FIGURE 4.20. Mediolateral projection of the radius and ulna of a dog with an early stage (a) and advanced stage (b) hypertrophic osteodystrophy. Image (a) shows an irregular radiolucent band in the metaphysis (arrows), parallel to the epiphyseal line. Image (b) shows a solid periosteal reaction (black arrow) and mineralised areas around the metaphysis and part of the diaphysis (white arrows).

- Remodelling of the affected areas takes place over time. Sometimes, the growth plate is prematurely or abnormally closed, thus causing deformation of the affected bone(s).

Panosteitis

This disease causes inflammation of the diaphyses of long bones in youngs large breed dogs. It affects more males than females, and German Shepherds could be more predisposed. It typically appears in animals between 5 and 18 months of age, but it has also been detected in dogs up to 7 years. It is clinically characterised by episodes of acute lameness, that may affect one or several limbs and it does not always appear simultaneously in all affected limbs (alternating lameness). During the examination, pain is observed at deep palpation of the affected limbs.

With regard to the radiographic signs (fig. 4.21):

- They may appear in one or several bones.
- Areas of focal increased density (sclerosis) are observed in long bone marrow, usually in the femur, humerus, radius, ulna and tibia.
- An irregular thickening of the cortical endosteum can be observed.
- A solid and smooth periosteal reaction can be appreciated.
- With time, resolution of bone marrow sclerotic lesions can make the bone trabecular pattern seem to be more marked than usual. Cortical thickness may persist.

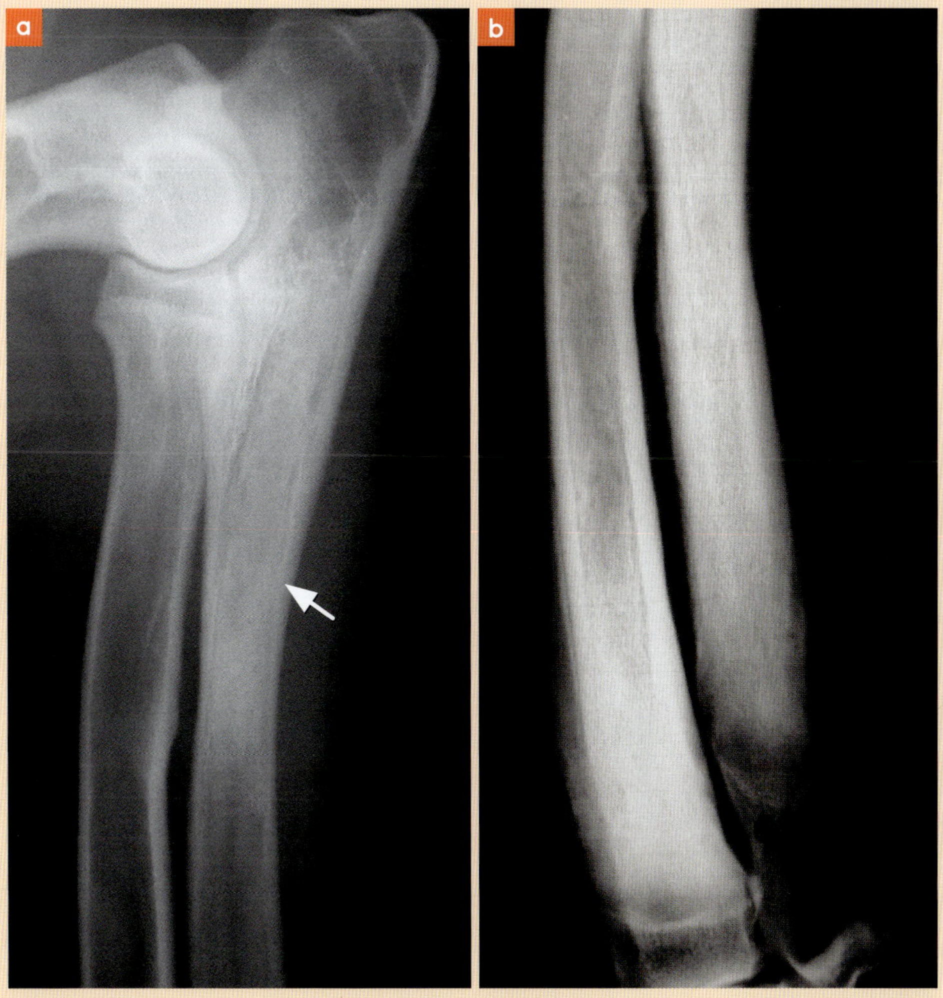

FIGURE 4.21. Images of the radius and ulna in mediolateral projection of two dogs with panosteitis. Image (a) shows a focal area of sclerosis in the proximal half of the ulna shaft (arrow). In image (b) increased bone marrow density is more diffuse and affects the radius and the ulna, that also present endosteal and periosteal growth of solid type.

Femoral head avascular necrosis

It is also called Legg–Calvé–Perthes disease or femoral head aseptic necrosis. It is a developmental disease that appears in young dogs between 4 and 11 months of age, of small or miniature breeds. Normally, the process is unilateral (fig. 4.22) and less frequently bilateral (fig. 4.23). It results from a deficit in vascular supply to the femoral head epiphysis that produces subchondral bone necrosis. In early stages of the disease, small radiolucent areas (osteolytic) are observed with an irregular morphology at the femoral head, which then evolves to deformation and flattening of the femoral head and neck, that may cause coxofemoral subluxation.

Incomplete ossification of the humeral condyle

It is a hereditary disease mainly affecting dogs from Spaniel breeds, although it has also been described in dogs from medium and large breeds. The two ossification centres that appear at the humeral condyle fuse at approximately 84 days from birth. Once skeletal maturation is complete, those animals with incomplete ossification will maintain a thin fissure between both halves of the condyle, thus predisposing them to pathological fractures at that site.

Spontaneous capital femoral physeal fracture in cats

Spontaneous femoral head fractures have been reported in young cats, with a mean age of 2 years. These fractures are not associated with trauma, are more frequent in males and may be unilateral or bilateral. If only one femur is fractured, the contralateral may show delayed physeal closure. They have been linked with obesity, early neutering and delayed capital femoral physeal closure (neutering could cause delayed physeal closure). The initial radiographic finding is a slipped capital femoral epiphysis, followed by different degrees of osteolysis (due to bone resorption) and sclerosis of the affected femoral head and neck (fig. 4.24).

Mucopolysaccharidosis

Mucopolysaccharidosis is a hereditary disease caused by a deficiency of a lysosomal enzyme responsible for breaking down glycosaminoglycans, which disrupts the development of the epiphyses of vertebrae and

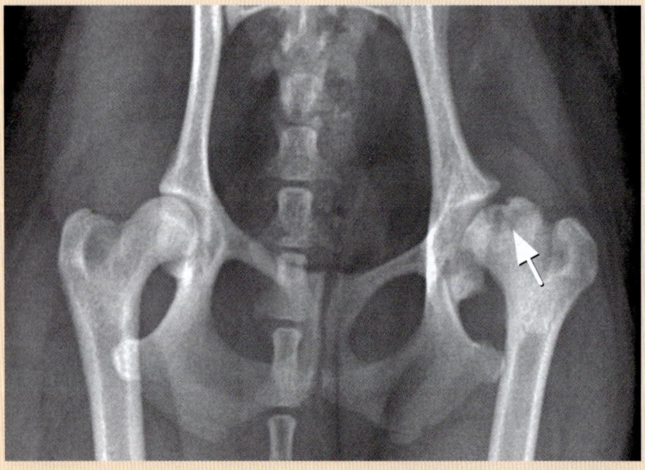

FIGURE 4.22. Enlarged image of the hip on a ventrodorsal radiograph of a dog with unilateral left avascular necrosis in the femoral head (Legg-Calvé-Perthes disease). Irregular radiolucent areas (arrow) due to necrosis are detected, as well as deformation of the femoral head and neck.

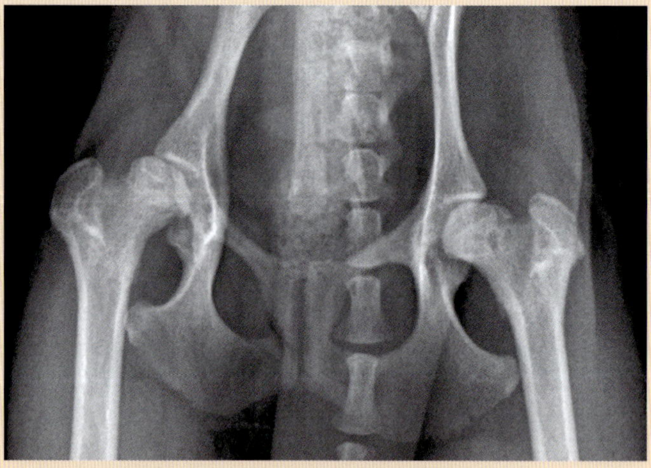

FIGURE 4.23. Enlarged image in ventrodorsal projection of the hip of a dog with bilateral avascular necrosis in the femoral head (Legg-Calvé-Perthes disease). Both femoral heads have small osteolytic areas and appear slightly deformed. Even when it is bilateral, radiological changes do not appear at the same time in both femurs in many cases.

long bones, as well as facial malformation. It is a very rare anomaly in dogs and cats, although the incidence in the latter is higher, especially in the Siamese breed. In long bones it causes malformation of the epiphysis with shortening and stiffness of the limbs. In the spine, it causes shortening and deformation of the vertebrae, bone neoformation around the articular processes and ankylosing spondylitis, which can present with paresis and paraplegia. Facial shortening and widening can be seen in the skull, with alteration of the pattern of the nasal turbinate. It also causes corneal abnormalities, and patients may have cardiac abnormalities and hydrocephalus.

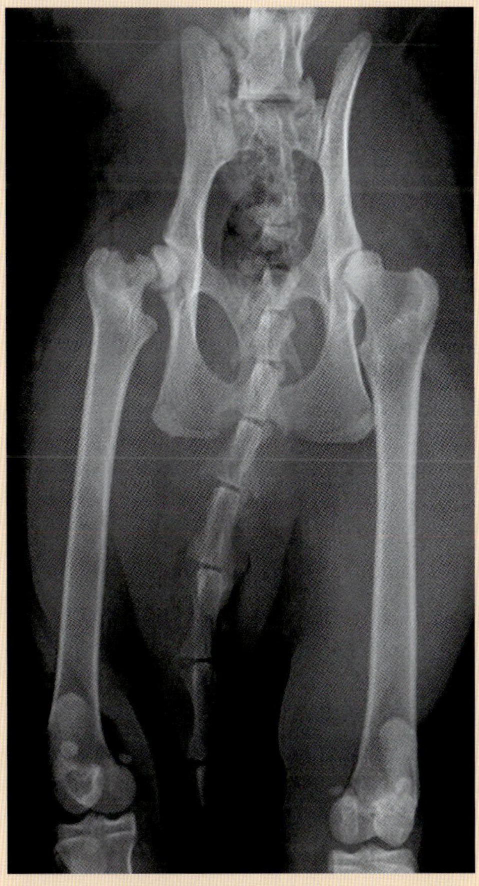

FIGURE 4.24. Ventrodorsal projection of the hip of a 2-year-old cat with right spontaneous femoral capital physeal fracture. Early neutering may be a predisposing factor for this injury in cats.

Fractures

Fractures are classified as:

- Closed (intact skin) or open (skin defect in the area) (fig. 4.25).
- Simple (single fracture line), comminuted (several fracture lines interconnect at one point or plane, thus dividing the bone in three or more fragments) or multiple (several fracture lines that do not interconnect, in the same or different bones).
- Transverse, oblique, spiral or irregular, depending on the fracture line direction.
- Complete (affects the whole bone diameter) or incomplete (e.g. greenstick fracture).
- Articular or nonarticular fracture, if it affects the joint or not.
- Avulsion fracture: it separates the insertion site of a muscle (fig. 4.26), ligament or tendon.
- Stress or fatigue fracture (caused by repeated mild trauma).
- Compression or impacted fractures: the end of one of the fragments jams into the other (fig. 4.27); shortening of the bone can be observed and it is more frequent in vertebrae.
- Salter–Harris fractures (see Box and fig. 4.28 and 4.29): they affect the physis.
- Pathological fractures: they are caused by another disease (processes that cause osteopenia, tumours, bone cysts, osteomyelitis) (fig. 4.30).

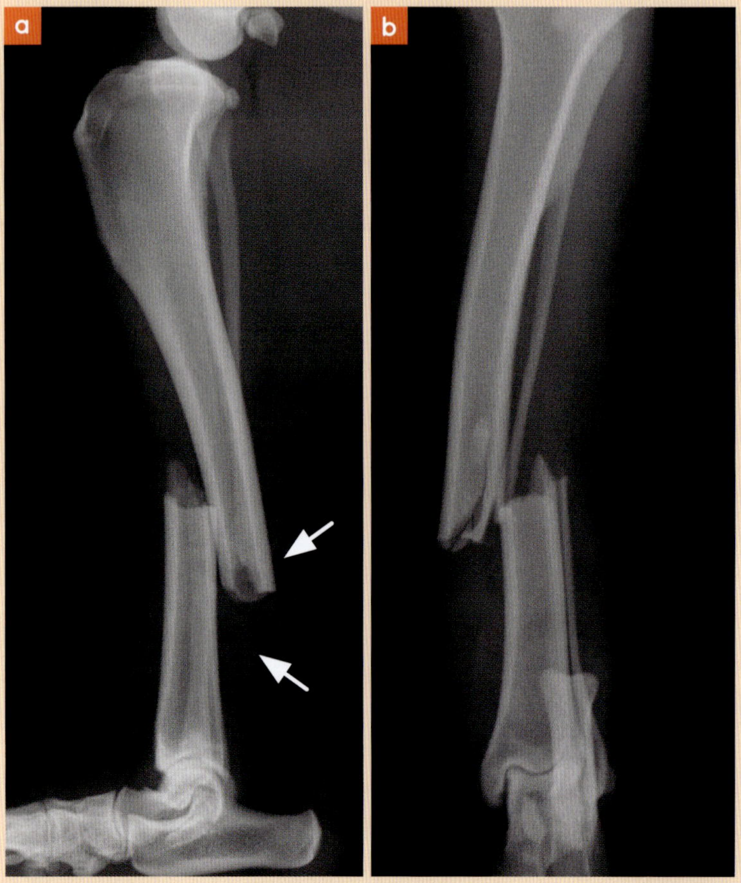

FIGURE 4.25. Mediolateral (a) and craniocaudal (b) radiographs of the tibia and fibula of a dog with an open fracture in both bones. The presence of small areas with gas density in surrounding soft tissues (arrows) is a radiological sign indicative of an open fracture.

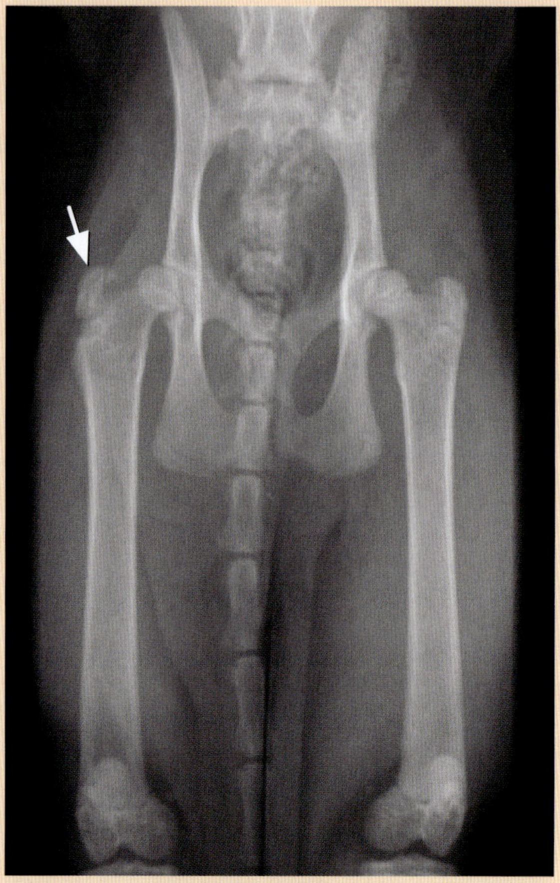

FIGURE 4.26. Ventrodorsal radiograph of the hip of a cat with an avulsion fracture in the greater trochanter of the right femur (arrow), in which the gluteus medius and profundus are inserted.

SALTER-HARRIS FRACTURES

Fractures that affect the physis are classified in 6 types (Salter-Harris classification) (fig. 4. 28):

- **Type I: t**he fracture occurs along the physis.
- **Type II:** the fracture line crosses the physis and also divides part of the metaphysis.
- **Type III:** the fracture line crosses the physis and also divides part of the epiphysis.
- **Type IV:** the fracture line crosses the physis and also divides part of the metaphysis and of the epiphysis (fig. 4.29).
- **Type V:** impacted or compressed fracture hat occurs at the physis level. It may completely or partially affect the physis. This is the type of fracture that may cause premature closure of the distal growth plate in the ulna.
- **Type VI (rare):** it is a consequence of trauma that only affects part of the physis thus causing its partial closure (asymmetric). This type has been added later to the classification and some authors think it should not be included.

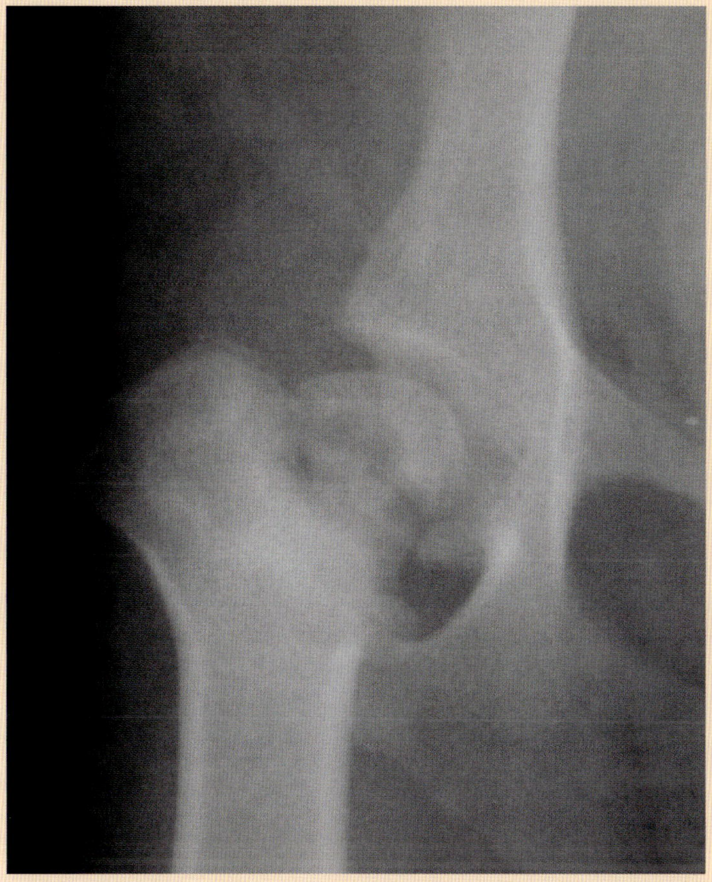

FIGURE 4.27. Enlarged image in ventrodorsal projection of the right coxofemoral joint of a dog with an impacted femoral neck fracture. Femoral neck shortening is caused by the fracture.

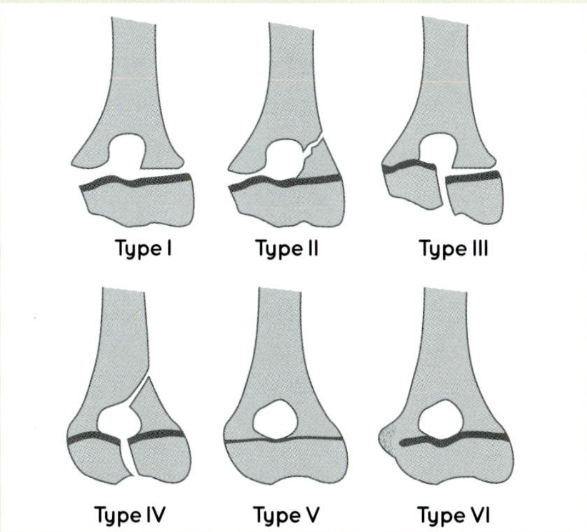

FIGURE 4.28. Diagram of the classification of Salter type fractures.

Immediately after surgical resolution of the fracture, a radiograph will allow the assessment of: the degree of fracture reduction (contact between the fragments); the alignment of the fragments; and the correct placement of the osteosynthesis material. In further radiological checks, the following will be examined: bone callus evolution; possible displacement of the fragments or the osteosynthesis material; rupture of the osteosynthesis material (fig. 4.31); and abnormalities in the adjacent soft tissues. The occurrence of radiolucent bands surrounding the osteosynthesis material indicates mobility of the material or infection (fig. 4.32). Nevertheless, an artefact with the same appearance (radiolucent lines surrounding metallic implants) has been described in digital radiography, due to overuse of the edge-enhancement tool. This has already been corrected in many modern equipment.

Follow-up X-rays of fractures are recommended every 2–4 weeks to evaluate progression and for the early detection secondary complications. In the first 2 weeks, a haematoma and a non-calcified callus form between the fragments, leading to an increase in soft tissue volume around the fracture. During this period, there is a certain degree of bone resorption at the ends of the fragments blurring their definition on the X-ray. The callus begins to calcify 10–12 days after the fracture and with this it can be identified in the images. From about 3 to 4 weeks, the calcification of the callus should already be marked and evident. This calcification usually progresses from the periphery toward the centre of the focus, with the fracture line gradually disappearing. Cortical remodelling occurs in the final phase, usually between 8 and 12 weeks after fracture reduction and stabilisation. These times spans are for general reference only. Progression in the resolution of a fracture depends on many factors, including bone type, fracture type, patient age, treatment methods and the existence of other systemic diseases.

Post-traumatic osteoporosis is a common sequela of many long bone distal fractures and can be especially acute in young animals. It is often wrongly called **disuse osteoporosis**. Post-traumatic osteoporosis develops distal to the fracture (fig. 4.33), whereas disuse osteoporosis (caused by limb immobilisation) affects the whole limb. Once the fracture has formed

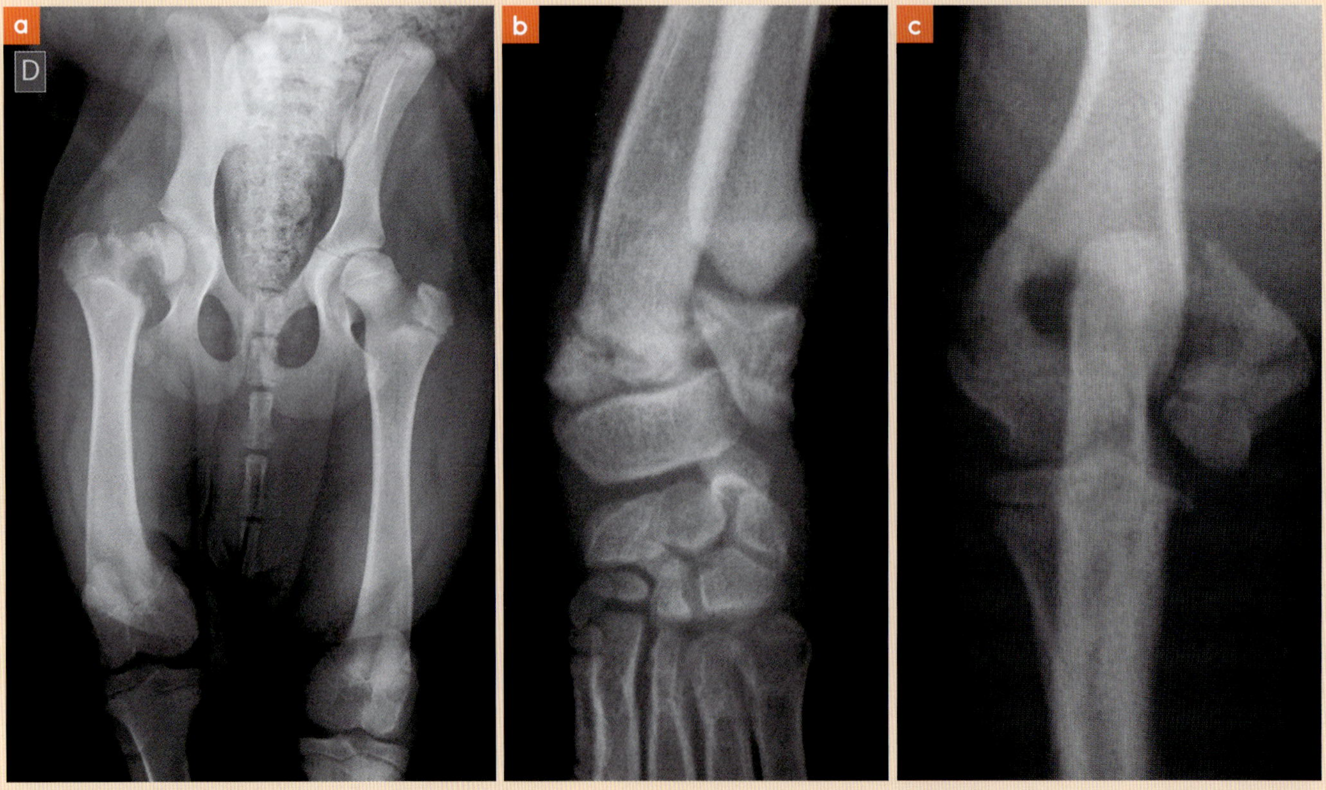

FIGURE 4.29. Radiographs of Salter-Harris-type fractures in three dogs. Type I Salter-Harris fracture of the right capital femoral epiphysis (a), causing secondary necrosis of the femoral neck. Type II Salter-Harris fracture of the epiphysis plus part of the distal radius metaphysis (b). Type IV Salter-Harris fracture of part of the epiphysis plus part of the distal metaphysis of the humerus (c).

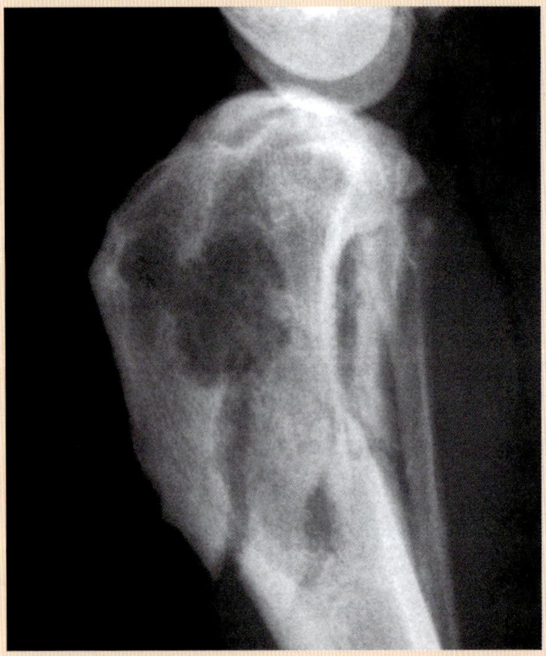

FIGURE 4.30. Enlarged image of the proximal tibia in mediolateral projection of a dog with a pathological fracture, caused by a markedly osteolytic aggressive bone lesion due to primary bone neoplasia.

FIGURE 4.31. Mediolateral radiograph of the tibia and fibula of a dog with a broken osteosynthesis plate, which was applied as treatment for a fracture of both bones. The central screw looks displaced and multiple small fragments can be identified surrounding the fracture focus. The shadow of the dressing can be observed in the image.

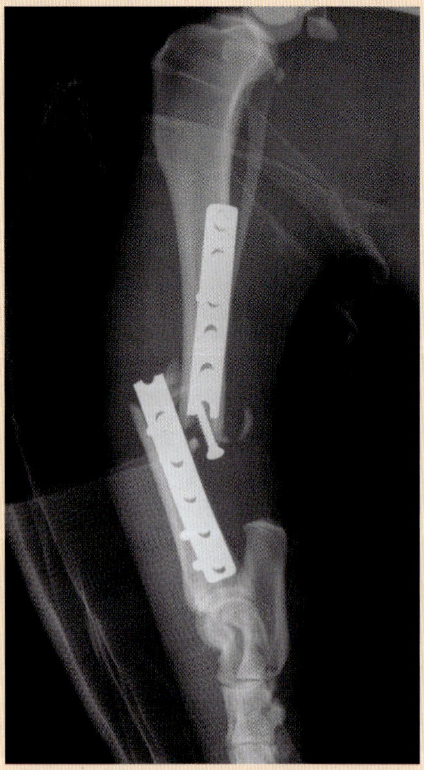

a solid callus and the bone is again rigid, bone density returns quickly to normal in both types of osteoporosis.

The main complications from fractures are:

- **Delayed union:** callus formation is slower than normal.
- **Non-union:** callus is not formed; it can be atrophic (end of fragments are pointed) (fig. 4.34) or hypertrophic (bone forms around the ends of the fragments, but they do not bind; the shape of the ends looks like an "elephant's foot" (fig. 4.35).
- **Defective consolidation:** fragments are bound, but not correctly aligned (fig. 4.36).
- **Exuberant callus:** splinters of bone incorporate to the callus, due to mobility of the fracture focus or to infection.
- **Osteomyelitis:** infection will be suspected when osteolysis is observed surrounding the material, together with an atypical periosteal reaction and marked soft-tissue tumescence, that may look like emphysema (focal gas accumulations) in some cases.
- **Neoplastic development:** it may appear after several years, especially if the osteosynthesis material was not removed or the fracture resolution was very complicated. Its cause is unknown but it could be related to chronic inflammation.

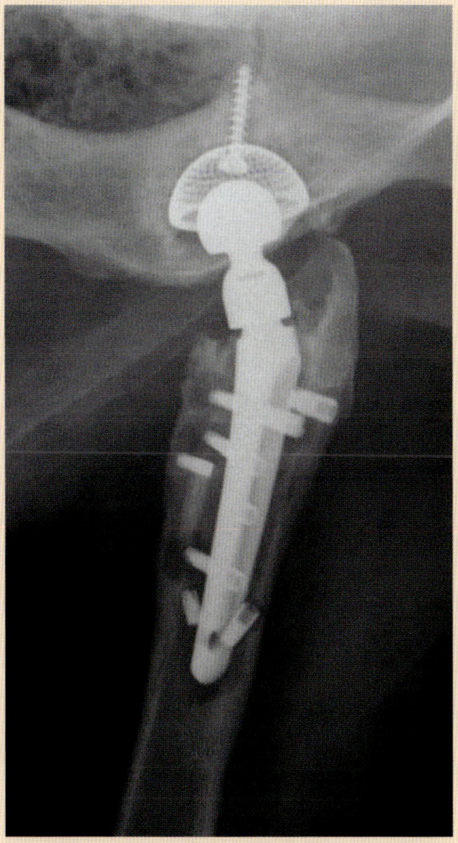

FIGURE 4.32. Enlarged image in mediolateral projection of the femur of a dog that shows some degree of mobility of a hip prosthesis. Radiolucent bands surrounding the rod can be seen, as well as rupture of several screws.

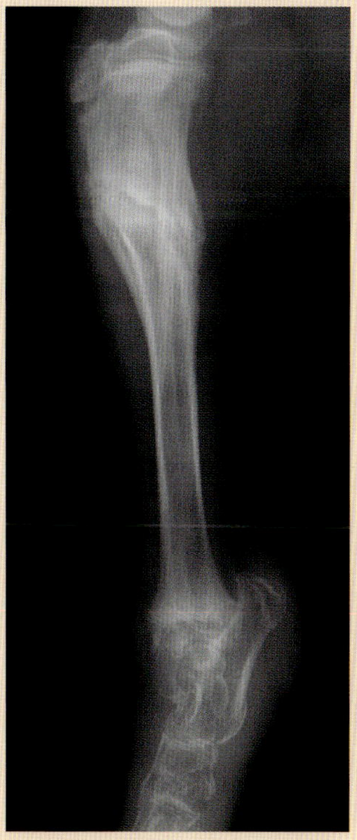

FIGURE 4.33. Mediolateral radiograph of the tibia and fibula of a dog with fracture of both bones in healing phase as well as post-traumatic osteoporosis. The osteoporosis develops distal to the fracture (in this case, more marked in the tarsus and metatarsals), unlike desuse osteoporosis that affects the whole limb.

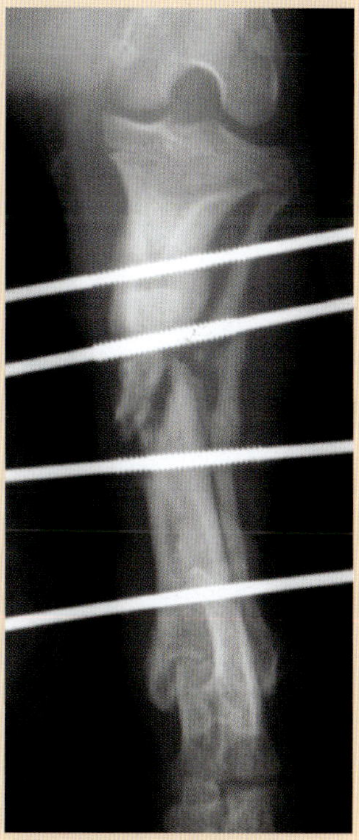

FIGURE 4.34. Craniocaudal radiograph of the tibia and fibula of a dog with atrophic nonunion of a tibial fracture. The fragment ends appear pointed. The external fixators and a double fibula fracture can be observed in the image.

Deformities due to growth plate alteration

Growth plate lesions cause slowed-down or arrested growth, and its consequences can be:

- Shortening of the affected bone(s).
- Angulation of the affected bone(s).
- Subluxation of adjacent joints.

The degree of bone shortening depends on the specific contribution that the damaged plate has in global bone growth and on the stage of growth when the lesion is produced (fig. 4.37).

Angulation or curvature of the affected bone takes place when the lesion affects more than one area in the plate, or when the affected bone is part of a pair (e.g. radius–ulna).

The most significant deformities occur by lesion of the proximal or distal growth plate of the radius and of the distal growth plates of the ulna, femur or tibia.

Due to its conical shape, the distal growth plate of the ulna is especially prone to lesions. Sometimes, premature growth line closure can be observed with no previous evident trauma. When distal growth of the ulna is slowed-down or arrested and the radius continues growing at a normal pace, cranial and medial curvature of the radius occurs, as well as valgus (lateral) deviation of the hand, elbow subluxation and proximal migration of the ulna styloid process (fig. 4.38). This deformity is called radius curvus.

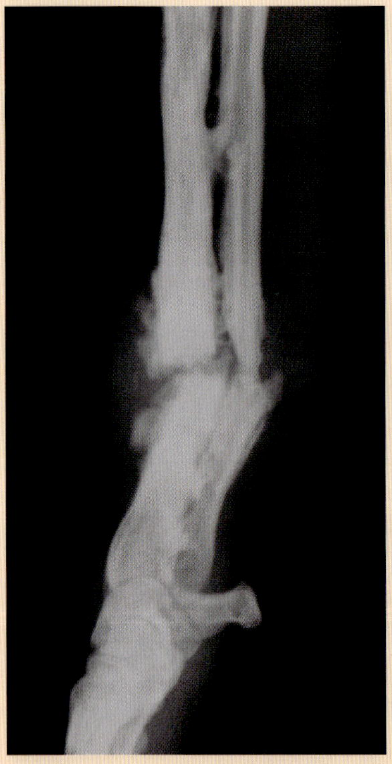

FIGURE 4.35. Mediolateral radiograph of the radius and the ulna of a dog with hypertrophic nonunion of the radial fracture. The fragment ends appear separated, sclerotic and new bone is forming around them. Nonunion of an ulnar fracture is also observed, with the proximal fragment looking atrophic and the distal, hypertrophic.

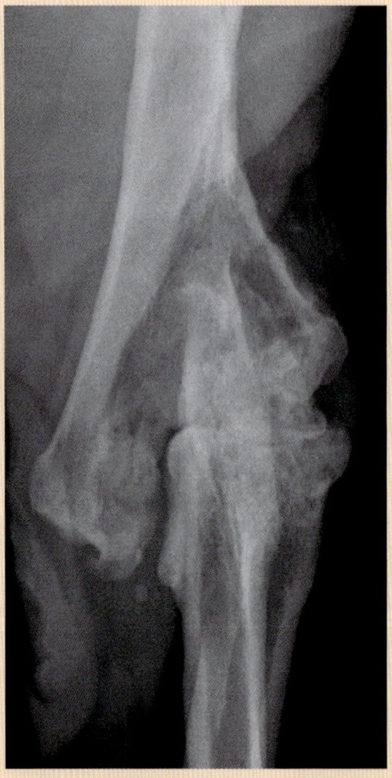

FIGURE 4.36. Craniocaudal radiograph of the elbow of a dog with poor consolidation of a distal humerus fracture.

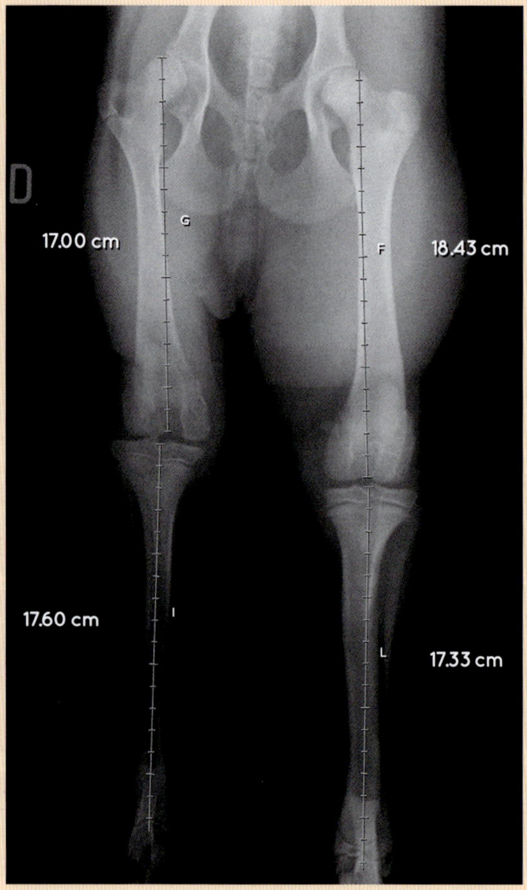

FIGURE 4.37. Craniocaudal projection of the femurs and tibias of a dog with premature closure of the distal growth line of the right femur, causing shortening of this bone (17 cm) compared with the left (18.43 cm).

When the lesion affects the distal radial growth plate, the radius is shortened with respect to the ulna, that keeps growing at a normal pace. The radial head separates from the humeral condyle, widening the joint space (fig. 4.39). Medial widening of the distal radial epiphysis occurs, which usually causes valgus deviation of the hand, although it is sometimes in the opposite direction (in varus, to the medial area).

Proximal growth plate lesions of the radius are much less frequent and cause similar radiographic signs to those of the distal plate, but the distal radius remains normal and there is no hand deviation.

Bone tumours and osteomyelitis

Bone tumours

Benign bone tumours are uncommon. They include osteomas, generally appearing as radiodense masses of amorphous bone; chondromas, with less radiopacity than osteomas; and osteochondromas, appearing as single cartilaginous exostoses.

Malignant bone tumours (osteosarcoma, fibrosarcoma, haemangiosarcoma, chondrosarcoma) appear as aggressive bone lesions, usually single, mainly located at the following metaphyses: proximal of the humerus, distal of the radius, distal of the femur and proximal or distal of the tibia (fig. 4.40). Chondrosarcomas usually affect the ribs, pelvis, or skull.

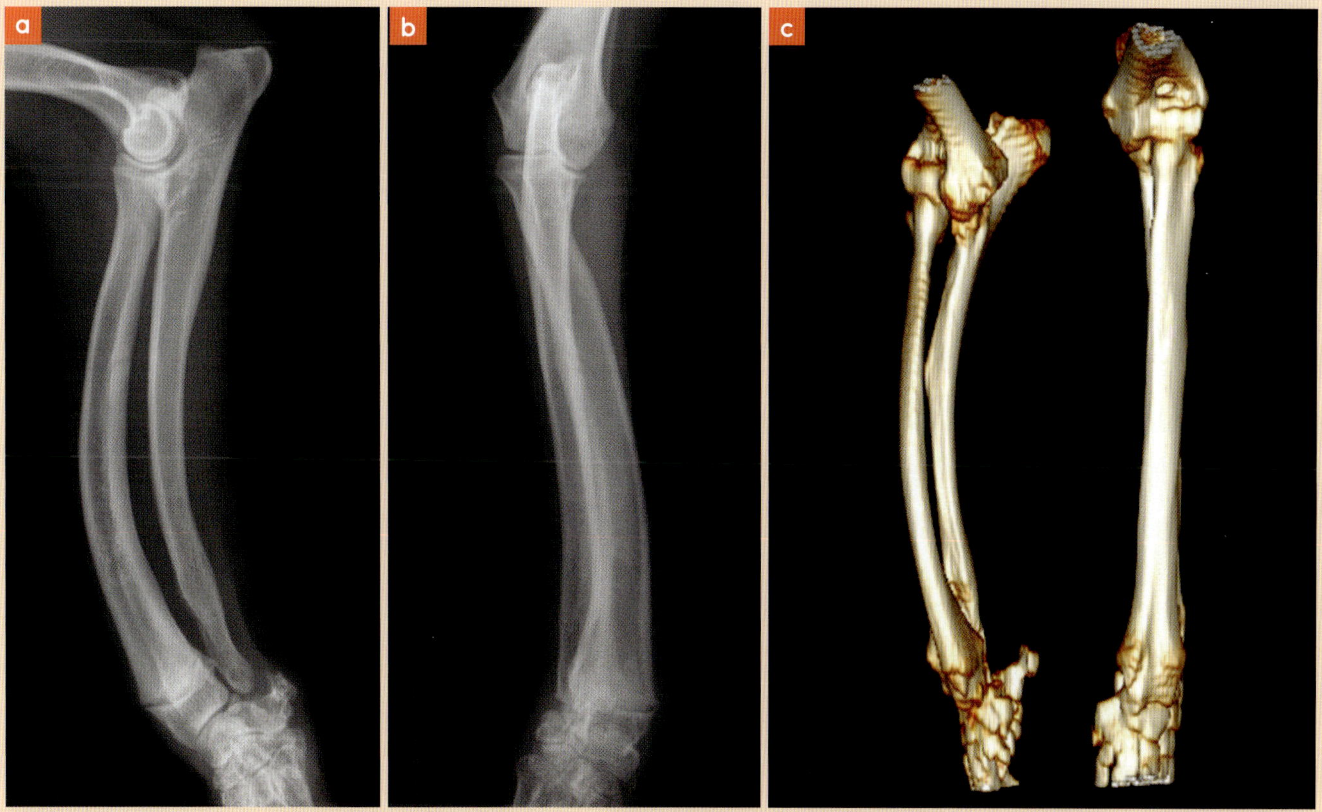

FIGURE 4.38. Radiographic images in mediolateral (a) and craniocaudal (b) projection of the radius and ulna of an 8-month old dog with radius curvus. Computed tomography image of the same patient (c). As previous trauma has caused premature closure of the distal growth line of ulna, the radius is curved cranially and medially. This causes elbow subluxation and valgus deviation of the hand. Accessory carpal bone deformity can be also observed, as well as a fragment caudal distal to the distal epiphysis of the radius. Both findings are related to the prior trauma. The image (c) shows computed tomographic-based volumetric reconstruction of both limbs, where the damaged limb can be compared in detail to the normal limb. The degree of deformity can therefore be easily assessed, as well as the degree of angulation of the affected limb. This is of special interest when planning surgical treatment.

Primary bone tumours can appear as lesions with various degrees of osteolysis and osteoproliferation. The zone of transition between the lesion and normal bone is usually wide and poorly defined, and the periosteal reaction of spiculated, sunburst or amorphous type. For years, tumours were thought to have a characteristic periosteal reaction that was called Codman triangle (fig. 4.41), and corresponds to a small triangular bone area located at the edge of the lesion. Today, it is known that it is formed when the periosteum gets broken and lifted "for any reason" and, although it is generally considered suggestive of malignancies, it can also be associated to subperiosteal haematoma and inflammatory processes.

Primary tumours do not normally "cross" the joint and extend to adjacent bone. They can be the cause for secondary pathological fractures. As lung metastases are frequent, it is advised to always perform a radiological thoracic study when these types of bone lesions are observed.

Bone metastases usually appear as multiple aggressive lesions (fig 4.42).

Multiple myeloma results from neoplastic proliferation of bone marrow plasma cells. It produces multiple focal lesions that affect long bones, ribs and vertebrae at the same time (see Chapter 5).

Malignant soft-tissue tumours adjacent to the bone may secondarily affect nearby bone structures. In these cases, the typical radiological finding is marked tumefaction of soft tissues together with osteolytic, rather than osteo-proliferative changes in the adjacent bone (it may affect several bones depending on the primary tumour extension) (fig. 4.43). Subungual squamous cell carcinoma is a typical example of a malignant tumour of soft tissues usually affecting adjacent bones (fig. 4.44), which appears more frequently in large breed dogs with black coat.

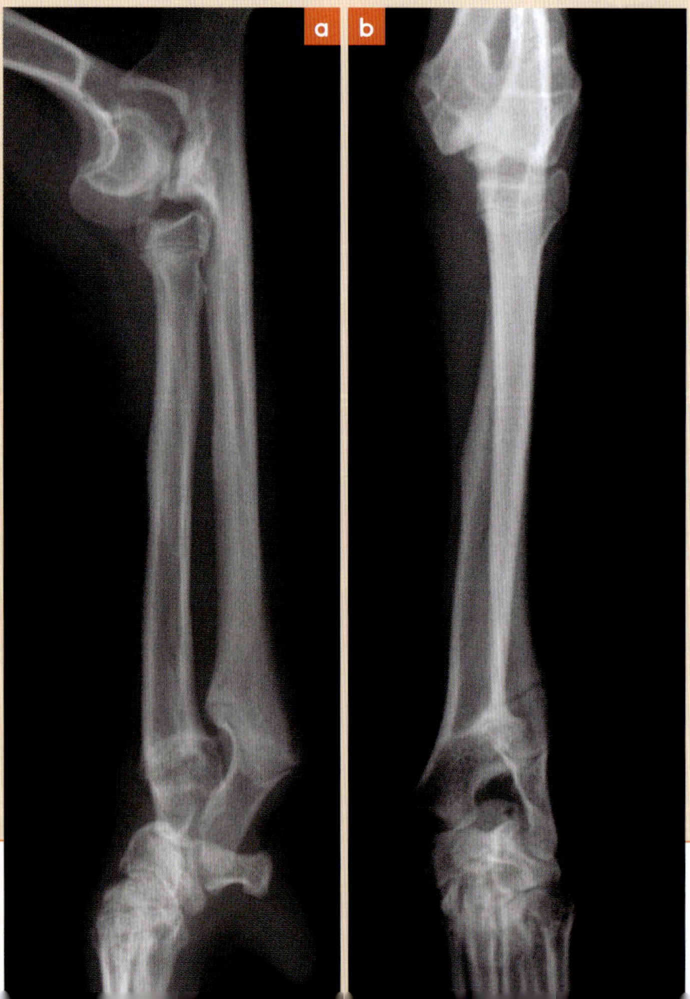

FIGURE 4.39. Mediolateral (a) and craniocaudal (b) radiographs of the ulna of a dog with a short radius. The radius is shortened by premature closure of the distal radial growth line, with the proximal epiphysis migrating distally, which causes elbow joint incongruity. The distal part of the ulna and the radius seems deformed.

Osteomyelitis

It is usually a sequela of surgical fracture repair (fig. 4.45), although it can also appear in open fractures. Sometimes the infection is produced haematogenously.

In the acute phase, aggressive periosteal reaction is observed, with some degree of cortical and trabecular osteolysis and inflammation of the adjacent soft tissues. In chronic phases, bone may proliferate around the lesion. A complication of osteomyelitis is the formation of **sequestra** (fig. 4.46), which are defined as avascular bone fragments that are isolated from the main bone and enclosed in a radiolucent area. Radiotranslucency of the bone surrounding the fragment is due to necrosis. This area is delimited by a peripheral sclerotic margin, referred to as **involucrum**. The appearance of sequestra is more common after the use of external fixation devices (fig. 4.46).

In practice, it is not possible to safely differentiate osteomyelitis from a bone neoplasm only by radiological imaging. A biopsy is always required to confirm diagnosis.

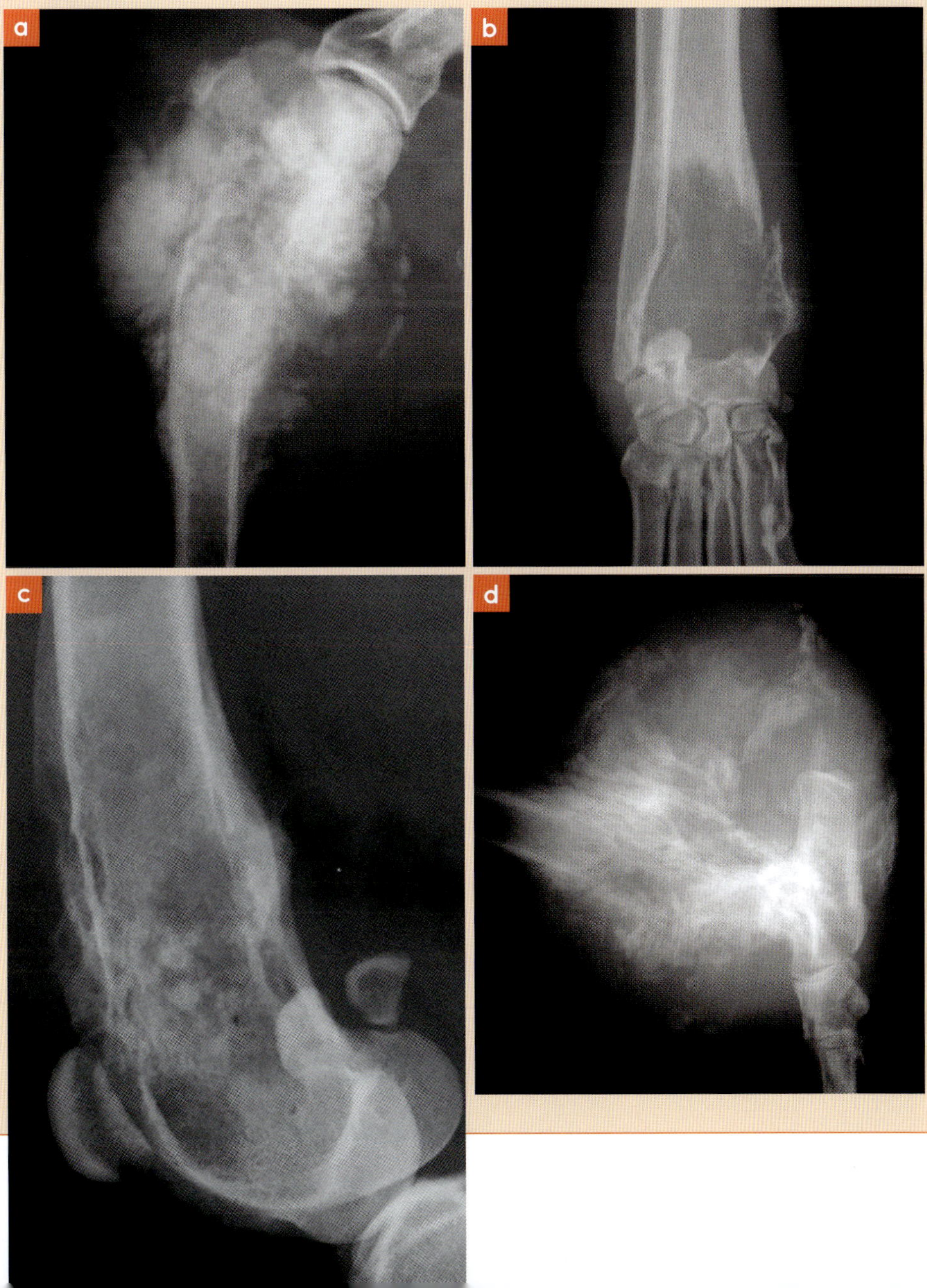

FIGURE 4.40. Images of the most common sites for bone neoplasms: proximal humerus (a), distal radius (b), distal femur (c) and proximal or distal tibia (d). The lesion in image (a) is mostly osteoproliferative with amorphous periosteal reaction, which is highly suggestive of malignancy. The lesion in image (b) is mostly osteolytic with mixed geographical pattern at its central area and infiltrating at its peripheral area. The cortex is interrupted at its medial margin. In image (c) the osteolytic pattern is mixed with partial cortical lysis, while the periosteal reaction is solid, with a more reactive appearance in the craniodistal area of the lesion. The marked mixed periosteal reaction (sunburst and amorphous) in image (d) makes it somewhat difficult to identify the pathological fracture in the patient's affected area.

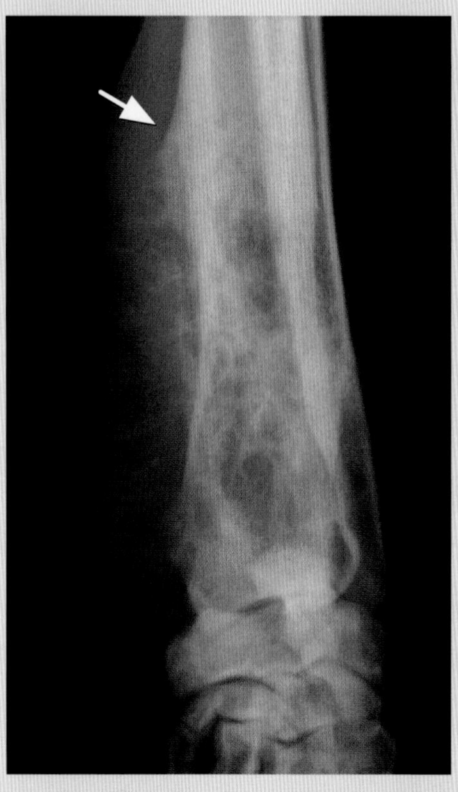

FIGURE 4.41. Enlarged image in craniocaudal projection of the radius and ulna of a dog with a bone neoplasm (osteosarcoma). The osteolysis pattern is moth-eaten, the zone of transition between the damaged and the normal bones is relatively wide, the periosteal reaction is spiculated, and a triangular bone overgrowth that corresponds to the so-called Codman triangle (arrow) can be identified at its medial and proximal edge.

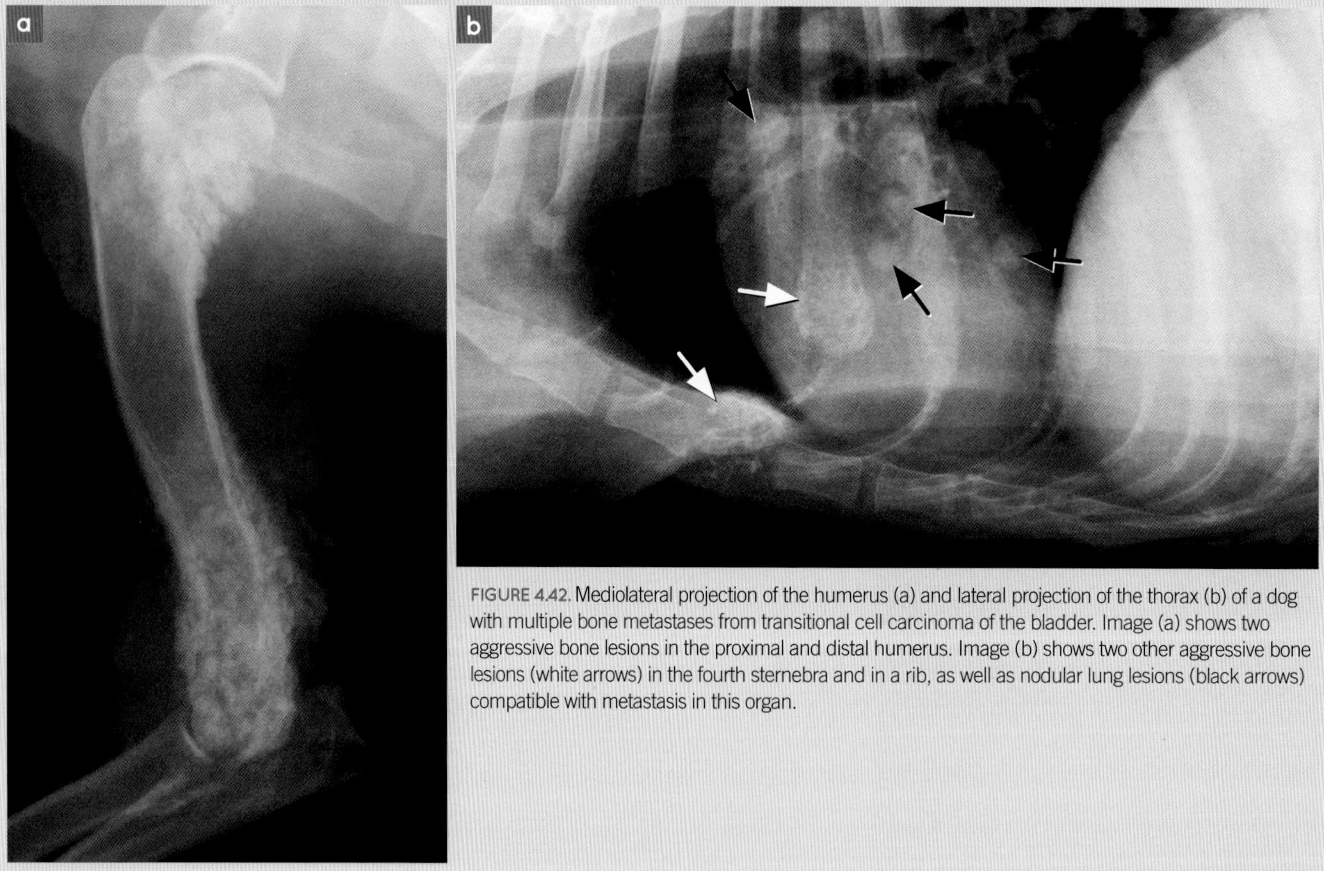

FIGURE 4.42. Mediolateral projection of the humerus (a) and lateral projection of the thorax (b) of a dog with multiple bone metastases from transitional cell carcinoma of the bladder. Image (a) shows two aggressive bone lesions in the proximal and distal humerus. Image (b) shows two other aggressive bone lesions (white arrows) in the fourth sternebra and in a rib, as well as nodular lung lesions (black arrows) compatible with metastasis in this organ.

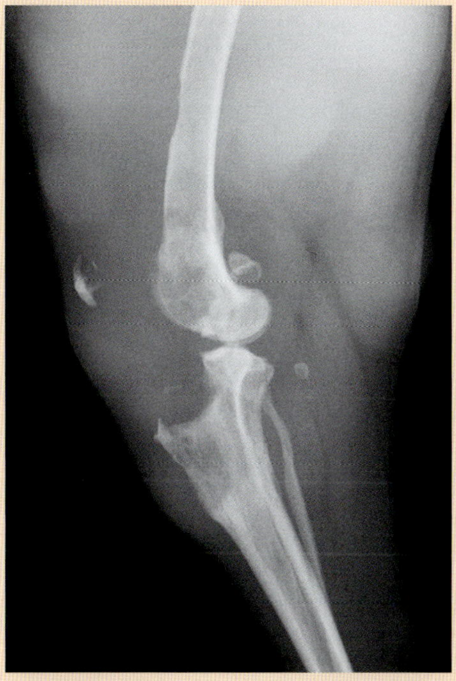

FIGURE 4.43. Mediolateral projection of the distal femur and proximal tibia of a dog with soft tissue sarcoma secondarily involving adjacent bone structures, causing osteolysis of the cranial margin of the femur, cranioproximal tibia and caudal portion of the patella.

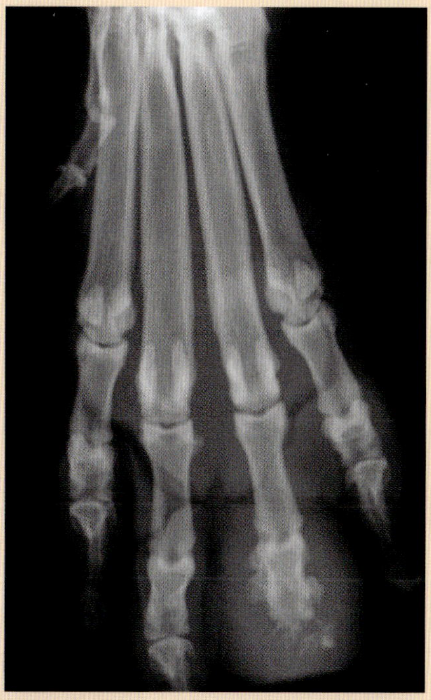

FIGURE 4.44. Dorsopalmar radiograph of the metacarpals and phalanges of a dog with a soft-tissue tumour that is secondarily affecting adjacent bones. The soft-tissue tumour is a squamous cell carcinoma that has destroyed the third phalanx of the fourth finger almost completely. It is also causing palisading periosteal reaction in the second phalanx of the same finger, thus indicating it is also affected.

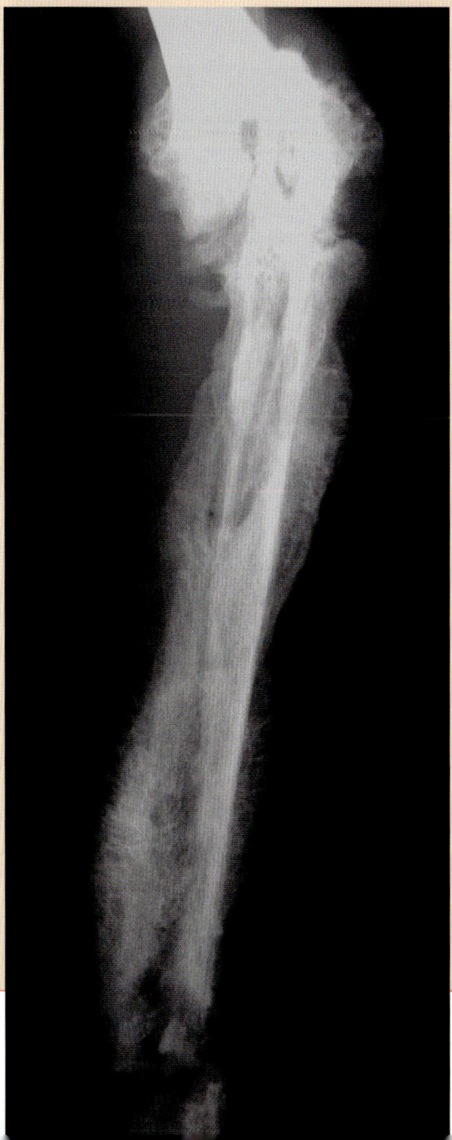

FIGURE 4.45. Craniocaudal radiograph of the radius and ulna of a dog with osteomyelitis that appeared after surgical fracture repair. The radiograph was taken after removing the osteosynthesis material and the fracture remains visible at the distal third of the diaphyses of both bones. Palisading periosteal reaction is observed.

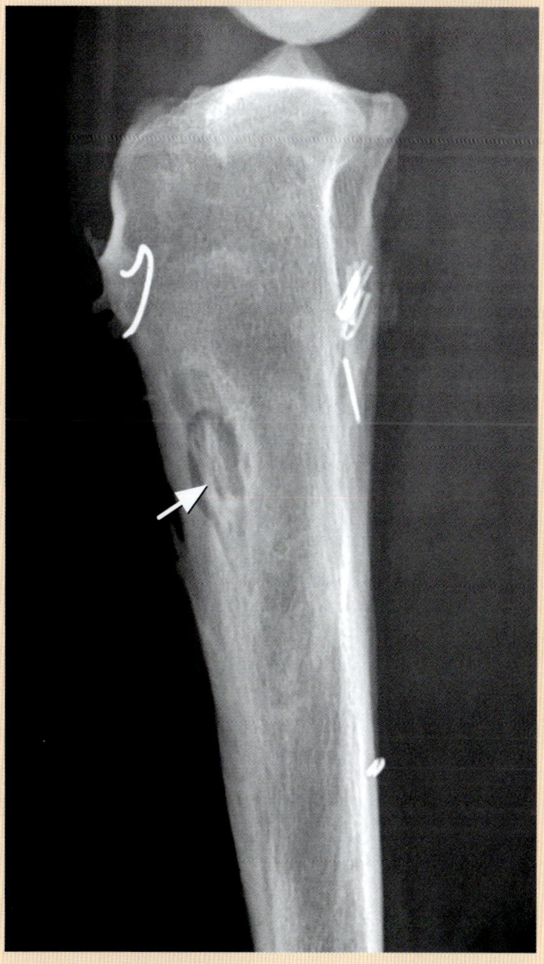

FIGURE 4.46. Enlarged image of the tibia in mediolateral projection of a dog with bone sequestration, which appears as an isolated fragment (arrow), surrounded by an osteolytic area with a sclerotic peripheral margin (*involucrum*). The lesion was identified after removal of the osteosynthesis material.

Nutritional and metabolic alterations

Balanced bone production and resorption is maintained in healthy adults. Numerous factors play a role to control this equilibrium, mainly the level of some hormones such as the parathyroid hormone and calcitonin (both are produced in the parathyroid gland), growth hormone, glucocorticoids and vitamin A, among others.

Bone is a living tissue that can reflect metabolic alterations and nutritional imbalances, that sometimes lead to increased bone production, although they more frequently cause increased resorption with subsequent bone density loss. Density changes in bone can be detected by conventional radiography but not at an early stage. In order to be evident on a radiograph, 30–50 % of bone calcium should be lost to reduce its opacity. Bone densitometry, a more sensitive and precise technique, is used in human medicine to evaluate changes in bone density.

Secondary nutritional hyperparathyroidism

It is also called nutritional osteodystrophy. It usually affects growing animals, especially cats, that feed on a low-calcium diet, or with an inappropriate calcium/phosphorus ratio (e.g. when they feed exclusively on meat, with a high phosphorus and low calcium content). Hypocalcaemia stimulates parathyroid hormone production. Radiographic signs are (fig. 4.47):

- Decreased bone radiopacity.
- Thinning of long bone cortex.
- A double cortical line caused by resorption of intracortical bone may be observed (rare).
- Secondary pathological fractures may be observed.
- Deformed bone limbs due to old pathologic fractures may be observed.
- Pelvic and vertebral deformity can appear.
- Fast calcification of bone structures after introducing a balanced diet.

Secondary renal hyperparathyroidism

It appears in animals with chronic renal failure. The reduction in the degree of glomerular filtration causes retention of phosphorus, which reduces calcium levels in blood. This stimulates the production of parathyroid hormone. It usually appears in older dogs, but it can also be detected in young patients with renal dysplasia. The radiographic findings in long bones are similar to those described in secondary nutritional hyperparathyroidism, but the most significant bone changes usually affect the skull (see Chapter 6).

Hypophyseal dwarfism

It mostly affects the German Shepherd and it is caused by abnormal growth hormone production (sometimes also with hypothyroidism). Unlike other metabolic or hereditary diseases also causing dwarfism, it causes proportional dwarfism. Radiographic signs are:

- Delayed calcification of the epiphyseal ossification centres.
- Delayed closure of growth lines.
- Incomplete epiphysis ossification when the skeletal maturation of the animal concludes.

Hypervitaminosis A

This disease affects cats that ingest excessive amount of vitamin A (usually in liver-based diets). Clinically these animals have spine stiffness, lameness and pain when the neck is being handled. In young animals, delayed development may occur. Radiographic signs are:

- Irregular bone growths in long bone metaphyses and around the joints (fig. 4.48).
- Exostosis in vertebrae, usually cervical and thoracic, sometimes causing the spinous processes to fuse.

It is important not to mistake the radiographic image for a neoplasm.

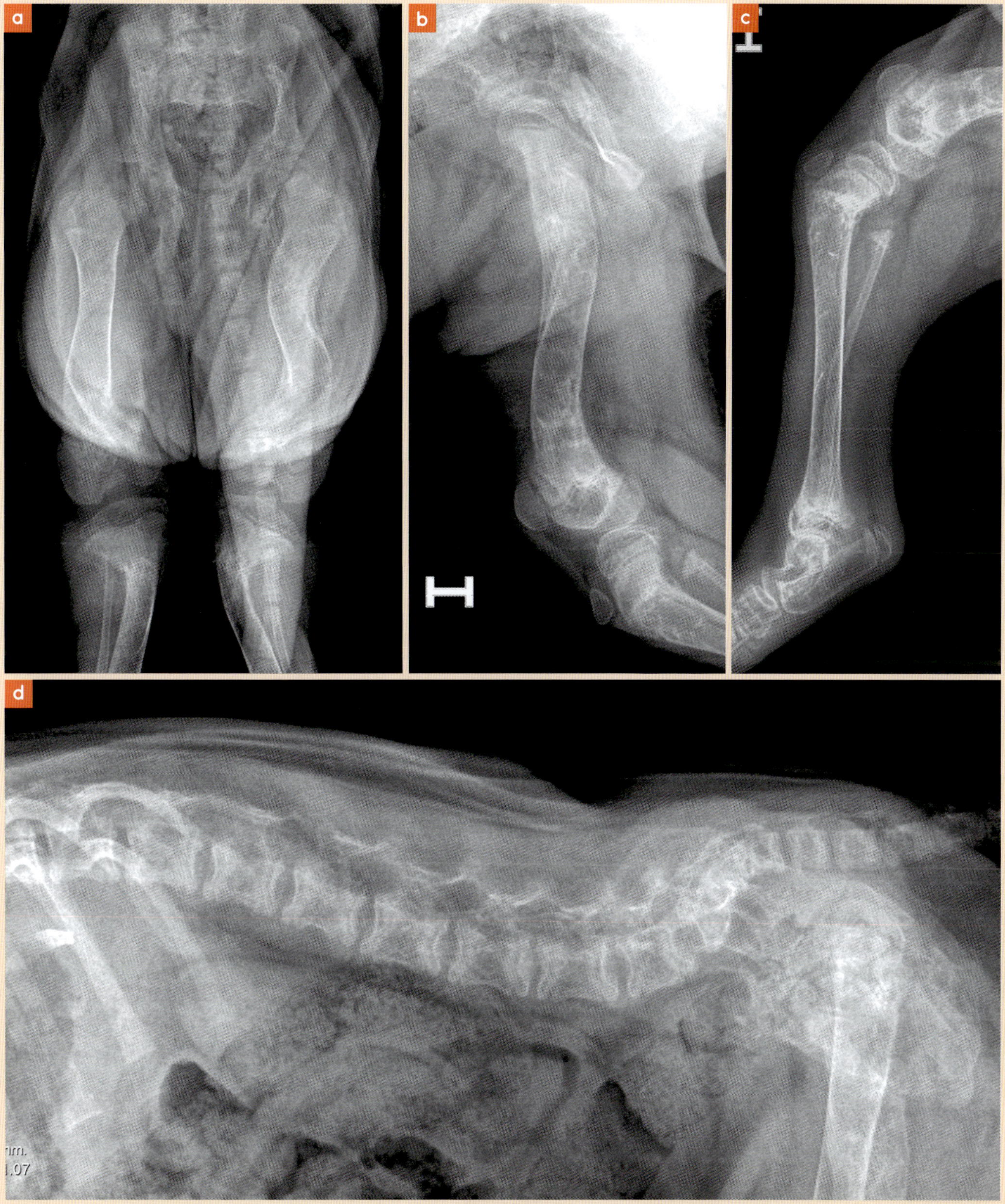

FIGURE 4.47. Ventrodorsal projection of the hip (a), mediolateral projection of the femur (b) and tibia (c) and lateral projection of the lumbar spine (d) of a young dog with nutritional secondary hyperparathyroidism. Osteopenia causes a loss of the radiopacity of the bones, thinning of the cortices, as well as secondary fractures that can lead to bone deformations. Image courtesy of María José Ruiz Fernández.

Joint disease

Joints are the regions of the locomotor system where movement takes place. Apart from this dynamic function, they are responsible for the skeleton functioning as an elastic set, and therefore, better prepared to bear pressure and stretching than a rigid block. The bones that integrate joints should keep interrelated in order to fulfil these functions.

Radiographic signs of joint disease

Numerous radiographic signs can be pinpointed on an X-ray that are indicative of joint disease as described below.

Increased synovial volume

The appearance of this sign is usually due to an increase in synovial fluid (synovial effusion), although this cannot be differentiated from the joint capsule, synovial membrane or articular cartilage on an X-ray as they are all of fluid/soft tissue density.

The joint in which increased synovial volume can most reliably be evaluated is the knee thanks to the anatomical landmark, the infrapatellar fat pad. This is located between the patellar ligament and the synovial components of fluid/soft tissue opacity in the joint, so a narrowing of its silhouette in the mediolateral projection is indicative of increased volume of synovial fluid and/or synovial soft tissues (fig. 4.49).

Altered thickness of the joint space

An actual increase in joint space width is usually due to an increase in the volume of the fluid/soft tissue opacity components of the joint (fig. 4.50), while a reduction in joint space usually appears in the advanced stages of degenerative joint disease. However, it is important to note that the radiographic assessment of joint space

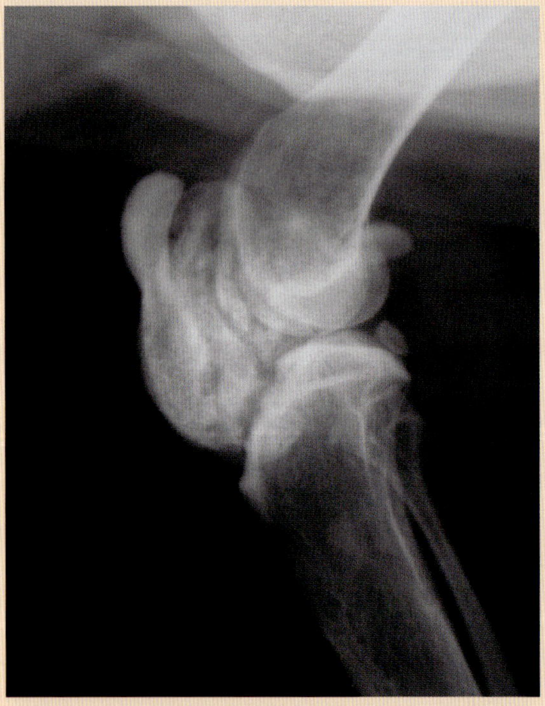

FIGURE 4.48. Mediolateral radiograph of the knee of a cat with hypervitaminosis A. The cat has a localised osteo-proliferative lesion on the cranial aspect of the joint. In these cases, similar lesions can be observed in long bone metaphyses and vertebrae.

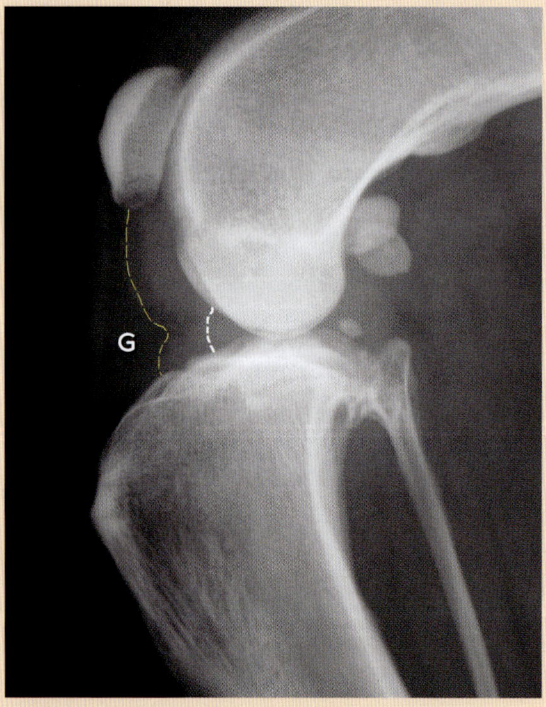

FIGURE 4.49. Mediolateral radiographs of the knee of a dog with signs of increased synovial volume. The narrowing of the silhouette of the infrapatellar fat (G) is a fairly reliable indicator of this increase in volume, which is usually due mainly to synovial effusion.

width is generally not very precise as it can vary significantly with patient positioning and depending on the fixation methods used.

Decreased subchondral bone opacity

The subchondral bone is located adjacent to the articular cartilage. Any pathology that causes the articular cartilage to erode can, secondarily, affect the integrity of the subchondral bone. When eroded, it shows radiolucent areas, which are called **subchondral defects** (fig. 4.51). These can appear in cases of severe or chronic degenerative joint processes and are also very typical in cases of inflammatory or infectious joint processes (inflammatory and infectious arthritis). Subchondral defects with rounded, well-defined morphology are described as subchondral cysts.

Increased subchondral bone opacity

The increased opacity of the subchondral bone is called **subchondral sclerosis**. This finding is usually associated with degenerative joint disease and usually occurs as a result of bone remodelling on the joint surface, caused by the degenerative process (fig. 4.52).

Osteophytes and enthesophytes

Osteophytes are defined as small new bone formations, which develop at the joint margin (periarticular osteophytes) or adjacent to the joint margin (extra-articular osteophytes). Periarticular osteophytes are the most characteristic finding in degenerative joint disease (fig. 4.53).

Enthesophytes are distinguished from osteophytes only by their location, since they appear at the point of

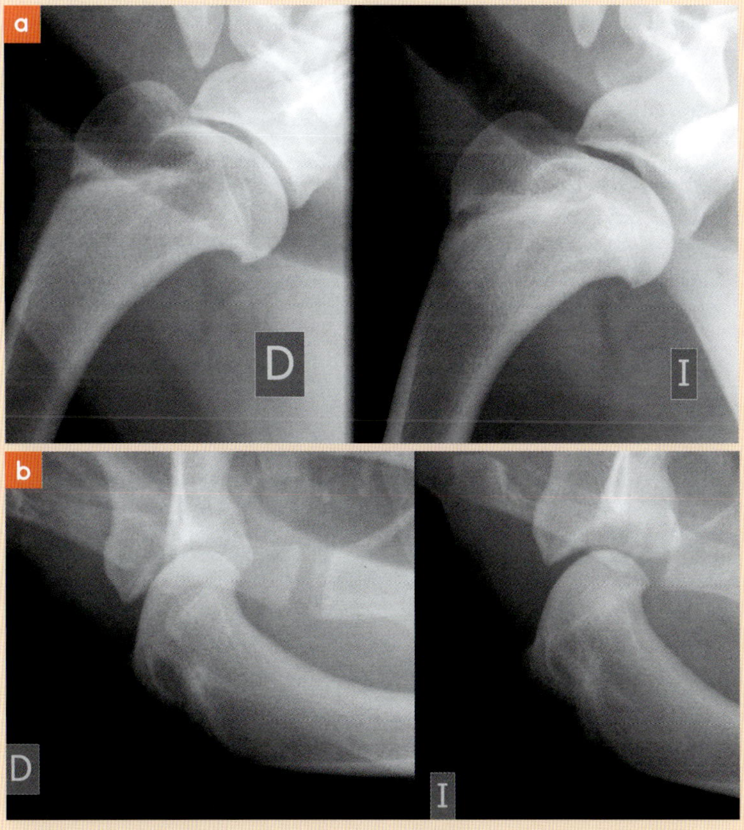

FIGURE 4.50. Standard mediolateral (a) and forced flexion mediolateral (b) projections of both scapulohumeral joints of a dog with increased left shoulder joint space width. It is important to be cautious when assessing joint space width, as the image can be significantly influenced by patient positioning and the degree of traction applied when taking the radiographs.

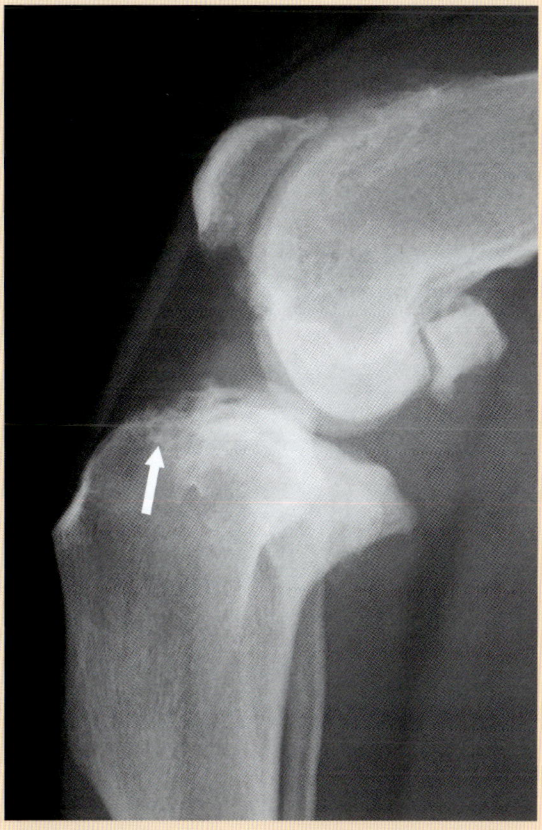

FIGURE 4.51. Mediolateral projection of the knee of a dog with severe degenerative joint disease. The arrow points to subchondral defects.

insertion of a ligament (fig. 4.54), tendon or joint capsule to the bone. On radiographs, they are often indistinguishable from osteophytes.

Soft tissue calcification

Calcification or mineralisation of intra-articular or periarticular soft tissues is a common finding in joint pathology. In the intra-articular components it may be due to calcification of the synovial capsule or synovial membrane (fig. 4.55). In some cases, especially in cats, meniscus calcification may be the cause (fig. 4.56). These findings are generally indicative of degenerative joint disease, although meniscus calcification in cats may be incidental. The appearance of calcification foci associated with various types of tendinopathy is also common.

The presence of very numerous and large areas of periarticular calcification may be due to what is called

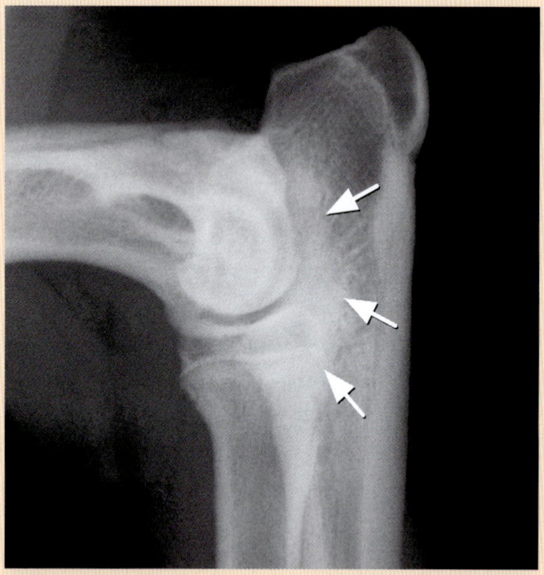

FIGURE 4.52. Medial-lateral projection of the elbow of a dog with sclerosis of the trochlear notch of the ulna (arrows) due to joint dysplasia.

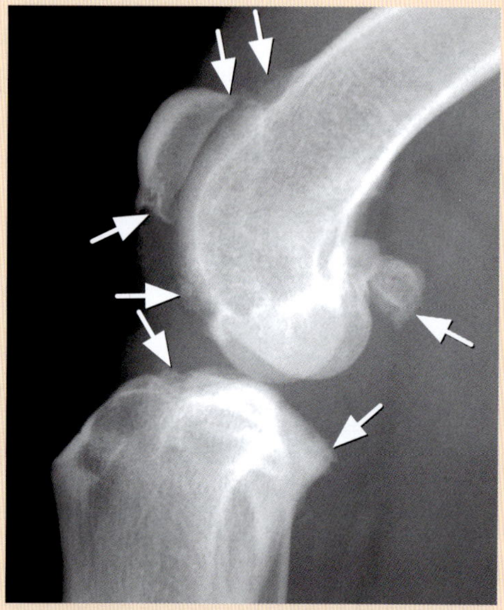

FIGURE 4.53. Mediolateral projection of the knee of a dog with moderate degenerative joint disease. The arrows point to osteophytes.

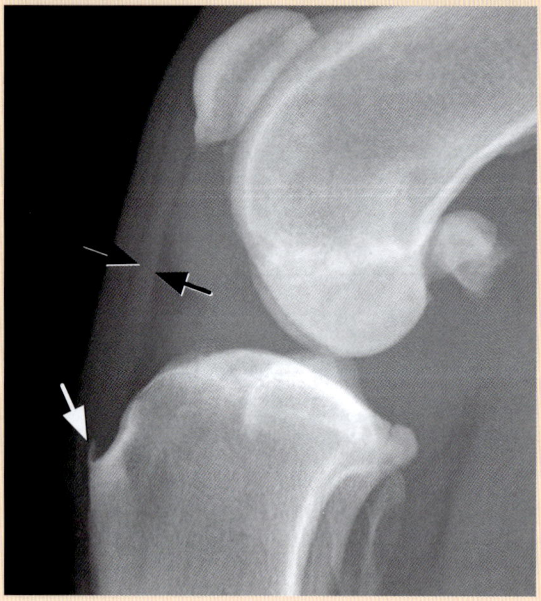

FIGURE 4.54. Mediolateral projection of the knee of a dog with mild degenerative joint disease. The white arrow points to an enthesophyte at the insertion of the patellar ligament (marked with black arrows).

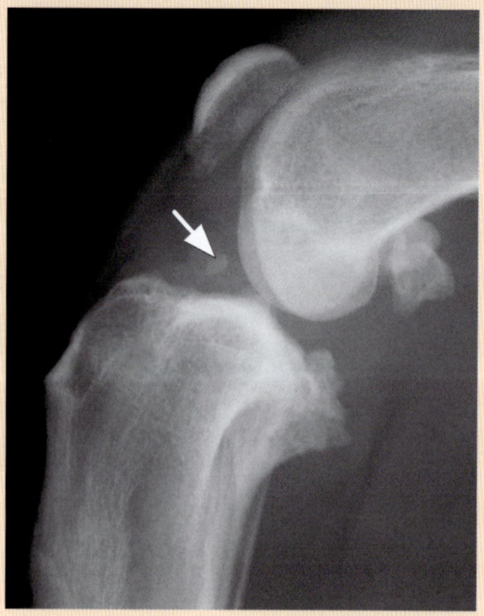

FIGURE 4.55. Mediolateral projection of the knee of a dog with moderate degenerative joint disease. The arrow points to intra-articular calcification.

synovial chondrometaplasia or osteochondromatosis, which may be primary or secondary to an underlying pathology. It usually appears on the hip (fig. 4.57), knee, tarsus or shoulder.

Intra-articular bodies (arthroliths)

Intra-articular loose bodies (arthroliths), more colloquially referred to as joint mice, are small fragments of bone that move around the intra- or peri-articular area (fig. 4.58). They usually come from the joint or peri-articular bone, although they may also correspond to osteochondral components from injured joint surfaces or small synovial osteochondromas.

Joint incongruence

The lack of congruence between the surfaces of the bones that form a particular joint is a clear sign of joint disease. A typical example is hip dysplasia, in which the articular surfaces of the acetabulum and femoral head are incongruent to a greater or lesser extent, depending on the degree of coxofemoral joint laxity (fig. 4.59).

Joint malformation

A morphological abnormality of the bone components of the joint is an obvious sign of joint pathology that can be easily diagnosed by X-ray (fig. 4.60).

Intra-articular gas

Intra-articular gas is most commonly associated with iatrogenic causes, following joint puncture, arthroscopy or arthrotomy, although it may also be associated with penetrating trauma or anaerobic joint infection.

The so-called "vacuum phenomenon" has also been described, in which intra-articular nitrogen gas accumulates spontaneously due to the negative pressure exerted by traction of the joint during radiographic positioning. It has been observed in dogs and cats when excessive distraction of the coxofemoral joint is applied, and it has also been described in 20 % of

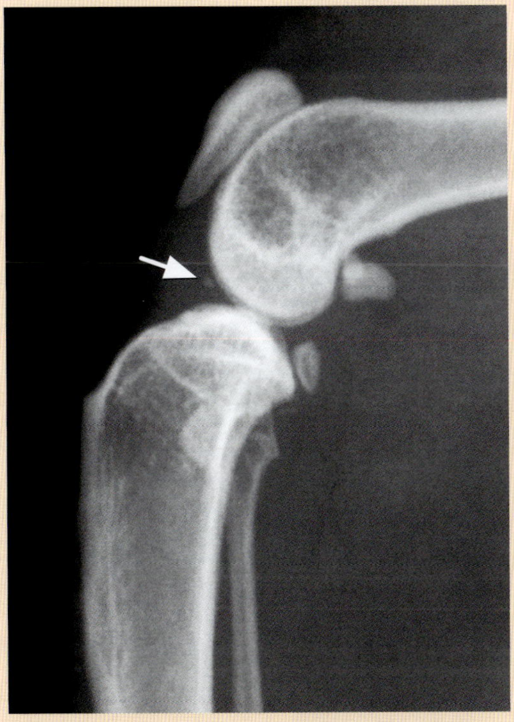

FIGURE 4.56. Mediolateral projection of the knee of a cat. The arrow points to possible intra-articular calcification of the meniscus, which is considered incidental in cats.

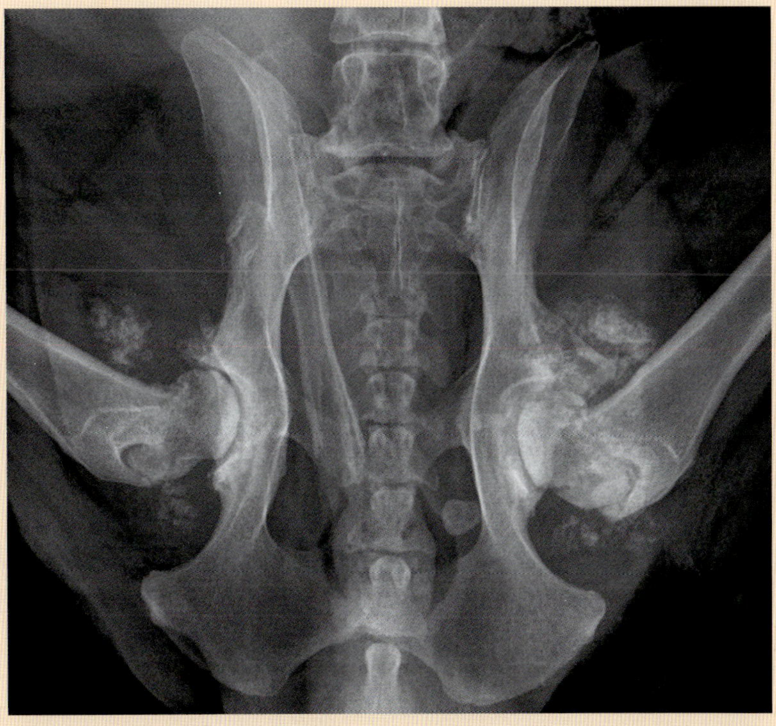

FIGURE 4.57. A frog-leg ventrodorsal projection of the hip of a dog with osteochondromatosis or synovial chondrometaplasia around both coxofemoral joints.

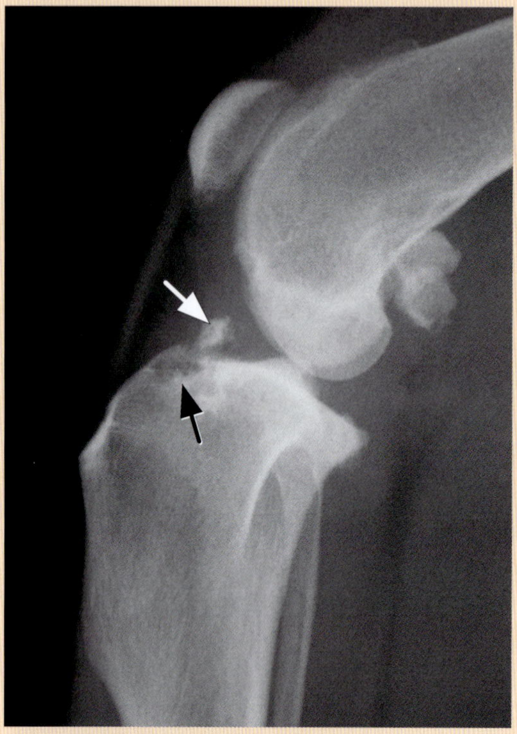

FIGURE 4.58. Mediolateral projection of the knee of a dog with moderate degenerative joint disease. The white arrow points to a joint body, which corresponds to a bone fragment from the radiolucent area, indicated by the black arrow.

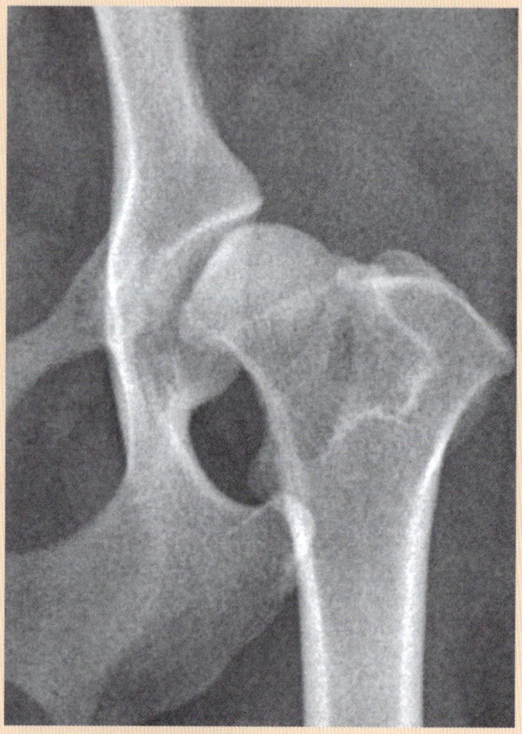

FIGURE 4.59. Enlarged view of the ventrodorsal projection of the left coxofemoral joint of a dog with hip dysplasia. The articular surfaces of the acetabulum and femoral head are not congruent.

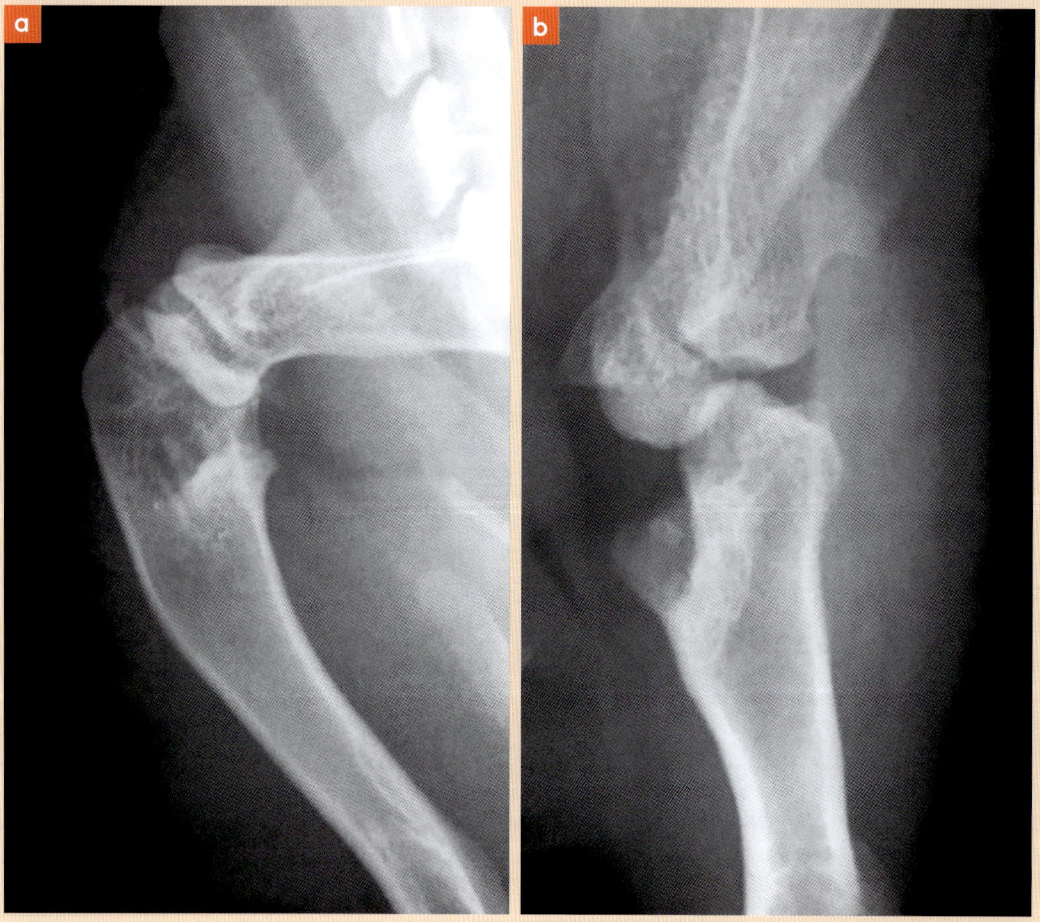

FIGURE 4.60. Mediolateral (a) and caudocranial (b) projections of the shoulder of a cat with malformation of this joint.

shoulder radiographs in dogs with osteochondritis dissecans of the humeral head. This sign is best appreciated on computed tomography scans.

Ligament injuries

In general, ligaments cannot be identified on X-rays because they have fluid/soft tissue density and, therefore, are indistinguishable from other joint components of similar radiopacity. The only exception is the patellar ligament of the knee, which is surrounded cranially by subcutaneous fat and caudally by infrapatellar fat, allowing its identification on the image.

When instability is observed in the orthopaedic examination of a joint, this would suggest the existence of some ligament injury, that is, a sprain. In these cases, X-rays in forced or stress projections are required, which must always be performed with patient under sedation. Some projections can be carried out without the operator in the room, using mechanical clamping (fig. 4.61), while others require the operator to be present. Lead gloves or mittens must be worn (fig. 4.62). Exposure to the main beam must be avoided whenever possible as the most energetic X-rays get through the leaded protection layer and irradiate the hands. When hyperextension, hyperflexion, valgus lateralisation or varus lateralization movements are forced, straps can be used to avoid hand exposure to the main X-ray beam. However, when radiographs are made with rotation of the joint, this movement cannot be performed with accessories so must be carried out by the operator.

Sprains are classified clinically as grade I (mild), grade II (moderate) and grade III (severe). Table 4.3 summarises the most common radiographic findings according to the sprain grade. These findings should

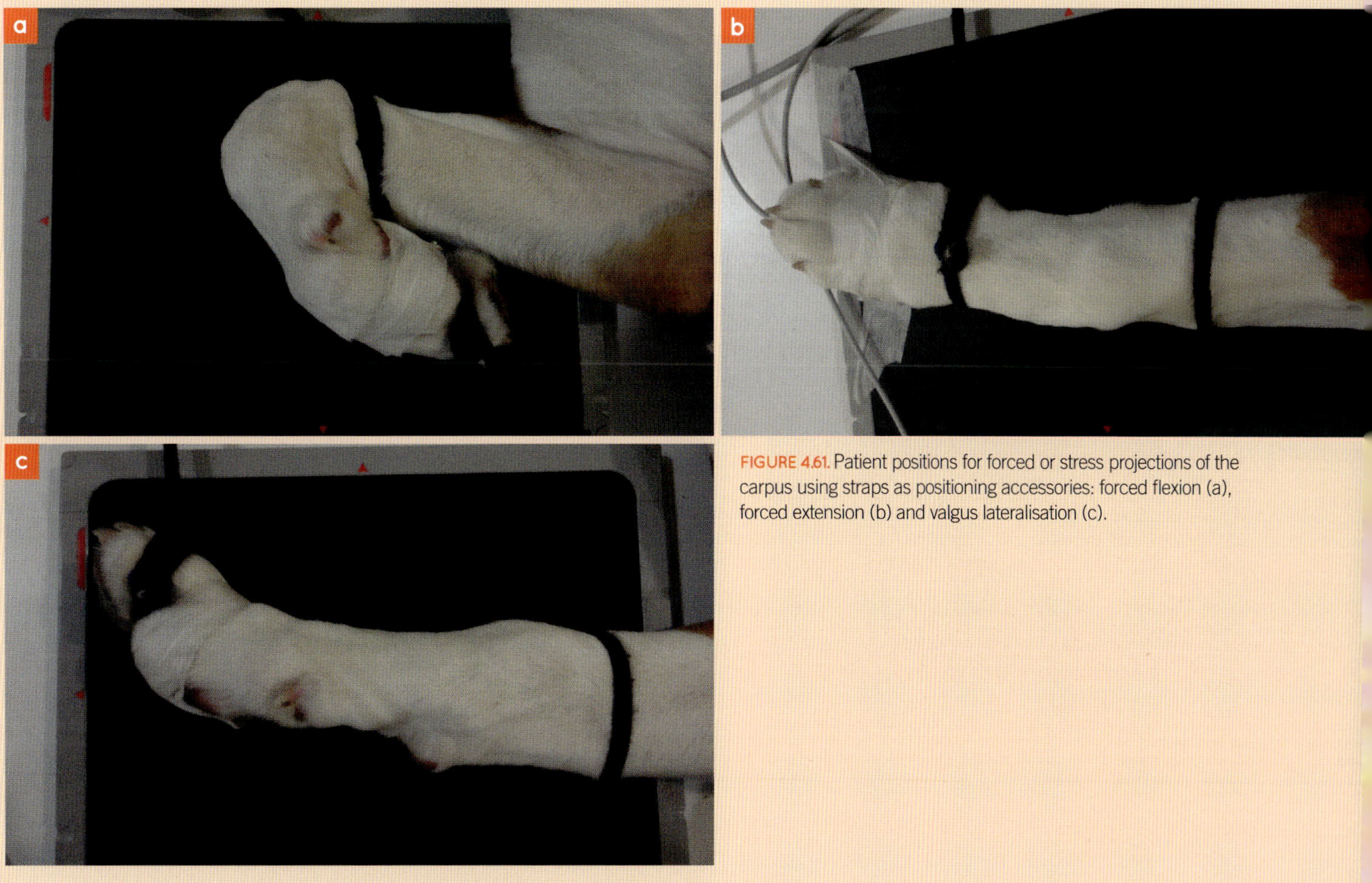

FIGURE 4.61. Patient positions for forced or stress projections of the carpus using straps as positioning accessories: forced flexion (a), forced extension (b) and valgus lateralisation (c).

always be correlated with orthopaedic examination. In these patients it is very important to compare the image of the injured limb with the contralateral limb and forced or stressed projections should always be performed (fig. 4.63).

The most common ligament lesion in clinical practice is the **cranial cruciate ligament rupture in the knee**. Although cranial tibial displacement or subluxation with respect to the femur is described as the typical radiographic sign of this pathology (fig. 4.64), in order to visualise this displacement on an X-ray a mediolateral projection forcing the displacement of the tibia is usually required and this often implies operator exposure. In practice, it is not necessary to perform a forced projection if the "cranial drawer sign" is evident in the orthopaedic examination. In a standard mediolateral projection in neutral position, we would rarely observe tibial subluxation. Radiological imaging of this joint would, however, allow us to assess whether signs of secondary degenerative joint disease have already developed at the time of diagnosis (fig. 4.65).

Tendon lesions

X-ray is usually not very useful for assessing diseases affecting tendons. Ultrasound, on the other hand, provides quite accurate diagnostic information but also requires extensive operator experience and very precise knowledge of the ultrasound anatomy of the musculoskeletal system.

A radiographic indicator of tendon pathology is the appearance of focal calcificated areas where the tendons are located, fundamentally at the insertion sites. For example, the appearance of mineralised areas immediately proximal to the greater trochanter of the femur, often bilaterally, is indicative of **calcific tendinitis of the gluteus medius** (fig. 4.66).

Biceps and supraspinatus tendinopathies in the shoulder may present with focal calcification of these tendons. Small calcifications may go undetected in a radiological study and be identified on an ultrasound.

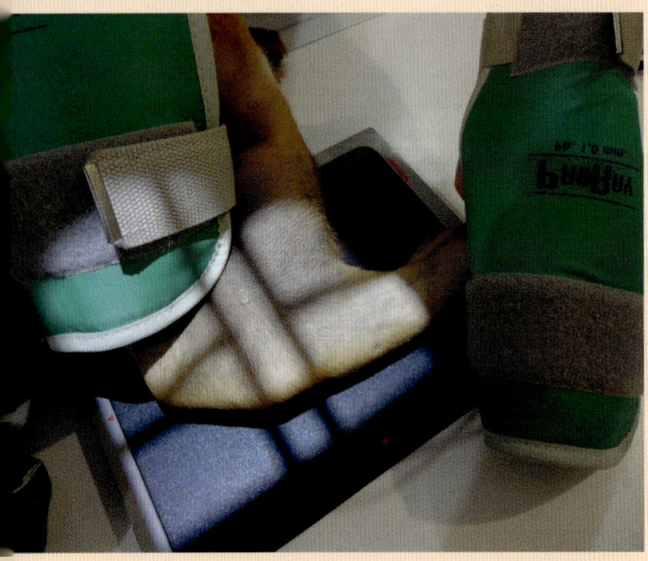

FIGURE 4.62. Patient positioning for forced cranial tibial displacement view for suspected rupture on cranial cruciate ligament in a dog. The operator wears protective lead mittens.

Table 4.3. Most common radiographic signs according to the sprain grade.

Sprain grade	Radiographic signs
Mild (Grade I)	▪ The only radiographic finding is usually an increase in soft tissue thickness at the ligament location, although this may not even be evident on the image. ▪ No associated bone lesions are observed. ▪ Forced projections show no abnormalities of joint spaces.
Moderate (Grade II)	▪ A moderate to marked increase in periarticular soft tissue thickness is generally seen. ▪ Associated bone lesions are rare. ▪ Abnormalities in joint spaces are usually not identified in neutral position projections but are identified in radiographs in forced projections.
Severe (Grade III)	▪ A marked increase in periarticular soft tissue thickness is usually observed. ▪ It is common for associated bone lesions to appear, which in many cases are small avulsion fractures. ▪ Abnormalities in joint spaces are usually seen in both neutral and forced positions.

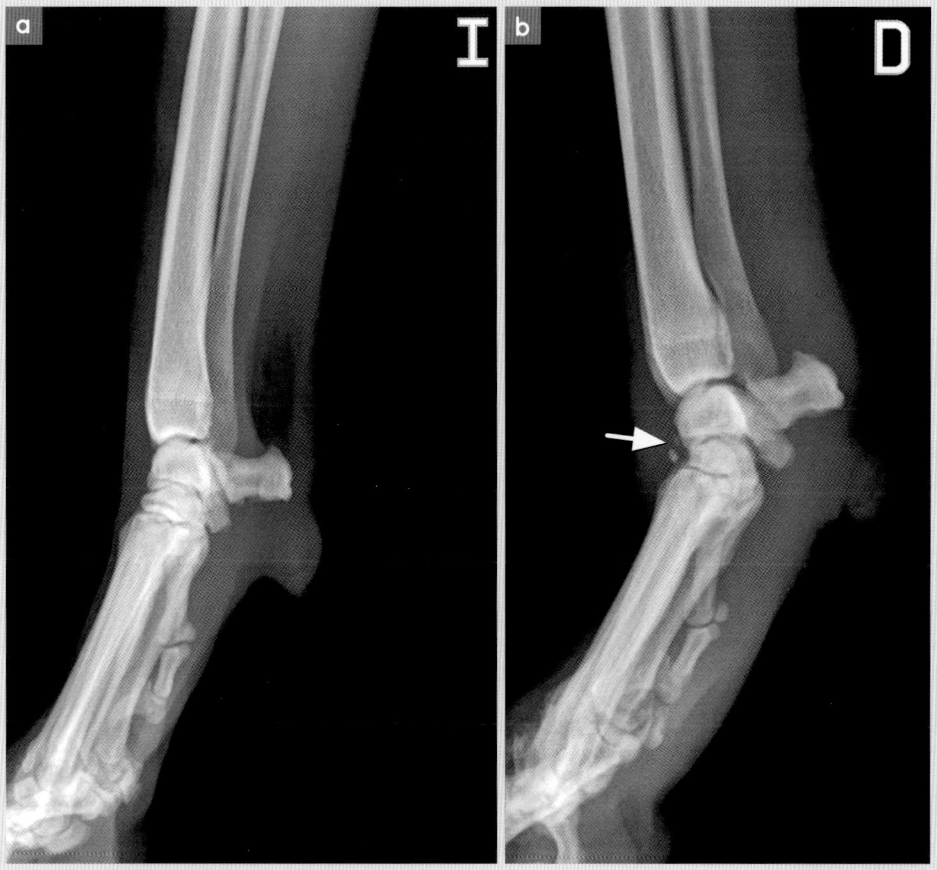

FIGURE 4.63. Mediolateral projection in forced hyperextension of both carpi of a dog with grade III right carpal sprain. The left carpus (a) shows no lesion and serves as a reference for normality in this projection. The right carpus (b) shows an increased extension angle and small bone fragments (arrow) on the dorsal aspect of the joint.

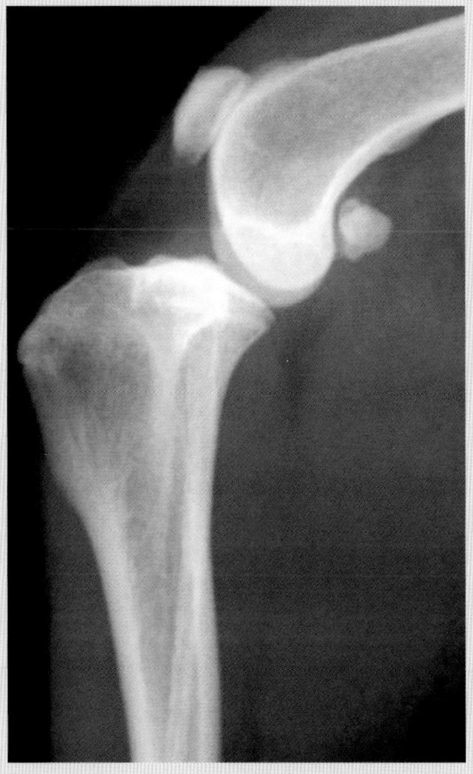

FIGURE 4.64. Forced mediolateral projection of the knee of a dog with a ruptured cranial cruciate ligament exhibiting cranial displacement of the tibia.

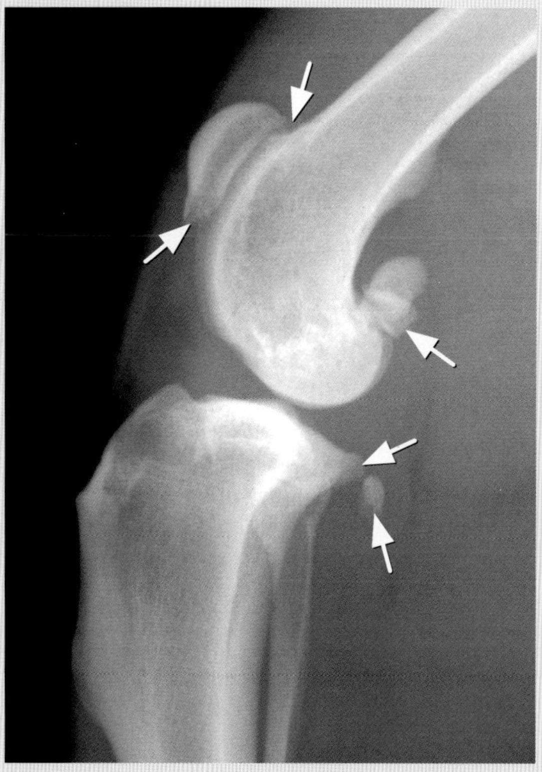

FIGURE 4.65. Mediolateral projection of the knee of a dog with a ruptured cranial cruciate ligament showing signs of secondary degenerative joint disease (osteophytes, white arrows). The narrowing of the infrapatellar fat silhouette is compatible with a marked increase in synovial volume, possibly due to moderate to severe synovial effusion.

The radiological image will suggest **biceps tendinopathy** when we observe areas of calcification at the location of this tendon, i.e. coinciding with the bicipital groove (fig. 4.67). Calcifications of this tendon may be confused with osteophytes located in the intertubercular groove of the humerus. The biceps tendon originates from the supraglenoid tubercle of the scapula, so an irregularity in the margin of this tubercle may also be indicative of pathology of this tendon.

The location of the supraspinatus tendon is more cranial, coinciding with the cranial part of the greater tubercle of the humerus. The appearance of mineralisations in this location further suggests **supraspinatus tendinopathy** (fig. 4.68). Tangential projections of the shoulder (fig. 4.69) may help distinguish them, since the location of the supraspinatus tendon is immediately cranial to the greater tubercle of the humerus, while that of the biceps is at the height of the sulcus intertubercularis and bicipital grooves. However, it is important to always correlate these radiographic findings with ultrasound examination of the joint.

Achilles or **calcaneus tendon lesions** usually cause soft tissue tumefaction at the insertion point, that is, around the proximal margin of the calcaneus, which may also present an irregular margin as a result of the tendon injury (fig. 4.70).

Sesamoids

Sesamoids that appear in the appendicular skeleton of dogs and cats are summarised in Table 4.4 (figs. 4.71 and 4.72). When a sesamoid divided into several parts is visualised, it may correspond to a **multipartite sesamoid** (fig. 4.73), which is considered an incidental finding of no clinical significance, or it may be a sesamoid fracture (fig. 4.74). A syndrome called **fragmented palmar metacarpophalangeal sesamoids** has been described which generally affects large dog breeds, with a greater incidence in Rottweilers. The fragmentation can be caused by bone necrosis (osteonecrosis), which in turn may be caused by developmental disorders, trauma or degenerative changes. The 2nd and 7th sesamoids, corresponding to the 2nd

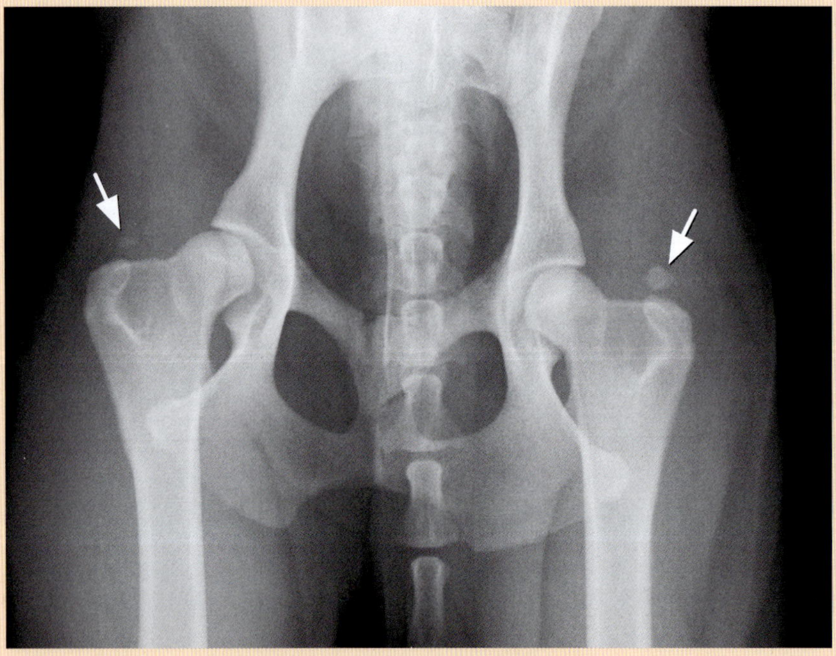

FIGURE 4.66. Ventrodorsal projection of the hip of a dog with calcific tendinitis of the gluteus medius. The arrows point to the calcifications at the muscle insertion area in both extremities.

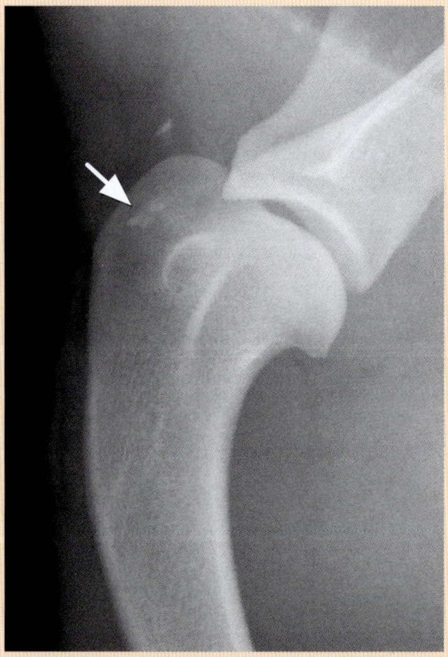

FIGURE 4.67. Mediolateral projection of the shoulder of a dog with biceps tendinopathy. The arrow points to mineralisation at the location of the tendon.

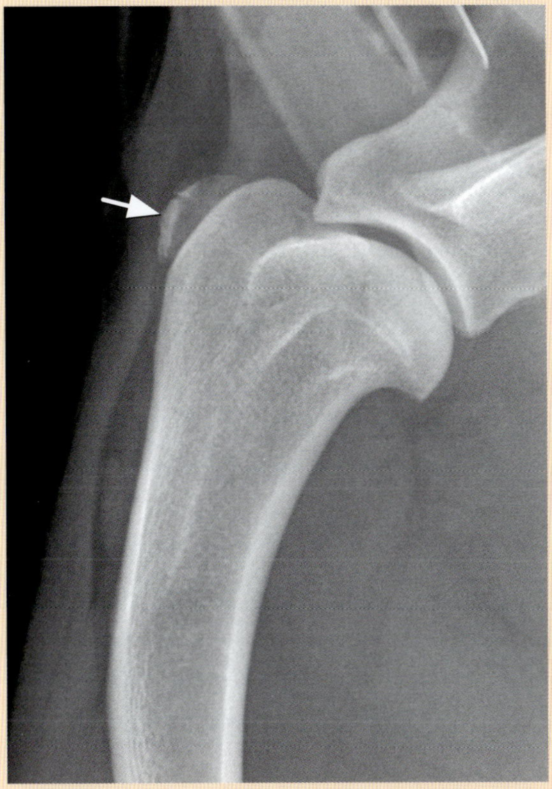

FIGURE 4.68. Mediolateral projection of the shoulder of a dog with supraspinatus tendinopathy. The arrow points to calcification at the location of the tendon.

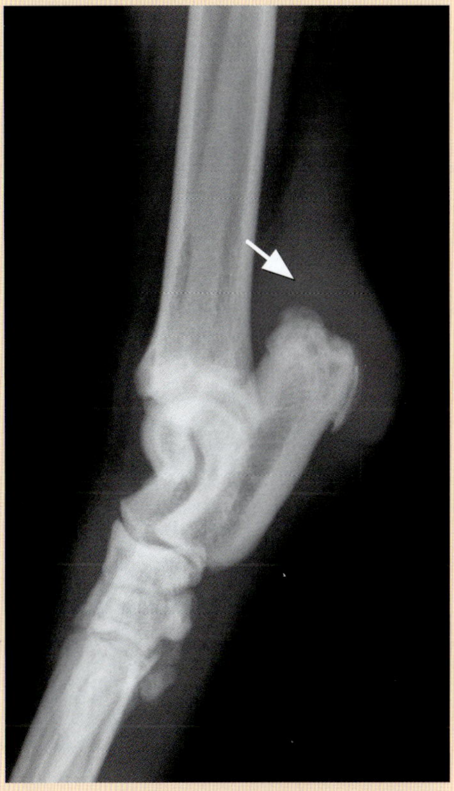

FIGURE 4.70. Mediolateral projection of the tarsus of a dog with a previous old rupture of the calcaneus tendon (Achilles tendon). Soft tissue thickening is observed in the location area, marked remodelling of the proximal calcaneus margin and small areas of mineralisation along the tendon (arrow).

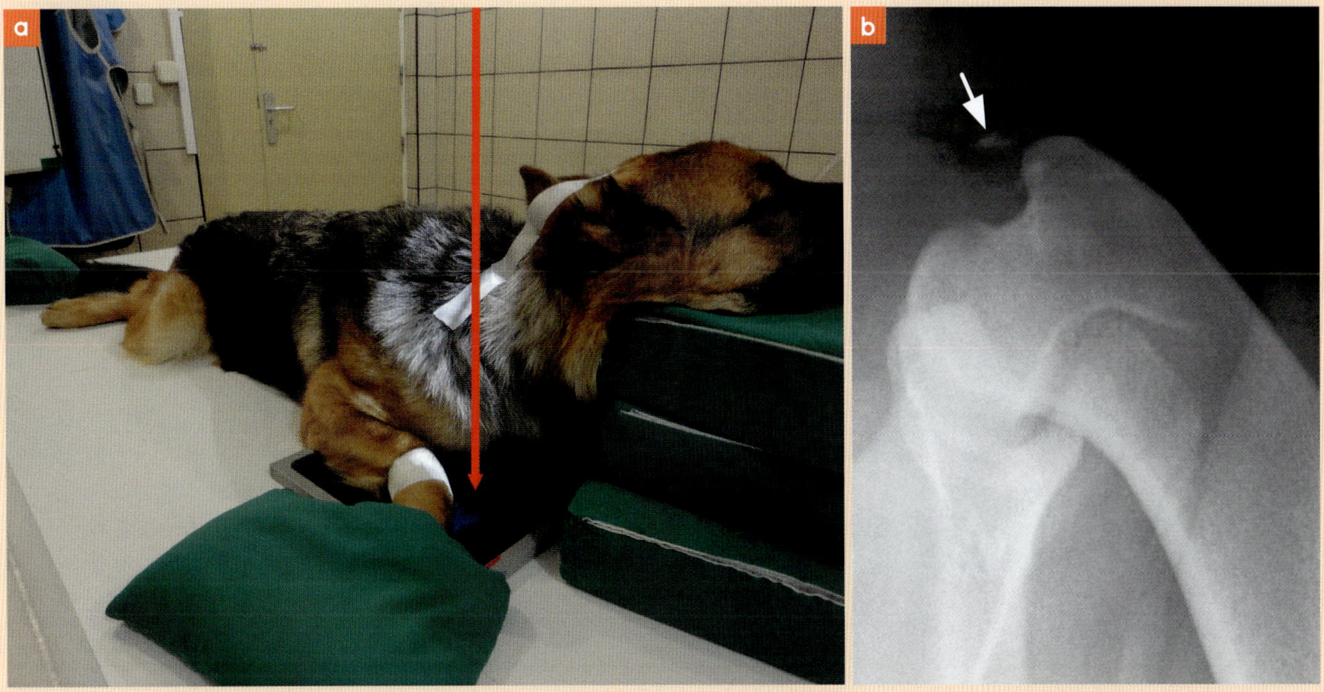

FIGURE 4.69. Patient position for tangential projection of the shoulder (a) and X-ray of the tangential projection of the shoulder (b) of a dog with supraspinatus tendinopathy (white arrow points to mineralisation in the area where the tendon is located). The red arrow on image (a) indicates the direction of the X-ray beam.

and 4th digits respectively, tend to be more affected. In the case of the Rottweiler, it has been shown that this syndrome can cause lameness in puppies in a very high percentage of cases. The margins of fragments of a multipartite sesamoid are usually smooth and regular, while those of a fragmented sesamoid usually have less defined or irregular edges, which would help differentiate them on an X-ray.

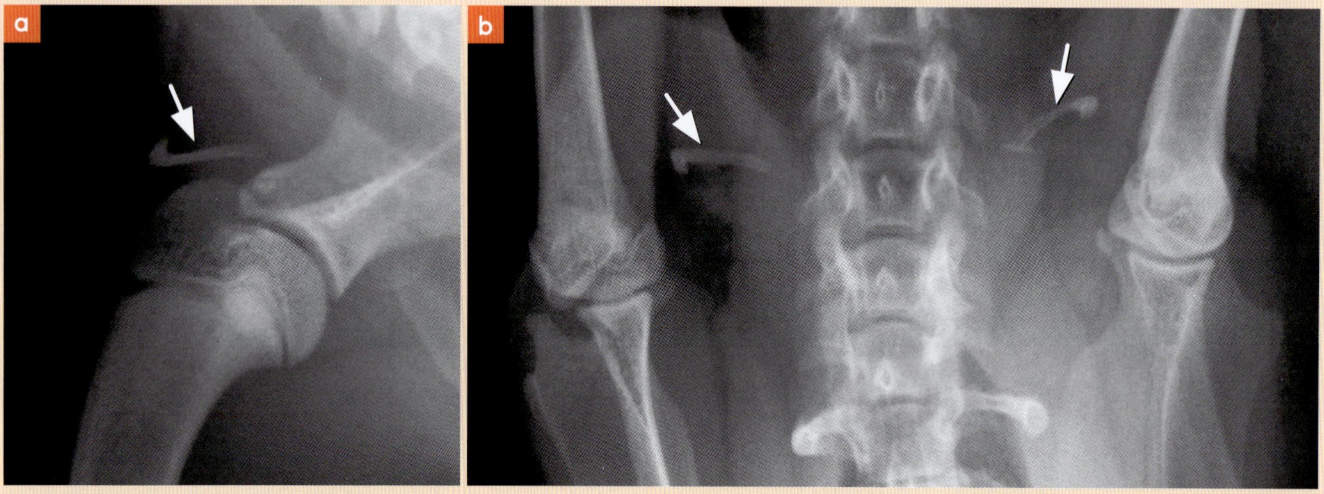

FIGURE 4.71. Mediolateral projection (a) of one shoulder and caudocranial projection (b) of both shoulders of a cat. Arrows point to the clavicles.

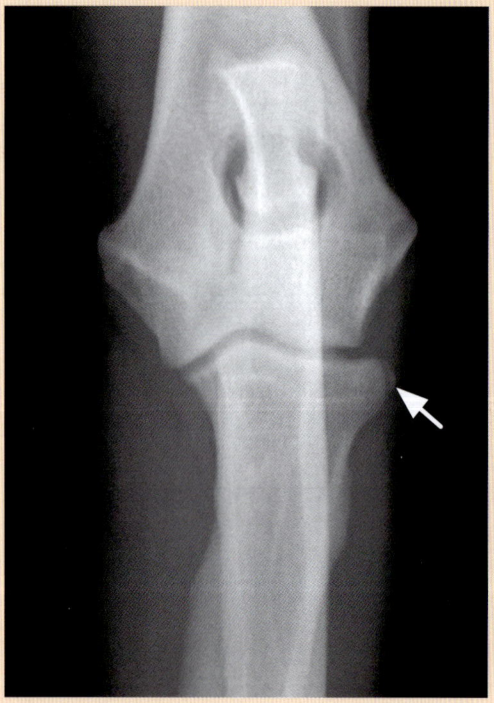

FIGURE 4.72. Craniocaudal projection of the elbow of a healthy dog. The arrow points to the sesamoid of the tendon of origin of the supinator muscle, located adjacent to the craniolateral surface of the radial head.

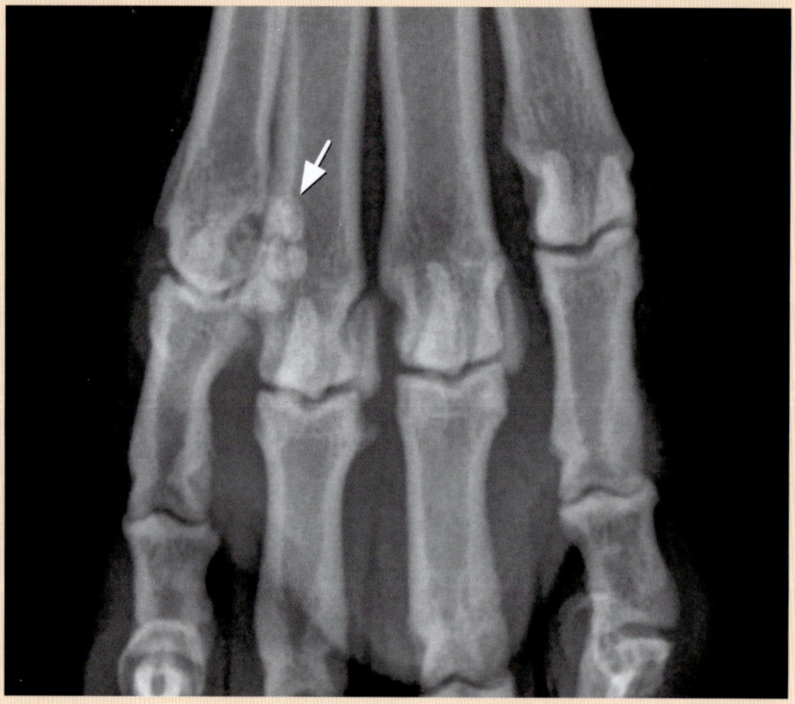

FIGURE 4.73. Dorsoplantar projection of the metacarpophalangeal joint of a dog with a multipartite sesamoid bone (arrow).

Variation in the position of sesamoids may be incidental or have pathological causes. For example, it is very common for the medial sesamoid of the gastrocnemius muscle to appear in a more medial and distal position than the lateral sesamoid. If this finding is bilateral, it is more likely to be incidental, due to anatomical variation in the patient (fig. 4.75). If it is unilateral, although it may also be incidental, injury to the gastrocnemius muscle may not be ruled out as a cause of this variation in location.

The most common example of sesamoid displacement is patella dislocation (luxation). Patellar luxation or subluxation may be of congenital or traumatic origin, with the former being much more common. The cause of patellar luxation is considered to be associated with conformational deformities and to

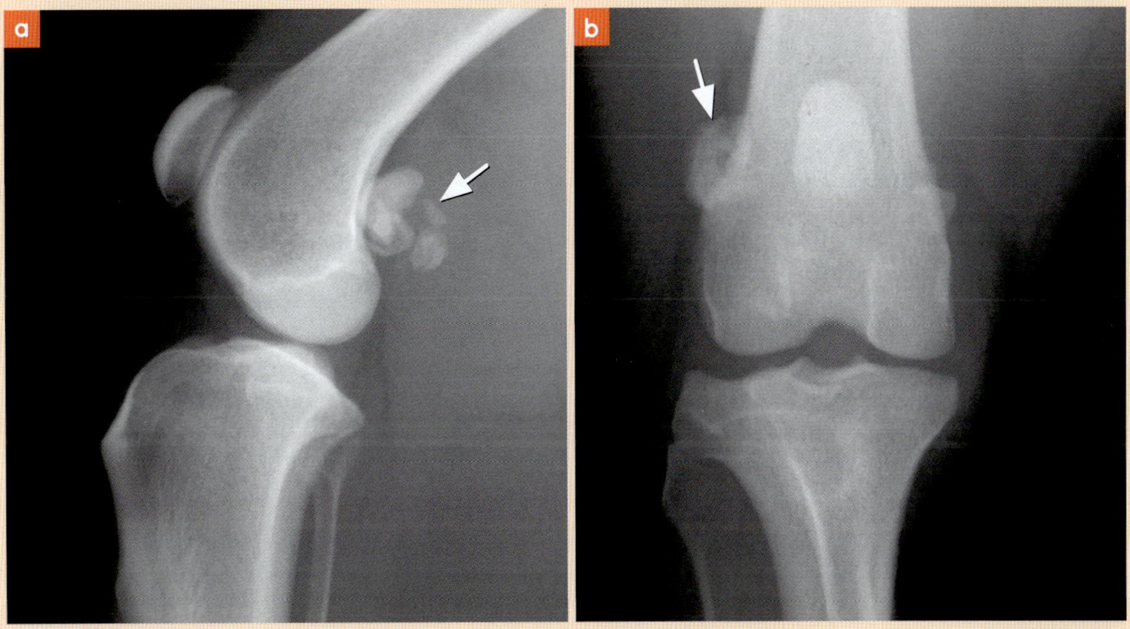

FIGURE 4.74. Mediolateral (a) and craniocaudal (b) projections of the knee of a dog with old fragmentation of the lateral sesamoid of the gastrocnemius muscle.

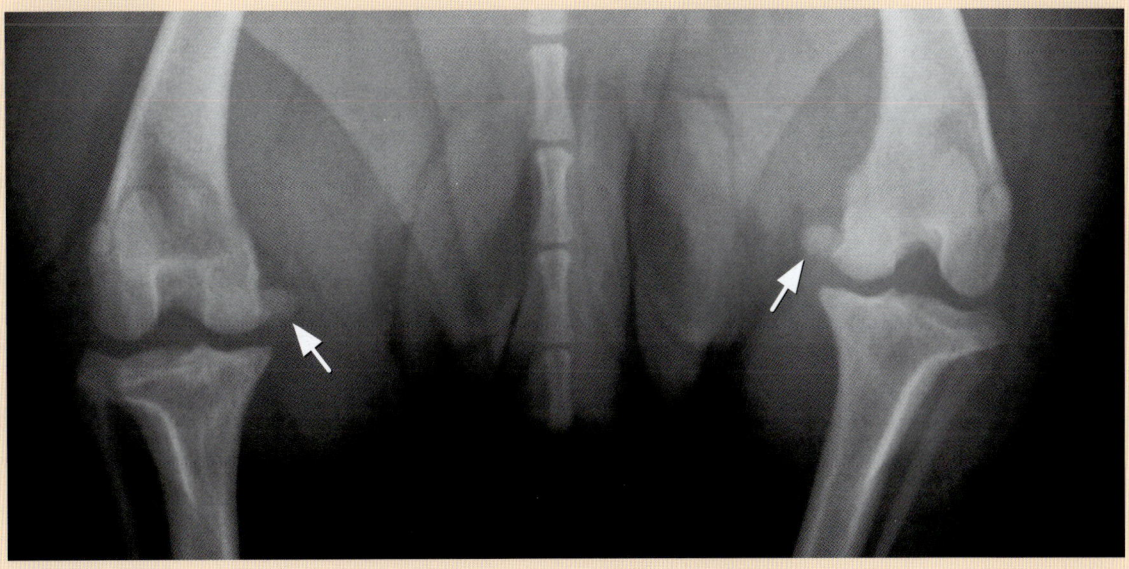

FIGURE 4.75. Enlarged image of the knees in a ventrodorsal projection of the hip, in which the arrows point to both medial sesamoids of the gastrocnemius muscle, which appear displaced medially and distally. This finding is usually incidental, especially if it is bilateral.

be multifactorial. The patellar extension mechanism is made up of the quadriceps muscles, patellar tendon, patella, patellar ligament and tibial tuberosity. This extension mechanism should form a straight line between the median plane of the proximal femur and the median plane of the tarsus. Most patients with patellar luxation have poor alignment of this extensor mechanism, which is considered a predisposing factor. Most dislocations are considered congenital because they occur in relatively young animals and are not associated with trauma. Although the patient may not have patellar dislocation at birth, it may well have some limb deformation that will cause this luxating at a later date. In these patients, the tibia appears curved medially. This alteration in the tibial conformation is believed to be compensatory, in other words, it was not always present, but this is not clear. In addition, the lack of pressure from the patella on the trochlear groove of the femur makes it appear more shallow or even flattened.

Medial dislocation of the patella is much more frequent than lateral. Approximately 75–80 % of knee dislocations occur medially (fig. 4.76). In general, patellar luxation is much more common in small or miniature dog breeds. In large breeds, in which this condition is much less common, lateral luxation is considered to be more frequent (fig. 4.77), although it appears that in recent years the diagnosis of medial luxation has increased significantly in large and giant breeds, especially in Labrador, Siberian Husky, Alaskan Malamute and Akita Inu. It has also been seen to occur concurrently with cranial cruciate ligament rupture in up to 20 % of cases.

Clinically, patellar dislocation has been classified into four grades based on orthopaedic examination and not radiographic findings. In fact, when a patient is classified as grades 1 and 2, on the craniocaudal or caudal projection of the knee, the patella may appear in its normal position. Apart from the standard projections, in some cases a tangential projection of the knee will be necessary (fig. 4.78), which will allow a more precise evaluation especially of the flattening of the trochlear groove, in addition to the position of the patella (fig. 4.79).

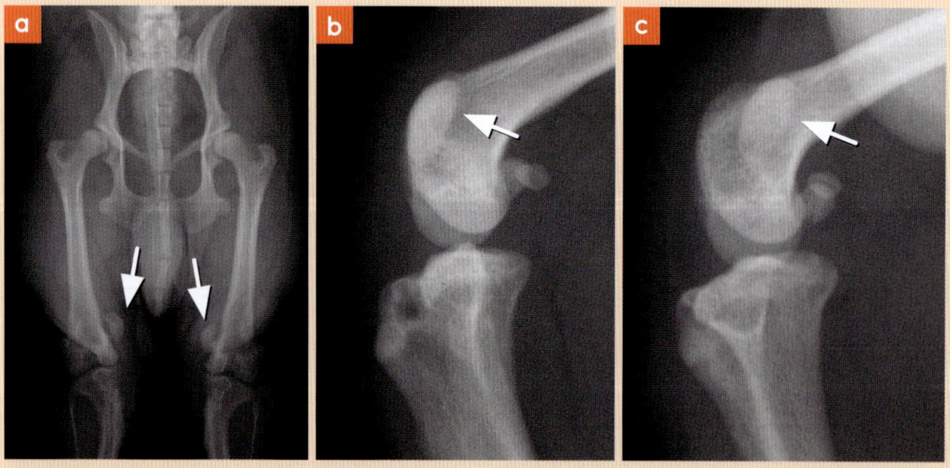

FIGURE 4.76. Ventrodorsal radiograph of the hip (a) and mediolateral radiograph of the left (b) and right knees (c) of a dog with bilateral medial patellar luxation (arrows). In image (a), the tibia looks curved medially. In images (b) and (c) the patella looks superimposed on the distal femur.

FIGURE 4.77. Ventrodorsal radiograph of the hip of a dog with lateral right patellar luxation. ▶

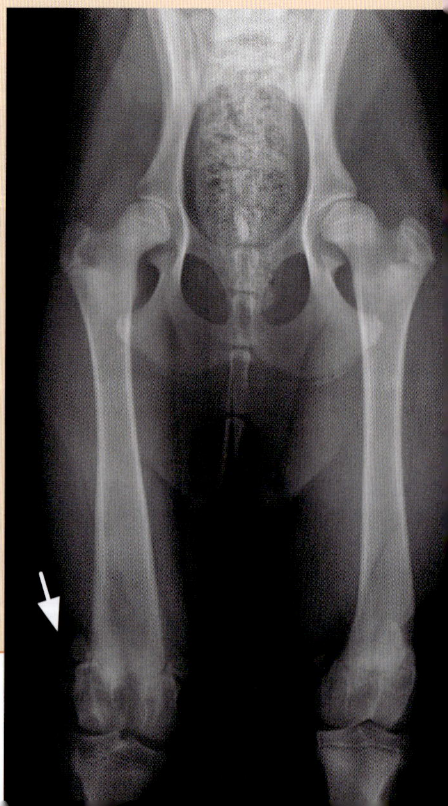

Table 4.4. Sesamoids in the appendicular skeleton in dogs and cats.	
Joint	**Name and location**
Shoulder	Clavicle (curvilinear and larger in cats and small or absent in dogs) at the medial tendon insertion of the brachiocephalic muscle, proximal to the greater tubercle of the humerus (fig. 4.71).
Elbow	Uncommon. It appears on the tendon of origin of the supinator muscle, adjacent to the craniolateral margin of the radial head (fig. 4.72). Usually bilateral if present.
Carpus	Often appears medial to the carpometacarpal joint, at the insertion of the tendon of the abductor pollicis longus muscle, near the proximal surface of the first metacarpal.
Metacarpophalangeal	Palmar sesamoids (paired) in the tendons of insertion of the interossei muscles. Individual dorsal sesamoids in the extensor tendons.
Coxofemoral	Very uncommon. It appears in the iliopubic cartilage, located cranially to the iliopubic eminence.
Knee	Patella on the femoral quadriceps tendon (the largest sesamoid). Two sesamoids in the lateral and medial tendons of the gastrocnemius muscle. A sesamoid bone of the popliteus muscle tendon.
Tarsus	Uncommon. Lateral-plantar tarsometatarsal sesamoids and intra-articular tarsometatarsal sesamoids. They can appear laterally or medially in the fibrocartilage.
Metatarsophalangeal	Plantar sesamoids (paired) in the tendons of insertion of the interossei muscles. Individual dorsal sesamoids in the extensor tendons.

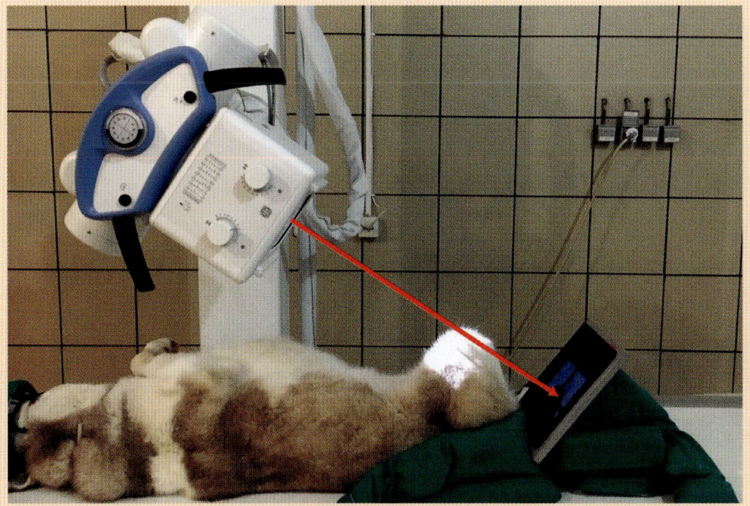

FIGURE 4.78. Patient position for a tangential projection of the knee.

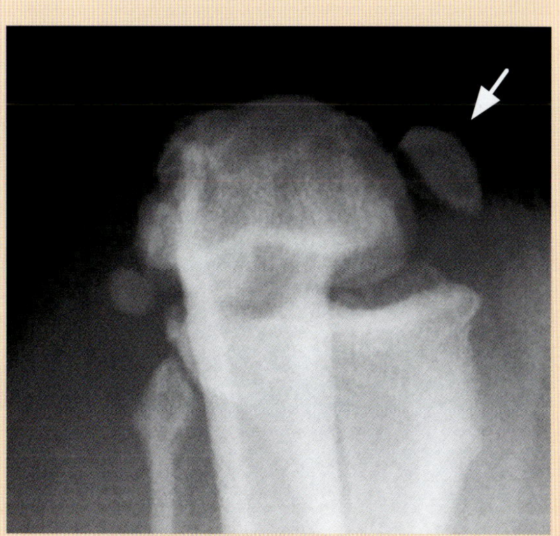

FIGURE 4.79. Tangential projection of the knee of a dog with medial patellar luxation, which appears markedly displaced medially (arrow). Degenerative changes in the femoral condyle can be observed, with marked trochlear groove remodelling.

Luxations and subluxations

Luxations are the complete loss of the normal congruity between the joint surfaces of two bones (fig. 4.80). When there is still a certain amount of apposition between them, the term subluxation is used (fig. 4.81). Luxations and subluxations are relatively easy to diagnose radiologically, although they are sometimes not evident on one of the orthogonal views. They may be caused by trauma, although they can also have a congenital origin or appear secondarily to developmental abnormalities. The most frequent congenital luxations are those affecting the elbow (fig. 4.82) and the shoulder, although they can affect other joints. They cause marked remodelling of the articular surfaces by degeneration.

Degenerative joint disease

The most common joint disease in dogs and cats is degenerative joint disease, also called **osteoarthritis** or **arthritis**. It can be primary (idiopathic) or secondary to other developmental or acquired diseases. Radiologically it is characterised by the appearance of increased volume of the joint fluid/soft tissue, formation of osteophytes and enthesophytes, increased or decreased subchondral bone opacity, appearance of intraarticular or periarticular soft tissue mineralisations (fig. 4.83) and, in advanced or severe cases, a decrease in the width of the joint space can be seen. It is, however, uncommon to observe the latter radiographic finding.

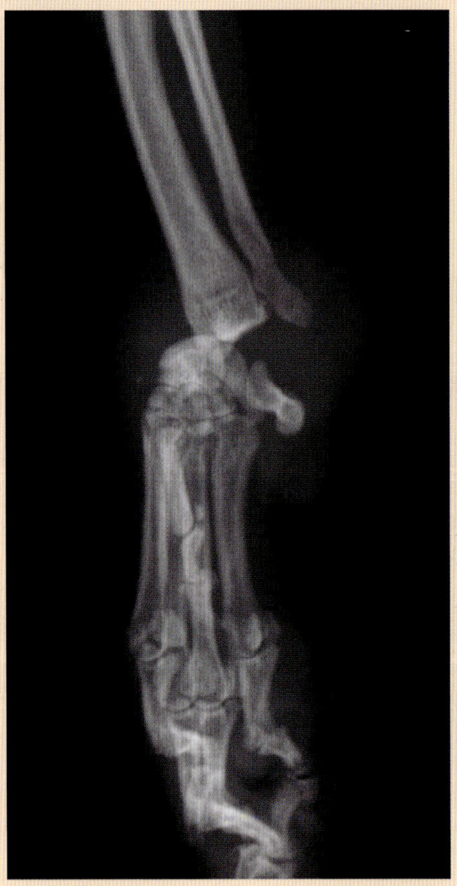

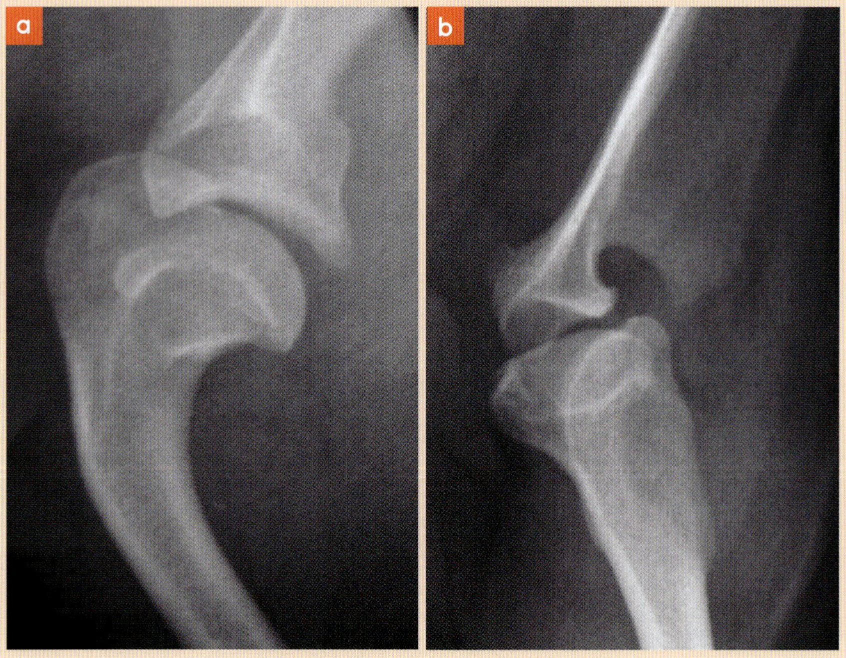

FIGURE 4.81. Mediolateral (a) and craniocaudal (b) radiographs of the elbow of a dog with scapulohumeral subluxation.

FIGURE 4.80. Mediolateral radiograph of the carpus of a dog with antebrachiocarpal joint luxation.

Infection

Septic arthritis may appear as a consequence of penetrating wounds affecting the joint, although they are also spread haematogenously. In the latter, one or several joints may be affected. Although the image could be mistaken for severe arthritis, the increase in the volume of joint fluid/soft tissue is normally higher, the appearance of subchondral bone defects is more frequent and the periarticular osteophytes and enthesophytes tend to have a more aggressive appearance (fig. 4.84). Secondarily, infection can spread to the bone. The diagnosis is confirmed by cytology and joint fluid culture.

Immune-mediated polyarthropathy

The term refers to the set of joint diseases with an immune-mediated origin. They are classified as erosive and non-erosive. It typically affects multiple joints, thus the term polyarthropathy. When inflammation of multiple joints is observed, haematogenous septic arthritis or immune-mediated polyarthropathy must be considered in the differential diagnosis.

In **non-erosive immune-mediated polyarthritis,** an increase in joint fluid/soft tissue volume is usually observed on radiographs, with no apparent bone abnormalities.

Erosive immune-mediated polyarthropathy is less frequent. In addition to the changes described in the non-erosive form, joint edge erosion is observed (fig. 4.85) and in many cases, aggressive periosteal reaction. The most common type of erosive polyarthropathy in the dog is rheumatoid arthritis. However,

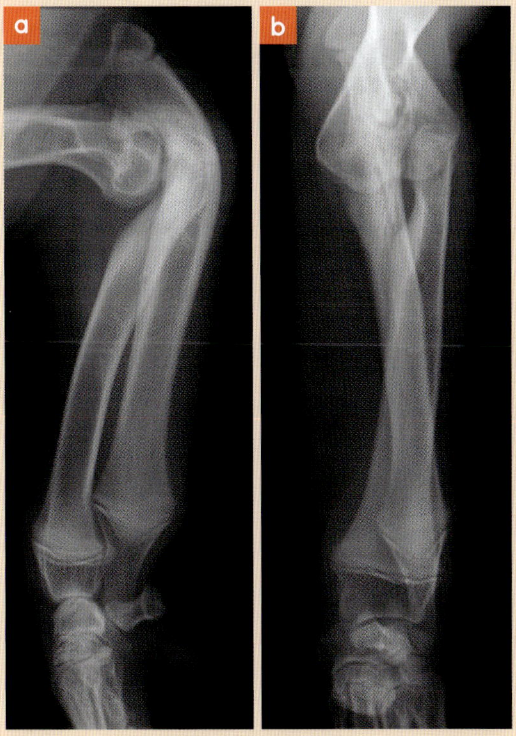

FIGURE 4.82. Mediolateral (a) and craniocaudal (b) radiographs of the radius and ulna of a dog with congenital luxation of the elbow. The proximal part of radius and ulna is very deformed and normal alignment between the humerus and the radial head is lost.

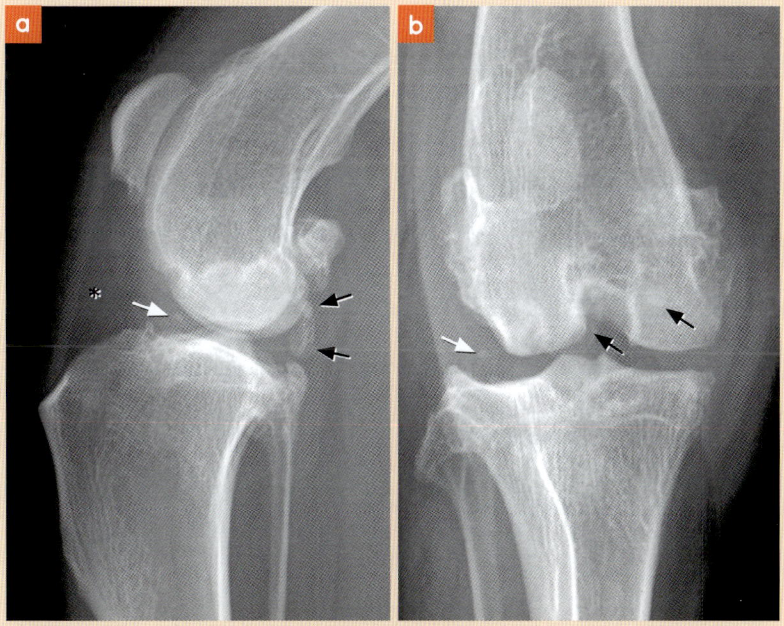

FIGURE 4.83. Mediolateral (a) and caudocranial (b) radiographs of the knee of a dog with moderate to severe degenerative joint disease. Osteophytes appear in the femoral trochlea, proximal and distal margins of the patella, sesamoids of the gastrocnemius and popliteus muscles, tibial plateau, medial margin of the medial epicondyles and lateral margin of the lateral epicondyles of femur and tibia, which are all typical locations of osteophytes appearing in this joint. In addition, intra-articular (white arrow) and peri-articular (black arrows) soft tissue mineralisations are identified. The mediolateral projection shows moderate narrowing of the infrapatellar fat pad (asterisk), which suggests the existence of moderate synovial effusion.

it is rare in dogs and cats. It usually affects the distal joints (mainly the carpus and tarsus, followed by metacarpus and metatarsus) of small and miniature breed dogs. In cats, the most striking radiographic finding is periosteal reaction and it has only been described in young male cats. Diagnosis is confirmed by the rheumatoid factor blood test, joint fluid analysis and synovial biopsy.

Joint tumours

Joint tumours are rare in dogs and very rare in cats. They most commonly affect medium or large dog breeds, and their most frequent location is the knee or elbow, although they can appear at any location. They usually cause a marked increase in volume of joint fluid/soft tissue, significant widening of the joint space due to soft tissue proliferation and marked erosion of the joint margins and subchondral bone, with well-defined osteolysis areas (fig. 4.86).

Other appendicular skeleton abnormalities

Pulmonary hypertrophic osteopathy

It is also called Marie's disease, hypertrophic osteopathy or pulmonary hypertrophic osteoarthropathy. This disease is usually associated with the presence of lesions in the thorax (generally masses), although it has also been described linked to abdominal diseases.

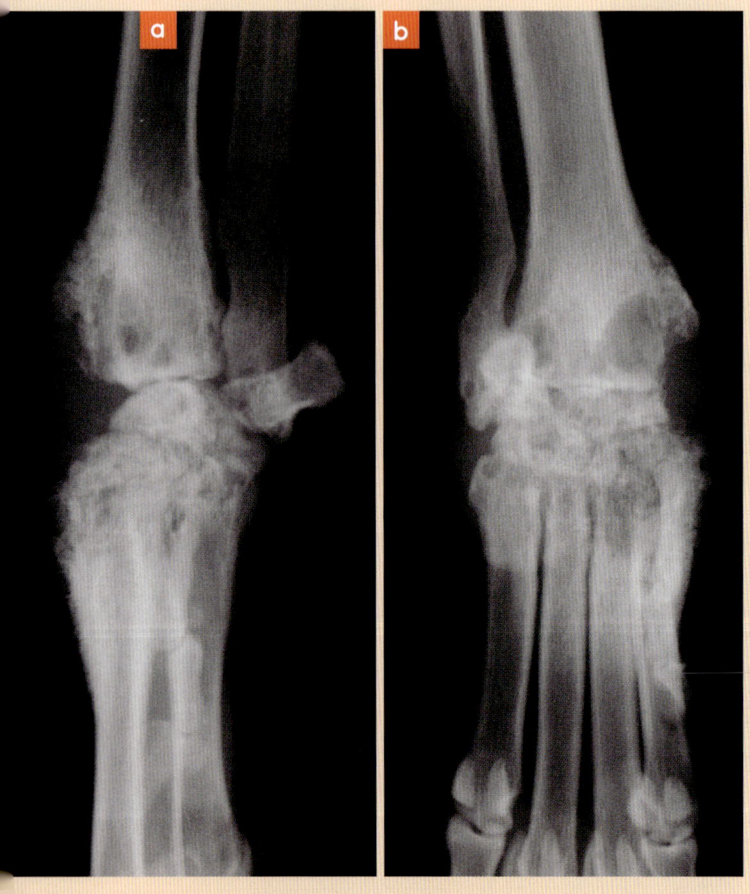

FIGURE 4.84. Mediolateral (a) and dorsopalmar (b) radiographs of the carpus of a dog with septic arthritis. Numerous osteolytic areas appear on the joint surfaces of every bone forming the joint. Periarticular osteophytes look more aggressive than those caused by degenerative joint disease.

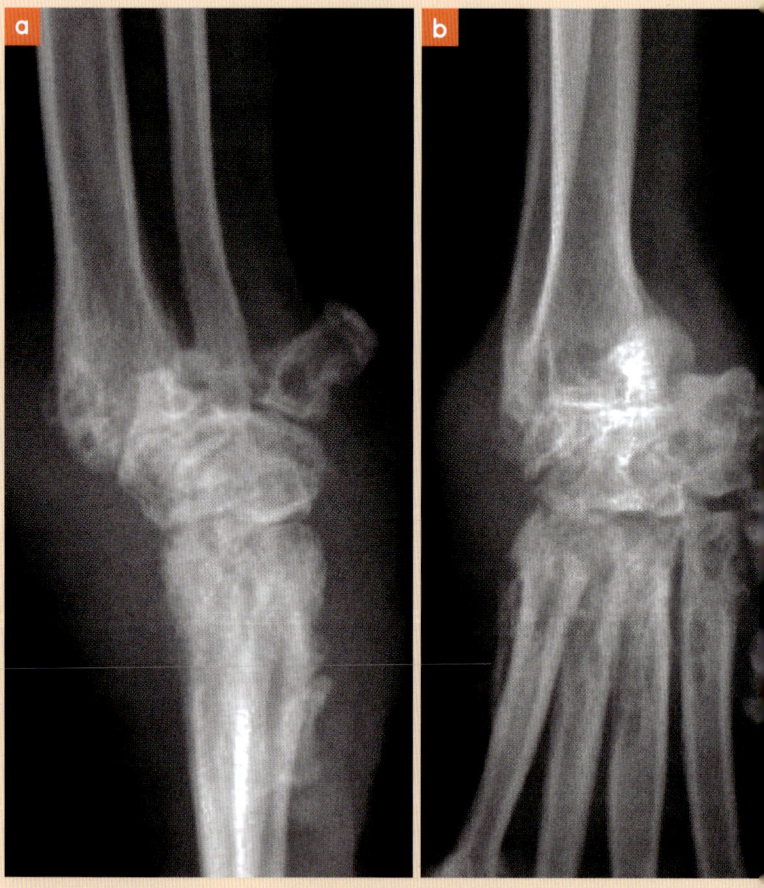

FIGURE 4.85. Mediolateral (a) and dorsopalmar (b) radiographs of the carpus of a dog with erosive immune-mediated polyarthropathy. Marked tumescence of the soft tissues surrounding the joint is observed, as well as osteolytic lesions (erosive) in the joint surfaces of all bones that make up the joint, extending even to the metacarpal diaphysis.

It is clinically characterised by affecting older dogs, that present with hot and painful inflammation of the distal limb area, as well as lameness. The first affected bones are the phalanges. If the primary cause is resolved, it is a reversible process. Radiographic signs are (fig. 4.87):

- Palisading periosteal reaction.
- Initial lesions tend to be distal and may affect the four limbs.
- Lesions may be bilaterally symmetrical.
- Marked soft-tissue inflammation.

To evaluate the presence of possible lesions in both anatomical regions, thoracic and abdominal radiographs should always be taken.

Circumscribed calcinosis

It presents as ectopic calcification foci in soft tissues, generally periarticularly located (fig. 4.88). It usually affects young large breed dogs, especially the German Shepherd.

Multiple cartilaginous exostoses

It is an benign osteoproliferative disease that appears in growing dogs. Exostoses in long bone metaphyses, vertebrae and ribs are evident on radiographs. It usually does not have clinical significance, unless the lesions cause excessive compression of certain anatomical structures such as the spinal cord, but this is rare. Lesions cease to grow when skeletal

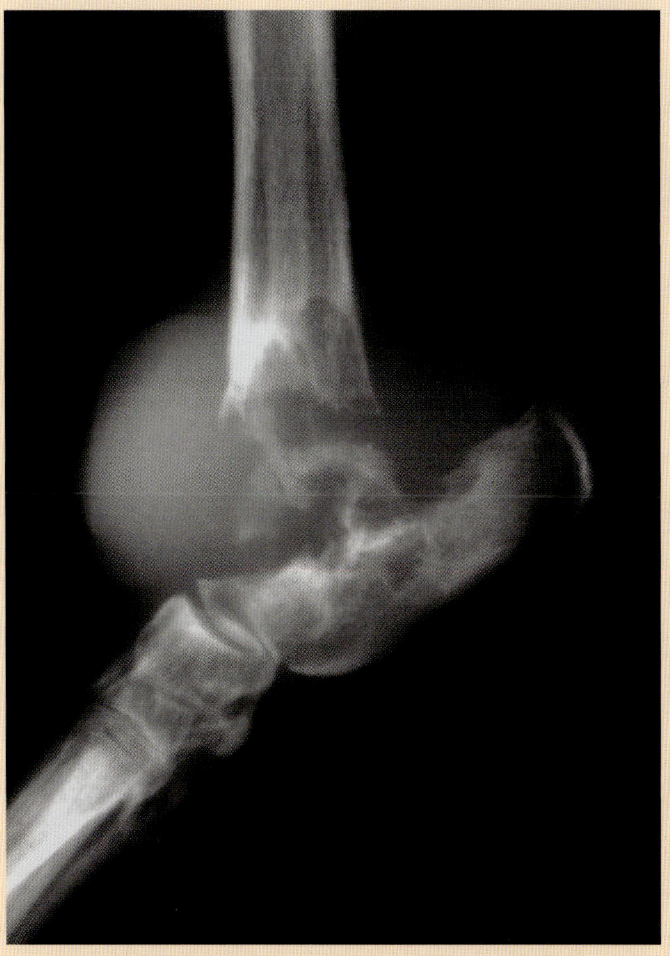

FIGURE 4.86. Mediolateral radiograph of the tarsus of a dog with a joint neoplasm. Marked soft tissue tumescence is observed, as well as great destruction (osteolysis) of the joint edges.

FIGURE 4.87. Dorsopalmar projection of the distal radius and ulna, carpus and metacarpals of a dog with hypertrophic pulmonary osteopathy (Marie's disease). Long bones exhibit a palisading periosteal reaction.

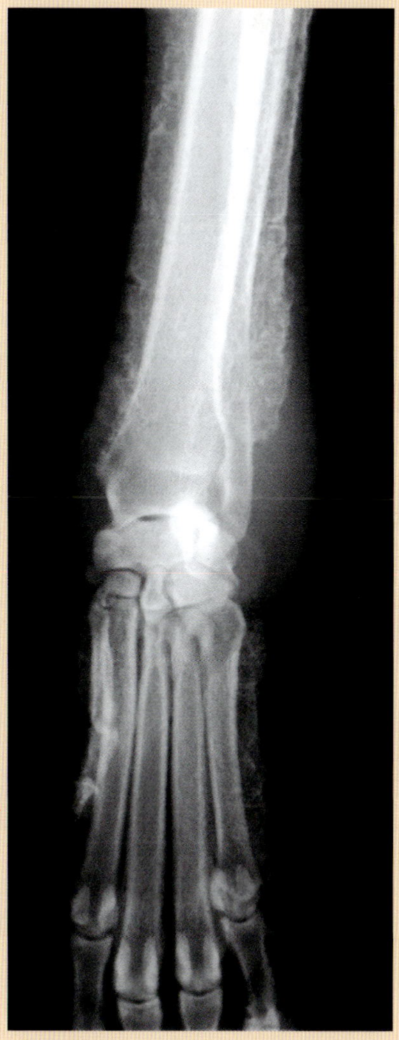

maturation of the animal concludes. Exceptionally, cases of affected adults and continued growth of the lesions after skeletal maturation have been described.

A similar disorder has been described in cats, although it may be of viral origin. Lesions appear in adult cats and they grow progressively. They are similar to those caused by hypervitaminosis A.

Cases for **self-assessment**

Case 4.1. Presentation Explanation

Case 4.2. Presentation Explanation

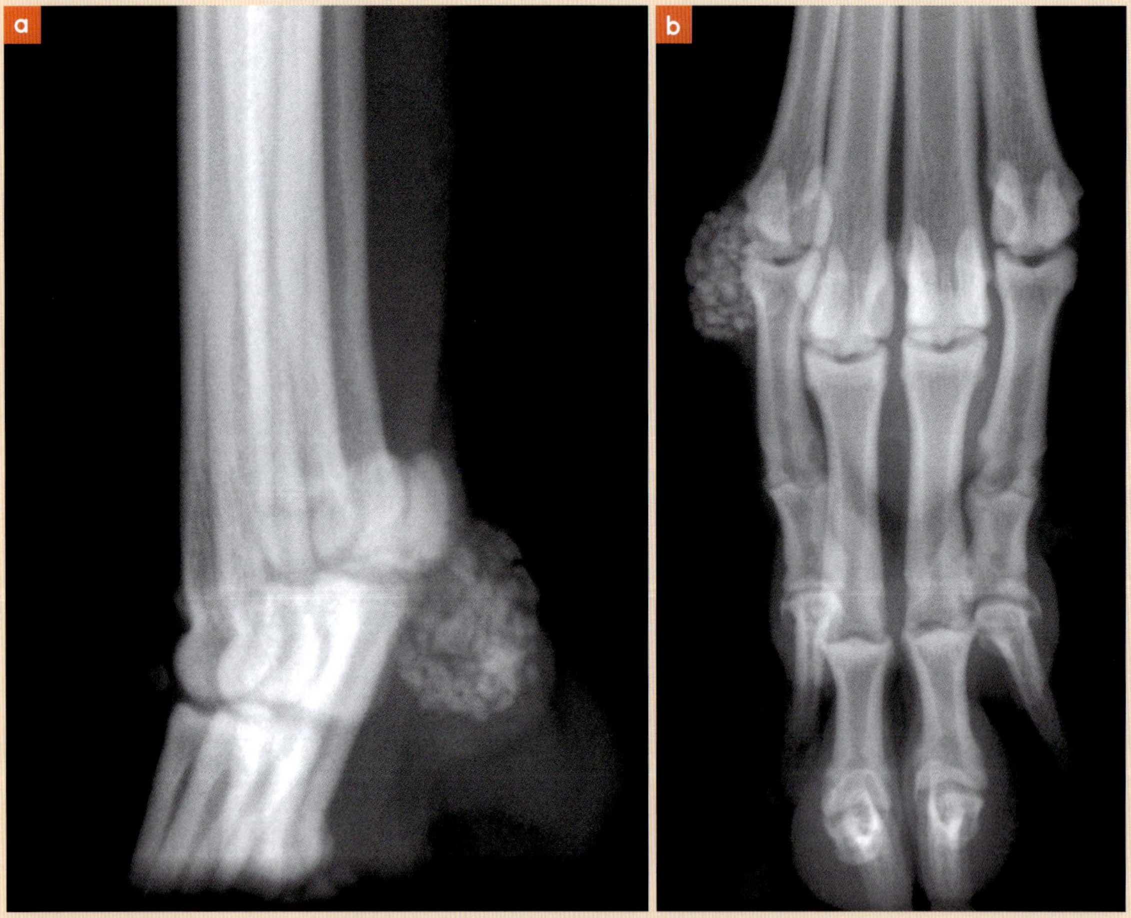

FIGURE 4.88. Mediolateral (a) and dorsoplantar (b) projections of the metatarsals and phalanges of a dog with calcinosis circumscripta, which appears as a lesion formed by multiple calcified foci in the medial and plantar area of the metatarsophalangeal joint. It is a benign lesion that is usually periarticularly located and it is more frequent in young dogs, especially in German Shepherds.

Spine 5

Normal radiographic anatomy of the spine
https://goo.by/Gspgz

Principles of interpretation

Both dogs and cats have 7 cervical vertebrae, 13 thoracic vertebrae, 7 lumbar vertebrae, 3 sacral vertebrae and a variable number of coccygeal vertebrae. Each anatomical region of the spine has different characteristics, and it is necessary to know them in order to interpret radiographs correctly. These are described in the following boxes.

Good-quality images are essential to carry out a thorough assessment of the spine. That is why it is recommended to take radiographs under sedation, using appropriate positioning accessories (radiolucent blocks, tape and sand bags).

In lateral projection, the longitudinal axis of the spine has to be parallel to the cassette, which is achieved

Thoracic spine

- T11 is the anticlinal vertebra (its spinous process is vertical instead of being directed caudally or cranially).
- T10–T1 is the anticlinal1 intervertebral space, which is the narrowest intervertebral space.
- The heads of the ribs appear cranial to their corresponding vertebrae.

Cervical spine

- C1 has a large transverse process (wings of the atlas).
- C2 is the largest vertebra and has a process in the cranioventral area of its body, called the odontoid process.
- The C2–C3 and C7–T1 intervertebral disc spaces are usually narrower than the rest.
- C6 has a large, characteristic ventral lamina.
- The spinous process of C2 must be adjacent to or superimposed on the arch of C1.

Lumbar spine

- The cat's lumbar vertebrae are longer than those of the dog.
- The ventral border of L3 and L4 can appear slightly blurry in dogs, especially in large breeds, which is due to the crura of the diaphragm being superimposed (this image should not be confused with that of a lesion).

Sacrum and coccygeal vertebrae

- The three vertebrae that form the sacrum are usually fused.
- Coccygeal vertebrae have haemal processes, which should not be confused with spondylosis deformans.

by placing a radiolucent block under the cervical area and another one under the lumbar area (fig. 5.1). To ensure that the sagittal plane of the vertebrae is parallel to the cassette, it is necessary to place blocks in order to slightly elevate the position of the limbs. If the spine is twisted when taking a lateral radiograph, the transverse processes of each vertebra will be separated in the image (fig. 5.2).

Lateral rotation of the spine should be avoided when taking a radiograph in ventrodorsal projection. If the position of the patient is correct, the spinous processes will be aligned and centred with the vertebral bodies in the image (fig. 5.3).

A complete study of the spine should include two cervical radiographs (one centred on C3–C4 and another one on C6–C7), a thoracic radiograph (centred on T6–T7) and a thoracolumbar radiograph (centred on T13–L1). Usually, the previous clinical assessment of the patient allows the location of the region or regions of the spine that may be injured, which narrows the radiographic study down to the affected area.

Spinal radiographs taken in forced flexion or extension may be useful for the diagnosis of certain diseases, such as atlantoaxial, cervical or lumbosacral instability. However, they should always be taken after standard radiographs in a neutral position. If these radiographs show an abnormal position of the vertebrae, radiographs in forced positions will not be recommended, since they can cause serious compressive lesions of the spinal cord. We should also always handle the patient very carefully when a fracture of luxation of the spine is suspected, since we could worsen the clinical picture.

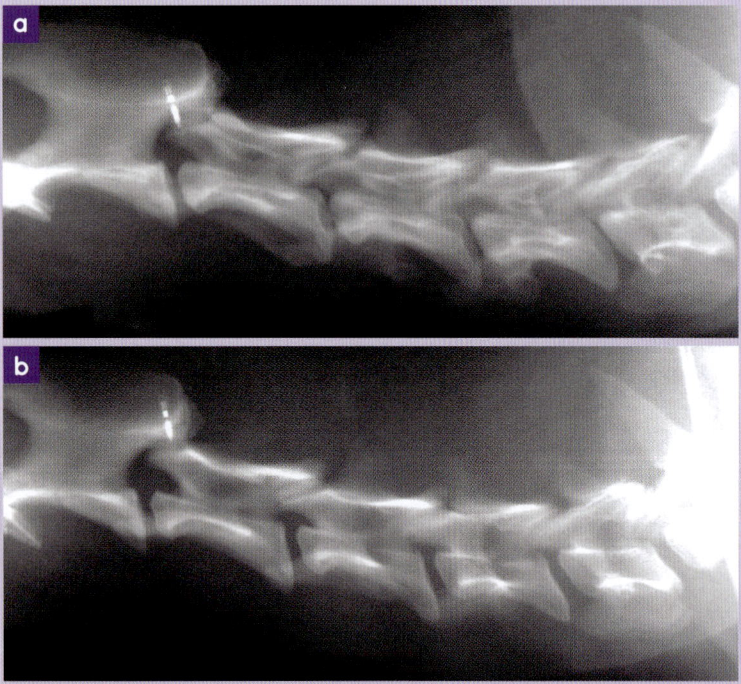

FIGURE 5.1. Poorly positioned lateral radiograph of the cervical spine of a dog (a) and lateral radiograph of the same region with correct positioning (b), after placing a radiolucent block under the neck so the longitudinal axis is parallel to the cassette. In the first radiograph, it is not possible to assess the intervertebral disc spaces in an appropriate way, since the X-ray beam penetrates obliquely through them.

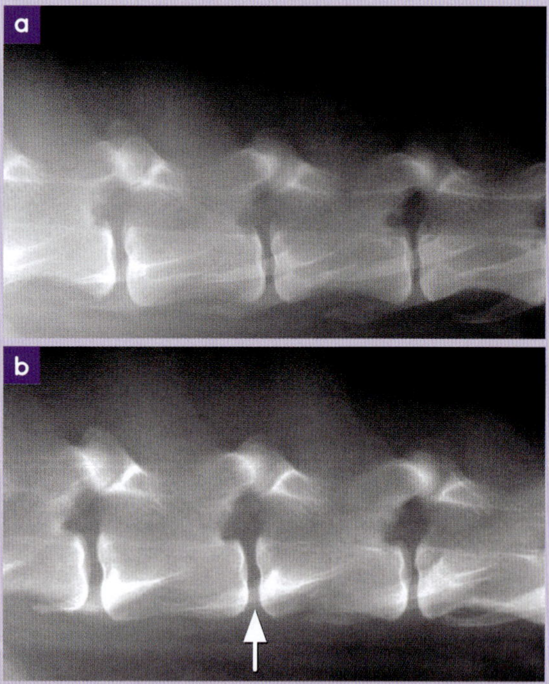

FIGURE 5.2. Enlarged images of the lumbar region of a dog, obtained in lateral projection, before (a) and after (b) placing a positioning block that slightly elevates the position of the limbs, so the sagittal plane of the vertebrae is parallel to the cassette. The perfect superimposition of the transverse processes of each vertebra (arrow) indicates that the radiograph was taken correctly.

Myelography

Myelography is the contrast technique most frequently used to assess the spine (fig. 5.4). It is based on the introduction of a contrast medium in the subarachnoid space. As it involves certain risks, it should be carried out only when considered absolutely necessary, generally when the choice of surgical treatment depends on the results of this test. Magnetic resonance imaging is an excellent alternative.

Myelograms must be performed under general anaesthesia. Before administering the contrast medium, it is necessary take plain radiographs with correct positioning. The contrast media of choice are low-osmolarity, nonionic iodinated contrast agents, such as iohexol or iopamidol, since they are less neurotoxic and remain longer in diagnostic concentrations in the subarachnoid space than other water-soluble agents. They are used at concentrations from 200 to 350 mg I/ml (the higher the concentration of iodine, the better defined the contrast columns will be in the images) and at doses of 0.3 ml/kg or 50 mg I/kg. The administered volume depends on the size of the animal and on the region that is going to be examined:

- **Small dogs and cats (1–5 kg):** 1.5–2 ml.
- **Medium-size dogs (5–15 kg):** 1.5–3 ml.
- **Large dogs (15–35 kg):** 3–5 ml.
- **Giant breed dogs (+ 35 kg):** 8–9 ml maximum.

The contrast medium may be introduced in the cisterna magna or in the lumbar area. Spinal needles

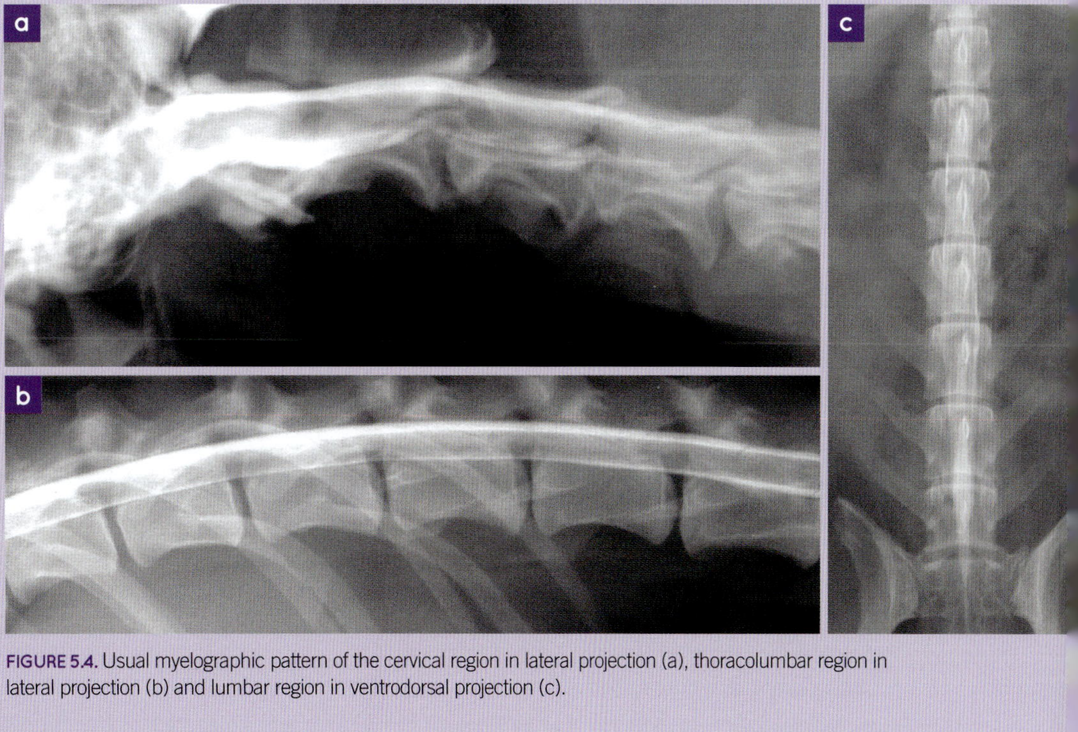

FIGURE 5.4. Usual myelographic pattern of the cervical region in lateral projection (a), thoracolumbar region in lateral projection (b) and lumbar region in ventrodorsal projection (c).

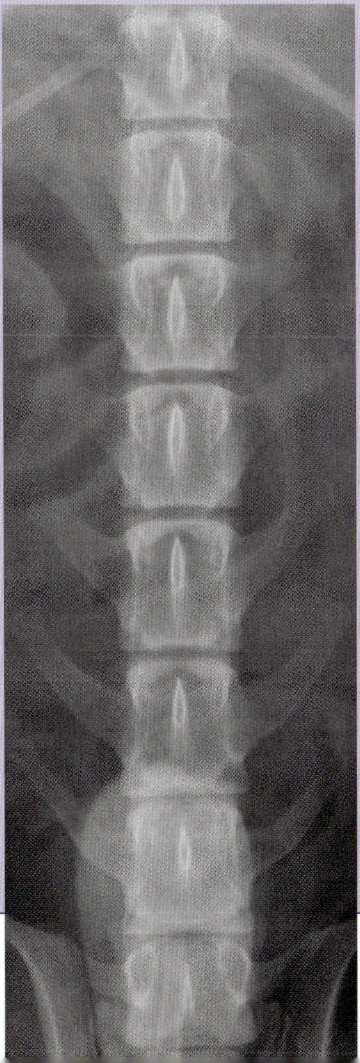

FIGURE 5.3. Ventrodorsal radiograph of the lumbar spine in a dog. The centred position of the spinous processes with respect to the vertebral bodies indicates that the radiograph was taken correctly.

are used for this purpose (25-mm needles for cats and small dogs, 40-mm needles for medium-size dogs and 75–90-mm needles for large dogs) and maximum asepsis should be maintained when performing the injection.

In order to perform a cisternal injection (cisternal myelography), the patient should be placed in lateral recumbency and its head bent at a 90º angle with respect to the neck. It is important to make sure this movement does not cause the obstruction of the airways. If the table can be inclined, it should be tilted 15º upwards approximately. Alternatively, radiolucent positioning blocks may be used to elevate the patient's head and neck. The technique is described in the box below.

It is recommended to allow an amount of cerebrospinal fluid similar to the volume of contrast medium that is going to be injected to flow out and analyse a sample. The injection of the contrast medium is performed slowly, in 2 to 3 minutes approximately. If the head has not previously been elevated, it is indispensable to do it at that moment, to ensure that the contrast material flows caudally and does not leak into the cerebral ventricles. If resistance is felt when administering the contrast medium, the injection should be stopped and the needle withdrawn.

If there is a compression site, the contrast column may fail to pass beyond the lesion, in which case it is not possible to determine the real extension of the area of compression.

In lumbar myelography, the contrast medium is injected in the subarachnoid space in the lumbar area. It is more difficult to perform and more traumatic, since the needle is inserted into the spinal cord. Two advantages of this technique are that the lumbar and thoracic areas are properly filled and that, in many cases, the contrast material can reach sites located cranial to an area of compression. The technique is described in the box below.

Puncture technique for cisternal myelography

In order to carry out the puncture, the depression between the external occipital protuberance and the dorsal lamina of the atlas should be palpated. The needle is inserted in the median line of this depression, at a slight angle in cranial direction and slowly moving forward. The bevel should be directed caudally. It is possible to feel some degree of resistance when going through the nuchal ligament. If the needle is positioned correctly, cerebrospinal fluid (CSF) will flow out. If blood flows out together with CSF, it is usual to carry on with the procedure. However, if only blood flows out, the needle must be removed and the injection should be attempted again with a new needle. In case of piercing through the bone, the needle should be redirected.

Puncture technique for lumbar myelography

In order to carry out a lumbar myelogram, the animal is placed in sternal recumbency, with the spine arched. This is achieved by extending the hind limbs forward. The spinal needle is inserted in the L5-L6 disc space in dogs and in the L6-L7 disc space in cats. The needle is moved forward, going through the spinal cord, until reaching the floor of the canal. The bevel of the needle should be directed cranially. When reaching the floor of the canal, the needle is removed slightly and the introducer needle is withdrawn. If CSF flows out, this indicates that the needle has correctly been placed. If no CSF flows out, the position of the needle may be checked by taking a radiograph or by means of fluoroscopy. An additional check can be made by introducing a small amount of contrast and examining its position in a radiographic image.

Attempting to enter in the dorsal subarachnoid space without going through the spinal cord is possible, by frequently removing the introducer needle to check if CSF flows out, but this is not easy.

The injection of a contrast medium in the spinal cord may be lethal (severe paresis or paralysis in lumbar injections cranial to L4–L5, or death of the animal in cisternal injections). If the contrast medium is injected in the epidural space, the contrast columns will be very irregular and difficult to analyse.

Although it would be recommended to inject the contrast agent as close as possible to the area where the lesion is suspected to be located, the simplest and safest technique is cisternal myelography, with which the area of most lesions can be determined. Lumbar myelography is usually reserved for the defining of the caudal margin of lesions that have been delimited cranially with a cisternal myelogram.

The subarachnoid space is larger in the cisterna magna. The spinal cord has a larger diameter in the cervical–thoracic region and in the central area of the lumbar region. The ventral column often appears slightly elevated at the intervertebral disc spaces, which should not be confused with spinal cord compression.

It should be borne in mind that the contrast medium is progressively absorbed, and will therefore no longer be evident in the image after approximately 50 minutes.

An **extradural lesion** causes the contrast column to be elevated or displaced at the site of compression. This is accompanied by a narrowing of the opposite column (fig. 5.5). This type of lesions includes herniated discs, thickening of the dorsal longitudinal ligament, thickening of the ligamentum flavum, haematomas, epidural fat deposits, deformations of the vertebral body, luxations, vertebral subluxations and fractures, cervical or lumboscral spondylopathy and abscesses, granulomas and extradural tumours.

An **intradural–extramedullary lesion** causes focal enlargement of the subarachnoid space (fig. 5.6). This type of lesions includes intradural tumours

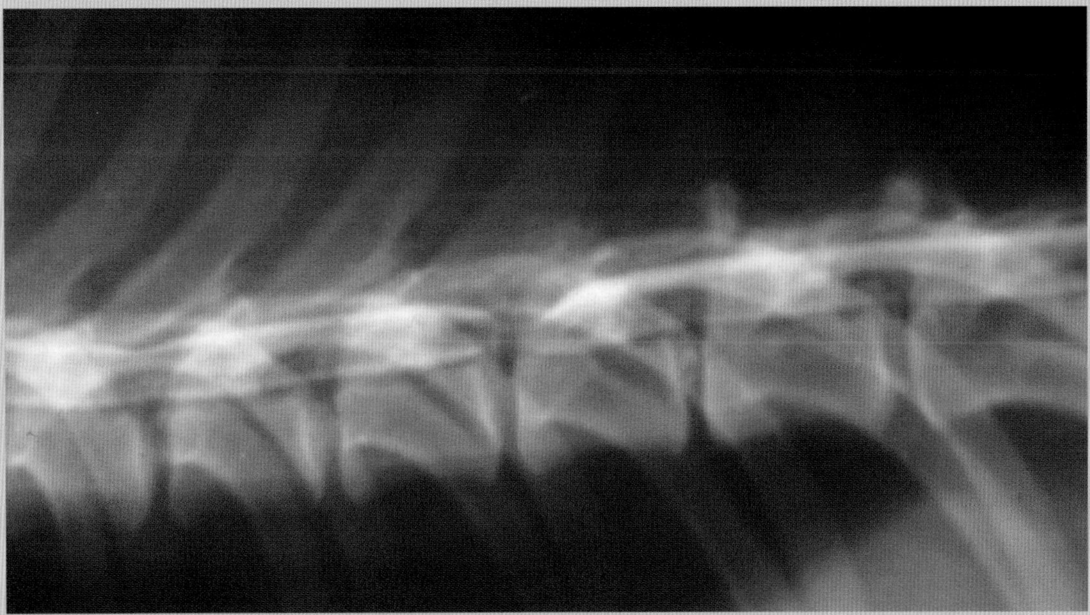

FIGURE 5.5. Myelographic pattern of an extradural lesion.

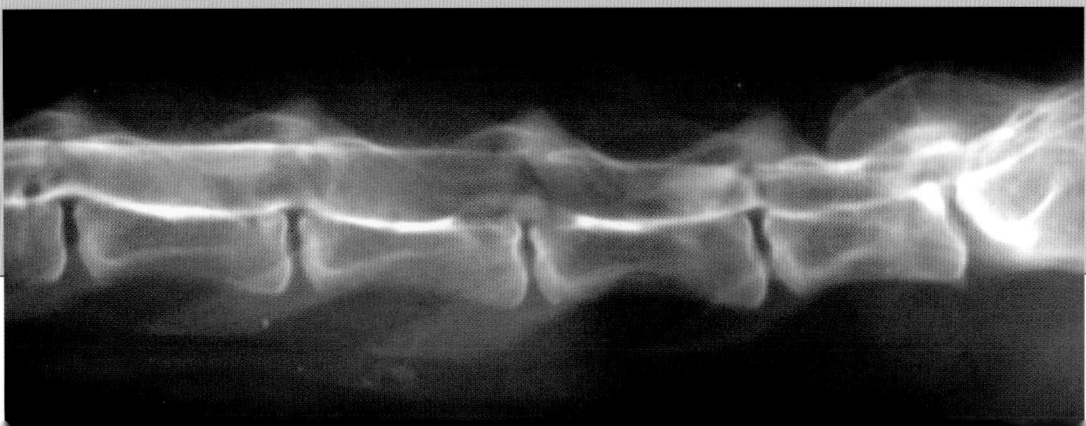

FIGURE 5.6. Myelographic pattern of an intradural-extramedullary lesion. The contrast medium surrounds the lesion located in the subarachnoid space.

(e.g. neurofibroma, meningioma), as well as haemorrhages, oedema or intradural granulomas.

An **intramedullary lesion** causes divergence of the contrast columns at the site of the lesion (fig. 5.7). There may be an interruption of the contrast column at the site of the lesion, cranial to the lesion in a cisternal myelogram, or caudal to the lesion in a lumbar myelogram. This type of lesions includes intramedullary tumours (e.g. ependymoma, astrocytoma), intramedullary haemorrhage or oedema, hydromyelia, syringomyelia and granulomatous meningoencepahlitis.

Other contrast techniques may be used to examine the spine instead of myelography, but their application is much more limited. Epidurography involves introducing the contrast medium (intentionally, not by mistake) in the epidural space, generally at the sacrococcygeal junction. It has been recommended for the detection of lesions in the cauda equina. The interpretation of the results of this technique is often difficult. Discography involves introducing a contrast medium in the intervertebral disc space, but is hardly used in cats and dogs.

Computed tomography offers excellent images of the bones that form the spine, but it is not as good as magnetic resonance imaging for the definition of its soft tissues.

Congenital disorders

Hemivertebra

It is due to an incomplete development of the vertebral body. It may affect one or several vertebrae. Hemivertebrae may have a butterfly shape on ventrodorsal

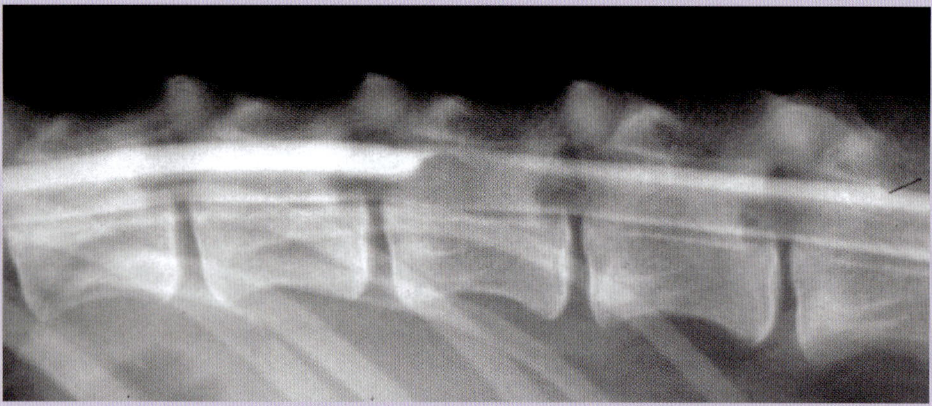

FIGURE 5.7. Myelographic pattern of an intramedullary lesion. The width of the contrast columns decreases around the spinal cord lesion. An enlargement of the dorsal contrast column, cranial to the site of the lesion, can be observed.

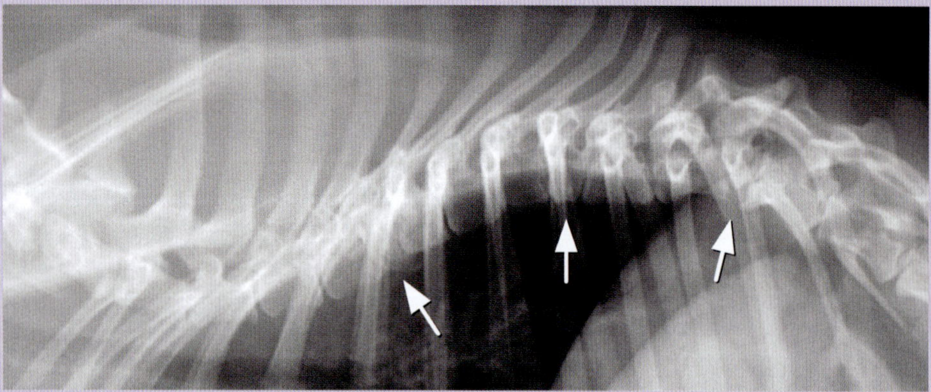

FIGURE 5.9. Lateral radiograph of the thoracic spine of a dog with several "wedge" vertebrae (arrows).

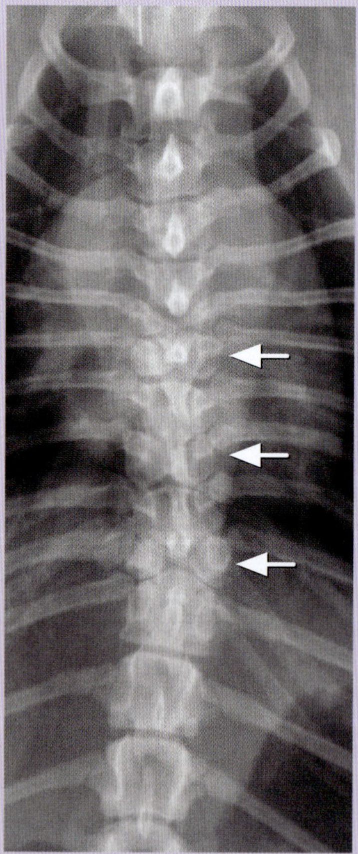

FIGURE 5.8. Ventrodorsal radiograph of the thoracic spine of a Bulldog with several "butterfly" vertebrae (arrows).

radiographs (fig. 5.8) or a "wedge" shape on lateral or ventrodorsal radiographs (fig. 5.9). Compensatory morphological changes in the adjacent vertebrae can usually be observed.

Hemivertebrae generally appear in the thoracic spine and are often associated with kyphosis and, to a lesser extent, lordosis or scoliosis.

Block vertebra

Two or more adjacent vertebral bodies appear partially or totally fused, with no intervertebral disc (fig. 5.10). The intervertebral space may be visualised as a thin radiolucent line or may not be visible at all if fusion is complete. Generally, this is not clinically significant, although some authors suggest that it may increase the risk of disc disease in adjacent intervertebral spaces.

Transitional vertebra

This occurs when the vertebrae of the atlantoaxial, cervical–thoracic, thoracolumbar, lumbosacral or sacrococcygeal junction have morphological characteristics of the vertebrae of both regions (they totally or partially have the shape of the previous or next vertebra):

- Lumbarisation: the S1 vertebra appears separated from the rest of the sacrum, and may have one or two transverse processes, similar to those of the lumbar vertebrae.
- Sacralisation: the transverse process of L7 is fused with the wing of the sacrum and may articulate with the ilium. This alteration may cause lumbosacral instability and degeneration of the intervertebral disc (fig. 5.12), leading to cauda equina syndrome. It may also make the correct positioning of the animal

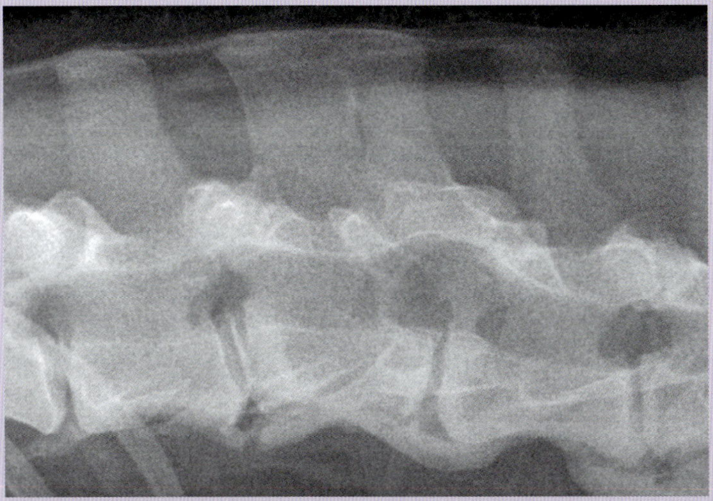

FIGURE 5.10. Lateral projection of the lumbar spine of a dog with partial L3 and L4fusion.

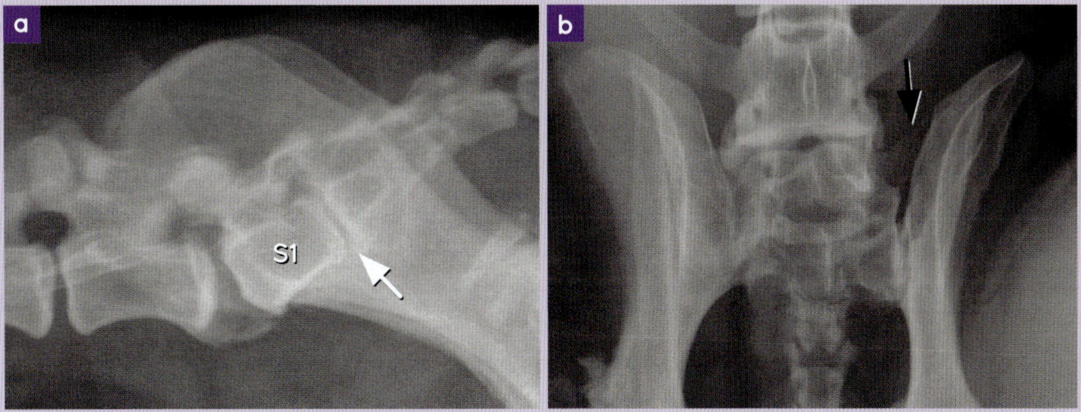

FIGURE 5.11. Lateral (a) and ventrodorsal (b) views of the lumbosacral area of the spine of a dog with lumbarisation of the sacrum. On the lateral view, a radiolucent line (white arrow) can be seen, which separates the S1 vertebra from the rest of the sacrum. On the ventrodorsal view, a transverse process (black arrow) can be identified on S1. Spondylosis at L7–S1 can be observed on both radiographs.

more difficult when taking a ventrodorsal radiograph of the hip.

- Partial or complete fusion of S3 with Cc1.
- A transitional T13 vertebra may have a transverse process instead of the rib (fig. 5.13). Vestigial ribs may be observed, and appear as structures with mineral density in soft tissues. This variation is relatively frequent. Therefore, when planning a spine surgery, it is recommended to always take radiographs in the two projections, since an image in lateral projection could lead to an error when locating the exact vertebra or intervertebral disc space.
- A transitional L1 vertebra may have one or two ribs instead of a transverse process.
- A transitional C7 vertebra may have ribs instead of a transverse process.
- Occipitalisation of the atlas.

Morphological changes may be unilateral or bilateral and, except for those affecting the lumbosacral junction, they do not usually have any clinical significance.

Spina bifida

It is a very uncommon anomaly. It is due to a failure in the closure of the neural arch and may affect one or more vertebrae. It can be associated with a protrusion of the meninges through the defect. It is best viewed on ventrodorsal radiographs. If there is a failure in the fusion of the spinous processes, the image will show a double spinous process in the affected vertebrae. In mild cases, the patient may not display any clinical signs.

Instability syndromes

They are associated with congenital anomalies that may worsen with growth, or with acquired lesions secondary to instability. They affect three anatomical regions: atlantoaxial, cervical and lumbosacral.

Atlantoaxial instability

Atlantoaxial instability or subluxation usually appears as a congenital anomaly in small and miniature breeds, such as Yorkshire Terriers, Chihuahuas, Pomeranians or Poodles. It may be due to agenesis or hypoplasia of the odontoid process, to a lack of fusion of this process with the axis, or to a stretching or rupture of the ligament holding it.

It may also have an acquired origin in any breed, due to trauma that fractured the apophysis or caused injury to the ligament.

On lateral radiographs, an increase in the distance between the dorsal arch of the atlas and the spinous process of the axis can be observed, accompanied by an angulation of the floor of the spinal canal at the atlantoaxial junction (fig. 5.14). Odontoid aplasia, hypoplasia or dorsal articulation with the axis may sometimes be identified. When this condition is suspected, the patient should be carefully positioned. Slightly bending the animal's neck can help identify these findings, although there is a risk of worsening the patient's clinical picture. Flexed positions should not be attempted if the patient has tetraparesis. The ventrodorsal projection is generally unhelpful for diagnosis and might exacerbate the patient's clinical condition in the presence of spinal cord compression. Some authors suggest using an oblique ventrodorsal projection to enhance the visualisation of the odontoid process.

Although the diagnosis is usually made by radiography, computed tomography or magnetic resonance imaging may provide additional diagnostic information useful for surgical planning.

Cervical instability

It is also called Wobbler disease, cervical spondylopathy, caudal cervical spondylomyelopathy, cervical vertebral malformation or cervical stenotic myelopathy. It is a developmental abnormality affecting young or middle-aged dogs, especially large breeds. It encompasses a series of alterations that manifest differently in each patient, including vertebral subluxation and malformation, deformation of joint apophyses, disc protrusion, and compensatory ligament hypertrophy. These changes culminate in the compression of the cervical spinal cord within the affected intervertebral spaces.

It particularly affects Great Dane and Doberman breeds, and to a lesser extent Basset Hound, although it has also been described in other breeds. The affected animals present with progressive discoordination of the hind limbs and, on occasions, of the forelimbs. The symptoms usually appear between 3 to 10 months

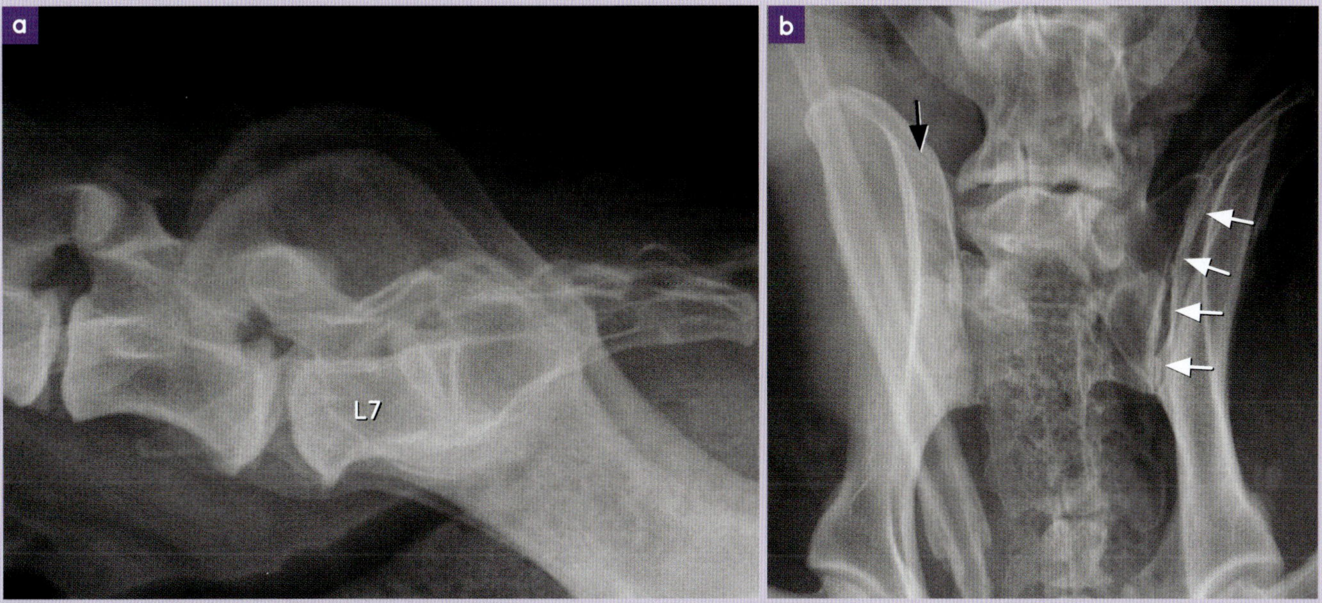

FIGURE 5.12. Lateral (a) and ventrodorsal (b) radiographs of the lumbosacral area of the spine of a dog with sacralisation of L7. On the lateral radiograph, L7 appears shortened. On the ventrodorsal radiograph, a fusion of the left margin of L7 with the sacrum may be observed (white arrows), while in the right side L7 has a transverse process.

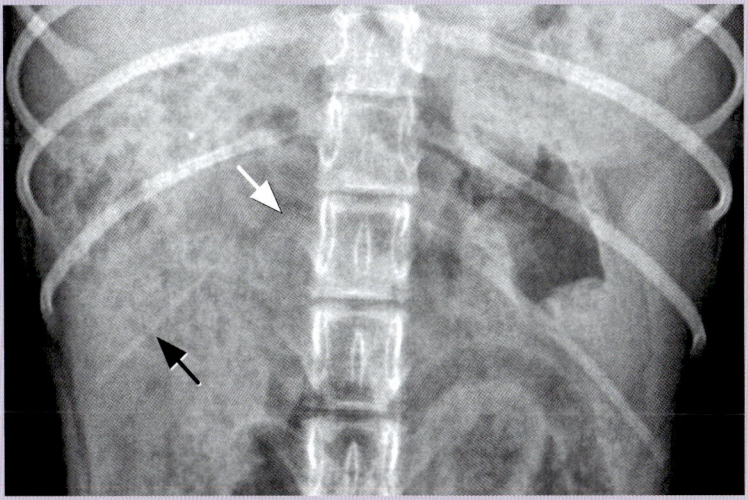

FIGURE 5.13. Ventrodorsal radiograph of the thoracolumbar spine of a dog with transitional T13. This vertebra has a right transverse process (white arrow), and a vestigial rib (black arrow) is observed lateral to the vertebra. It is important not to confuse the vestige with a foreign body when performing abdominal radiographs.

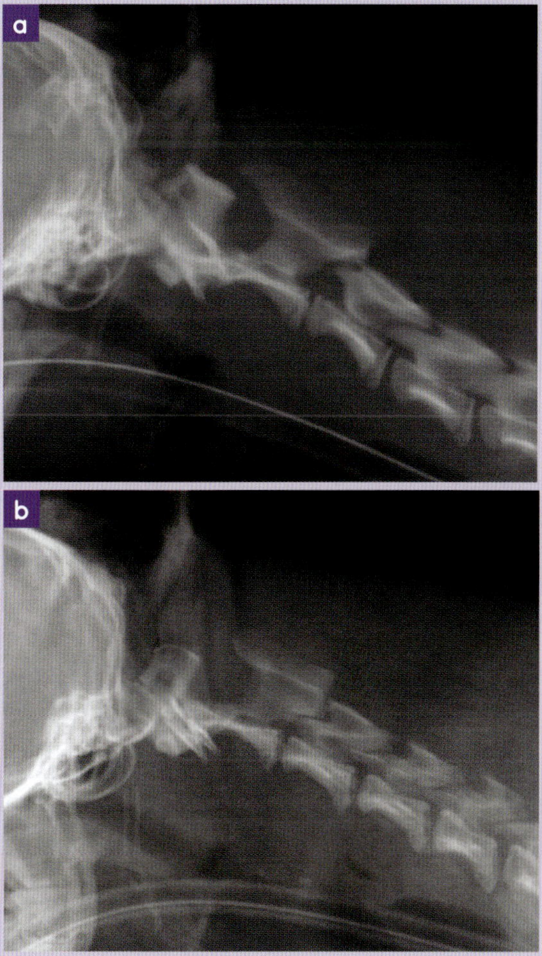

FIGURE 5.14. Enlarged image of the cervical spine on a lateral radiograph of a Yorkshire Terrier with no vertebral anomalies (a) and of a dog of the same breed with atlantoaxial subluxation (b).

of age, although they may also appear at a later age, especially in the Doberman breed. The C2–C4 location is more common in the Basset Hound, C3–C7 in young and C4–C7 in older Great Dane dogs, while in young and middle-aged Doberman the segment usually affected is C5–C7.

The general radiographic signs that may be observed are:

- Alteration in the shape of the affected vertebra or vertebrae.
- Narrowing of the cranial part of the affected vertebra or vertebrae, which gives the spinal canal the aspect of a "funnel" or triangle.
- The cranial articular processes may appear deformed or be absent.
- If there is subluxation (fig 5.15), lateral images obtained with the neck flexed will show the cranial end of the affected vertebra protruding dorsally towards the spinal canal. It should be taken into account that, when the neck is flexed, the cranial end of the vertebrae is always raised to some degree, which should not be confused with a pathological subluxation.
- The intervertebral disc space cranial to the affected vertebra may be enlarged and the affected discs may be calcified.
- There may be new bone formation and sclerosis of the end-plates of the vertebral bodies.
- The myelogram may show spinal cord compression. This should not be confused with the normal image obtained with the neck flexed, in which a certain degree of elevation of the contrast column is observed in the areas located on the intervertebral disc spaces.
- Ventral compression indicates a prolapsed disc or hypertrophy of the dorsal longitudinal ligament, while dorsal compression indicates hypertrophy of the ligamentum flavum.

Taking radiographs in flexion, extension or with cervical traction can reveal subluxations undetected in a neutral position. These lesions are termed dynamic lesions. In the case of adynamic lesions, there are no differences with the image obtained in neutral position. These neck movements should be performed with care, especially the forced flexion and extension, as they can aggravate the patient's clinical picture. Traction is also useful and poses less risk.

Although radiological findings may be sufficient to establish the diagnosis, advanced imaging tests (computed tomography or magnetic resonance imaging) are necessary to establish the exact location and severity of the spinal cord compression causing the clinical symptoms.

Lumbosacral instability

Lumbosacral instability is also called lumbosacral stenosis or lumbosacral malarticulation. Cauda equine syndrome is a broader term, which applies to numerous degenerative, inflammatory, traumatic or neoplastic disorders that affect the lumbosacral junction causing pain and neurological dysfunction in the hind limbs. The most common causes are degenerative, including degenerative disc disease at L7–S1 and bone remodelling causing spinal canal or foraminal stenosis at L7–S1. However, fractures, discospondylitis, osteochondrosis and neoplasms in lumbosacral locations may also cause the clinical signs that are included under cauda equina syndrome.

The radiographic findings most commonly identified with lumbosacral instability or stenosis are the associated degenerative changes, particularly spondylosis deformans and sclerosis of the caudal end of L7 and cranial end of the sacrum (fig. 5.16). The intervertebral space may be narrower or collapsed. It is sometimes possible to identify a reduction of the spinal canal dorsoventral diameter at the level of L7 or of the sacrum, or a ventral displacement of the sacrum relative to the position of L7 (fig. 5.17). This latter finding may be constant or inconstant, and may appear alone, or become more noticeable when a radiograph is taken in hyperflexion or hyperextension.

There is no direct correlation between the clinical signs and the radiological findings. In fact, some patients with symptoms show a normal image of the lumbosacral junction on plain radiographs while many patients with radiographic evidence of L7-S1 spondylosis do not present with any clinical signs. Myelography, epidurography or discography may help with the diagnosis, although computed tomography and, above all, magnetic resonance imaging are the most appropriate techniques to evaluate this disease (fig. 5.18).

Degenerative intervertebral disc disease

Each disc is formed by an annulus fibrosus (fibrous ring) and a nucleus pulposus. This latter is composed of a homogeneous gelatinous material. The annulus

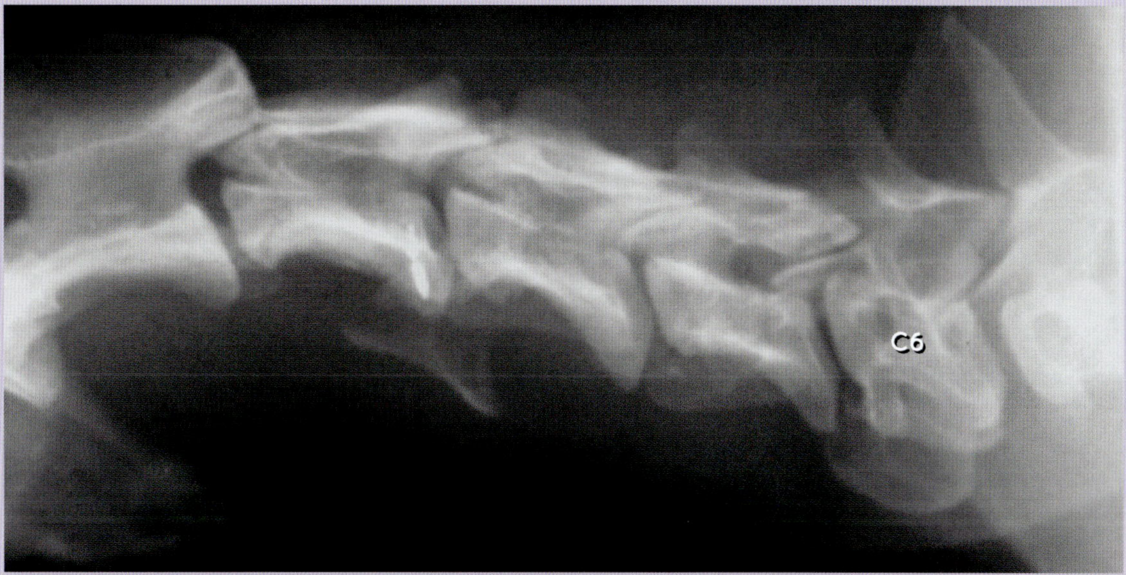

FIGURE 5.15. Lateral radiograph of the cervical spine of a Great Dane with Wobbler disease. The C6 vertebra is subluxated, which causes a marked narrowing of the spinal canal in this area.

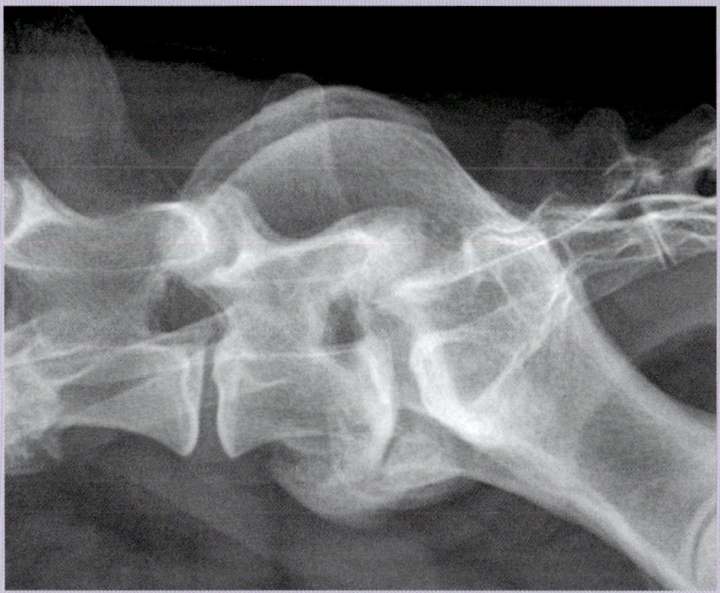

FIGURE 5.16. Lateral radiograph of the lumbosacral area of the spine of a dog with spondylosis deformans at L7–S1 and sclerosis of the caudal end of L7 and of the cranial end of the sacrum. These findings of a degenerative nature are suggestive of lumbosacral instability.

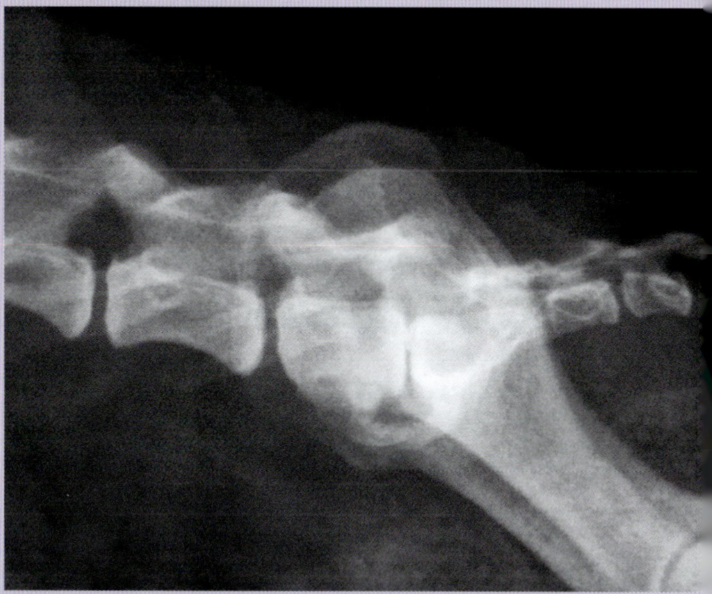

FIGURE 5.17. Lateral radiograph of the lumbosacral area of the spine of a dog with ventral displacement of the sacrum with respect to L7, a marked reduction of the L7–S1 intervertebral space and spondylosis deformans at L7–S1. These findings indicate lumbosacral instability.

fibrosus is much thicker in its ventral part than in its dorsal part (this is why ventral protrusions are rare, and would not affect the spinal cord in any case). Discs are covered dorsally by the longitudinal ligament, which runs through the floor of the spinal canal. This ligament is reinforced by other ligaments in the area between T1 and T10, so herniated discs in this area are rare.

The most appropriate projection to examine intervertebral disc spaces (IVDS) is the lateral one. Radiolucent positioning blocks or wedges should be placed under the cervical and lumbar spine in an attempt to align the spine parallel (not curved) to the cassette. The obliquity of the peripheral X-rays of the beam makes it necessary to centre the radiograph appropriately on the IVDS where a lesion is suspected (fig. 5.19). On each radiograph, it is only possible to assess the centred IVDS and the spaces immediately cranial and caudal to it. If the area that we are going to examine is wider, several radiographs should be taken, centring the images on different sites.

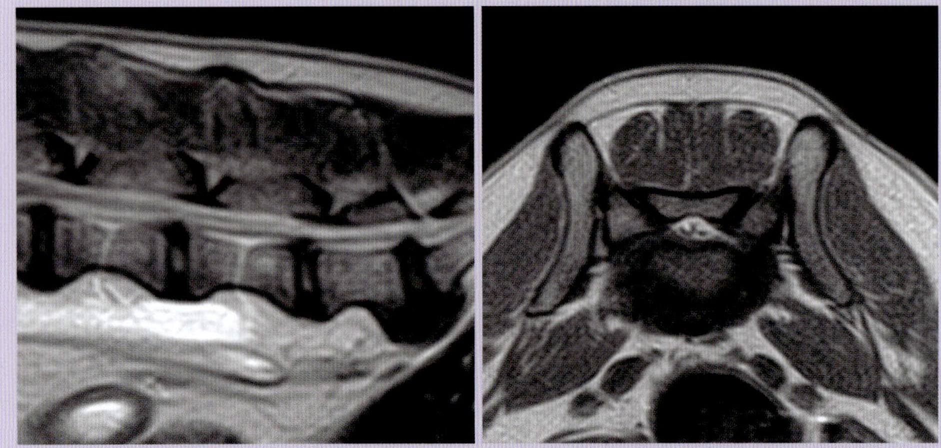

FIGURE 5.18. Magnetic resonance images in sagittal and transverse plane of the L7–S1 disc in a dog with lumbosacral instability. The images show degenerative changes and protrusion of the disc, which causes a compression of the cauda equina.

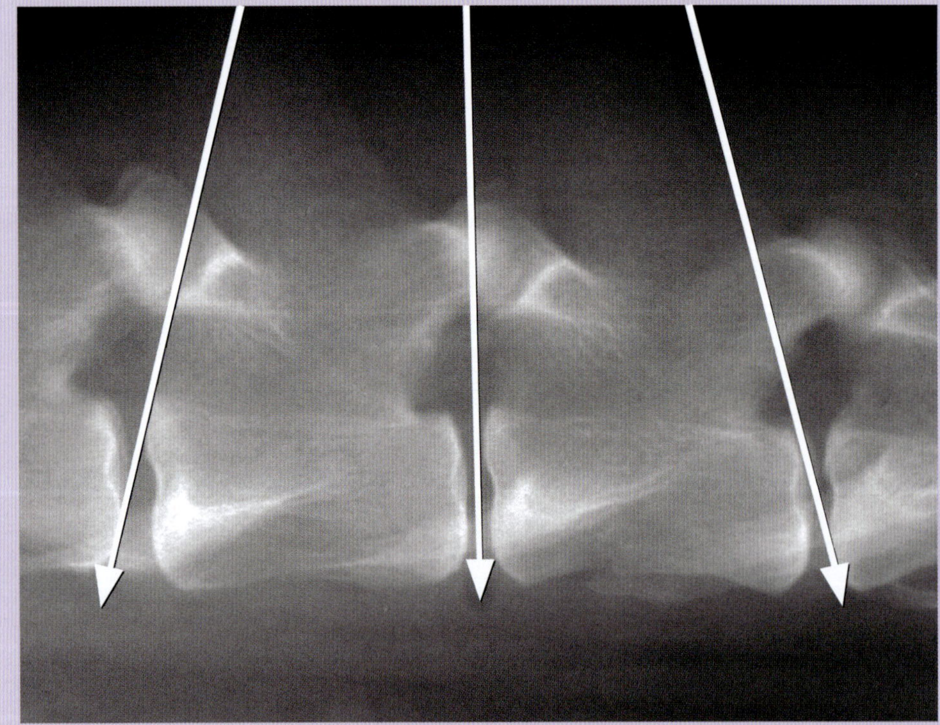

FIGURE 5.19. Representation of the direction of entry of the X-ray beam through the intervertebral spaces. Since the X-ray beam is divergent, only the central rays of the beam are aligned with the intervertebral disc space on the radiograph. The entrance direction of X-rays into other intervertebral spaces will be more oblique the farther away the spaces are from the center of the beam.

The IVDS at the cervicothoracic junction and at the lumbosacral junction are slightly narrower than the others. The IVDS located between T10 and T11 may also be slightly narrower in normal conditions. If no radiolucent positioning blocks are placed under the cervical or lumbar spine, the width of the IVDS may appear falsely reduced, due to the curvature of the spine.

Disc degeneration is a phenomenon related with age. Problems occur when the degeneration process is faster than usual. Two types of degeneration are distinguished:

- **Hansen type I:** it is generally observed in chondrodystrophic breeds, in which a degeneration of the nucleus pulposus at early ages is frequently observed (many animals have calcified discs, with no clinical significance). With time, the annulus fibrosus also degenerates, which can cause its rupture and subsequent bulging out of the nucleus pulposus into the spinal canal, which is called extrusion of the disc material.
- **Hansen type II:** more common in non-chondrodystrophic breeds, in which degenerative changes occur more slowly, and rarely cause calcification. A protrusion of the disc (with no rupture of the annulus fibrosus) usually occurs. The disc moves to a greater or lesser extent towards the spinal canal and may cause different degrees of spinal cord compression.

In cases of type I extrusion, clinical signs appear in an acute manner, with pain, neurological deficiency and paralysis. In cases of type II protrusion, the clinical picture is less dramatic, and progressive ataxia and neurological deficiency are usually observed.

A variant of type I extrusion, described later, is that which occurs acutely from a non-degenerated disc. This variant is also known as high-velocity low volume or type III disc extrusion. It is due to a rupture of the annulus caused by the exit of disc material of low volume, and presumably at high speed, towards the vertebral canal. Secondary spinal cord damage is caused by the impact and haemorrhage (spinal contusion).

The radiological signs that may appear in degenerative intervertebral disc disease are:

- Disc calcification (more frequent in chondrodystrophic breeds). This finding alone is not diagnostic of disc prolapse, but does indicate its degeneration (fig. 5.20).
- Narrowing of the affected IVDS (fig. 5.21).
- Observation of calcified disc material in the spinal canal (fig 5.22). It is also sometimes possible to identify non-calcified disc material when this is located in the area of the intervertebral foramen.
- Appearance of a pattern of ventral or ventrolateral extradural lesion on the myelogram.

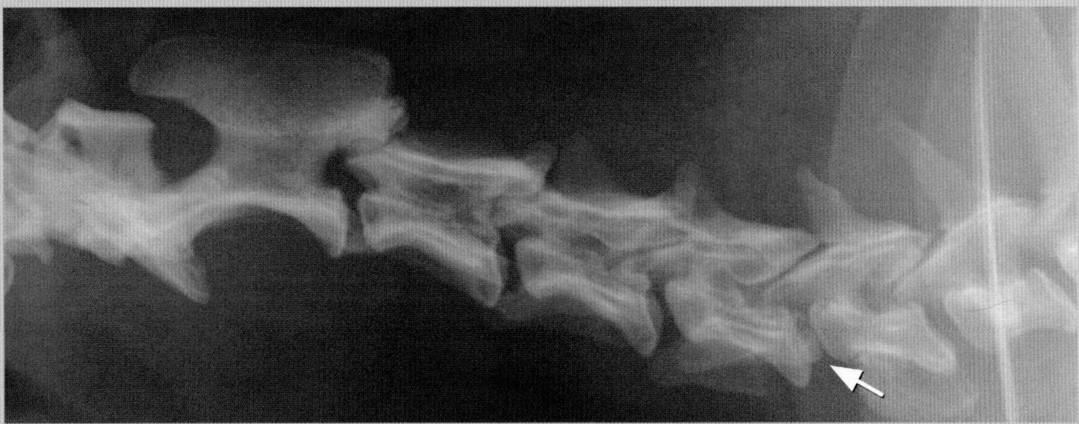

FIGURE 5.20. Lateral radiograph of the cervical spine of a dog with calcification of the C5–C6 intervertebral disc (arrow). Calcification is a finding that indicates disc degeneration.

The radiological signs should always correlate with the clinical symptoms, although the finding of spinal cord compression on the myelogram is always significant. Computed tomography and magnetic resonance imaging provide much more precise diagnostic information about this condition. An acute disc protrusion may produce a normal image in plain radiographs. Old lesions may not have any clinical significance, and may be accompanied by sclerosis of the end-plates of the adjacent vertebral bodies and spondylosis deformans (fig. 5.23).

Other disorders of the spine

Scoliosis, kyphosis and lordosis

Scoliosis is defined as an abnormal curvature of the spine in lateral direction, and is therefore best visualised on ventrodorsal radiographs (fig. 5.24). Kyphosis is defined as an abnormal curvature of the spine in dorsal direction (fig. 5.25), while lordosis occurs in ventral direction (fig. 5.26). These are therefore best observed on lateral radiographs.

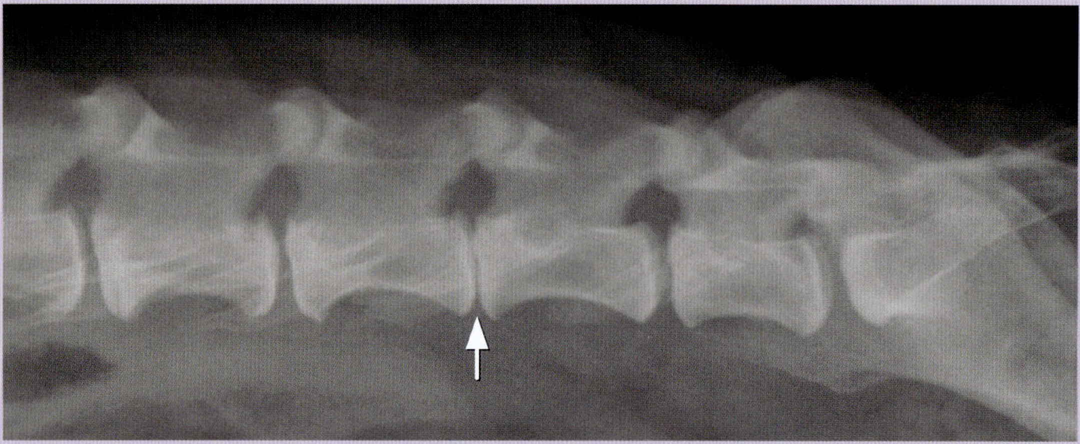

FIGURE 5.21. Lateral radiograph of the lumbar spine of a dog with a narrowing of the L5–L6 intervertebral disc space (arrow), which indicates disc disease.

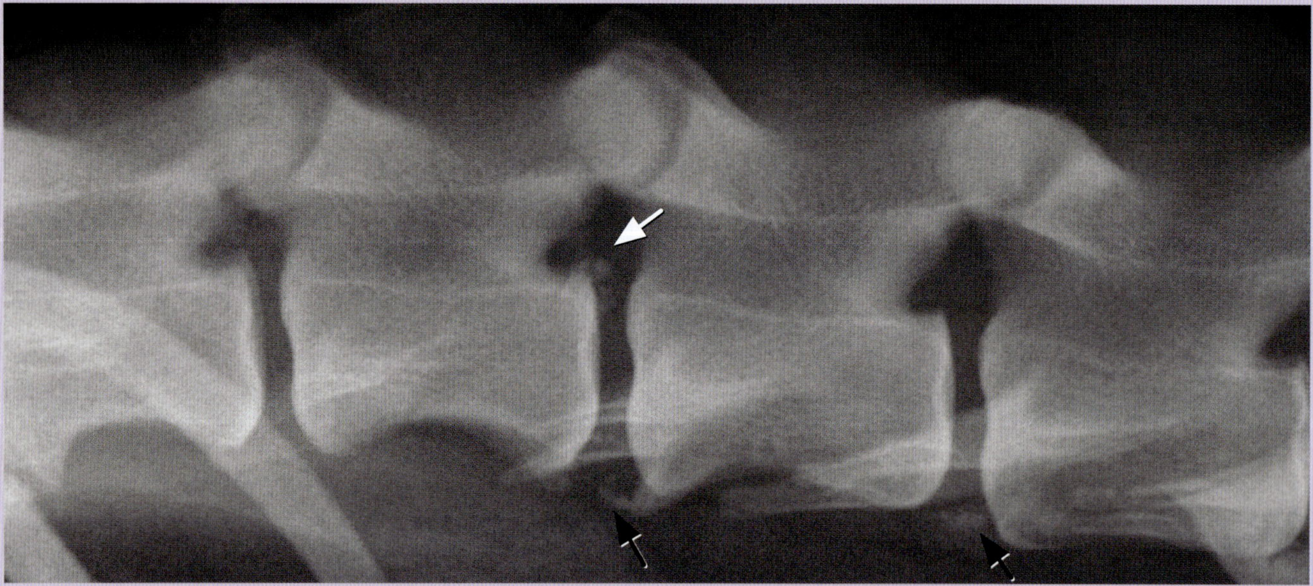

FIGURE 5.22. Enlarged image of the lumbar spine of a dog in lateral projection, in which calcified disc material is observed, immediately dorsal to the L2–L3 intervertebral disc space (white arrow), as well as in the ventral areas of the L2–L3 and L3–L4 disc spaces (black arrows).

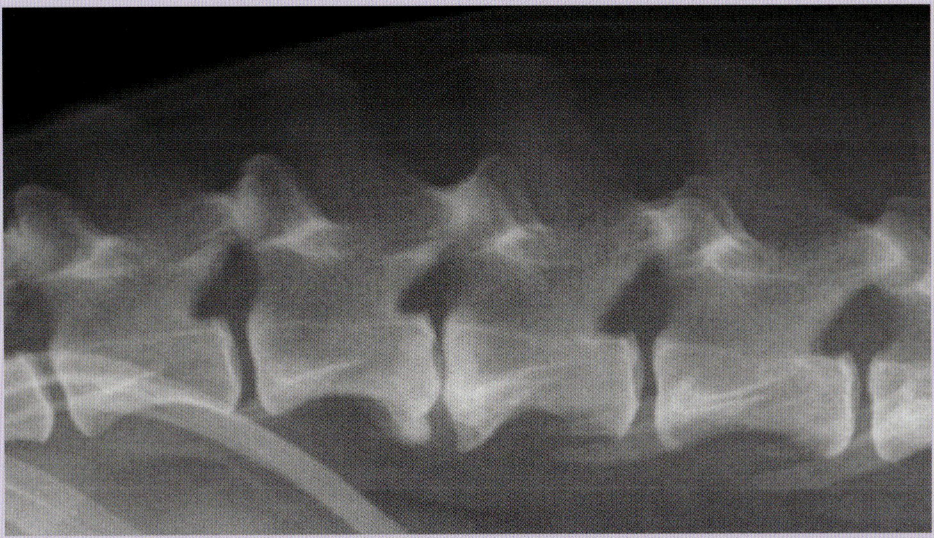

FIGURE 5.23. Enlarged image of the lumbar spine on a lateral radiograph of a dog with a narrowing of the L2–L3 intervertebral disc space, sclerosis of the caudal margin of L2 and cranial margin of L3 and spondylosis deformans at L2–L3. The sclerosis and spondylosis suggest a possible old disc lesion.

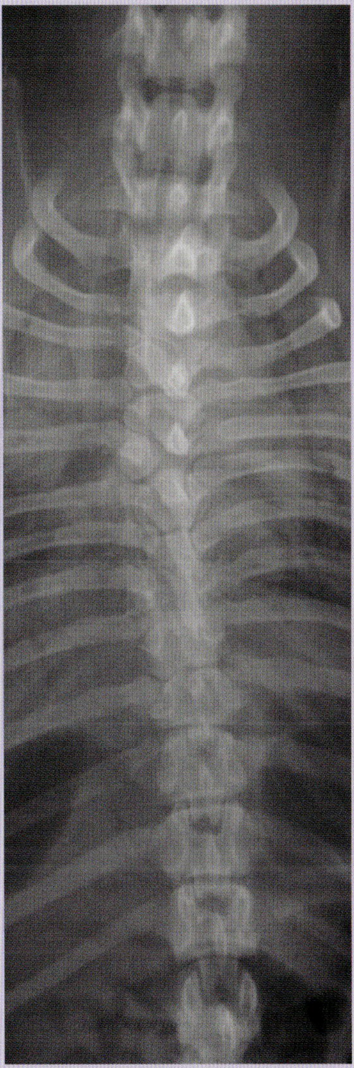

FIGURE 5.24. Ventrodorsal radiograph of the thoracic spine of a dog with scoliosis (displacement of the spine in lateral direction). Lordosis commonly appears associated with multiple vertebral deformations.

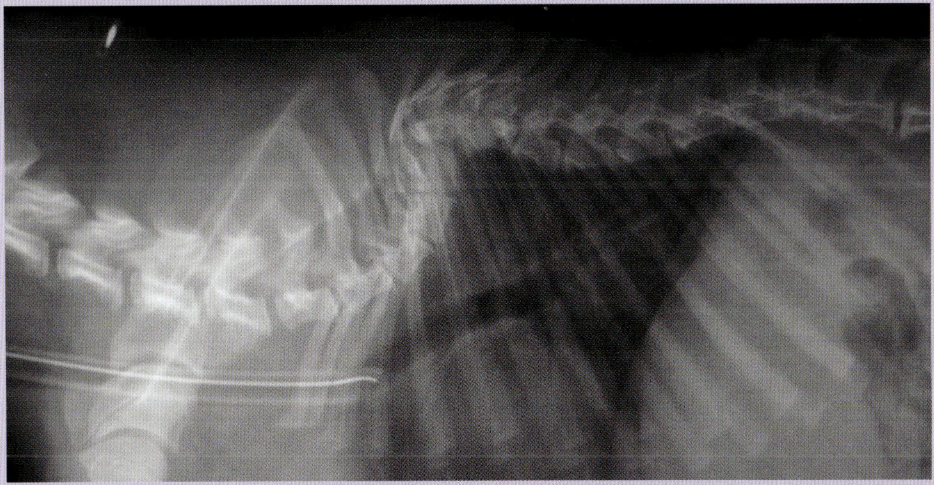

FIGURE 5.25. Lateral radiograph of the thoracic spine of a dog with kyphosis (displacement of the spine in dorsal direction). Lordosis commonly appears associated with multiple vertebral deformations.

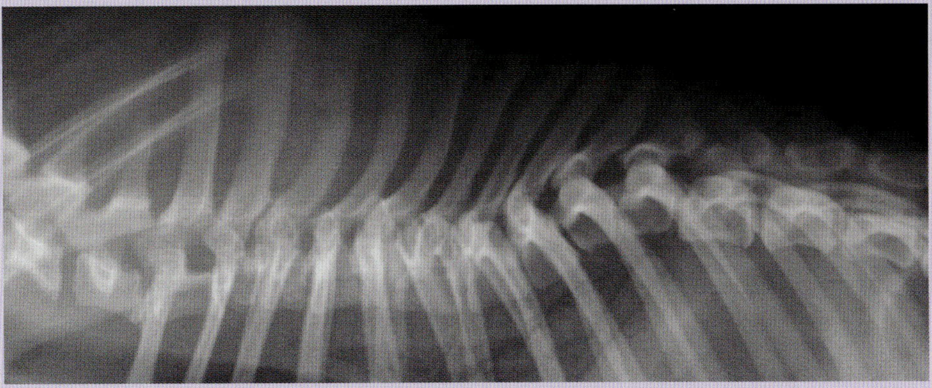

FIGURE 5.26. Lateral radiograph of the thoracic spine in a dog with lordosis (displacement of the spine in ventral direction). Lordosis commonly appears associated with multiple vertebral deformations.

These disorders may be congenital, idiopathic or may appear associated with other diseases affecting the spine. As in people, the degree of kyphosis determines the likelihood that secondary neurological dysfunction may occur, usually due to progressive myelopathy as a result of spinal canal stenosis or spinal instability in the affected segment. Scoliosis, on the other hand, is not usually associated with significant neurological dysfunction.

The degree of angulation of the spine in dogs with kyphosis can be quantified using the Cobb angle which is formed by the intersection of two lines: one parallel to the cranial margin of the vertebra immediately cranialward of the malformed vertebra and the second line parallel to the caudal margin of the vertebra immediately caudally to the malformed vertebra. This can be calculated more accurately with post-processing tools in digital radiography. If the patient has several non-contiguous affected vertebrae, the angle is measured for each of them. On the other hand, if several contiguous malformations appear, the angle is measured considering the vertebra with the most marked malformation (fig. 5.27). A Cobb angle greater than 35 ° has been associated with a high probability of the appearance of secondary neurological deficits. The angle may vary progressively in these animals, so monitoring in patients with measurements less than 35° may be useful for early detection of potential secondary neurological dysfunctions.

Magnetic resonance imaging provides very precise information on the secondary involvement of the spinal cord and nerve roots in patients with vertebral malformations (fig. 5.28), while computed tomography allows the obtaining of 3D images with excellent anatomical detail, especially of the bone components of the affected segment. These 3D images can also be used to print 3D anatomical models, which can be invaluable in surgical planning for patients requiring surgery.

Spondylosis deformans

It is a degenerative alteration, characterised by the development of bony growths in the ventral area of the cranial and/or caudal end-plates of the vertebral bodies (fig. 5.29). These growths are considered enthesophytes that form on the vertebral epiphysis. Over time they tend to increase in size and even to fuse with adjacent vertebrae, forming bony bridges (fig. 5.30).

They can also grow on the lateral surface of the end-plates of the vertebral bodies, although this is less common (fig. 5.31). When growth occurs laterally, it rarely causes compression at the exit of the nerve roots, except in the case of lumbosacral instability, where the impingement of the roots is caused by narrowing of the foramen caused by the dorsal extension of the enthesophytes.

Dural ossification

It is characterised by the formation of bony plaques in the dura mater, which may be visible or not on a plain radiograph. When they are observed, they appear as thin lines of mineral density running parallel to the floor of the spinal canal (fig. 5.32). It is more common in large breed dogs. It is considered an incidental finding of degenerative origin. If it coincides with the presence of an extradural lesion, meningeal deviation can be seen if the lesion is compressing the spinal cord ("automyelogram").

Spondyloarthrosis

The degenerative joint disease involving intervertebral joints is called spondyloarthrosis. It causes remodelling of the joint process margins, with osteophyte formation and, occasionally, joint space narrowing (fig. 5.33). It is observed more frequently in the lumbar region and occasionally, in the cervical region. It should not be confused with spondylosis deformans, even if both are of a degenerative origin.

Diffuse idiopathic skeletal hyperostosis

It is a rare idiopathic condition in dogs and very rare in cats. It mainly affects Boxers and Great Danes. It is characterised by the appearance of abundant new linear bone formations on the ventral and lateral surfaces of the spine (fig. 5.34), which causes ankylosis. It does not usually produce clinical signs apart from stiffness when walking, although it could be a predisposing factor for disc disease in the intervertebral spaces adjacent to the affected segment. The image is similar to that of advanced spondylosis deformans, but at present they are considered to be different pathologic entities. It is diagnosed when at least four of the following X-ray findings occur at the same time in a patient:

- Formation of ventrolateral bony bridges in at least three contiguous vertebral bodies.
- Normal width of the intervertebral spaces in the affected segment with no obvious signs of disc degeneration (disc calcification or sclerosis of the end-plates of the vertebral bodies).
- Signs of spondyloarthrosis in the joints of the affected segment.
- Pseudoarthrosis of the spinous process.
- Appearance of enthesophytes in the axial and appendicular skeleton.
- Presence of osteophytes, sclerosis and ankylosis of sacroiliac unions.
- Ankylosis of the pubic symphysis.

Inflammation and infection

The inflammation of the vertebrae is called spondylitis, and may be accompanied or not by an infection. It usually causes new bone formation in the ventral area of the body of the affected vertebra or vertebrae (fig. 5.35). It is important to remember that the ventral margin of L3 and L4 may appear poorly defined due to the crura of the diaphragm being superimposed. This should not be confused with spondylitis.

Vertebral infection is termed osteomyelitis or spondylopyosis. It is characterised by the appearance of an aggressive lesion, which may affect one or several vertebrae, with an osteolytic and osteoproliferative component (fig. 5.36). The infection may extend to the spinal canal, causing meningitis and myelitis. In many cases, it is related to the penetration of foreign bodies (e.g. grass awns), although it may also be associated with penetrating wounds or infections through the haematogenous route.

Vertebral physitis affects young dogs initially causing osteolysis of the physes of the affected vertebrae, with reduction in the size of the epiphyses. With progression, there is collapse of the cranial and caudal aspect of vertebral body and end-plate sclerosis. The most likely cause is a disseminated haematogenous infection.

The term discospondylitis is used when an infectious process affects the intervertebral disc and the end-plate of the adjacent vertebral bodies. The infection may extend to the meninges and spinal cord. The radiograhic image varies according to the moment at which the diagnosis is carried out (fig. 5.37):

- In the early stages, it is possible to observe osteolysis and irregularity of the end-plates of the vertebral bodies adjacent to the affected disc or discs (fig. 5.38), which may cause a widening of the intervertebral disc space.
- Bone growths form on the ventral and lateral surfaces of the affected vertebrae, which is similar to spondylosis deformans. However, if they are secondary to discospondylitis, they tend to present greater extent and a more aggressive appearance.
- Over time, bone is produced in the areas where it had been destroyed, resulting in a narrowing of the intervertebral disc space (fig. 5.39). Sclerosis of the end-plates of the affected vertebral bodies is observed and the ventral new bone acquires a more regular and well-defined image (similar to that of spondylosis).

Discospondylitis is often caused by the haematogenous spread of genitourinary infections, although it can also be associated with the presence of paraspinal abscesses or foreign body migration. It affects mostly middle-aged dogs and large breeds, and one or more intervertebral spaces may be involved (fig. 5.40). In the early stages of the infection, no obvious abnormalities may appear on the radiograph. A normal image of the vertebrae does not rule out early stage discospondylitis, which can be detected early with magnetic resonance imaging, computed tomography and even ultrasound in young animals.

A study of 10 dogs under 6 months of age indicated that the radiographic image of discospondylitis in these animals may differ from that of adults in the initial phase of the process. In these puppies, the initial radiographic finding was a decrease in the width of the affected intervertebral space, with no evidence of osteolysis at this early stage, although it did appear later on follow-up radiographs with an osteolytic pattern similar to that of adults. Some of these animals also presented subluxation of the affected vertebrae at the time of diagnosis or during follow-up.

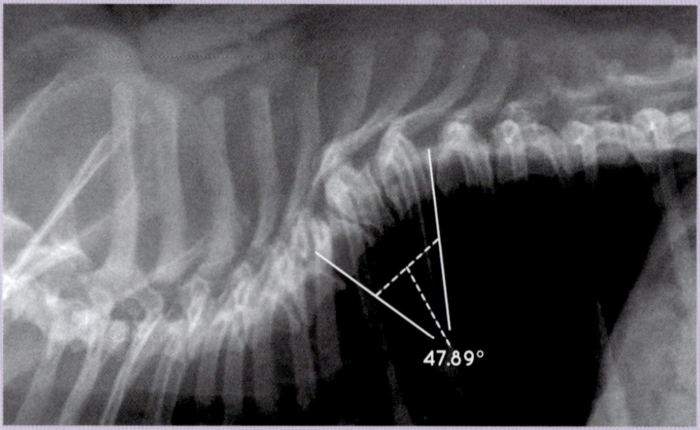

FIGURE 5.27. Lateral projection of the thoracic spine of a dog with kyphosis showing the Cobb angle measurement method (it can also be measured on the ventrodorsal view). In this patient the angle measures 47.9°, indicating a high probability of secondary neurological deficits.

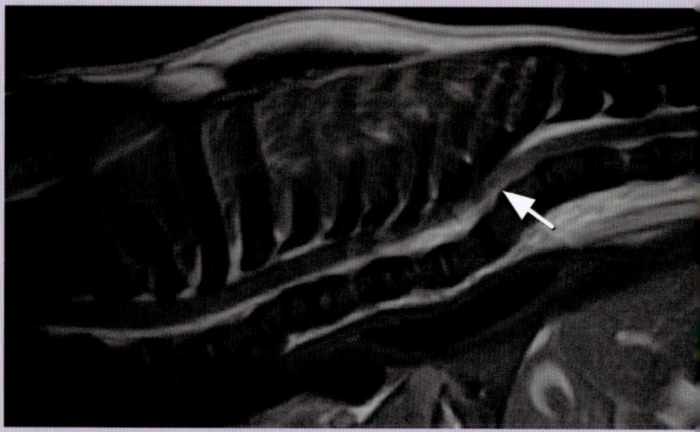

FIGURE 5.28. Magnetic resonance image of the thoracolumbar spine of a dog with multiple vertebral deformations causing angulation of the spinal canal and spinal cord compression (arrow).

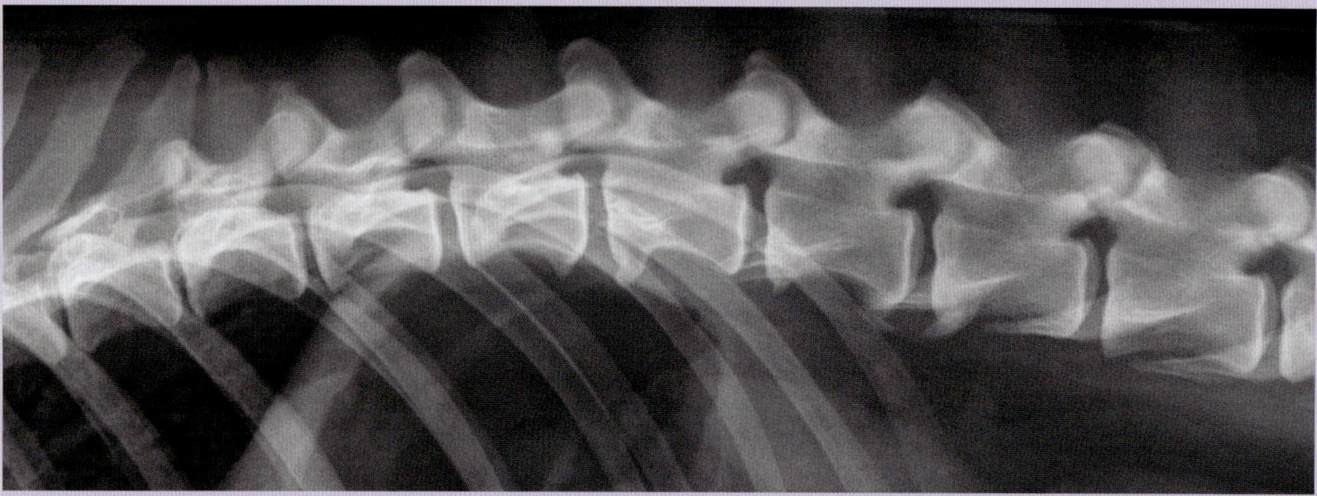

FIGURE 5.29. Lateral radiograph of the thoracolumbar spine of a dog with mild spondylosis deformans at T13–L1, L1–L2 and L2–L3.

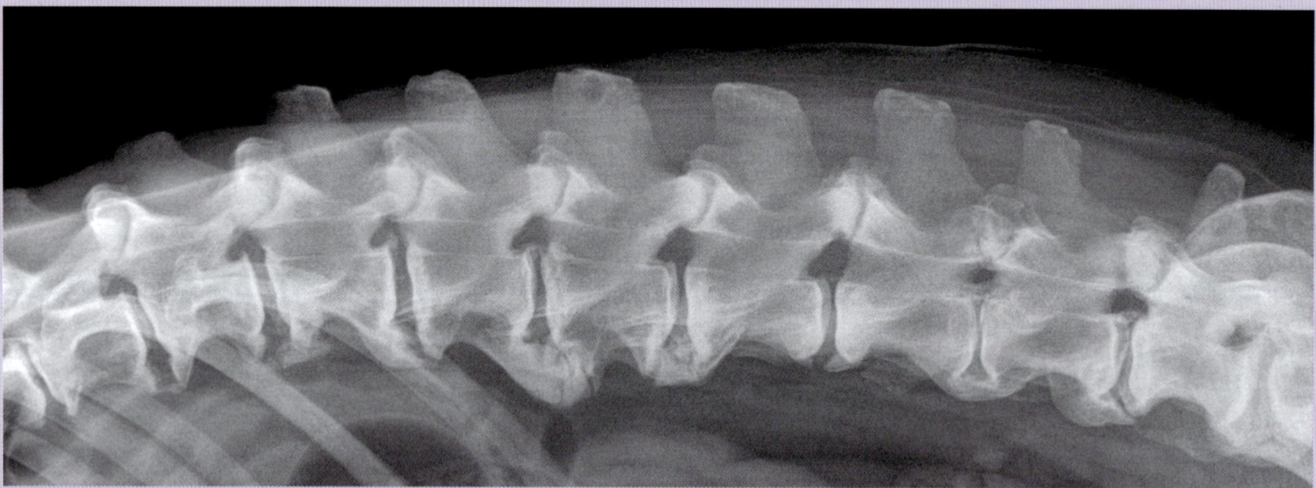

FIGURE 5.30. Lateral projection of the lumbar spine of a dog with marked spondylosis deformans affecting all lumbar and thoracic caudal vertebrae.

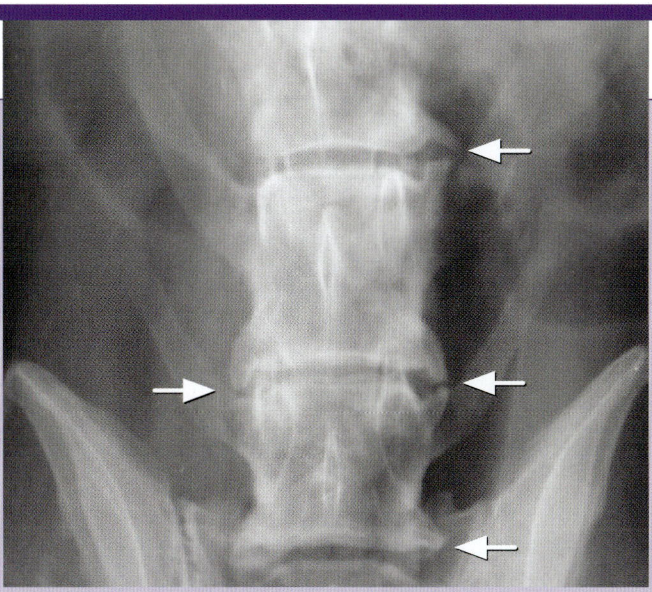

FIGURE 5.31. Enlarged image of the lumbar spine on a ventrodorsal radiograph of a dog with lateral spondylosis deformans at L5–L6, L6–L7 and L7–S1 (arrows).

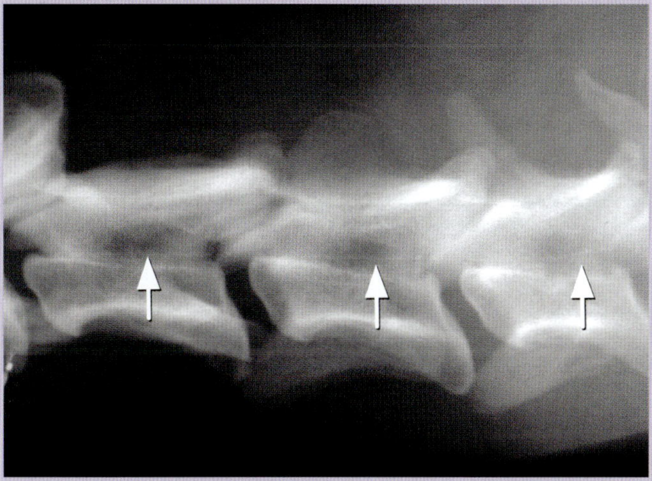

FIGURE 5.32. Enlarged image of the cervical spine on a lateral radiograph of a dog with dural ossification (arrows).

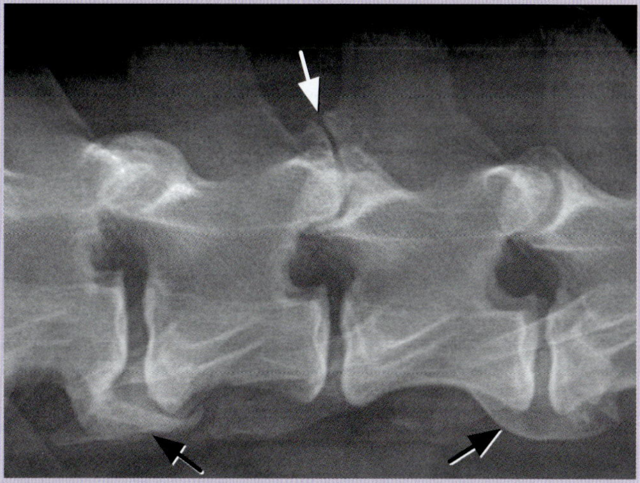

FIGURE 5.33. Enlarged image of the lumbar spine on a lateral radiograph of a dog with spondyloarthrosis (white arrow). The joint facets appear deformed, and the joint space is diminished. The patient also presents spondylosis deformans (black arrows).

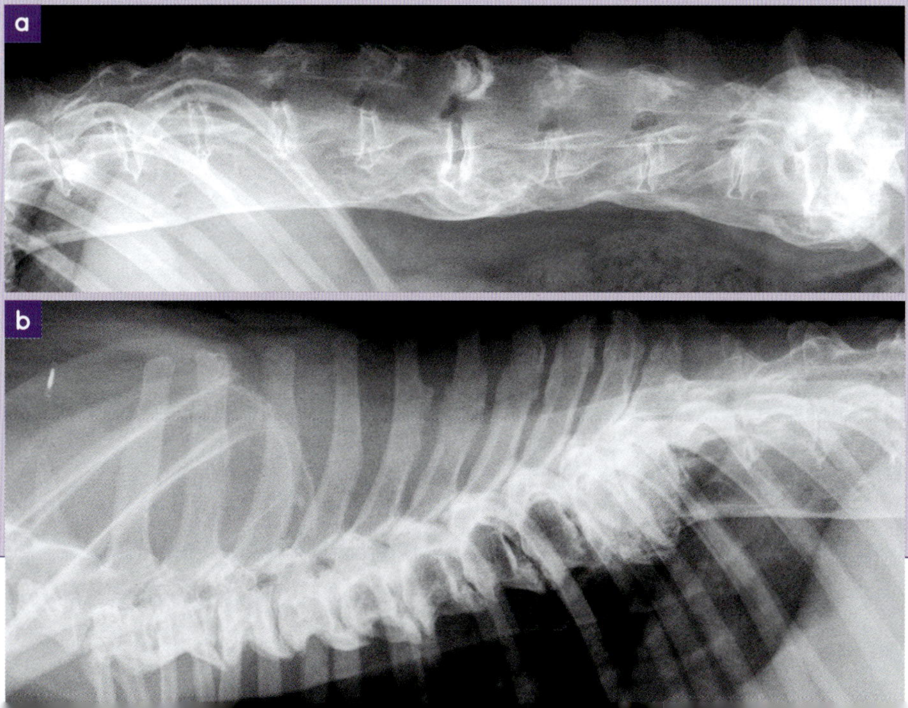

FIGURE 5.34. Lateral projection of the lumbar spine (a) and thoracic spine (b) of a Boxer dog with diffuse idiopathic skeletal hyperostosis.

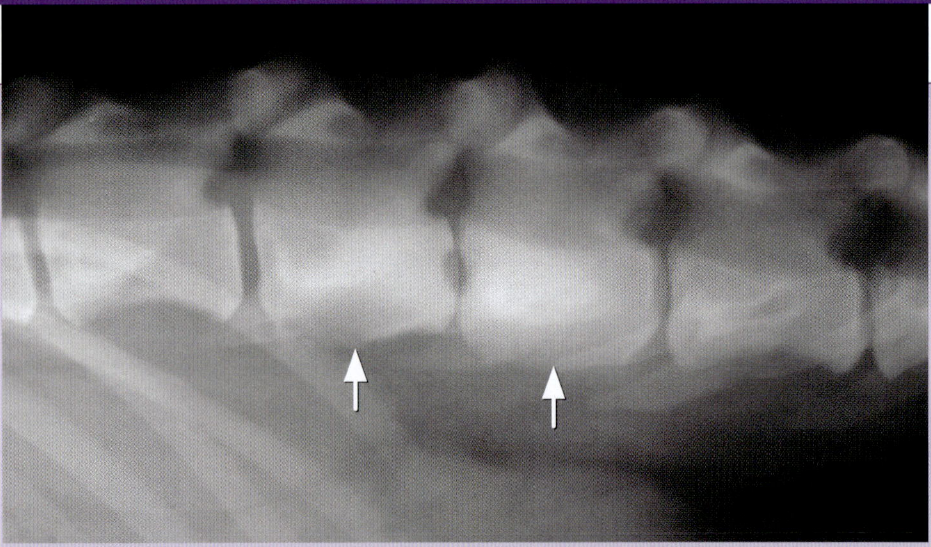

FIGURE 5.35. Enlarged image of the lumbar spine on a lateral radiograph of a dog with spondylitis at L2 and L3. The regular overgrowth of the ventral margin of both vertebrae (arrows) indicates inflammation of the vertebral bodies. In addition, the L2–L3 intervertebral disc space appears reduced and with initial signs of osteolysis of the caudal margin of L2 and cranial margin of L3, which suggests a disc infection at initial stage.

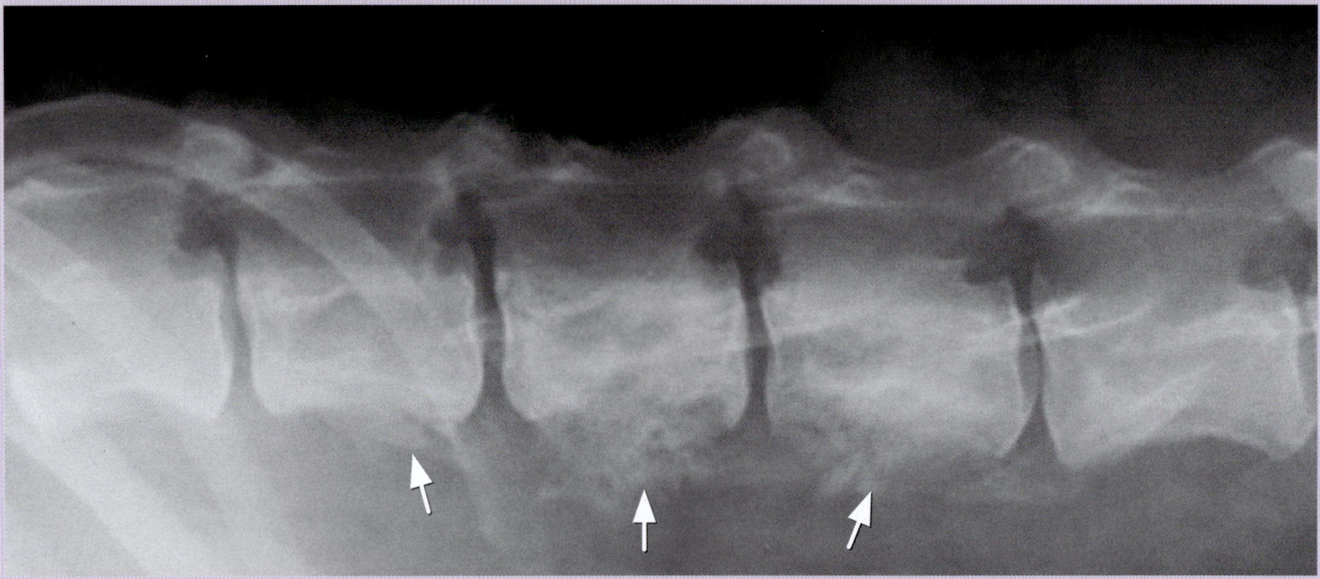

FIGURE 5.36. Enlarged image of the thoracic spine of a dog with spondylopyosis (vertebral osteomyelitis). An aggressive-looking periosteal reaction at the ventral margin of affected vertebrae (arrows) is indicative of spinal infection.

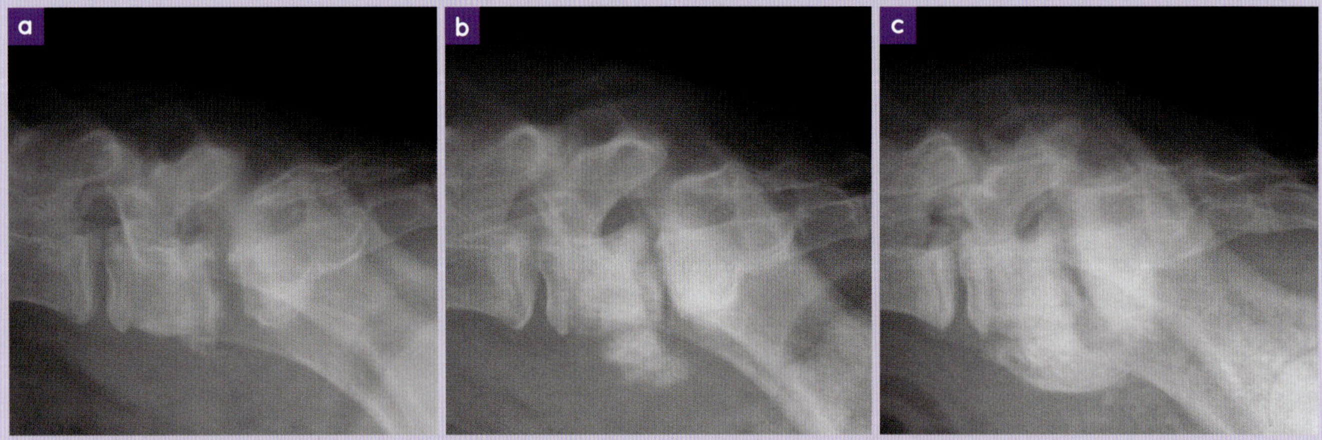

FIGURE 5.37. Images of the lumbosacral area of the spine on a lateral radiograph of a young dog with discospondylitis at an initial (a), intermediate (b) and advanced or chronic (c) stage.

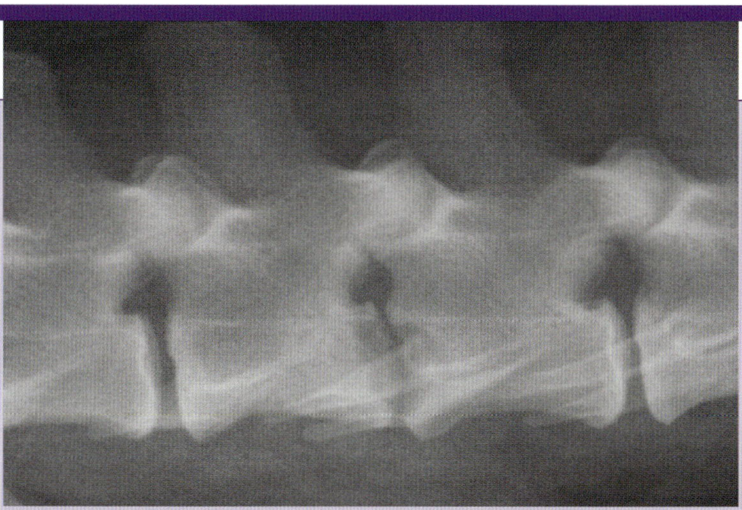

FIGURE 5.38. Enlarged image of the lumbar spine on a lateral radiograph of a dog with discospondylitis at L2–L3 at an initial stage.

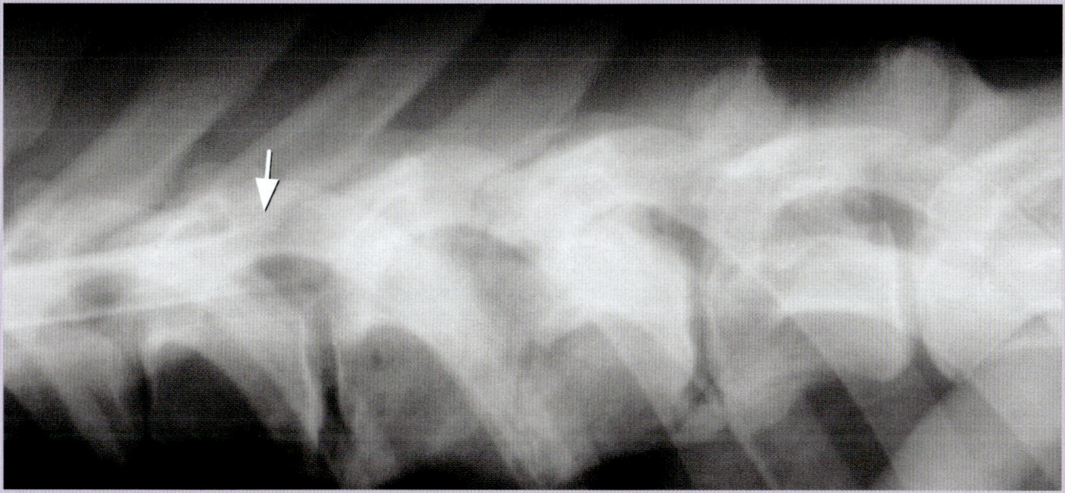

FIGURE 5.39. Enlarged lateral cisternal myelogram showing the thoracic spine of a dog with discospondylitis at an advanced or chronic stage. The affected vertebrae appear fused, with ventral overgrowths with regular margins. The lesions cause an interruption of the contrast columns (arrow) located cranial to the lesion.

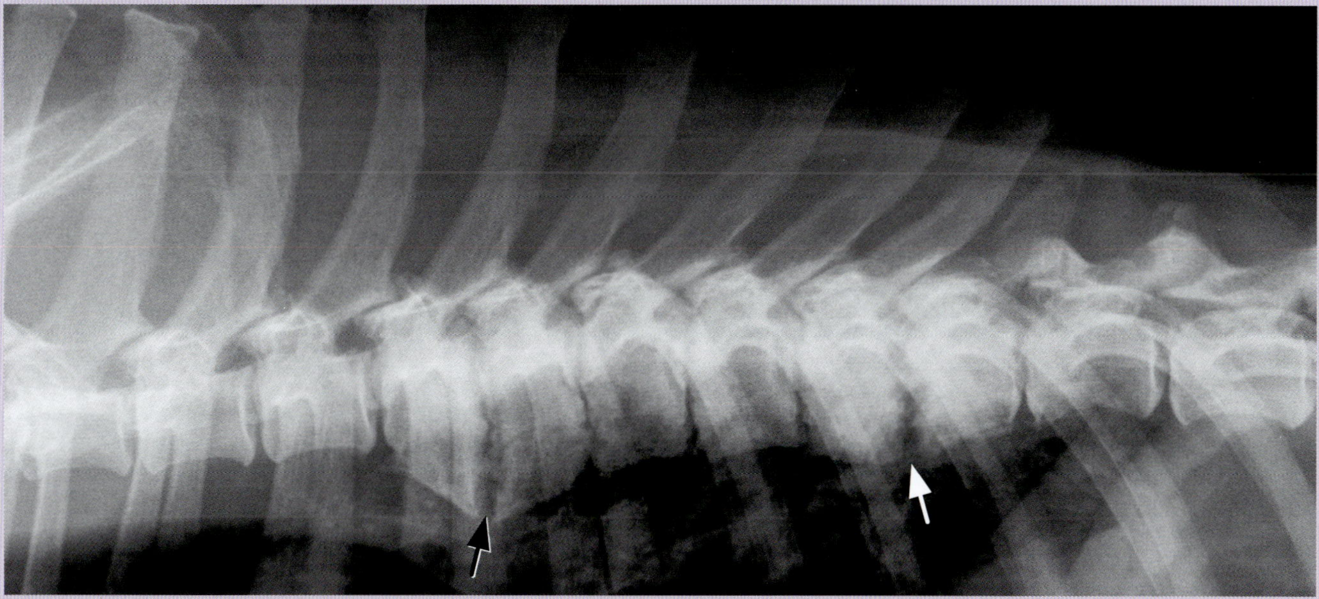

FIGURE 5.40. Enlarged image of the thoracic spine in lateral projection of a dog with multiple discospondylitis. The most cranial intervertebral space of the affected segment (black arrow) shows signs of advanced stage discospondylitis, while the more caudal (white arrow) is indicative of the earlier stages. The intervertebral spaces between the two show different degrees of intermediate stage involvement. These findings suggest that the infection spread from cranial to the caudal area.

Fractures and luxations

They are generally caused by trauma, although they may also be secondary to other lesions (pathological fractures). The ease with which a vertebral fracture is identified on radiographs depends on the degree of displacement of the fragments (fig. 5.41). In cases of fractures by compression, the image shows an apparent loss of vertebral body height. If a vertebral fracture is suspected, the patient should be handled with extreme care. A lateral projection should be taken first, as positioning the patient in dorsal recumbency for a ventrodorsal projection poses an increased risk of aggravating possible spinal cord damage. When working with X-ray machine that allows the tube to be rotated to deliver the beam horizontally, the X-ray cassette can be positioned adjacent to the spine, perpendicular to the table, while the animal is in lateral recumbency. Emitting the beam horizontally, a ventrodorsal projection is obtained without moving the patient.

During a fracture recovery period, it must be taken into account that the bone callus can produce spinal cord compression.

Fractures of spinous or transverse processes are not usually clinically significant (fig. 5.42).

Complete luxations are easily identifiable on plain radiographs. The ease with which a vertebral subluxation is identified depends on the degree of displacement of the affected vertebrae (fig. 5.43). In normal conditions, the body of L4 may have a position that is slightly ventral to that of L3, which should not be confused with pathological subluxation.

Both in spinal fractures and luxations, a vertebral displacement of more than 2/3 of the diameter of the spinal canal is considered a sign indicating severed spinal cord (fig 5.44).

In patients with spinal trauma, computed tomography is considered superior to magnetic resonance imaging to determine the degree of bone injury, although magnetic resonance imaging offers more precise information on secondary spinal cord damage.

Tumours

Tumours in vertebrae are quite rare. The tumours that usually affect vertebrae are osteosarcomas, chondrosarcomas and mestastases of primary tumours of a different origin. While usually only a single vertebra is involved, it can sometimes spread to adjacent vertebrae in advanced stages. Lesions are usually predominantly osteolytic (fig. 5.45) or have a mixed osteolytic and osteo-proliferative pattern (fig. 5.46). Secondary pathological fractures can occur (fig. 5.47). Given the morphological complexity of the vertebrae, tumours are not usually identified on radiographs until the advanced stages of disease.

The spine is a site of predilection for myelomas, which have a radiographic pattern that is characterised by the appearance of numerous small, round osteolytic areas (3–5 mm, although they can be larger in diameter when several lesions converge) in long bones and spine (fig. 5.48). Bone lymphoma may also present a multifocal pattern, with lesions that are predominantly osteolytic.

Metastases usually appear as single or multiple aggressive bone lesions located in the spine and other bones. Bone metastases of some pelvic tumours, especially prostate and transitional cell carcinomas, have a peculiar image, since they affect the surrounding bones (last lumbar vertebrae, sacrum and pelvis), causing lesions that are fundamentally proliferative (fig. 5.49). These lesions are sometimes detected before the primary tumour.

Soft tissue tumours adjacent to the spine may also secondarily affect the vertebrae (e.g. post-vaccination sarcomas in cats, retroperitoneal tumours, etc.). They can involve several vertebrae adjacent to the tumour (fig. 5.50).

Hypervitaminosis A

It usually affects cats from 2 to 4 years old that ingest excessive amounts of liver. It is much less frequent in dogs. The excess of vitamin A causes the growth of subperiosteal bone. In young animals, an asymmetric longitudinal growth of the long bones occurs. In adults, bone exostoses develop essentially in the cervical and thoracic spine, ribs and around the limb joints, and can lead to ankylosis of these joints and of the vertebrae.

Mucopolysaccharidosis

Mucopolysaccharidosis can cause vertebral lesions in cats similar to those caused by hypervitaminosis A, as well as alterations in vertebral morphology and spondylosis deformans in young animals.

Osteopetrosis

Osteopetrosis, also known as myelofibrosis, is rare in cats and extremely rare in dogs. It causes generalised increased radiopacity of the skeleton, including the spine (fig. 5.51). It has been associated with feline leukaemia and lymphoma in cats and with pyruvate kinase deficiency in dogs. Other possible causes are excessive intake of dietary calcium, hypervitaminosis D and myelosclerotic neoplasia.

Multiple cartilaginous exostoses

It is an uncommon anomaly, which is characterised by osteo-proliferative benign lesions in the metaphyses of the long bones, ribs and vertebrae of young dogs (fig. 5.52). The growth of the lesions generally stops when skeletal maturity is reached. It is not usually clinically significant, unless the lesions invade the spinal canal or the intervertebral foramina, causing compression of the spinal cord or nerve roots. Exceptionally, a late evolution to osteosarcoma or chondrosarcoma has been described.

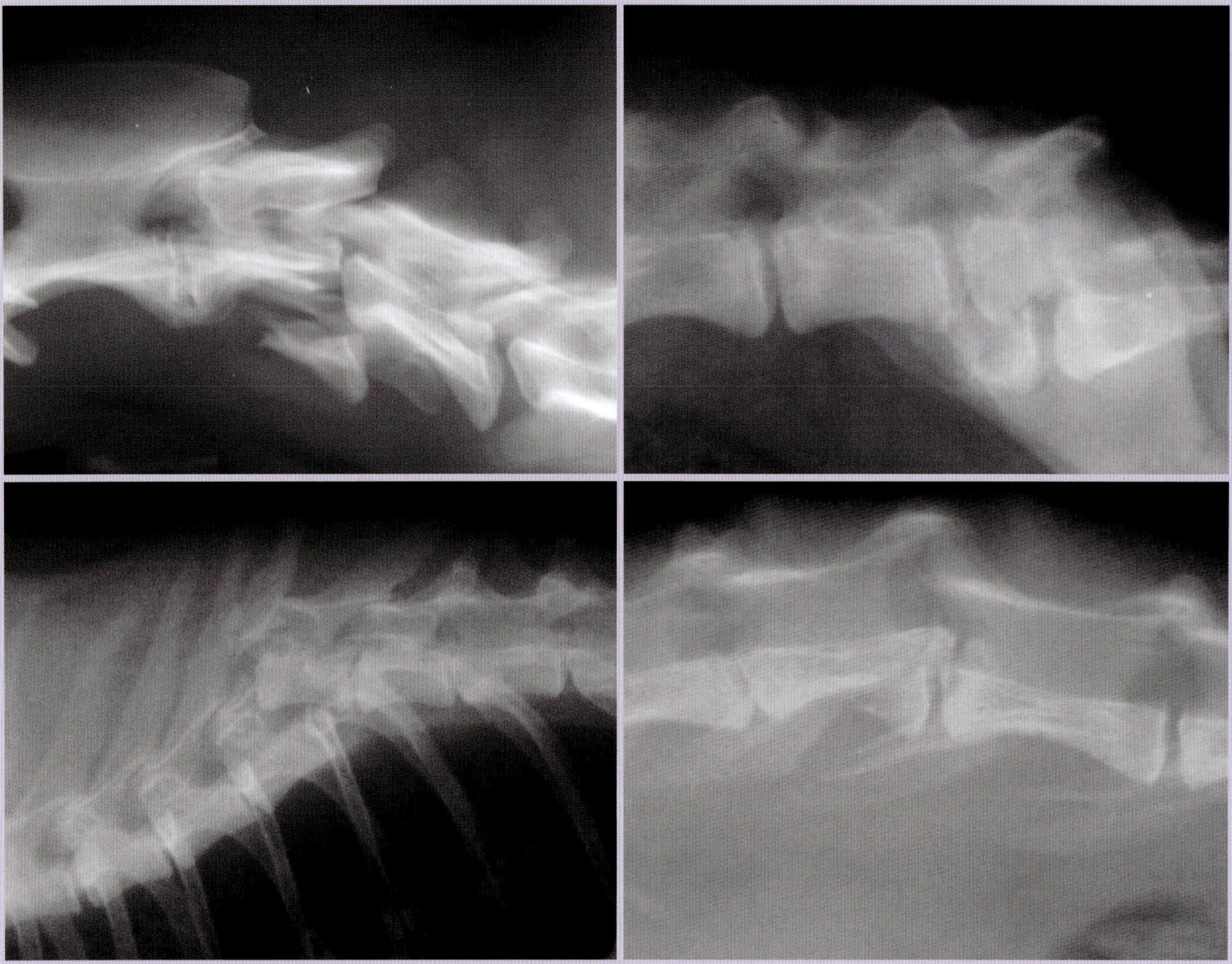

FIGURE 5.41. Images of various vertebral fractures.

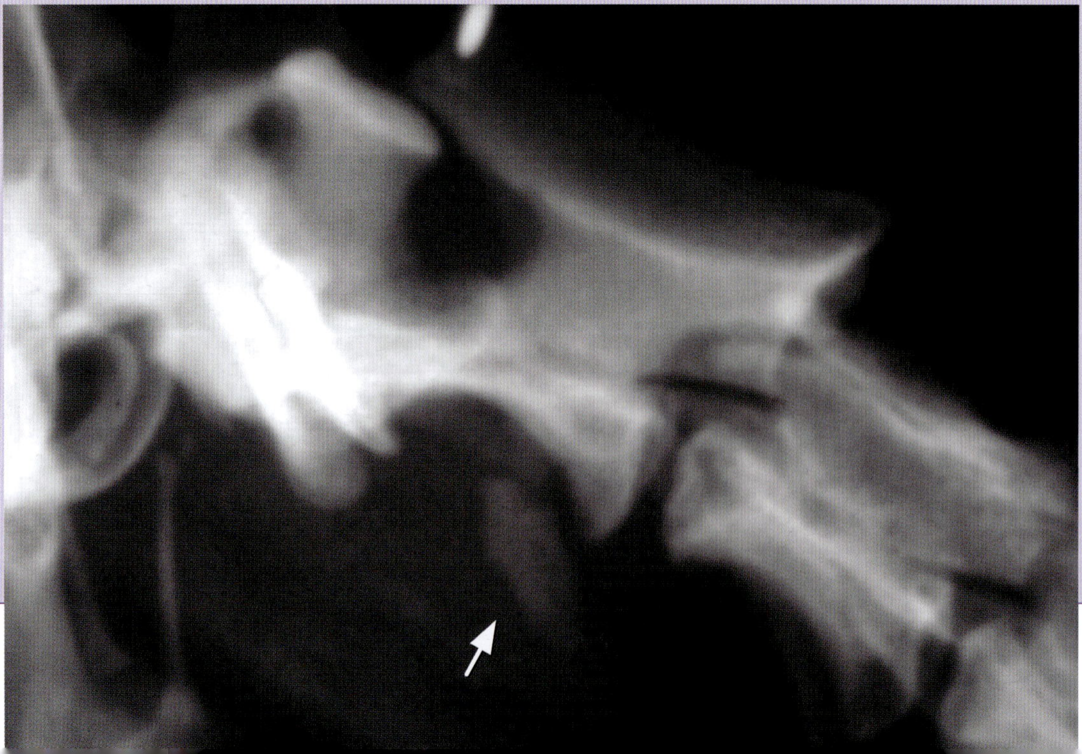

FIGURE 5.42. Enlarged image of the cervical spine on a lateral radiograph of a dog with a fracture of the transverse process of the axis (arrow).

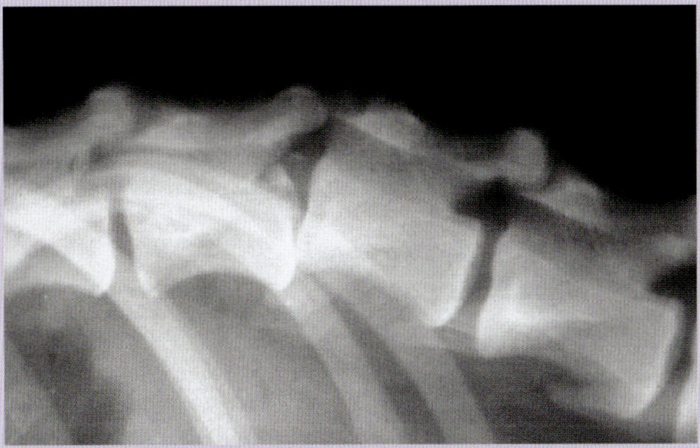

FIGURE 5.43. Enlarged image of the lumbar spine on a lateral radiograph of a dog with L1–L2 subluxation.

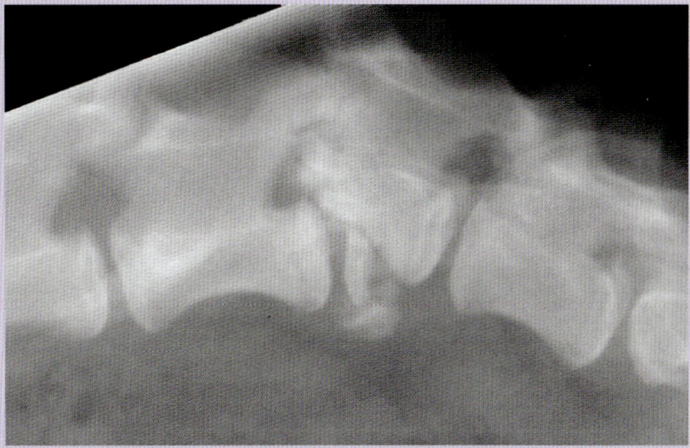

FIGURE 5.44. Enlarged image of the lumbar spine on a lateral radiograph of a dog with a comminuted fracture of L6. The displacement of L6 exceeds 2/3 of the diameter of the spinal canal, which indicates a severed spinal cord.

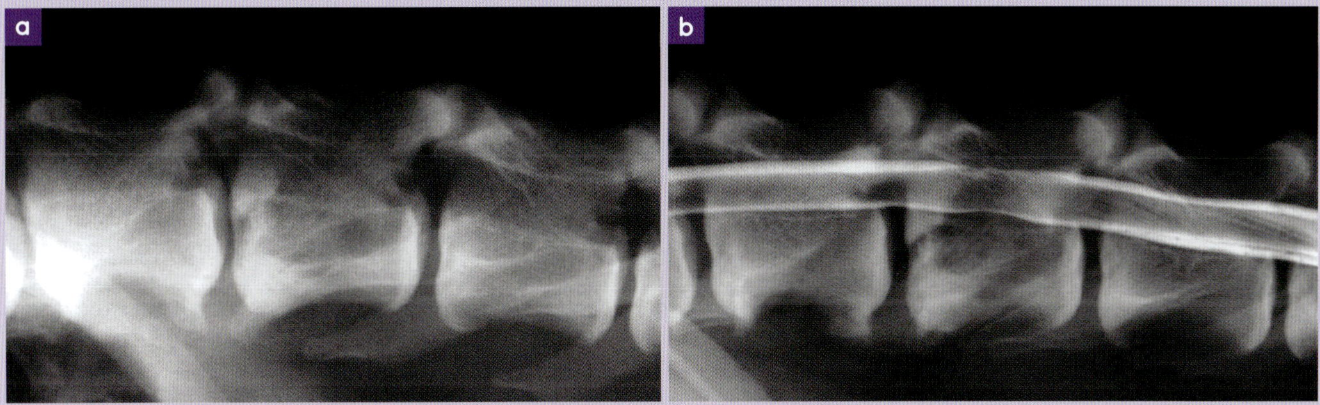

FIGURE 5.45. Enlarged image of the lumbar spine on a lateral radiograph of a dog with osteorsarcoma of L2. The tumour appears as an osteolytic geographic lesion on the plain radiograph (a). On the myelogram (b), it has an extradural pattern.

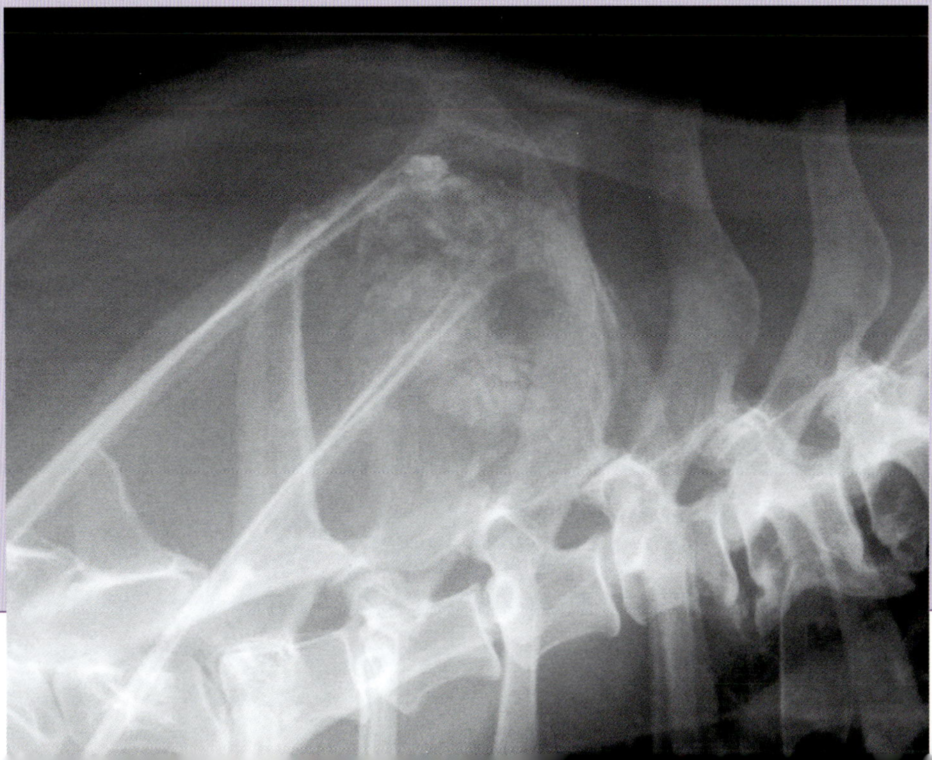

FIGURE 5.46. Enlarged image of the thoracic spine in lateral projection of a dog with a chondrosarcoma located in the spinous process of T2. The lesion presents a mixed osteolytic and osteo-proliferative pattern.

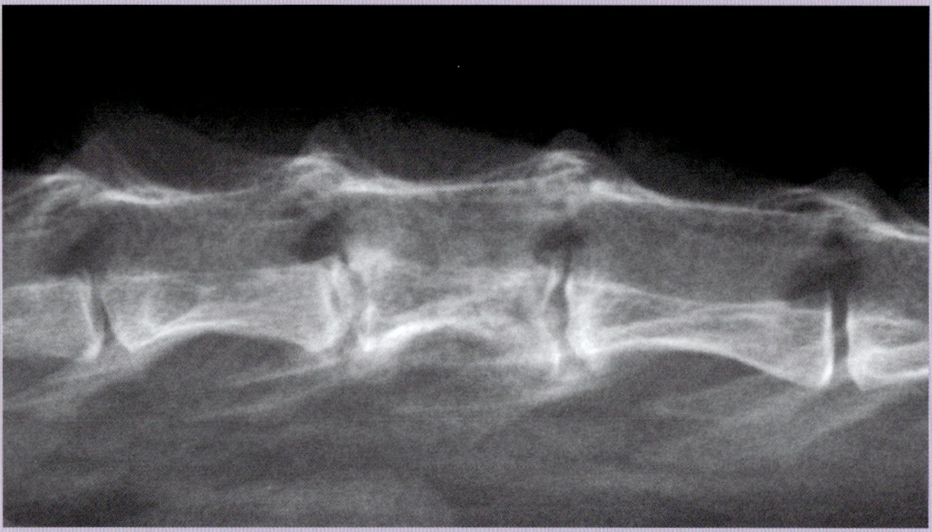

FIGURE 5.47. Enlarged image of the lumbar spine in lateral projection of a cat with pathological L4 fracture caused by a bone lesion with an infiltrating osteolytic pattern. The shortening of the vertebra coupled with the alteration in the cranial and caudal margins were suggestive of a fracture, later confirmed by computed tomography. The histological diagnosis of the primary bone lesion was a fibroblastic osteosarcoma.

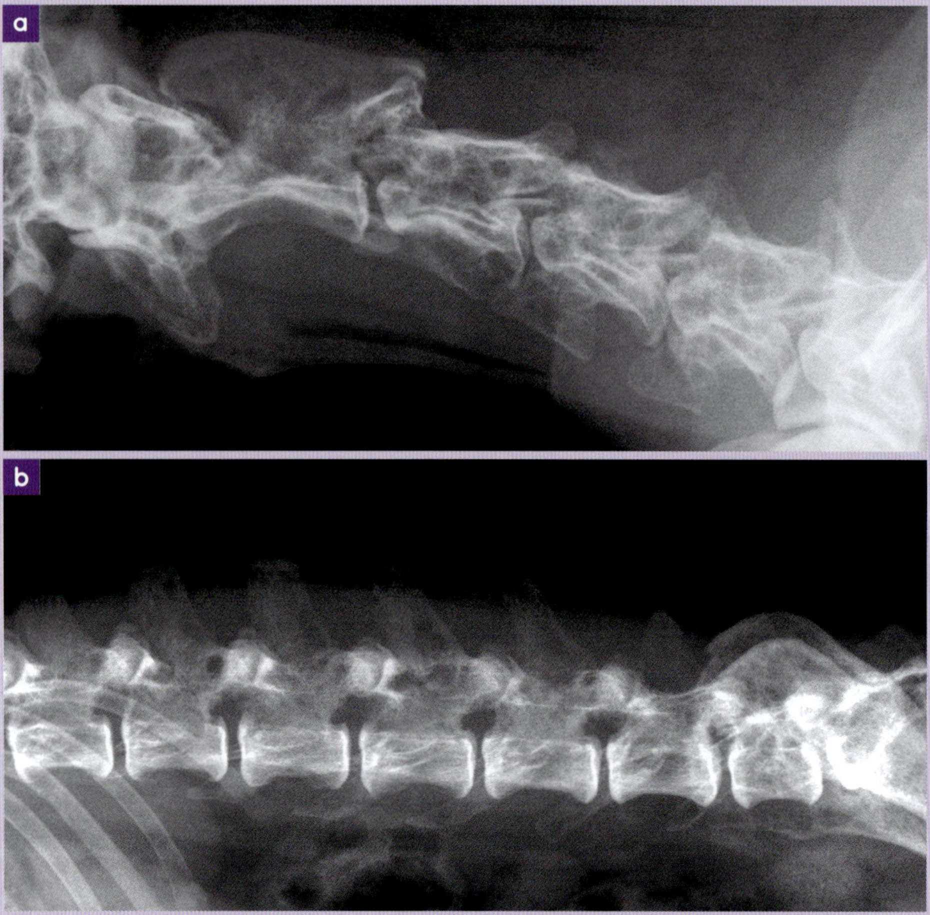

FIGURE 5.48. Lateral projections of the cervical (a) and lumbar (b) spine of a dog with multiple myeloma, showing the typical moth-eaten osteolytic pattern of this type of neoplasm in all the vertebrae visible in both images. The patient also presented involvement of the rest of the spine, ribs, sternum and long bones.

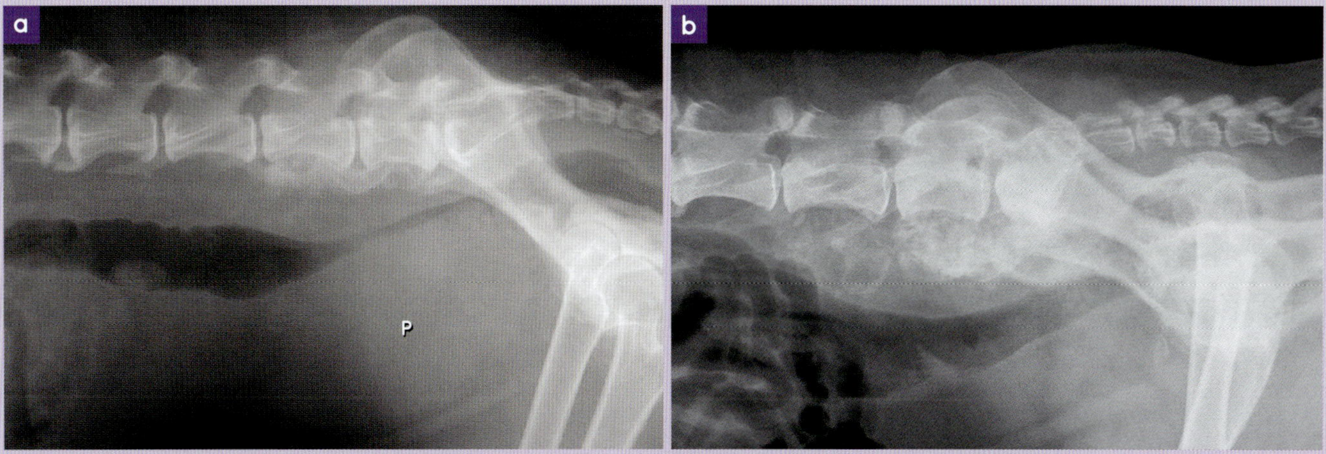

FIGURE 5.49. Lateral projection of the abdomen of a dog with prostate carcinoma and spinal metastases (a) and enlarged image of the caudal area of the lumbar spine of a dog with transitional cell carcinoma and spinal metastases (b). In image (a) the prostate (P) appears greatly enlarged and L6 presents an irregular overgrowth on its ventral margin, which corresponds to a prostate tumour metastasis; spondylosis deformans also appears in L6–L7 and L7–S1 as bony bridges of regular morphology and smooth margins, which differentiates them from the metastatic lesion. In image (b), aggressive-looking bone overgrowths from the ventral margin of L6, L7, and the cranial part of the sacrum corresponded to metastases of transitional cell carcinoma.

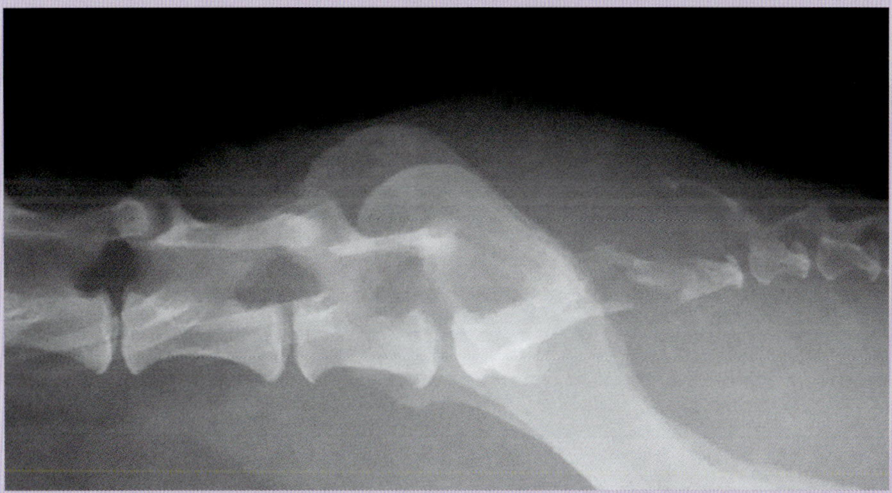

FIGURE 5.50. Enlarged image of the lumbosacral area of a dog with superficial soft tissue sarcoma with secondary involvement (osteolysis) of the L7, sacrum and first coccygeal vertebra.

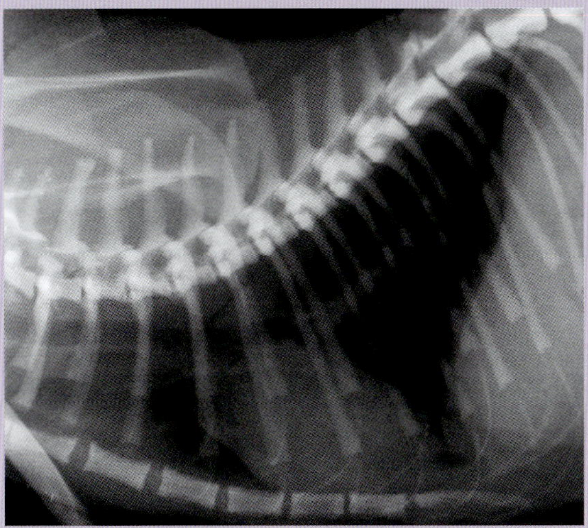

FIGURE 5.51. Lateral projection of the thorax of a cat with osteopetrosis, which causes increased radiopacity of the entire skeletal structures. The radiopacity of the vertebrae, ribs, sternebrae and the visible part of the humerus image is increased, with loss of distinction of the normal trabecular pattern and differentiation between cortical bone and bone marrow.

Cases for **self-assessment**

Case 5.1.

Presentation Explanation

Case 5.2.

Presentation Explanation

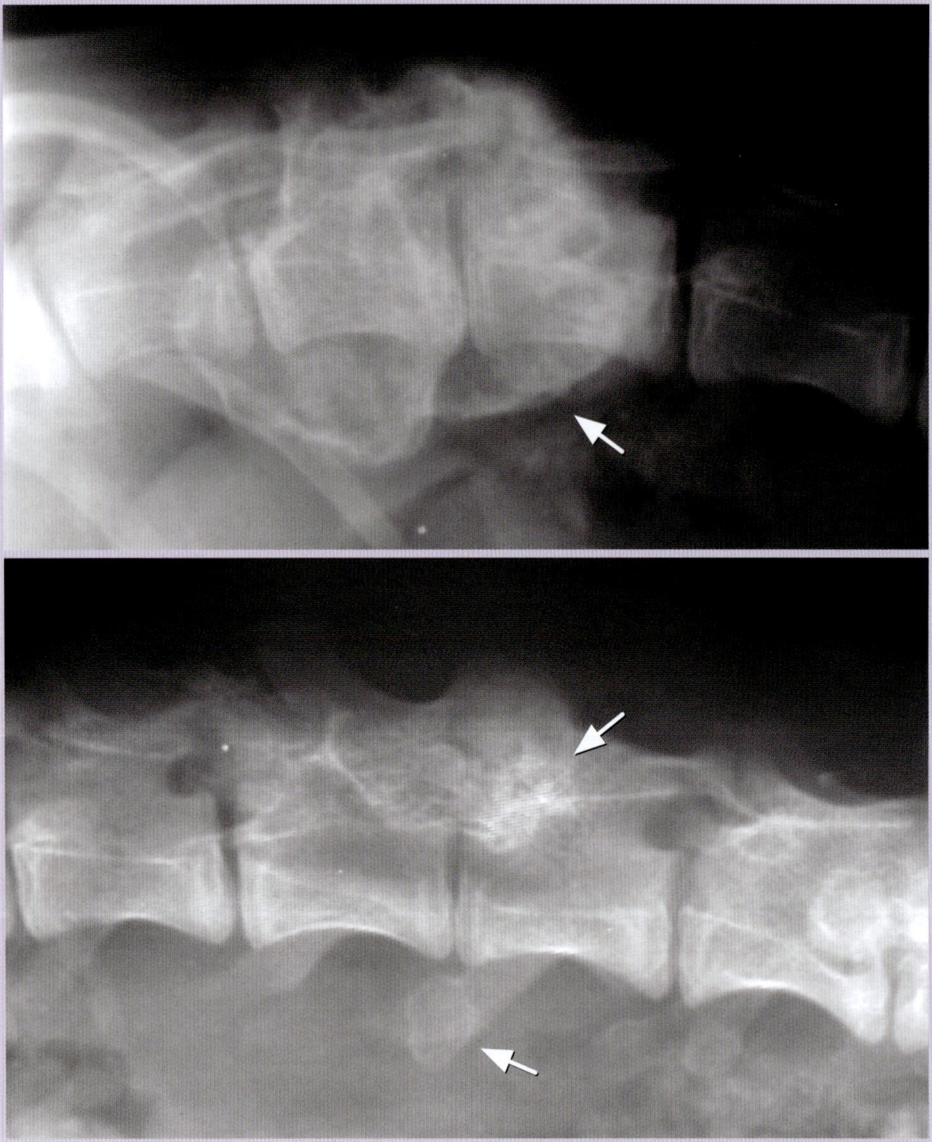

FIGURE 5.52. Enlarged images of the lumbar spine on lateral radiographs of a young dog with multiple cartilaginous exostoses, which appear as benign osteoproliferative lesions in the vertebrae (arrows).

Head

6

Normal radiographic anatomy of the head

https://goo.by/BOjKw

Principles of interpretation

The head is an extremely complex anatomical region, formed by approximately 50 bones, numerous teeth and various soft tissues. Furthermore, its morphological characteristics vary greatly among species and, within the canine species, among different breeds. Three basic conformations of the skull have been described:

- **Dolichocephalic:** nasal area longer than the cranial cavity.
- **Mesaticephalic:** the nasal area has approximately the same length as the cranial cavity.
- **Brachycephalic:** nasal area shorter than the cranial cavity.

Brachycephalic breeds have a series of anatomical features distinctive from other breeds, including a smaller size of the nasal cavity, the vomer bone may by slightly wavy in the dorsoventral and ventrodorsal projections, smaller or absent frontal sinuses, common mandibular prognathism and variations in the dentition.

In order to correctly interpret radiographs of the head, it is essential for the animal to be correctly positioned, since the radiological interpretation will often be based on the symmetrical image of the skull. Performing the radiological study under sedation or anaesthesia is recommended to obtain good-quality images. If an endotracheal tube is used, it will sometimes be necessary to remove it at the moment of taking the radiograph, so that it is not superimposed with the anatomical structures that are going to be assessed in the image. In some cases, it will also be necessary to change the position of the tongue, especially when taking a ventrodorsal open-mouth radiograph.

As it is an extremely complex anatomical region, comparing the images obtained with those that are included in atlases of normal radiographic anatomy is very useful. When the lesions affect only one side of the head, the contralateral half may also be used as reference for normality.

A wide variety of projections may be used to assess the different clinically important regions of the head. The choice of projections will be made according to the region that is to be examined.

- Cranial vault: lateral and ventrodorsal projections.
- Nasal cavity and frontal sinuses: lateral, ventrodorsal open mouth (ventral 20º rostral-dorsocaudal) or dorsoventral intraoral (occlusal) and rostrocaudal tangential (also termed "skyline") projections of the frontal sinuses.
- Mandible: lateral, dorsoventral, ventrodorsal intraoral and lateral oblique with open mouth (left 20º dorsal-right ventral to assess the right mandibular arcade and right 20º dorsal-left ventral to assess the left mandibular arcade).
- Maxilla: lateral, dorsoventral, dorsoventral intraoral and lateral oblique with open mouth (left 20º ventral-right dorsal to assess the right maxillary arcade and right 20º ventral-left-dorsal to assess the left maxillary arcade).
- Temporomandibular joint: dorsoventral and oblique lateral (with a 20 to 45º inclination of the rostral part of the head).
- Teeth: lateral oblique open mouth (those indicated above for the mandible and maxilla) and intraoral.

- Auditory apparatus: dorsoventral, lateral oblique, rostrocaudal with open mouth in dogs and rostral 10º ventral–caudodorsal in cats and brachycephalic dogs.
- In many cases it will be useful to take radiographs centred on the lesion, which will provide complementary information to that provided by standard projections.

Radiographs provide valuable information of the bone structure of the head, but are usually not very useful to assess soft tissues in this anatomical region. Ultrasonography may help to characterise lesions located in superficial soft tissues and is of great interest for the study of the eyeball and retrobulbar space. However, the diagnostic imaging techniques that offer more comprehensive diagnostic information about the head are computed tomography and magnetic resonance imaging. Both provide tomographic images of the patient (with no superimposition of structures) with excellent detail of intra- and extracranial anatomical structures. In general, magnetic resonances imaging is more appropriate to assess soft tissues, while computed tomography offers more detailed images of bone structures.

Cranial vault

Congenital hydrocephalus

It is more common in miniature breeds such as Chihuahua, Pomeranian and Yorkshire Terrier, among others. It can be asymptomatic or present with various neurological disorders. The radiological signs that may be associated with this disease are excessive enlargement of the cranial vault, thinning of the bones that form it, persistence of the fontanelles in the adult animal and relatively homogeneous appearance of the intracranial content (fig. 6.1a and b).

Ultrasound examination can be very useful to assess the degree of dilation of the ventricular system when the fontanelle is large enough to allow good transducer contact and ultrasound beam penetration (fig. 6.1c), although magnetic resonance imaging is the technique of choice to accurately assess this condition.

Occipital dysplasia

As with hydrocephalus, this congenital alteration also mainly affects miniature breeds and can have little clinical significance. Rostrodorsal–caudoventral radiographs are particularly useful for its radiological assessment. The main radiological sign is the abnormal dorsal enlargement of the foramen magnum, which acquires a "lock" shape (fig. 6.2). In some cases, this malformation appears associated with other abnormalities such as deformation of the C1 vertebra (shortened and with prominent dorsal arch), hypoplasia of the occipital condyles or atlantoaxial subluxation. Computed tomography is the preferred advanced imaging technique for its evaluation. Occipital dysplasia is considered a normal morphological variation in brachycephalic breeds.

Fractures

Fractures located in the cranial vault are generally difficult to visualise on radiographs, since the displacement of the fragments is usually minimal (fig. 6.3). The areas of greater inflammation of the soft tissues are a useful guide and the patient should be positioned so that these areas are centred on the radiograph (fig. 6.4).

Computed tomography is an excellent option to assess patients in which a skull fracture is suspected, since in addition to providing detailed information about bone structures, it also allows the evaluation of possible associated intracranial lesions.

Infection

Infections in the cranial vault are uncommon. They can present with an osteolytic pattern, an osteoproliferative pattern or a combination of both, similar to what is observed in other bone locations (fig. 6.5).

Tumours

Osteosarcomas are the bone tumours that most frequently appear in the cranial vault (fig. 6.6), followed by chondrosarcomas and multilobular osteochondrosarcomas. These tumours usually have a greater osteoproliferative than osteolytic component. Multilobular osteochondrosarcomas generally appears as well-defined masses, characterised by a pattern of granular ossification with minimal or no associated osteolysis.

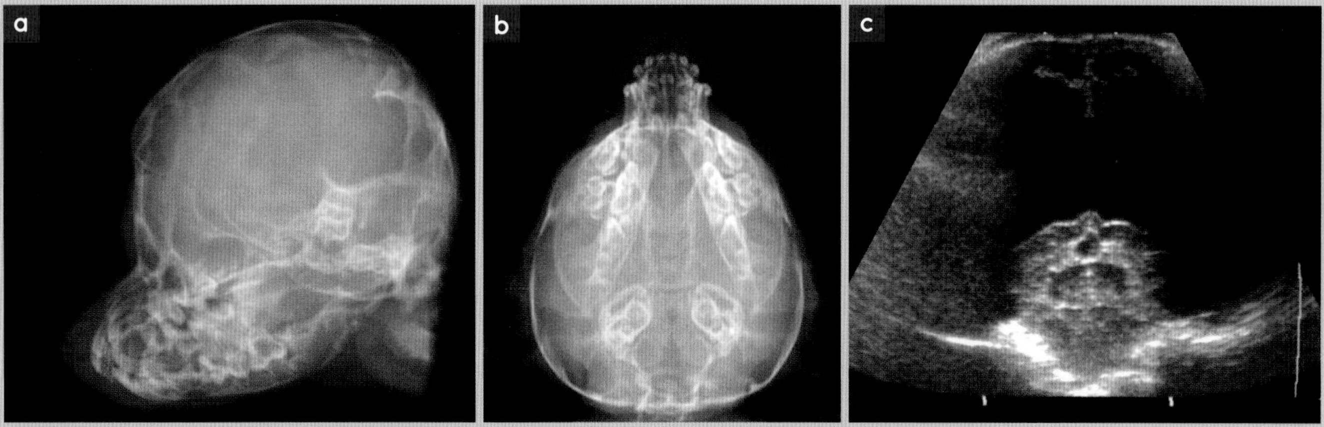

FIGURE 6.1. Lateral (a) and dorsoventral (b) radiographs of the head of a dog with congenital hydrocephalus. The radiographs show enlargement of the cranial vault and thinning of the bones. The ultrasound scan (c) shows marked dilatation of the lateral ventricles.

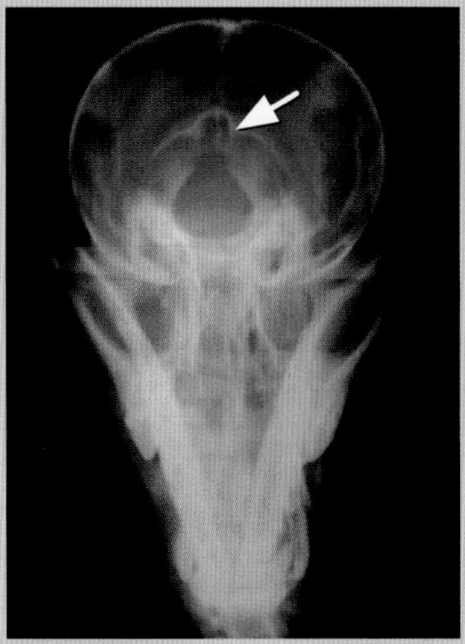

◀ FIGURE 6.2. Rostrodorsal-caudoventral view of the head of a dog with occipital dysplasia. The foramen magnum has an abnormal dorsal extension (arrow).

▼ FIGURE 6.3. Dorsoventral (a) and dorsoventral oblique views centred on the lesion (b) of a dog with a comminuted fracture of the temporal bone and mandible, involving the left temporomandibular joint. The patient presents marked swelling of the soft tissues adjacent to the lesion, causing narrowing of the left external auditory canal. Some fragments and the defect in the temporal bone are better appreciated (arrow) in the projection centred on the lesion.

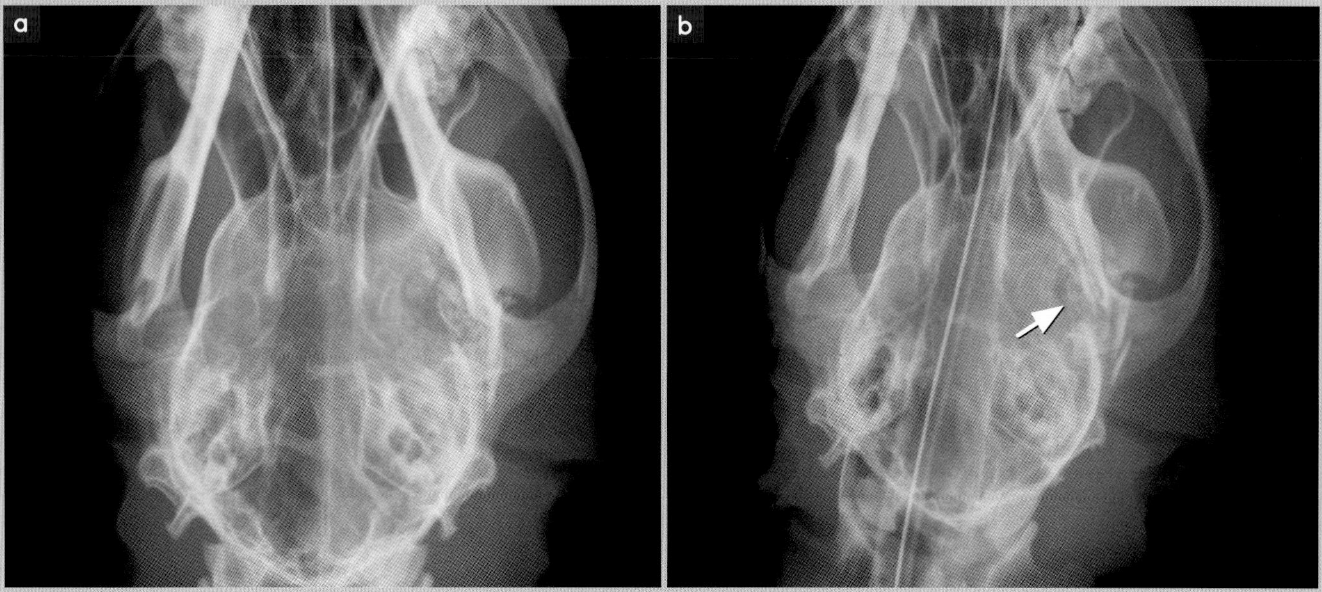

The most common location is the occipito–temporal region (fig. 6.7), although they have also been described in the orbit, maxilla, mandible, tympanic bulla, zygomatic arch and hard palate. Osteomas are less common and tend to be more sclerotic and delimited than osteosarcomas, and sometimes have a "cauliflower" shape (fig. 6.8).

As in other anatomical regions, aggressive soft-tissue neoplasms (e.g. squamous cell carcinomas, melanomas, fibrosarcomas, etc.) may also secondarily affect the bones of the skull (fig. 6.9).

Nasal cavity and sinuses

The complete radiological study of the nasal cavity and the sinuses must be carried out under sedation or anaesthesia and should include lateral, ventrodorsal open mouth with oblique orientation of the X-ray beam and rostrocaudal tangential (skyline) projections of the frontal sinuses. Standard dorsoventral and ventrodorsal projections offer very limited information due to the overlapping of the mandible with the rostral and lateral area of both nasal cavities. The main limitation

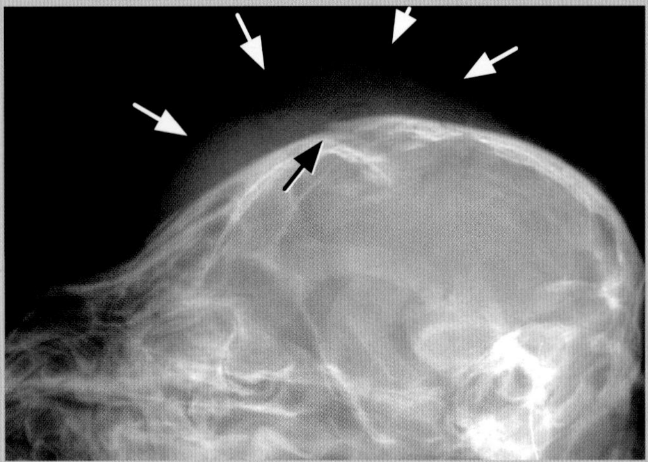

FIGURE 6.4. Enlarged image of the cranial vault of a young dog in lateral oblique projection. The radiograph was centred on the area of inflammation of the soft tissues (white arrows), which allowed the identification of a cranial fracture (black arrow), which was not visible on the standard lateral radiograph.

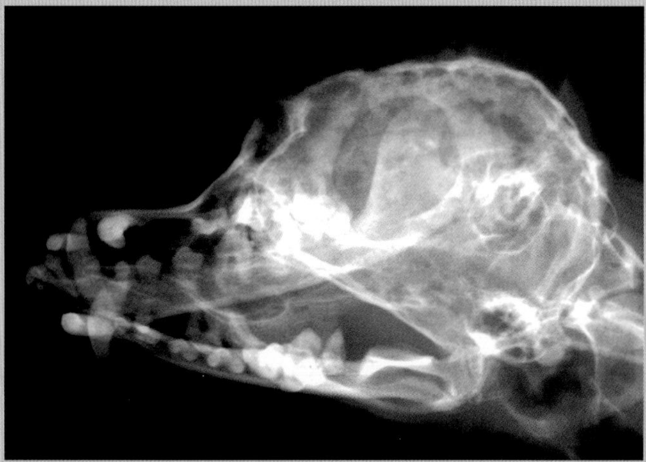

FIGURE 6.5. Oblique lateral radiograph of the head of a small breed dog with osteomyelitis of the cranial vault caused by a bite from another dog. The vault presents numerous osteolytic lesions of various sizes with partial lysis of the cortex.

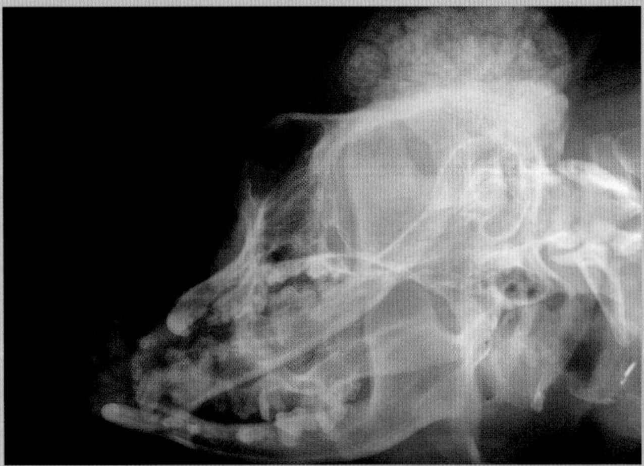

FIGURE 6.6. Lateral oblique radiograph of the head of a dog with a markedly osteoproliferative bone lesion located in the cranial vault. The radiograph was centred on the lesion to improve its visualisation. Histological diagnosis: osteosarcoma.

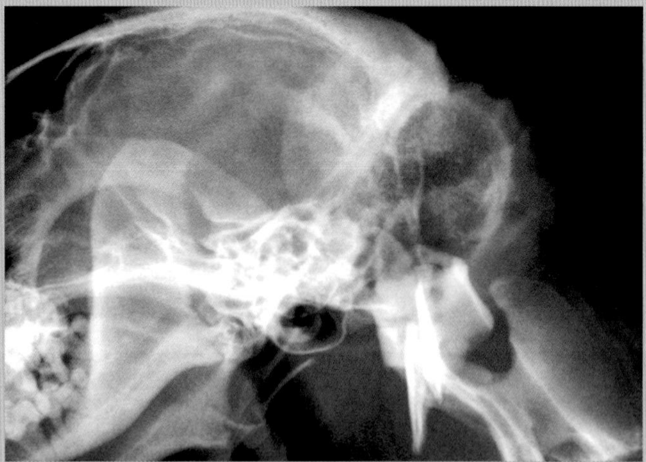

FIGURE 6.7. Enlarged image of the occipital region on a lateral radiograph of the head of a dog with a multilobular osteochondrosarcoma. This appears as an expansile lesion of the occipital bone with tiny spots of mineral opacity and a granular appearance.

of the lateral projection is that both nasal cavities and the two frontal sinuses overlap on the image. However, it is particularly useful when assessing the integrity of the dorsal nasal bone in patients with advanced-stage nasal neoplasms.

The ventrodorsal view performed with the mouth open and the X-ray beam at a 20º angle (ventral 20º rostral–caudodorsal) circumvents or minimises overlapping of the mandible with the nasal cavity. If it is not possible to tilt the X-ray tube, it will be technically more difficult to obtain this projection. A syringe case (or another object of low radiopacity) placed between the upper and lower canines can be used to keep the mouth open. It is important to remove the tongue and endotracheal tube from the radiographed area, as far as possible, to avoid overlapping with the region of interest.

The rostrocaudal tangential view is taken by positioning the long axis of the patient's head parallel to the direction of the X-ray beam, aligning the centre of the beam with the frontal sinuses. In this way, both sinuses can be visualised in the same image, avoiding their overlapping with each other, as happens in the standard lateral projection.

In radiographic images obtained in dorsoventral or ventrodorsal projection, the nasal cavity appears divided into two halves by the nasal septum, formed by the vomer bone and nasal cartilage. The nasal conchae appear as thin lines of mineral density in the rostral part of the cavity (dorsal and ventral nasal conchae) and as thicker swirls of mineral density in the caudal area of the cavity (ethmoid labyrinth or ethmoid conchae). The morphologic pattern of the nasal conchae is highly symmetrical in dogs but may be slightly asymmetrical in cats with no nasal pathology.

In both dogs and cats, the paranasal sinuses include the frontal sinuses, the lateral maxillary sinuses or recesses and the small sphenoid sinuses. The frontal sinuses are the most clearly observed on radiographs and their morphology can vary greatly depending on the patient's cranial conformation. They appear delimited by a bone wall and contain air. In dolichocephalic breeds, they may be very flattened which limits their evaluation in the tangential rostrocaudal projection, while in brachycephalic breeds, they may be smaller or absent.

Fractures

Fractures affecting the nasal bone (fig 6.10) or the frontal sinuses (fig. 6.11) may be difficult to diagnose. There is usually depression of the bone fragments, which is accompanied by inflammation of the adjacent soft tissues and, in many cases, subcutaneous emphysema as air escapes to the adjacent tissues.

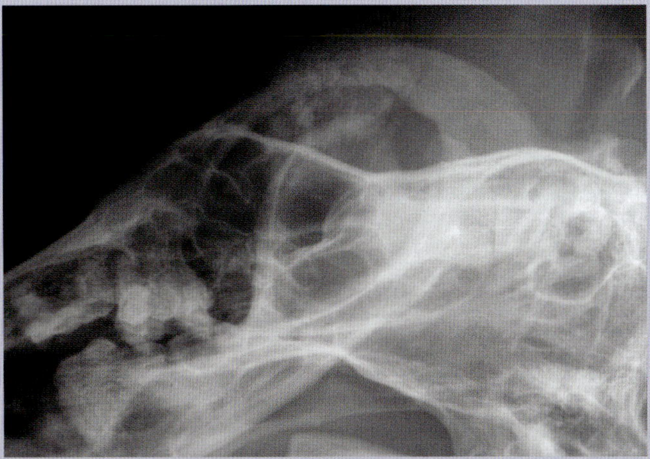

FIGURE 6.8. Enlarged image in lateral oblique projection of the region of the zygomatic bone of a dog with an osteoproliferative lesion in the central area of the zygomatic arch. The radiograph was centred on the lesion to improve its visualisation. Histological diagnosis: osteoma.

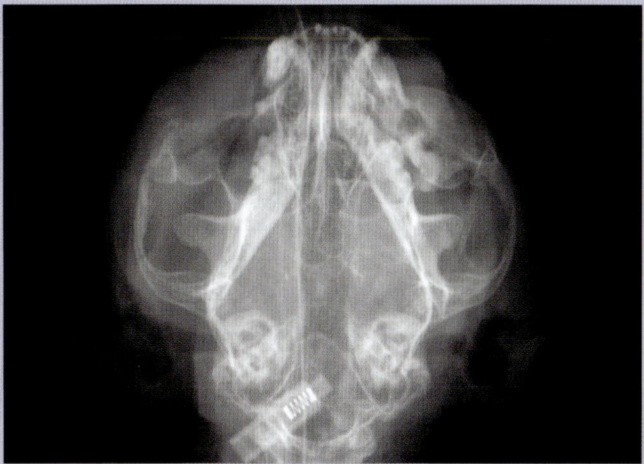

FIGURE 6.9. Dorsoventral radiograph of the head of a cat with a soft-tissue neoplasm (squamous cell carcinoma) that affects the adjacent bone and partially destroys the rostral part of the right zygomatic arch and the lateral area of the maxilla of the same side.

Rhinitis

Rhinitis secondary to bacterial infections and lymphoplasmatic rhinitis usually lead to increased radiographic density of the nasal cavity, accompanied or not by increased density of the frontal sinuses, although the nasal conchae are usually still well-differentiated in the image (fig. 6.12). In acute processes, there may not be any evident alterations of the cavity in the radiographic image.

Hyperplastic chronic rhinitis may cause, together with an increase in the radiopacity of the cavity, a loss of differentiation of the nasal conchae due to a thickening of the mucosa and the presence of exudate between them (fig. 6.13).

It is more difficult to assess the image of the nasal conchae in cats, since under normal conditions they have a more irregular pattern than in dogs. It is important to bear this aspect in mind when assessing

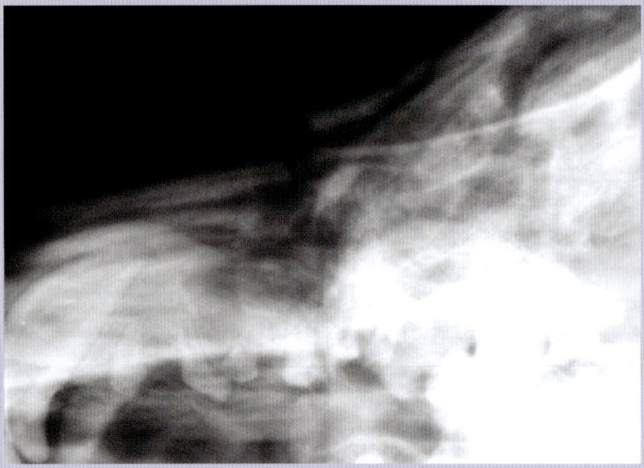

FIGURE 6.10. Enlarged image of the nasal region on a lateral oblique radiograph of a dog with a fracture of the nasal bone. The radiograph was centred on the lesion to improve its visualisation.

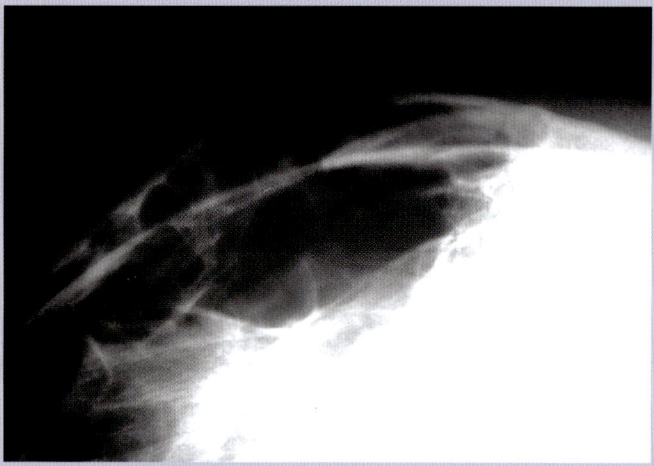

FIGURE 6.11. Enlarged image of the frontal region on a lateral oblique radiograph of a dog with a fracture of the frontal bone. The radiograph was centred on the lesion to improve its visualisation.

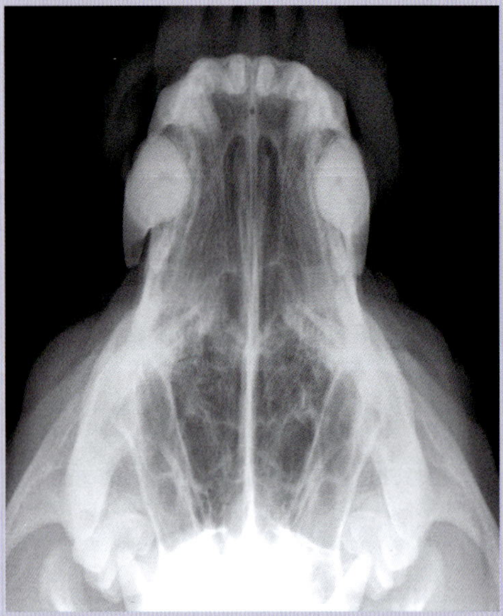

◀ **FIGURE 6.12.** Enlarged image of the nasal cavity on a ventrodorsal open-mouth radiograph of a dog with bacterial rhinitis. A generalised increase in the radiopacity of both nasal cavities is observed without evident alteration of the radiological pattern of the nasal conchae.

FIGURE 6.13. Enlarged image of the nasal cavity on a ventrodorsal open-mouth radiograph of a dog with chronic hyperplastic rhinitis. An increase in the radiopacity of the left nasal cavity is observed, especially in the middle third, where the nasal conchae are difficult to differentiate (this is attributed to the thickening of the mucosa and the presence of exudate between them). ▶

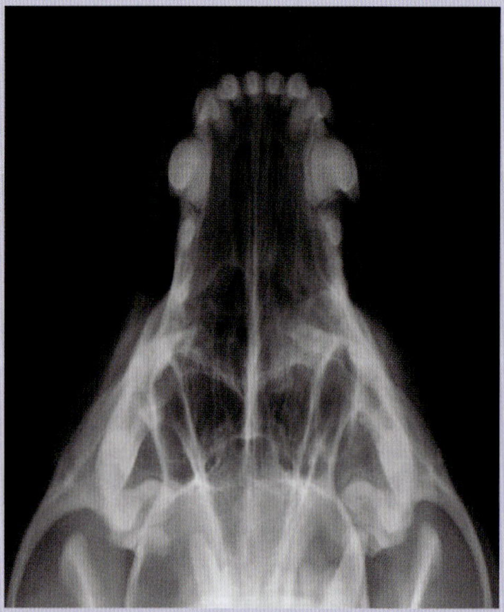

a possible case of feline chronic rhinitis, since it may cause a disorganisation or destruction of the conchae (fig. 6.14).

Fungal rhinitis, especially when caused by *Aspergillus*, is a destructive or aggressive type rhinitis. It usually presents a mixed radiological pattern in which areas of osteolysis (where there is a loss of differentiation of the conchae) are combined with areas of increased focal opacity (fig. 6.15). In advanced stages of the disease, a deviation or erosion of the vomer bone may appear, as well as lysis of the bones adjacent to the nasal cavity, although these findings are more common in cases of nasal neoplasia than in fungal rhinitis. The latter can also cause secondary involvement of the frontal sinuses, with increased intraluminal opacity and thickening and/or lysis of its wall.

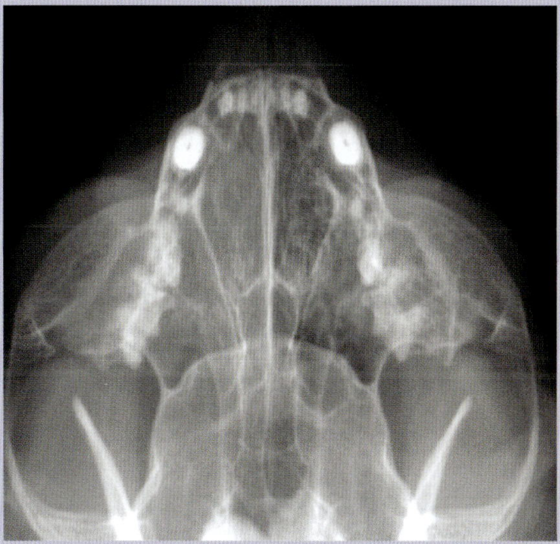

FIGURE 6.14. Enlarged image of the nasal cavity on a ventrodorsal open-mouth radiograph of a cat with chronic rhinitis. It is possible to observe an increase in the radiopacity of the right nasal cavity with a loss of differentiation of the nasal conchae.

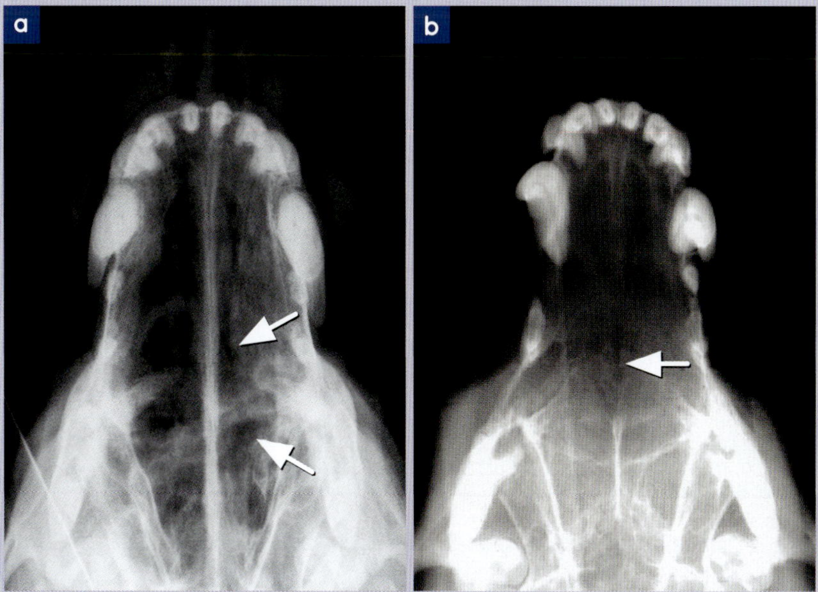

FIGURE 6.15. Enlarged images of the nasal cavity on ventrodorsal open-mouth radiographs of two dogs with fungal rhinitis caused by *Aspergillus*. The radiograph (a) shows large areas of osteolysis in the right nasal cavity mainly involving the middle and rostral thirds of the nasal cavity, and smaller focal areas adjacent to the septum in the left nasal cavity (arrows). The radiograph (b) shows multiple osteolytic areas in the middle third of the right nasal cavity (arrow), an increase in the radiopacity of both nasal cavities and disappearance of a great part of the vomer bone.

Foreign bodies

Mineral or metallic density foreign bodies located in the nasal cavity are usually easy to identify on radiographs. However, those with a radiographic density similar to that of soft tissues and fluids (radiolucent foreign bodies), such as grass awns, sticks, small plastic objects, etc., usually cannot be visualised in the image, although in many cases the underlying signs of focal rhinitis are identified (fig. 6.16).

Intranasal foreign bodies that remain in the cavity for a long time can cause atrophy of the conchae in the affected area, which could be mistaken for osteolysis.

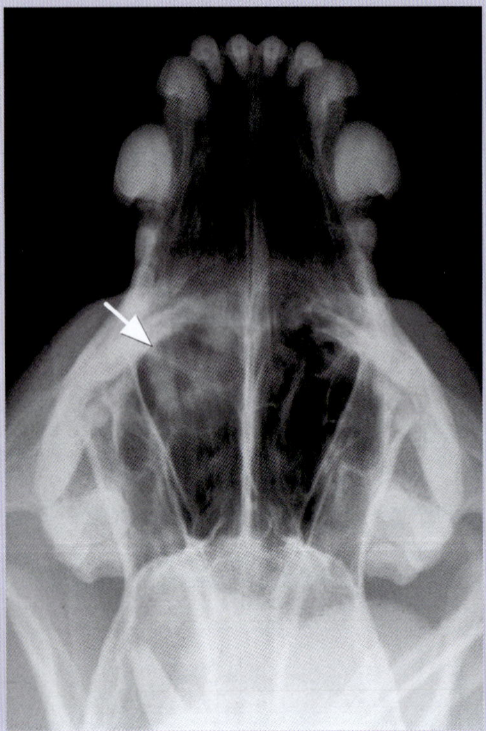

FIGURE 6.16. Enlarged image of the nasal cavity on a ventrodorsal open-mouth radiograph of a dog with focal rhinitis due to penetration of a foreign body. The arrow points to an area of increased soft tissue opacity with a radiolucent centre, located in the middle third of the right nasal cavity, due to focal inflammatory changes associated with the presence of the foreign body (grass awn, not identifiable in the image).

Tumours

In small animals, approximately two thirds of nasal tumours are carcinomas and the other third are sarcomas. Nasal lymphoma, which is more common in cats, has also been described.

The radiographic image of a nasal neoplasm varies depending on the type of tumour and its stage of development (fig. 6.17). In the early phase, it can cause an increase in soft tissue opacity in the affected nasal cavity, which could be confused with the radiological changes caused by inflammatory rhinitis. As the disease progresses, the tumour may cause displacement or destruction of the nasal septum and osteolysis of the conchae and paranasal bones. In cats, the loss of teeth adjacent to the lesion is also common. Radiographic identification of osteolysis is more indicative of neoplasia than of aggressive rhinitis, but it can occur in both cases. It is usually not possible to establish a differential diagnosis based solely on radiographic findings.

Nasal tumours sometimes cause osteolysis of the nasal bone which can spread to the superficial planes leading to the formation of an external soft-tissue mass which in turn can produce facial deformities (fig. 6.18). This is more typical in cases of tumours than in cases of rhinitis. Nasal neoplasms may also invade the cribriform plate and penetrate into the cranial cavity. They may thus affect the brain. The cribriform plate can be identified in the ventrodorsal and dorsoventral radiographs in the caudal area of the nasal cavity as a C or V shape. However, confirmation of possible erosion or destruction of the plate is usually difficult. This type of lesion can be evaluated more precisely with computed tomography or magnetic resonance imaging. Although extension of the tumour to the frontal sinus is also possible, the increase in density that is often observed in the ipsilateral sinus is usually due to the development of obstructive sinusitis, more than to a neoplastic invasion of the sinus (fig 6.19).

Nasal lymphoma in cats may cause an increase in the radiographic density of the nasal cavity, accompanied or not by bone destruction (fig. 6.20).

Regarding advanced imaging diagnostic techniques, computed tomography should be selected to analyse the involvement of the bone structures with greater precision, while magnetic resonance imaging is more appropriate if the animal had neurological signs that would suggest a secondary spreading of the tumour to the brain through the cribriform plate.

Tumours affecting the frontal sinuses are not uncommon; the most common is squamous cell carcinoma. They generally cause increased radiopacity in one or both frontal sinuses, which is often accompanied by lysis of the frontal bone as the process progresses. Extensive destruction and/or expansion of the frontal bone and invasion of other adjacent bones and soft tissues may be observed in more advanced stages (fig. 6.21).

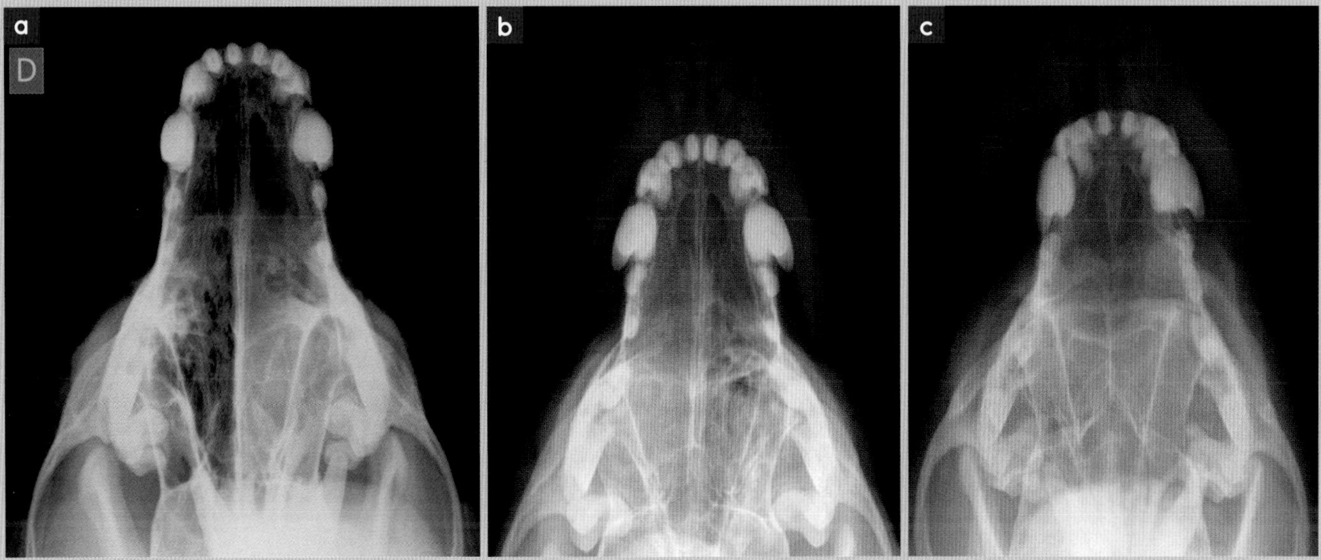

FIGURE 6.17. Enlarged image of the nasal cavity on a ventrodorsal open-mouth radiograph of three dogs with nasal neoplasms. Image (a) shows a slight increase in radiopacity in the rostral third, moderate increase in the middle third and very marked increase in the caudal third of the left nasal cavity, with osteolytic areas of irregular morphology in its middle third and loss of the normal pattern of the nasal conchae in the caudal third and especially in the middle third. Image (b) shows increased radiopacity of both nasal cavities, with marked loss of differentiation of the nasal conchae on the right. Image (c) shows increased radiopacity of both nasal cavities, with partial destruction of the vomer bone and loss of the normal pattern of the nasal conchae. The histological diagnosis of the three lesions was nasal carcinoma.

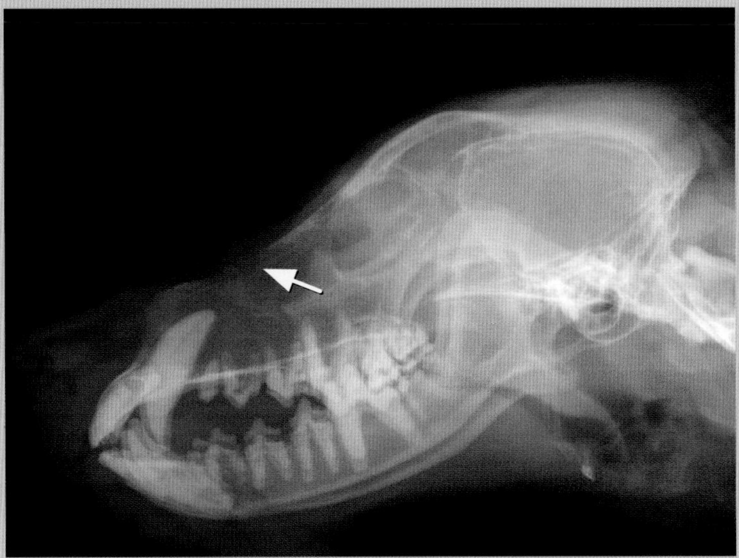

FIGURE 6.18. Lateral radiograph of the head of a dog with a nasal neoplasm. Partial destruction of the nasal bone (arrow) and inflammation of the adjacent soft tissues may be observed.

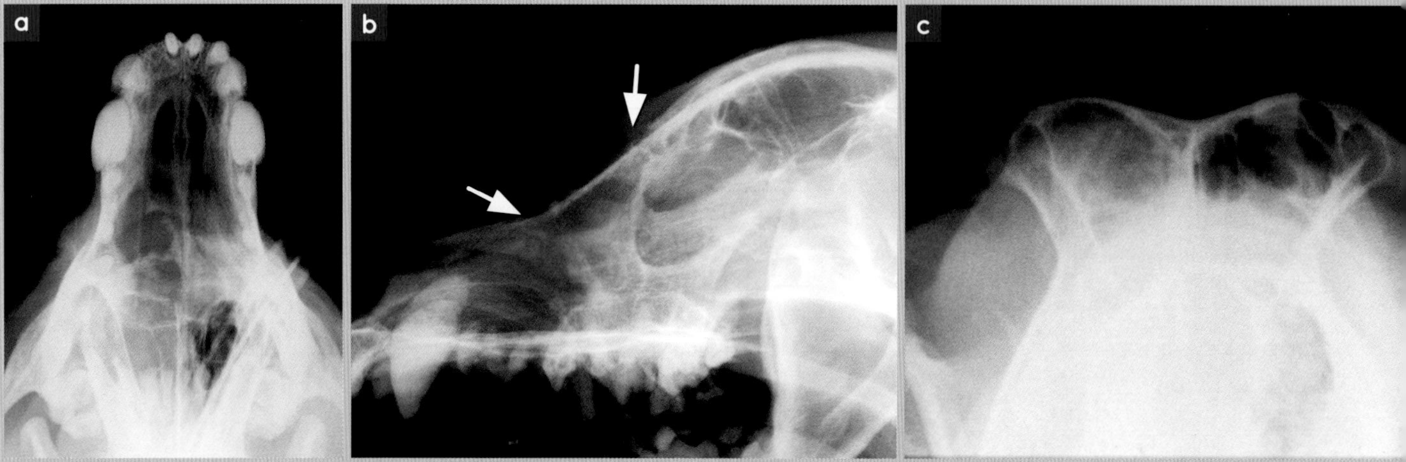

FIGURE 6.19. Enlarged image of the nasal cavity on a ventrodorsal open-mouth radiograph (a), lateral radiograph of the head (b) and rostrocaudal tangential radiograph of the frontal sinuses (c) of a dog with a nasal neoplasm. On the open-mouth ventrodorsal view, marked osteolysis is seen in the middle third and caudal third of the right nasal cavity, with partial destruction of the vomer bone, incipient osteolytic changes in the rostral third of the left nasal cavity and marked enlargement of focal opacity in the middle third of this cavity. Tooth 102 is missing (possibly unrelated to the nasal tumour). The lateral radiograph shows osteolysis of the nasal bone (the arrows point to the affected segment) and an increase in radiopacity in the frontal sinuses, although it is not possible to determine whether it is unilateral or bilateral on this view. The rostrocaudal tangential radiograph allows us to determine that the increase in radiopacity only affects the right frontal sinus. This can be attributed to obstructive sinusitis secondary to the presence of the mass in the ipsilateral nasal cavity, or to a neoplastic invasion of the sinus.

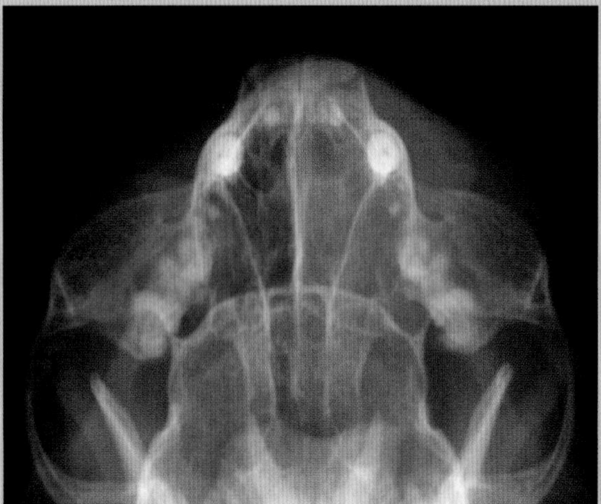

FIGURE 6.20. Ventrodorsal open-mouth radiograph of the head of a cat with a nasal neoplasm. An increase in the radiopacity of the left nasal cavity, with displacement of the rostral third of the vomer bone to the right, may be observed. Histological diagnosis: nasal lymphoma.

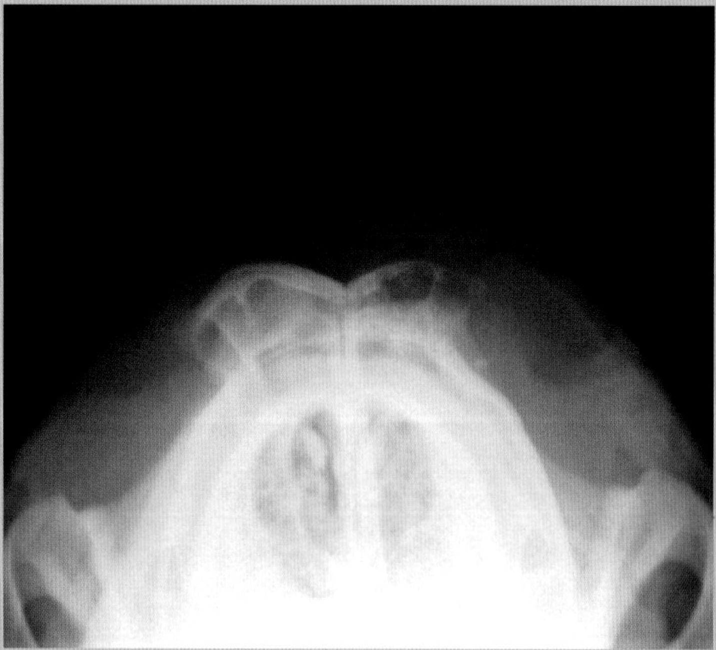

FIGURE 6.21. Rostrocaudal tangential radiograph of the frontal sinuses in a dog with a soft-tissue neoplasm in the left frontal area. Marked swelling of the soft tissues and partial destruction of the left frontal sinus may be seen. Histological diagnosis: carcinoma.

Mandible, maxilla and temporomandibular joint

Fractures

Fractures of the mandible usually appear in the symphysis (especially in cats) (fig. 6.22) or in the body of the mandible (fig. 6.23). They are identified with greater or lesser difficulty depending on the degree of displacement of the fragments. The lateral oblique and ventrodorsal intraoral projections (fig. 6.24) are the most appropriate to examine these fractures. Fractures may be secondary to marked bone loss due to severe periodontitis or neoplasms.

In order to assess fractures of the maxilla, the ventrodorsal open-mouth or dorsoventral intraoral projections are used (fig. 6.25). Fragments of the maxillary bone are often minimally displaced, which makes radiographic identification of this type of fracture difficult.

Mandibular and maxillary fractures may be accompanied by tooth injuries, so dentition should also be carefully examined in these patients.

The fractures that affect the components of the temporomandibular joint are often difficult to accurately assess using X-rays. Computed tomography offers an excellent alternative for the diagnosis of this type of lesion.

Temporomandibular joint luxation

In addition to performing the standard views to examine the temporomandibular joint, when a temporomandibular luxation is suspected, it will be useful to compare the image obtained with the closed-mouth and open-mouth lateral and lateral oblique projections.

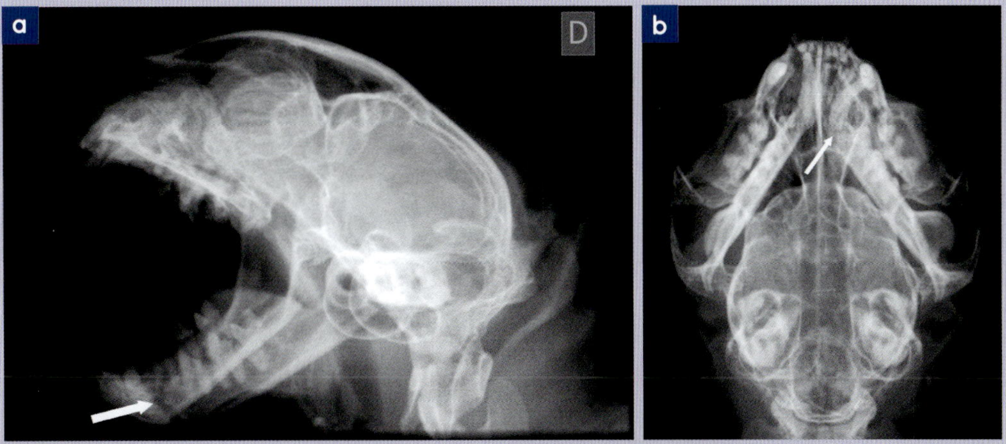

FIGURE 6.22. Lateral (a) and dorsoventral (b) radiographs of the head of a cat with a fracture of the mandibular symphysis and of the rostral end of the left mandibular body. The arrows point to the fracture line of the rostral part of the mandibular body.

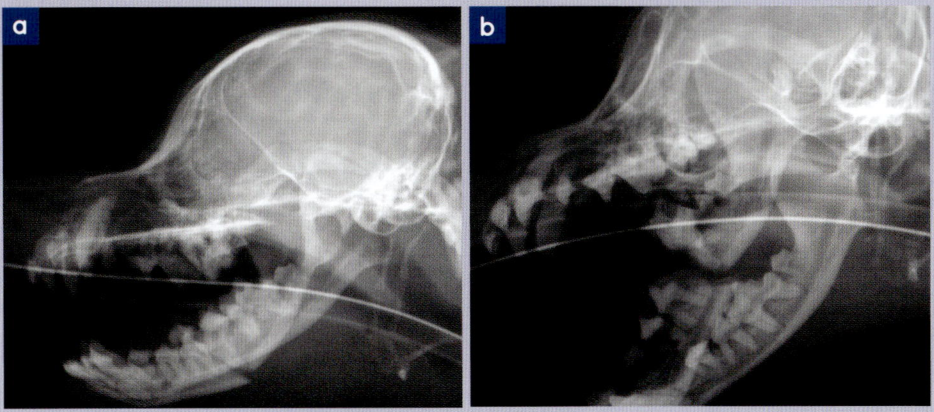

FIGURE 6.23. Lateral (a) and lateral oblique (b) radiographs of the head of a dog with an oblique fracture of the body of the right mandible. The fracture is better visualised on the oblique radiograph.

The luxation of the temporomandibular joint is more frequent in cats than in dogs. It usually appears as a sequela of trauma, may be uni- or bilateral and is often associated with a fracture of the mandible. Clinically, the affected animals cannot close their mouth completely, have poor dental occlusion with lateral displacement of the mandible and suffer from excessive salivation. This problem may be difficult to identify on radiographs. The condyloid or condylar process of the mandible usually appears displaced in rostral and dorsal direction (fig. 6.26). Associated fractures of the condyloid process of the mandible or of the mandibular fossa of the temporal bone may also be observed.

Temporomandibular subluxations are difficult to identify on radiographs (fig. 6.27). Computed tomography is an excellent alternative for the diagnosis of this type of lesion.

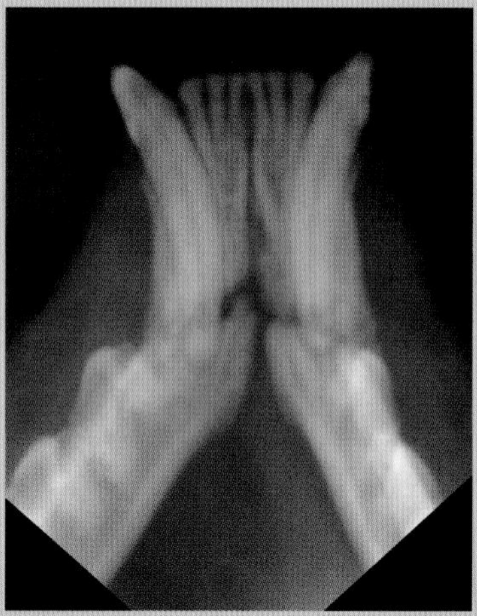

FIGURE 6.24. Ventrodorsal intraoral radiograph of the mandible of a cat with a fracture of the symphysis and rostral area of the body of both mandibles.

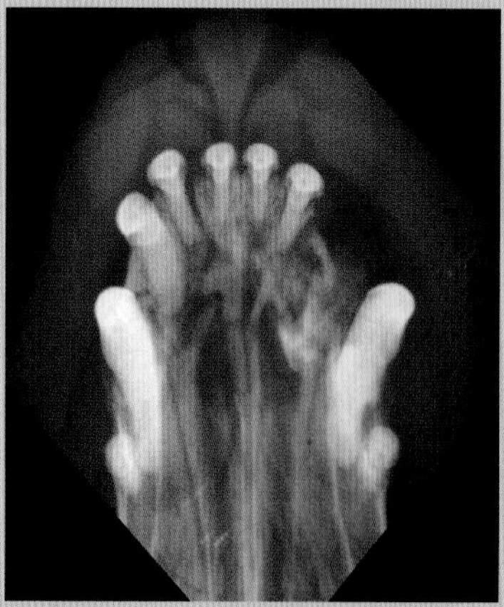

FIGURE 6.25. Dorsoventral intraoral radiograph of the maxilla of a dog with a comminuted fracture of the rostral area of the maxilla. Several lines of fracture may be observed and the upper left third incisor is missing (tooth 203).

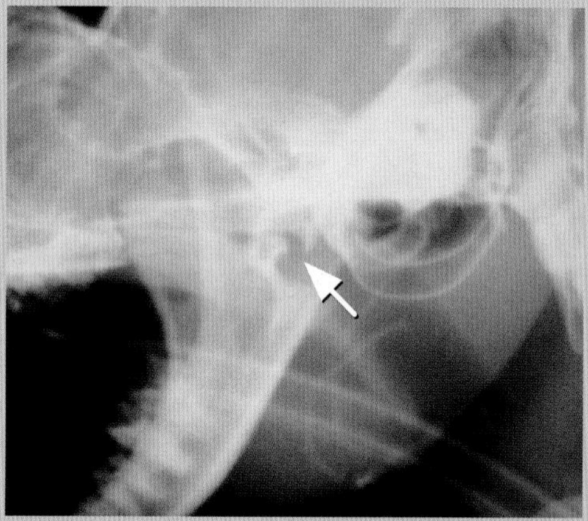

FIGURE 6.26. Lateral oblique radiograph with elevation of the rostral part of the head of a cat with luxation of the temporomandibular joint (arrow).

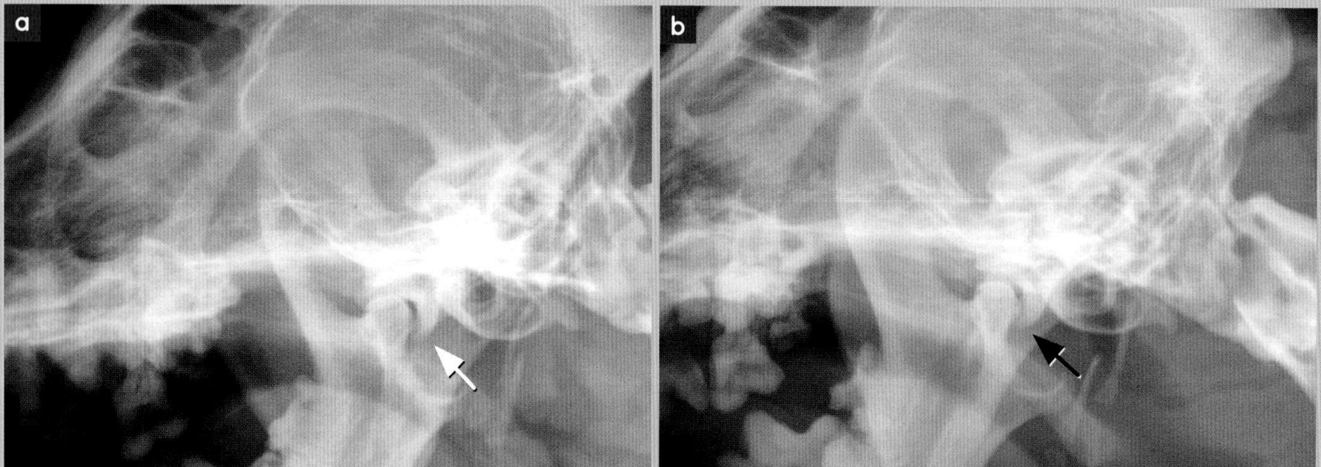

FIGURE 6.27. Right (a) and left (b) lateral oblique radiographs with elevation of the rostral part of the head of a dog with temporomandibular subluxation. The right temporomandibular joint (white arrow) is better visualised on the right lateral oblique radiograph, and the left joint (black arrow) is better visualised on the left lateral oblique radiograph.

Temporomandibular dysplasia

This is a rare congenital abnormality that has been described more frequently in the Basset Hound, although it can appear in many other breeds. Radiographs may show alterations in the bone such as flattening of the condyle, shallow fossa and the joints may be angled more obliquely than normal rostromedially (fig. 6.28). Oblique projection both with the mouth closed and open may show subluxation of the mandibular condyle, causing joint space narrowing.

The technique of choice to confirm the diagnosis is computed tomography, which can be used for three-dimensional volume rendering that can greatly enhance the surgical planning for these patients.

Temporomandibular joint ankylosis

Ankylosis involves a reduction in the mobility or complete immobility and consolidation of the joint. It usually occurs as a result of untreated intra-articular (true ankylosis) or extra-articular (false ankylosis) trauma. The latter may be due to untreated mandibular and zygomatic fractures, mandibular or zygomatic masses, marked new bone formation in patients with severe

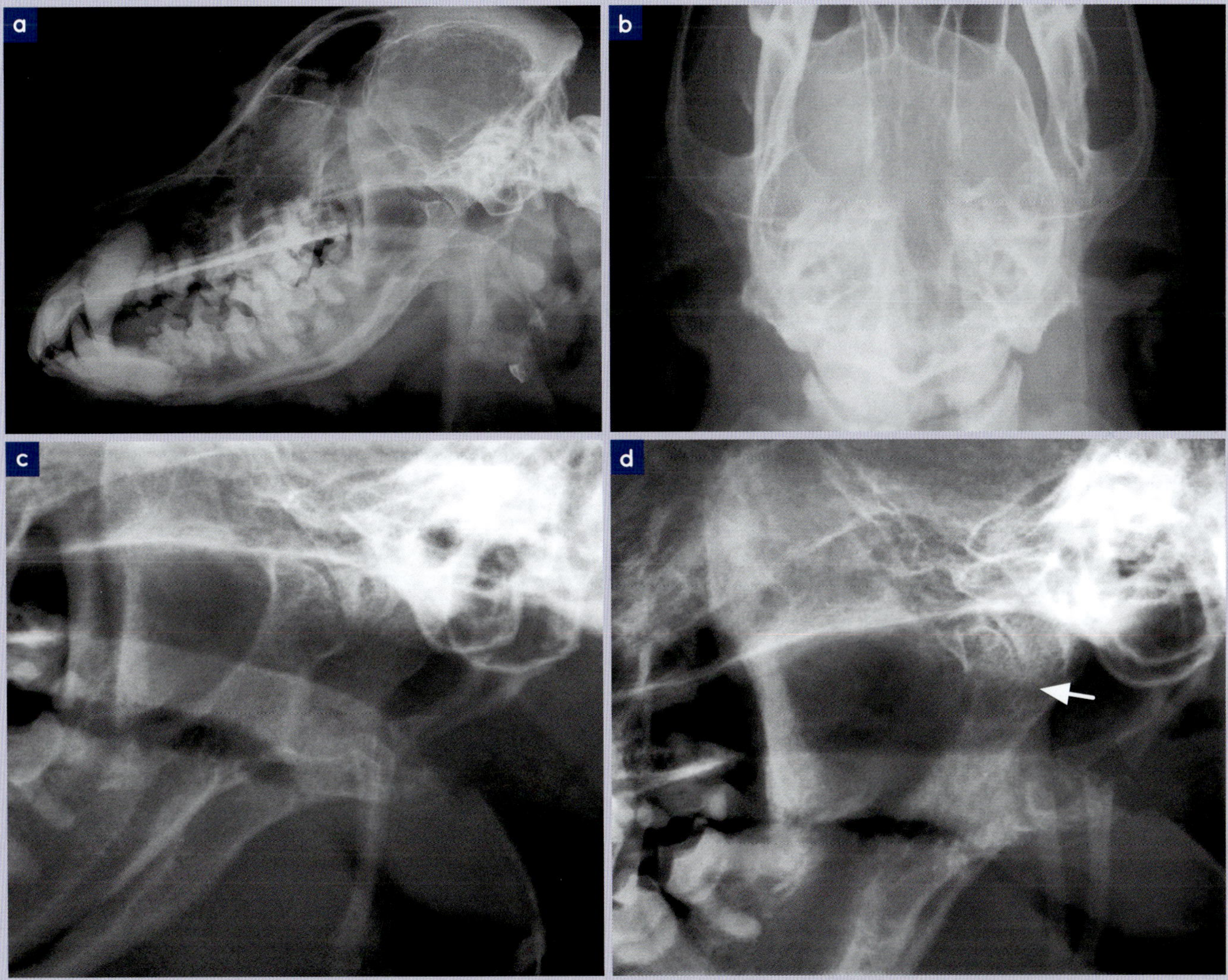

FIGURE 6.28. Lateral (a), dorsoventral (enlarged image) (b), right lateral oblique (c) and left lateral oblique (d) radiographs of a 9-year-old Basset Hound with temporomandibular dysplasia. Images (c) and (d) are the most useful to evaluate the degree of deformation of both temporomandibular joints, which show flattening of the condyle and condylar fossa, as well as partial fusion of the left joint (arrow).

chronic otitis media or craniomandibular osteopathy, or it may be due to the presence of abscesses close to the temporomandibular joint. True ankylosis is more common in cats and is characterised radiographically by the appearance of irregularities in the joint space and contour of the mandibular condyle, with periarticular new bone formation.

Degenerative joint disease

Degenerative joint disease (arthritis) of the temporomandibular joint may appear as a sequel to trauma, dysplasia or contralateral mandibulectomy. Radiographic signs include joint space narrowing, subchondral sclerosis and periarticular osteophyte formation. Involvement is usually bilateral.

Infection

Osteomyelitis of the maxilla and mandible are usually secondary to fractures of these bones or infections that primarily affect the teeth. They usually appear as osteoproliferative reactions in the periphery, with thickening of the cortical bone and medullary lysis, which can give the appearance that the teeth are surrounded by soft tissue instead of bone.

Infections of the temporomandibular joint are rare. They usually occur from the spreading of osteomyelitis involving the ipsilateral tympanic bulla or from bites in this region. Hence, they are usually unilateral. The radiographic image may be similar to that of osteoarthritis, with bone-forming alterations, although bone lysis may also be evident.

Tumours

Primary bone tumours of the maxilla and mandible are rare, with the most common being osteosarcomas (fig. 6.29), multilobular osteochondrosarcomas, fibrosarcomas and undifferentiated sarcomas.

Most maxilla and mandible tumours originate in the adjacent soft tissues and are, therefore, identified in the physical examination. A radiograph is then useful to determine possible secondary involvement of the adjacent bones. The most common malignant oral tumours in dogs are melanomas (fig. 6.30), squamous cell carcinomas and fibrosarcomas (fig. 6.31). In cats, the most common are squamous cell carcinomas (fig. 6.32) and fibrosarcomas. They appear on radiographs as masses of soft-tissue opacity which, when infiltrating the adjacent bone, cause the appearance of an aggressive bone lesion with both bone-lytic and bone-forming components. The osteolytic lesions may present a moth-eaten pattern, while bone proliferative lesions usually present a spiculated or sunray pattern. The tumour can cause tooth displacement or loss. When a radiographic image is suggestive of an oral tumour, osteomyelitis should also be included in the differential diagnosis, especially in cats as the periosteal reaction can be proliferative and poorly defined.

Craniomandibular osteopathy

It is also known as "lion's jaw". This disease appears in young dogs, of 3 to 18 months of age, especially in the West Highland White Terrier, although it has also been described in the Boston Terrier, Cairn Terrier, Scottish Terrier and, exceptionally, in the Labrador Retriever and Doberman Pinscher. Clinically, it is possible to observe inflammation of the mandible, difficulty to pick up food, pain when opening the mouth or when chewing, and fever. On radiographs, a marked bone proliferative reaction is observed in the affected areas, which could involve the mandible (fig. 6.33.), the tympanic bullae and the petrous part of the temporal bone (fig. 6.34). The temporomandibular joint, and therefore its mobility, may also be affected. The changes may be uni- or bilateral. The dorsal area of the cranial vault may also appear enlarged, although its aspect is usually not as irregular as in other regions (fig. 6.35). Bone proliferation usually ceases upon completion of skeletal growth, and occasionally, a remodeling of the lesions occurs.

Secondary renal hyperparathyroidism

It is also called renal osteodystrophy or "rubber jaw". The reduction in the degree of glomerular filtration causes retention of phosphorus, which reduces calcium levels in blood. This stimulates the production of parathyroid hormone. This disease seems to affect the mandible and maxilla. It usually appears in older dogs, but can also be detected in young patients with congenital renal dysplasia. Clinically, it may be characterised by the appearance of dental disease, excessive salivation, loss of teeth or respiratory problems due to maxillary collapse. The radiographic signs include

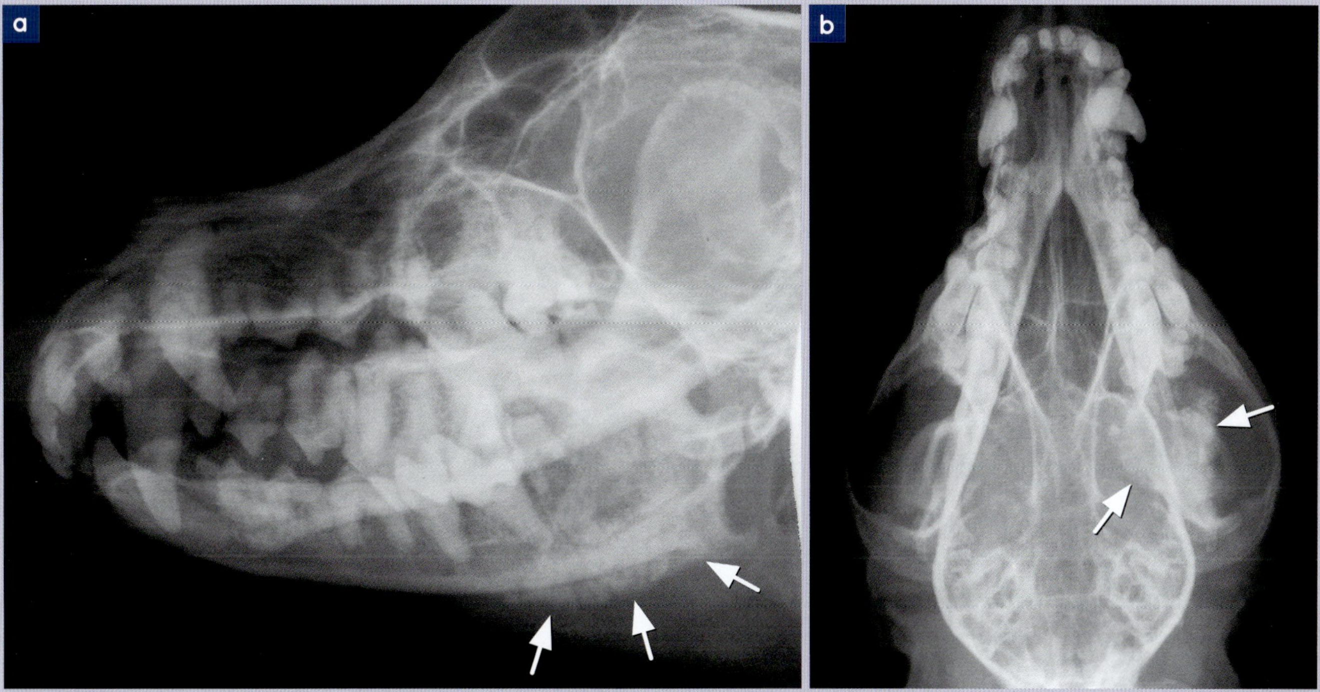

FIGURE 6.29. Lesion-centred lateral oblique (a) and dorsoventral (b) radiographs of a dog with an osteosarcoma in the caudal third of the left mandible. The lesion is exceedingly bone-forming. **Video 6.1** presents the volume rendering computed tomography images of this patient.

Video 6.1.
Volumetric rendering of a computed tomography images of a dog with an aggressive bone lesion with osteolytic and osteoproliferative components in the left mandible.

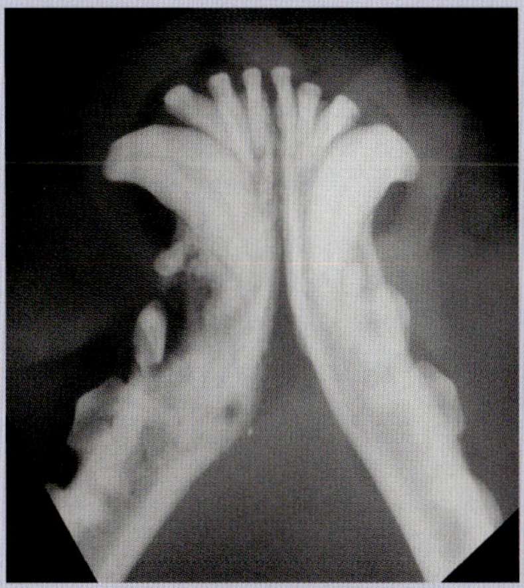

FIGURE 6.30. Ventrodorsal intraoral radiograph of the mandible of a dog with an oral soft-tissue neoplasm. Osteolysis is observed in the rostral end of the right mandibular body, with displacement of the lower right first and second premolars (teeth number 405 and 406), which is indicative of secondary bone involvement. Histological diagnosis: melanoma.

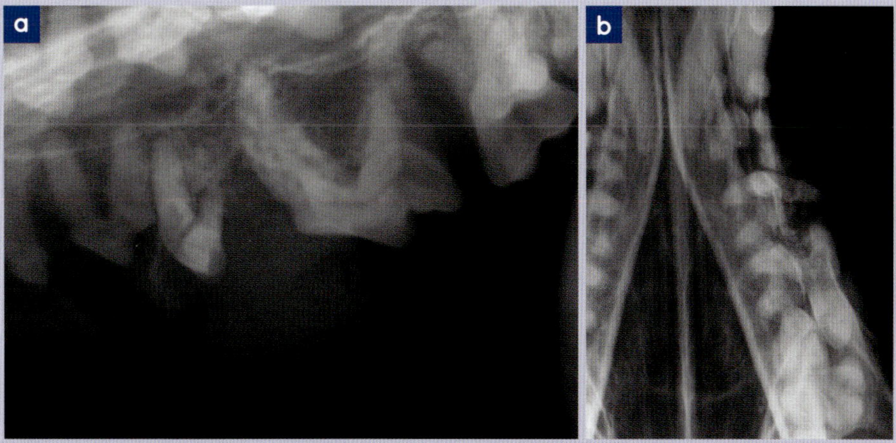

FIGURE 6.31. Enlarged images of the left maxillary area on left lateral oblique (a) and ventrodorsal (b) radiographs of the head of a dog with an oral soft-tissue neoplasm. It is possible to observe a mass of soft tissue located between the upper left third and fourth premolars (teeth 207 and 208), which causes the rostral displacement of the third premolar and the loss of the normal bone structure in the area adjacent to the lesion. This is compatible with secondary bone involvement. Histological diagnosis: fibrosarcoma.

demineralisation of the mandible and/or maxilla, loss of the lamina dura and formation of radiolucent halos around the dental roots. At advanced stages, the mineral density of teeth markedly contrasts with the demineralised surrounding bone (fig. 6.36). In chronic processes, there may be demineralisation of the long bones of the limbs.

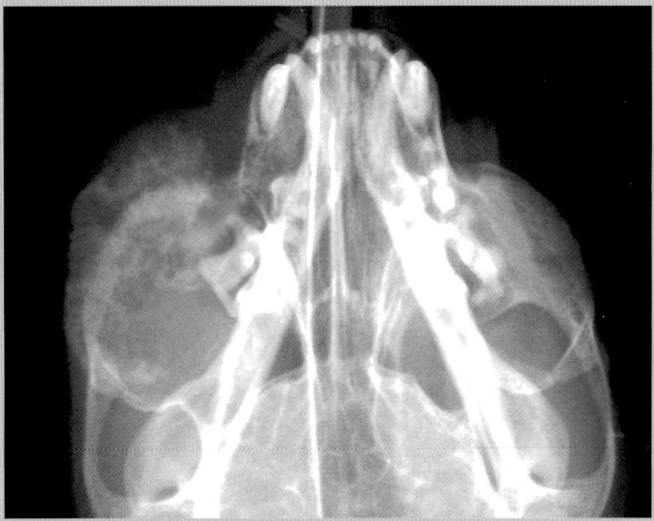

FIGURE 6.32. Enlarged image of the rostral area in dorsoventral radiograph of the head of a cat with a right maxillary squamous cell carcinoma. The lesion produces osteolysis of the lateral zone of the right maxillary bone and the rostral part of the right zygomatic bone, in which it also produces osteoproliferative changes.

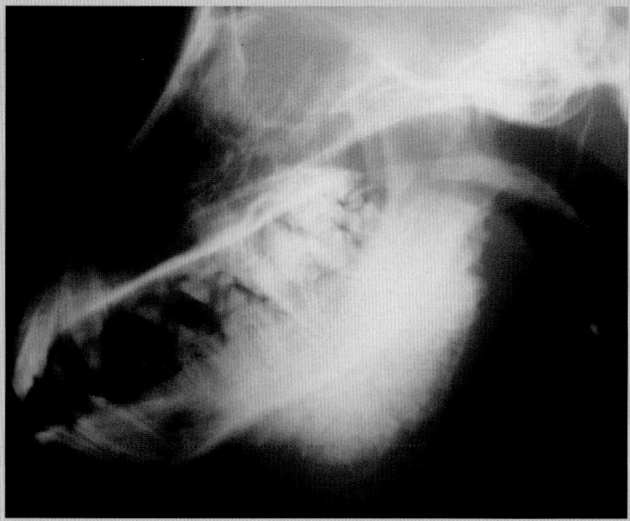

FIGURE 6.33. Enlarged image of the mandibular region on a lateral radiograph of the head of a dog with craniomandibular osteopathy affecting the mandible.

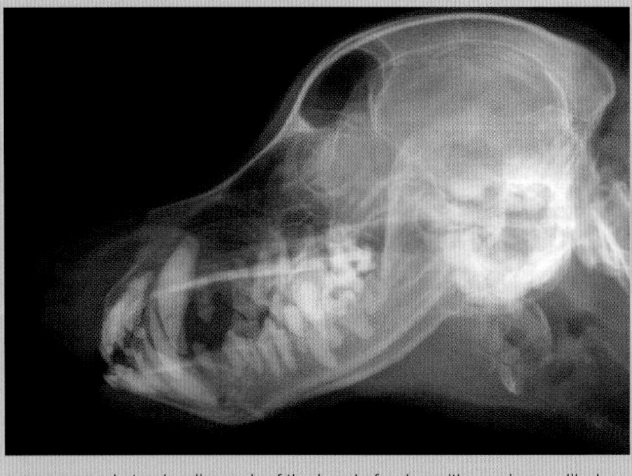

FIGURE 6.34. Lateral radiograph of the head of a dog with craniomandibular osteopathy that affects the tympanic bullae and the petrous region of the temporal bone.

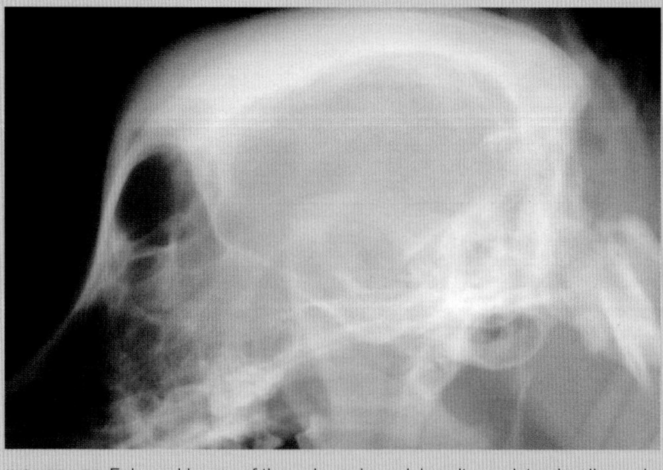

FIGURE 6.35. Enlarged image of the enlarged cranial vault on a lateral radiograph of a dog with craniomandibular osteopathy.

Teeth

The tooth (fig. 6.37) is divided into crown, neck and root or root canal. A distinction is made between the anatomical crown and the clinical crown. The latter is defined as the visible part of the tooth, that is, the part that protrudes above the gum line. The hard tissues of the tooth are dentin, enamel (covering only the crown) and cementum (covering only the root), which are of mineral density. Dental enamel is the most highly mineralised tissue in the body, so it appears slightly more radiopaque than dentin. In contrast, dentin cannot be radiographically distinguished from cementum. The pulp cavity is of soft tissue density, is larger in young animals and diminishes with age. The periodontium, also referred to as periodontal tissues, is the tooth's connective tissue, that is, it is the supporting structure that surrounds the tooth. It is composed of the cementum (dentists consider the cementum part of the periodontium rather than a part of the tooth itself), the periodontal ligament, the alveolar bone and the gingiva. The periodontal ligament is made up of collagen fibres that anchor the tooth to the alveolar bone and is of soft tissue opacity. The more radiopaque margin of alveolar bone, which is in contact with the periodontal ligament, is the lamina dura. The socket in the bone where the teeth are inserted is called the alveolus. The gingiva covers the alveolar bone and has soft tissue opacity.The dental formulas of the dog and cat are shown in table 6.1. The Triadan numbering system is used (fig. 6.38) in which each tooth is identified by a three-digit number. The first digit denotes the quadrant of the mouth and indicates whether the tooth is part of the primary or permanent dentition:

Permanent teeth:

1. Upper right arcade.
2. Upper left arcade.
3. Lower left arcade.
4. Lower right arcade.

Temporary or deciduous teeth:

5. Upper right arcade.
6. Upper left arcade.
7. Lower left arcade.
8. Lower right arcade.

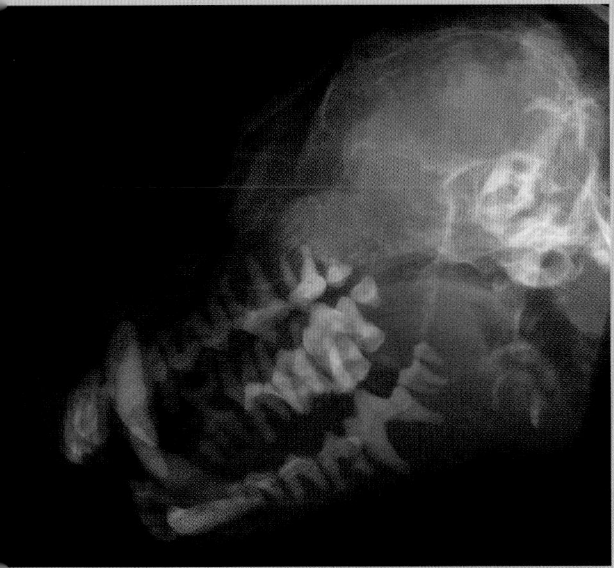

FIGURE 6.36. Lateral oblique radiograph of the head of a dog with secondary renal hyperparathyroidism ("rubber jaw"). Marked demineralisation of the mandible, maxilla, zygomatic arches and cranial vault may be observed. The frontal bone appears depressed. The density of the teeth contrasts to a large extent with that of the demineralised bone.

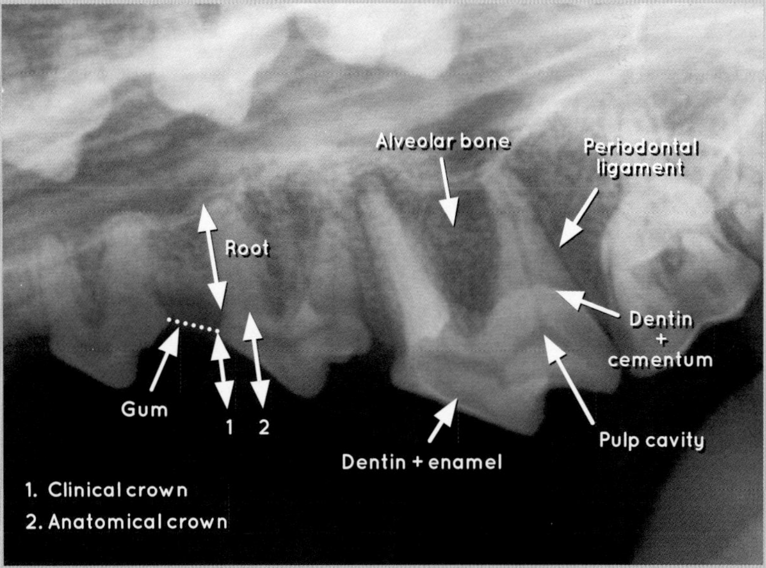

FIGURE 6.37. Enlarged image of the maxillary region in a lateral oblique radiograph of a healthy dog showing the radiographic anatomy of the teeth.

TABLE 6.1. Dental formulas of the dog and cat.

Species	Deciduous teeth	Permanent teeth
Cat	2 × (I 3/3 C 1/1 PM 3/2) = 26	2 × (I 3/3 C 1/1 PM 3/2 M 1/1) = 30
Dog	2 × (I 3/3 C 1/1 PM 2/2 M 1/1) = 28	2 × (I 3/3 C 1/1 PM 4/4 M 2/3) = 42

The second and third digits indicate the type of tooth, with the incisors beginning at 01, the canines are 04 and molars starting at 09.

Although some dental abnormalities can be identified using conventional X-ray equipment and standard cassette-film or digital radiography systems, the use of dental X-ray equipment or at least dental film or intraoral digital radiography systems (direct digital sensors and photostimulable phosphor plates) is preferable.

Projections with X-ray equipment and standard digital film, screen or detector systems are open-mouth lateral oblique of maxilla and mandible, open-mouth ventrodorsal (ventral 20° rostral–caudodorsal), intraoral dorsoventral to evaluate the rostral portion of the maxillary arch and the intraoral ventrodorsal to evaluate the rostral portion of the mandibular arch.

To perform intraoral projections, a distinction is made between the paralleling and bisecting angle techniques. The **paralleling technique** (fig. 6.39) is used to examine the mandibular molars and premolars (excluding the first premolar) by positioning the dental digital detector or cassette medially to the body of

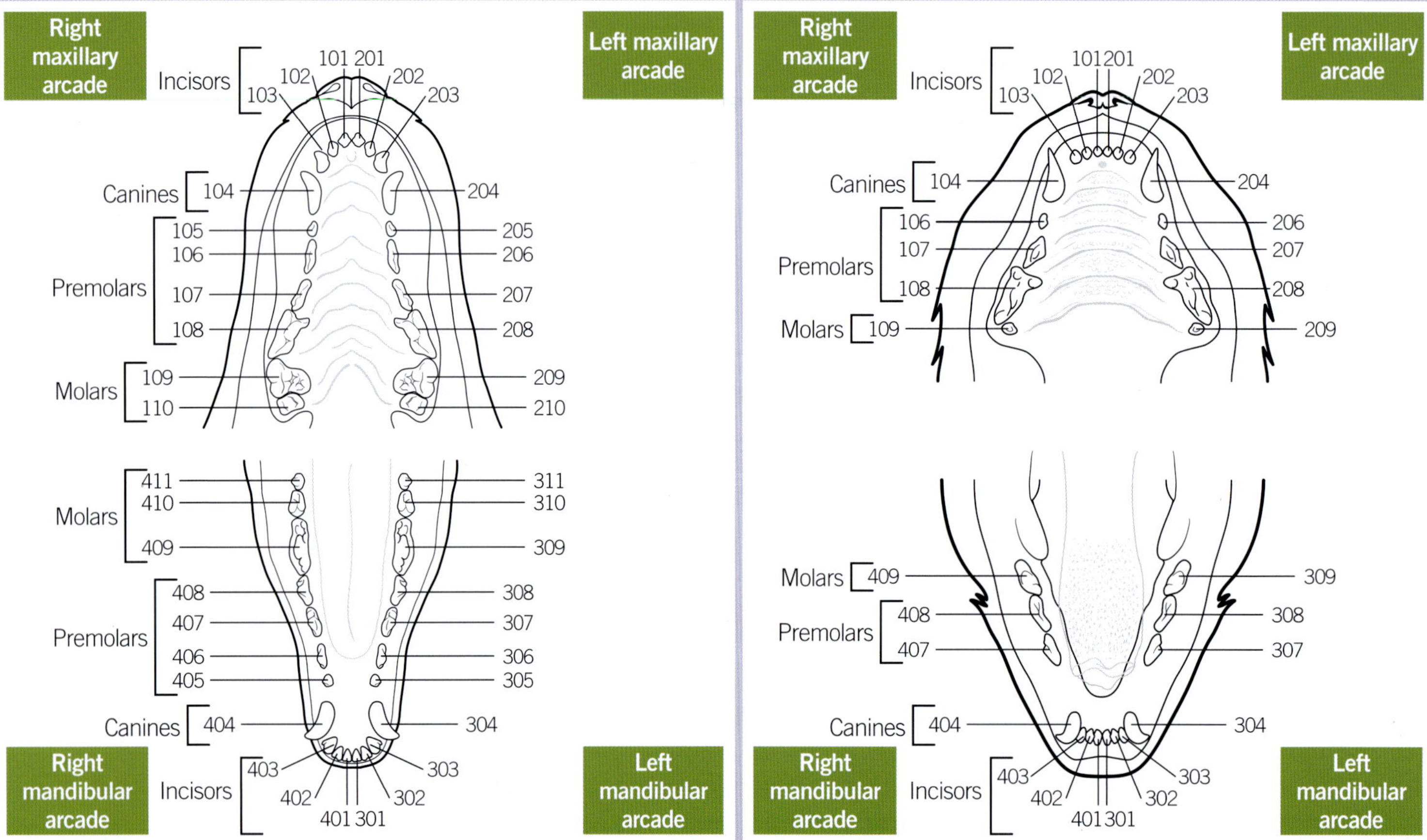

FIGURE 6.38. Schematic diagram of the Triadan permanent tooth numbering system in the dog (left) and the cat (right).

the mandible, as parallel as possible to the tooth to be examined so that the X-ray beam is oriented perpendicular to the tooth and the film/detector. The **bisecting angle** technique (fig. 6.40) permits correction of the distortion in the radiographic silhouette of the tooth due to the angle of the X-ray beam (fig. 6.41). It is used to evaluate the maxillary and mandibular incisors and canines, as well as the maxillary premolars. For this, the X-ray beam must be directed perpendicular to the imaginary line that divides the angle formed by the cassette/detector and the long axis of the tooth in two. In this way, the silhouette of the tooth presents less geometric distortion in the image.

Periodontal disease

This is the most common dental disease in dogs and cats. The incidence is very high in small and miniature breed dogs. Initially, radiographs reveal loss of visualisation of the lamina dura and later progressive lysis (resorption) of the alveolar bone. This creates an image of progressive widening of the periodontal space (fig. 6.42). Two resorption patterns can be distinguished: a **horizontal pattern**, in which there is a somewhat homogeneous loss of alveolar bone height, which generally affects several teeth (fig. 6.43), and a **vertical pattern**, in which alveolar bone height loss affects more of a localised area (fig. 6.44). It is very common for both radiological patterns to appear together. As the process progresses, external resorption of the roots may also be observed. Also, periodontal disease can secondarily affect the pulp cavity causing it to widen, and this would indicate pulpitis.

In severe cases of periodontal disease, significant bone loss can lead to pathologic fractures.

Periapical abscess

These abscesses may appear associated with periodontal disease, caries or fractures of dental roots. They give rise to the formation of a radiolucent halo around the root of the tooth affected by the destruction of the alveolar bone. Reabsorption of the dental root, which appears thinner and with an irregular outline, may also be observed (fig. 6.45). In dogs, infections of the fourth maxillary premolar (carnassial) may lead to the formation of a fistulous tract that usually opens to the outside under the eye.

Periapical abscesses sometimes progress to chronic osteomyelitis, which can cause more extensive bone lytic and proliferative lesions that can resemble a tumour. A biopsy would be required for a definitive diagnosis.

Tooth resorption

Tooth resorption develops progressively and is caused by the activation of odontoclasts. It begins on the surface of the root, from there spreads to the root dentin and then into the crown dentin, where it can cause enamel defects. Two types of dental resorption have been distinguished: inflammatory and idiopathic. Idiopathic tooth resorption is very common in cats (fig. 6.46), although it can also occur in dogs. A complete radiological examination of the mouth is recommended for the evaluation of this pathology in feline patients. The number of lesions increases with the patient's age. The American Veterinary Dental College has established a classification based on the severity of the lesions (stages 1 to 5) and on their location (types 1 to 3).

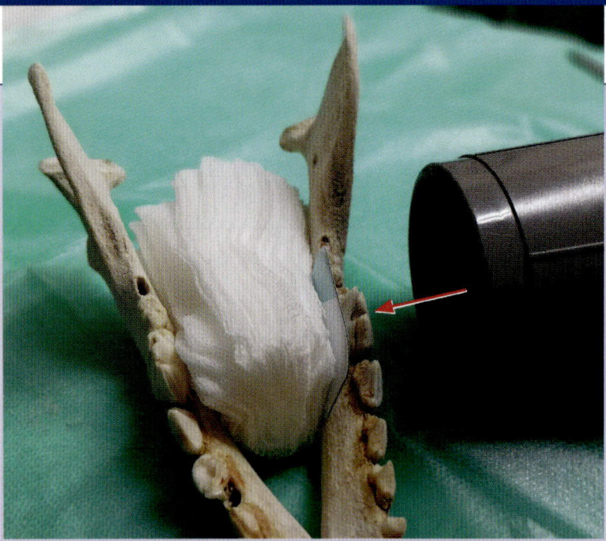

FIGURE 6.39. Representative image of the paralleling technique performed with an anatomical mandible, intraoral dental film and the X-ray tube of a dental X-ray machine. The red arrow represents the direction of the X-ray beam. The film is positioned parallel to the tooth to be radiographed and the beam is oriented perpendicular to the film and the tooth.

FIGURE 6.40. Representative image of the bisecting angle technique performed with an anatomical skull, intraoral dental film and the X-ray tube of a dental X-ray machine. The X-ray beam, represented by the red arrow, is oriented perpendicular to the imaginary line that bisects the angle formed by the film (P) and the long axis of the tooth (blue line) to be radiographed, in this case tooth number 103. The green line corresponds to the bisector between the film and the long axis of the tooth.

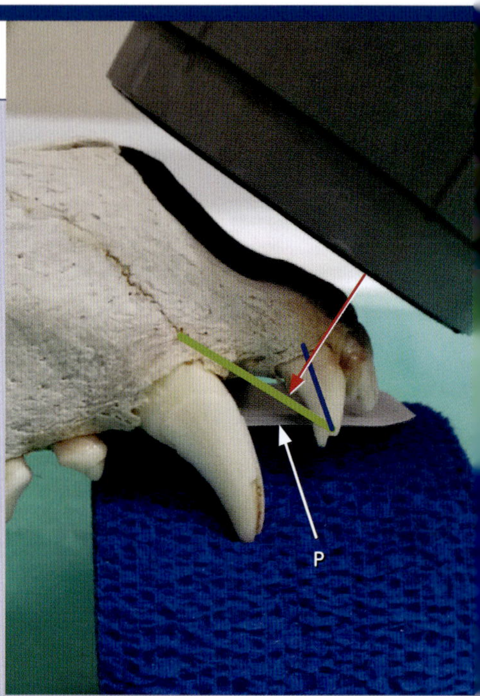

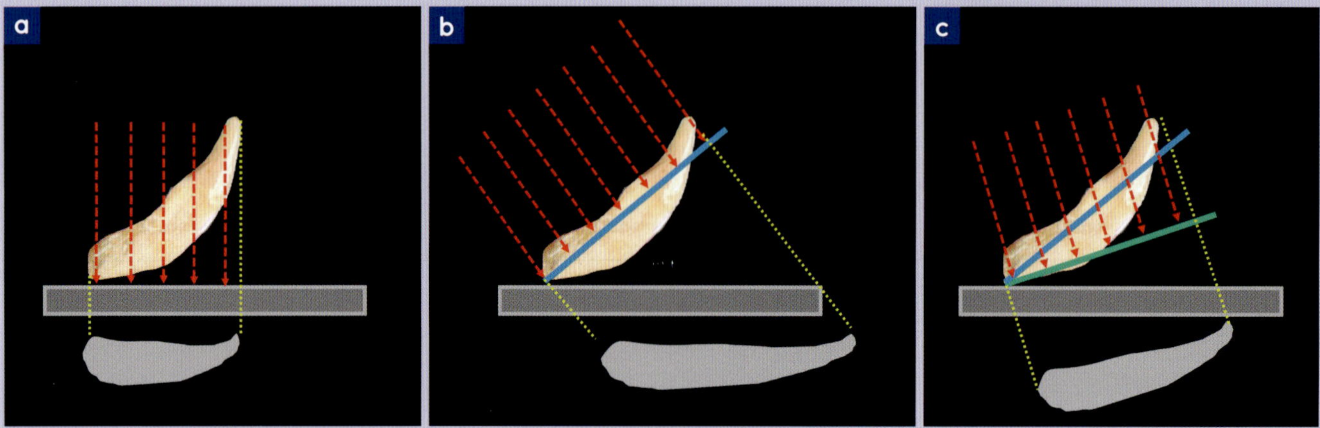

FIGURE 6.41. Schematic representation of the suitability of using the bisecting angle technique whenever the intraoral film or digital system cannot be placed parallel to the tooth. Diagram (a) shows the shortening of the radiographic silhouette of the tooth if the X-ray beam is oriented perpendicular to the film/detector. Diagram (b) shows the elongation of the radiographic silhouette of the tooth if the X-ray beam is oriented perpendicular to the long axis of the tooth. Diagram (c) shows the bisecting angle technique, in which the X-ray beam is oriented perpendicular to the imaginary line that bisects the angle formed by the film/detector and the long axis of the tooth, thus minimising the geometric distortion of the radiographic image.

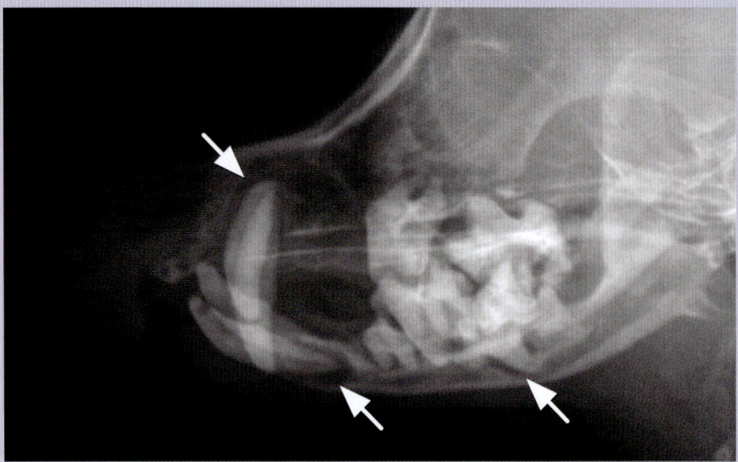

FIGURE 6.42. Enlarged image of the maxillary and mandibular region on a lateral radiograph of the head of a dog with periodotontal disease. Radiolucent halos around several dental roots (arrows) and the absence of numerous teeth may be observed.

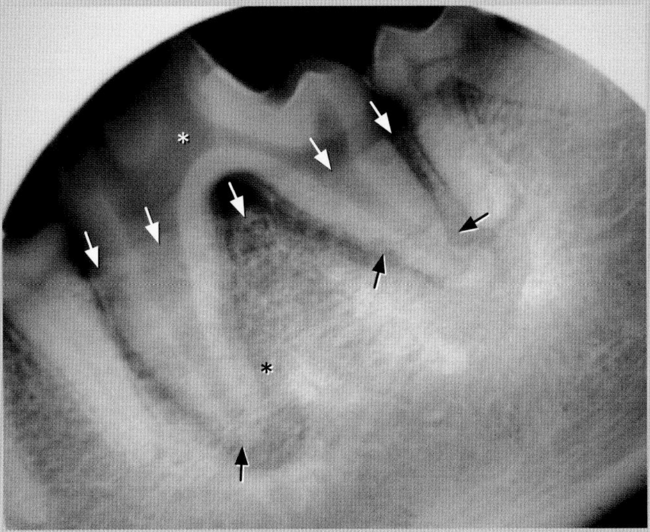

FIGURE 6.43. Intraoral dental radiograph of a patient with a horizontal resorption pattern due to periodontal disease. The alveolar bone presents a somewhat uniform loss of height affecting several teeth (white arrows). There is also widening of the periodontal space (black asterisk) and widening of the pulp (white asterisk), and areas of root resorption (black arrows) can be observed. Image courtesy of Pilar Llorens Pena and Fidel San Román Ascaso.

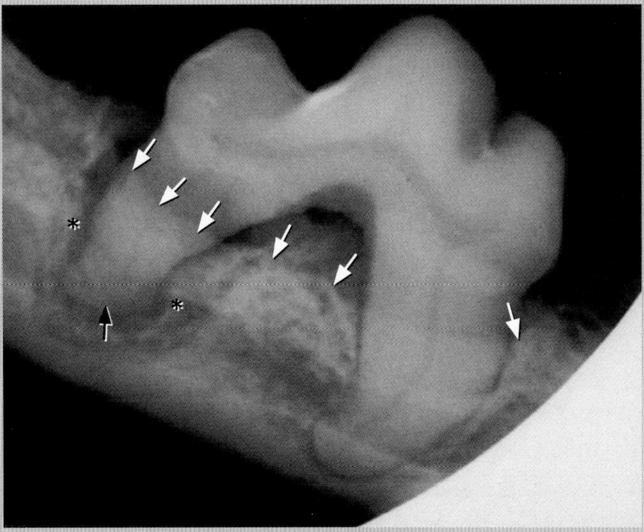

FIGURE 6.44. Intraoral dental radiograph of a patient with a vertical resorption pattern due to periodontal disease. The alveolar bone show a loss of height that locally affects this tooth (white arrows). There is also widening of the periodontal space (black asterisks) and root resorption (black arrow). Image courtesy of Pilar Llorens Pena and Fidel San Román Ascaso.

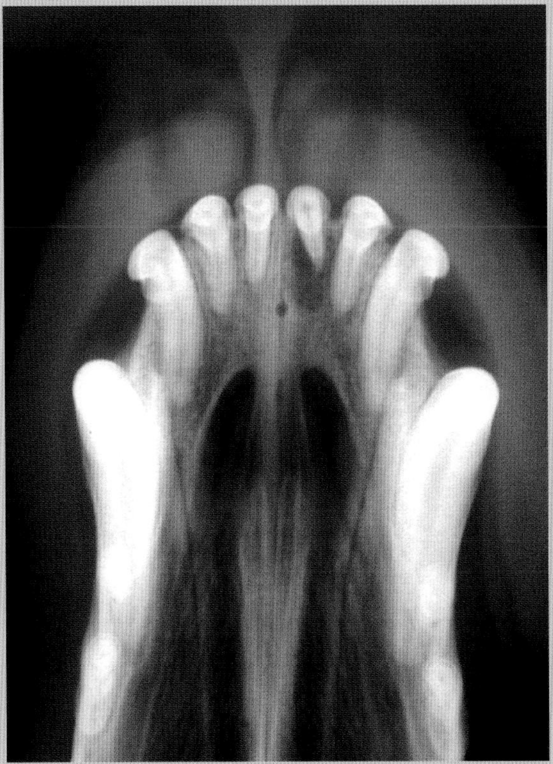

◀ **FIGURE 6.45.** Enlarged image of the maxillary region on a ventrodorsal open-mouth radiograph of the head of a dog with a periapical abscess. A radiolucent area is observed around the root of the upper left first incisor (tooth 201), with partial resorption of this dental root.

▼ **FIGURE 6.46.** Intraoral radiographs of a cat with idiopathic tooth resorption (also called feline osteoclastic resorptive disease). Image courtesy of Pilar Llorens Pena and Fidel San Román Ascaso.

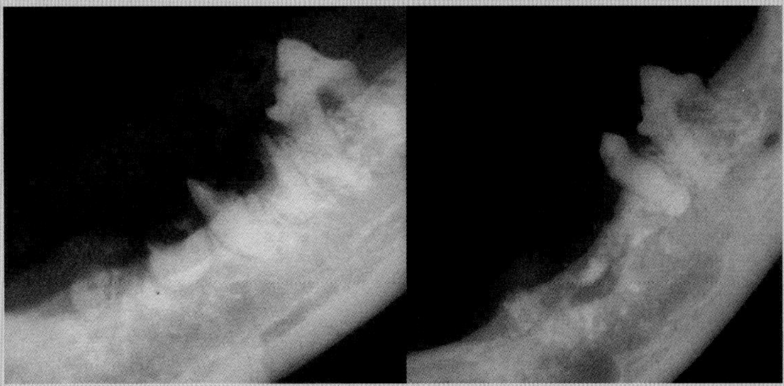

Tumours

The most common tumours are peripheral odontogenic fibromas (formerly known as fibromatous epulis, arising from the periodontal ligament), odontomas and acanthomatous ameloblastomas.

Peripheral odontogenic fibromas are very common oral growths in dogs and can be either fibromatous or ossifying types. They arise from the periodontal ligament and create localised firm swellings. They contain variable amounts of bone and osteoid substances, dentinoid or even cementum-like material. The radiographic image depends on the degree of calcification and can range from the appearance of small lesions starting from the bone margin to single or multiple lesions, as islets of bone, with a trabecular pattern. The teeth may be displaced but there is usually no osteolysis.

Odontomas are made up of regular dental tissue that has grown in an irregular fashion (hamartomas). Compound odontomas are hamartomas that contain numerous complete tooth-like structures (fig. 6.47). Complex odontomas contain structures derived from individual dental components: enamel, dentin, cementum and pulp. They can form close to the crown or root of normal teeth so can be confused with a displaced or extra tooth. On radiographs they appear as expansile masses with regular borders that cause lytic changes to adjacent bone by compression atrophy. They may present mineralised dental elements.

Acanthomatous ameloblastomas are locally invasive and generally cause tooth displacement (fig. 6.48). They most often form around the canines and incisors. On radiographs they usually appear as slow-growing, expansive lesions.

Auditory system

In order to assess the auditory system, it is recommended to take a ventrodorsal radiograph, which allows the examination of the ear canals, a rostrocaudal open-mouth radiograph, in which the two tympanic bullae may be observed, and right and left oblique lateral radiographs, which improve the visualisation of the bulla closest to the chassis.

Although the standard open-mouth rostrocaudal view can also be performed in the cat, it is preferable

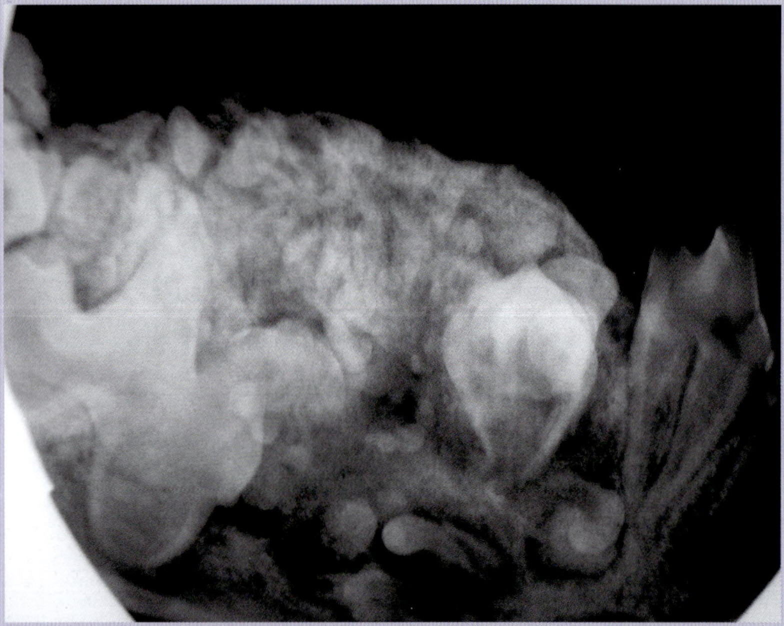

FIGURE 6.47. Intraoral dental radiograph of a patient with a compound odontoma. Image courtesy of Pilar Llorens Pena and Fidel San Román Ascaso.

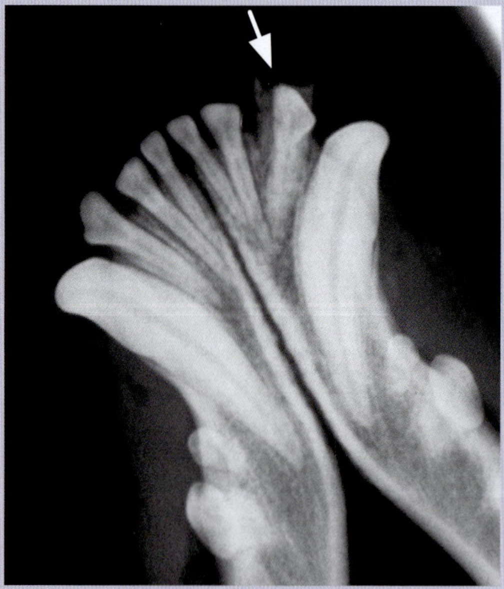

FIGURE 6.48. Ventrodorsal intraoral radiograph of the mandible of a dog with an acanthomatous ameloblastoma. The tumour produces an osteoproliferative reaction with displacement of the affected incisor (tooth 203) and swelling of the adjacent soft tissues (arrow).

to obtain the rostroventral–oblique caudodorsal at a 10° angle (rostral 10° ventral–caudodorsal) to visualise and compare both tympanic bullae on the image (fig. 6.49).

The ear canals appear as gas density tracts lateral to the tympanic bullae on ventrodorsal radiographs. On lateral oblique and rostrocaudal open-mouth radiographs, the tympanic bulla appears as an approximately round structure containing air, limited by a thin wall of mineral density (fig. 6.50). The image is slightly different in cats, since they have a bone division that creates two compartments, one internal and the other external (fig. 6.51).

Otitis externa

Otitis externa is diagnosed clinically and, in many cases, does not cause any evident alteration of the radiographic image of the patient's ear canals. Obstruction of the affected canal or canals is sometimes observed and it is common to find calcification of the walls in chronic processes (fig. 6.52).

Otitis media

It is usually secondary to chronic otitis externa. The left and right lateral oblique views, as well as the rostrocaudal open-mouth view, are the most appropriate to assess this alteration. The radiological signs indicative of otitis media are thickening and/or irregularity of the bone wall of the tympanic bulla, as well as increased radiographic density in its interior (fig. 6.53). The process may be uni- or bilateral (fig. 6.54). If the osteoproliferative reaction is very marked, it may eventually affect the temporal bone and temporomandibular joint. A normal radiographic image of the bullae does not rule out otitis media. Both computed tomography and magnetic resonance imaging are excellent techniques for the evaluation of this disease.

In young cats, inflammatory polyps can form in the middle ear that can extend into the external auditory canal or into the nasopharynx, producing masses of soft tissue opacity that can be identified on the lateral projection with some degree of difficulty depending on their size. Usually, the cranial margin of these nasopharyngeal polyps is masked by the overlapping of other structures, while its caudal margin is more easily identified as it contrasts with the air contained in the nasopharynx.

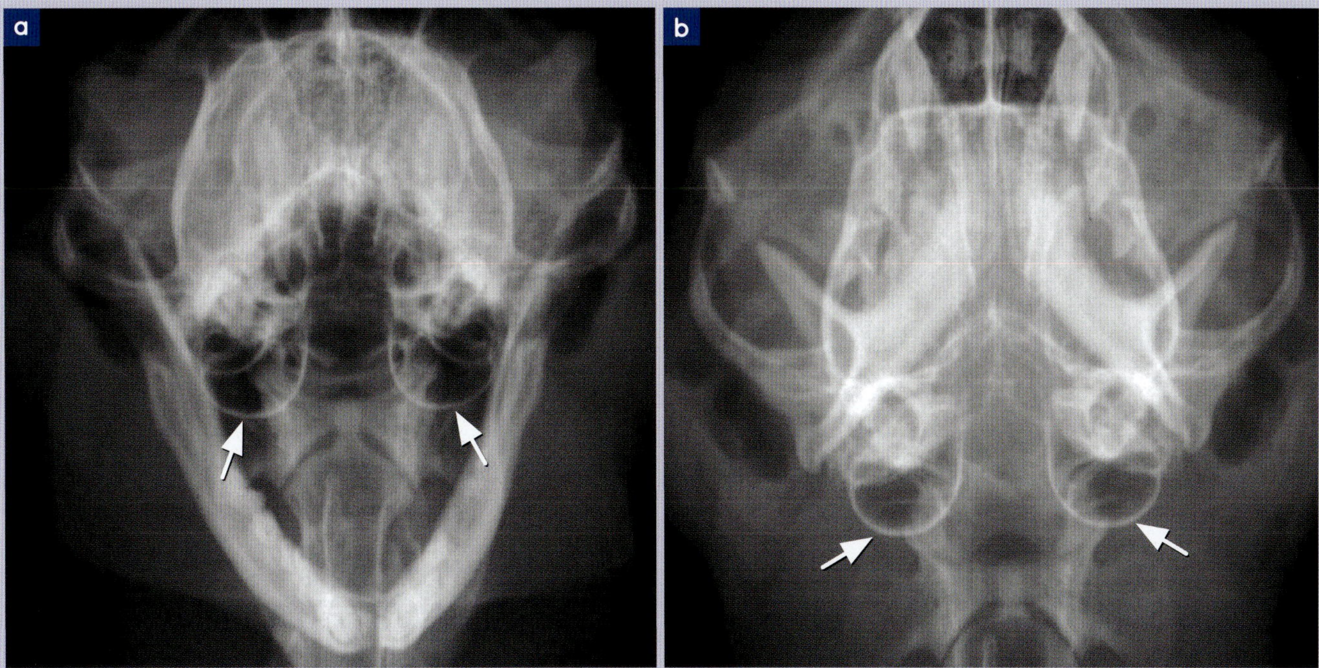

FIGURE 6.49. Rostrocaudal open-mouth (a) and rostroventral-dorsoventral oblique (b) radiographs of the head of a healthy cat. Both views are appropriate for the assessment of the tympanic bullae (arrows) in cats.

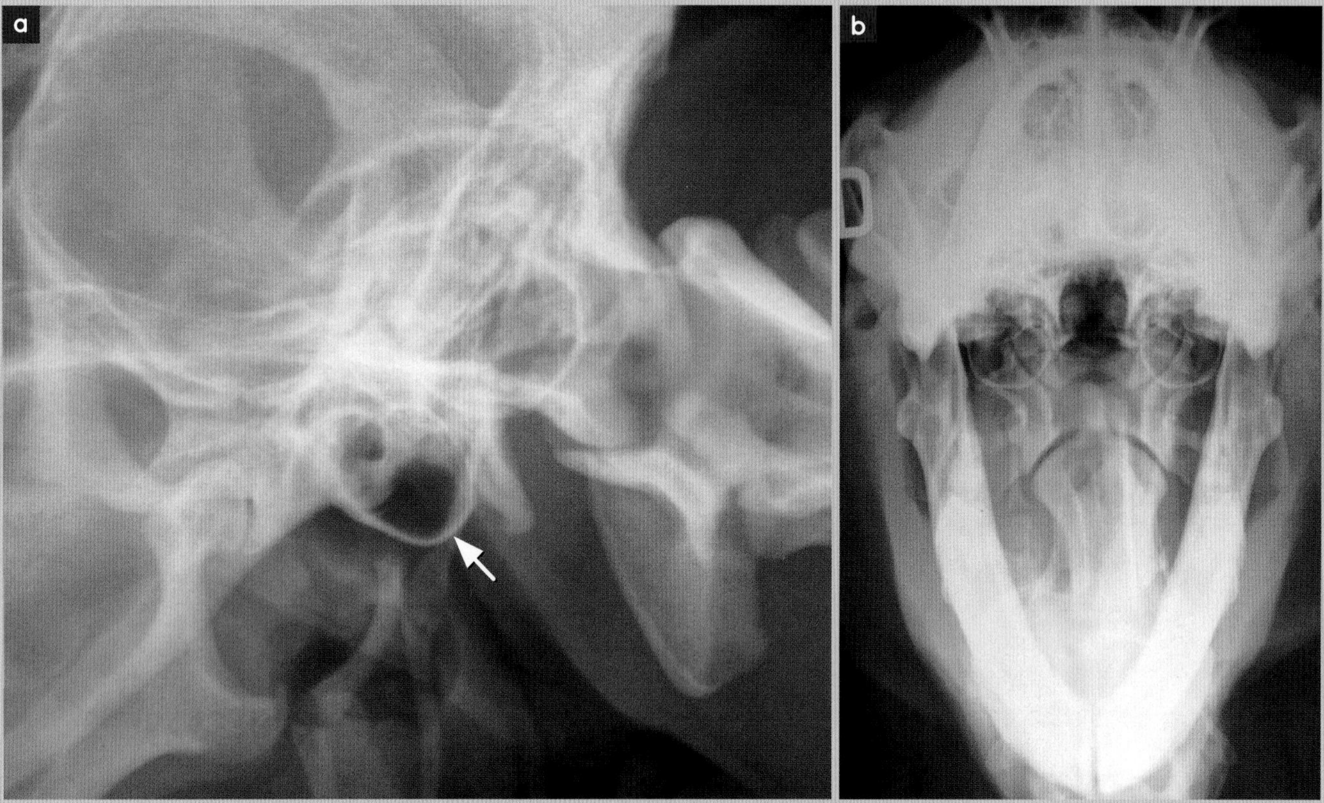

FIGURE 6.50. Enlarged image of the left tympanic bullae (arrow) on lateral oblique (a) and rostrocaudal open-mouth (b) radiographs of the head of a healthy dog.

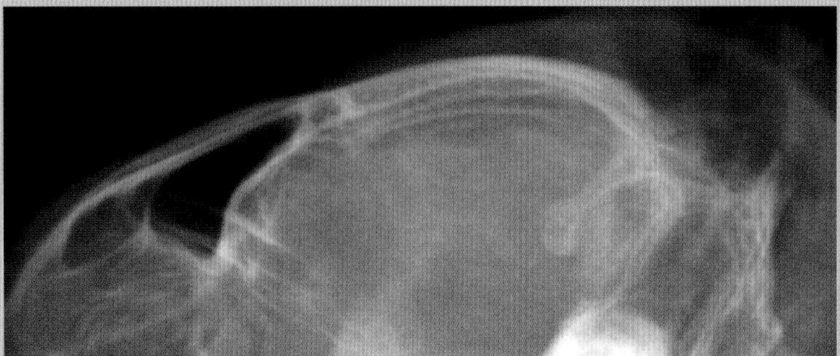

FIGURE 6.51. Lateral radiograph of the head of a healthy cat. In cats, the tympanic bullae have a bone division that separates an internal compartment (white arrow) from an external compartment (black arrow).

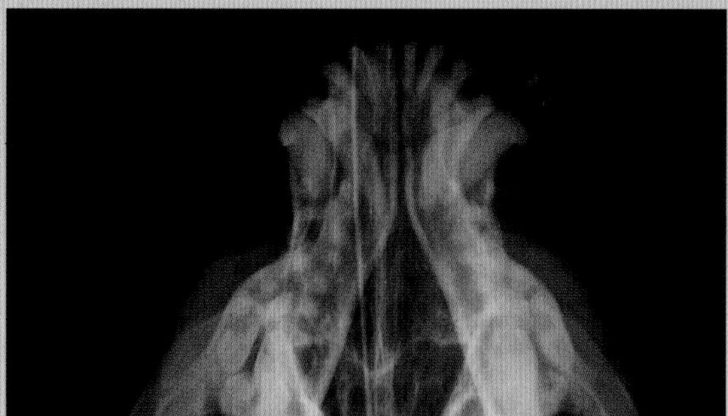

FIGURE 6.52. Dorsoventral radiograph of the head of a dog with otitis externa. Calcification of the ear canals is observed (arrows).

Tumours

Neoplasms involving the tympanic bulla are rare. External auditory canal tumours (ceruminous gland adenomas, ceruminous gland adenocarcinomas and squamous cell carcinomas) are more common and may extend to secondarily involve the bulla. Primary or secondary middle ear tumours often cause bulla wall lysis, bone proliferation and soft tissue swelling. An increase in the opacity of the affected bulla is generally observed, either due to accumulation of exudate or to proliferation of tissue it contains. Neoplasms can also cause lysis of other bone structures adjacent to the bulla (fig. 6.55).

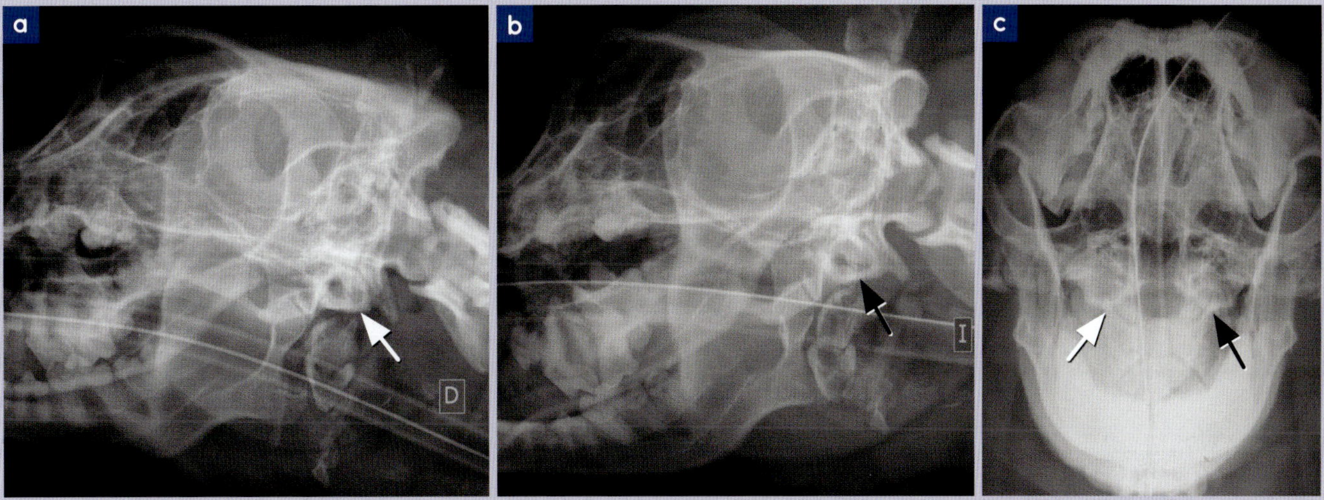

FIGURE 6.53. Enlarged images of the tympanic bullae on right (a) and left (b) lateral oblique radiographs and on a rostrocaudal open-mouth radiograph of the head of a dog with bilateral otitis media. Both the right tympanic bulla (white arrows) and the left tympanic bulla (black arrows) have a thickened wall and increased radiographic density in their interior. Both ear canals are calcified.

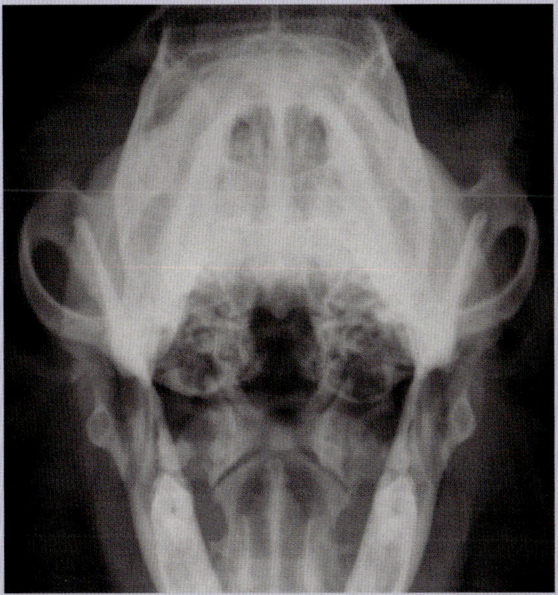

FIGURE 6.54. Enlarged image of the tympanic bullae on a rostrocaudal open-mouth radiograph of the head of a dog with right unilateral otitis media. Thickening and irregularity of the wall of the right tympanic bulla may be observed.

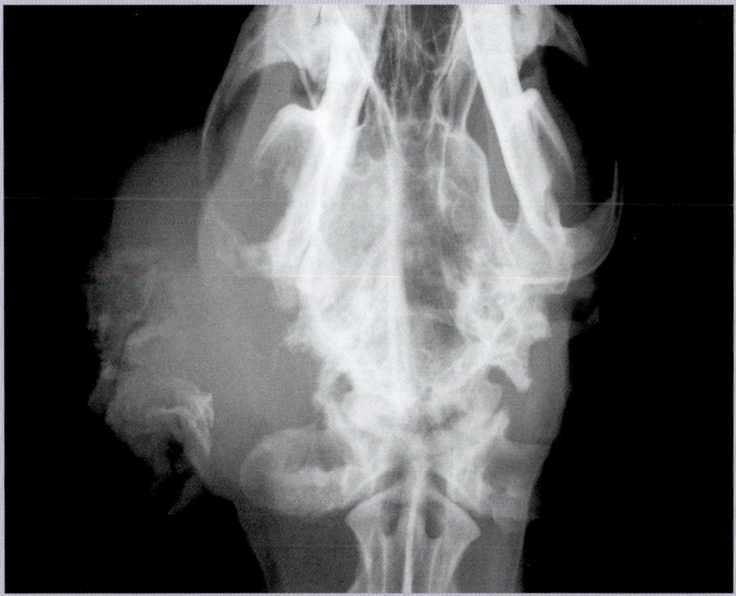

FIGURE 6.55. Dorsoventral radiograph of the head of a dog with an external auditory canal tumour. A large mass is observed in the area of the right external auditory canal with soft tissue density and some areas of irregular calcification, which causes osteolysis of numerous adjacent structures (temporal bone, occipital bone, mandible, zygomatic bone and C1 vertebra). Image courtesy of María José Ruiz Fernández.

Cholesteatoma

Middle ear cholesteatomas are non-neoplastic lesions that can appear similar to aggressive tumours in that they can cause expansion and lysis of the bone components of the ear (fig. 6.56). These are epidermoid cysts that accumulate hyperkeratotic material. As they progressively increase in size, they can cause compression and destruction of the adjacent tissues. Sometimes they break, causing inflammation and in some cases infection of the surrounding tissues.

They may be primary acquired associated with Eustachian tube dysfunction and chronic poor ventilation of the ear canal, or secondary to chronic otitis media, middle ear trauma or previous surgeries of the external auditory canal or middle ear.

X-rays may show features similar to those of otitis media. If bulla wall lysis appears, chronic otitis media, cholesteatoma and neoplasia should be considered as differential diagnoses. Enlargement of the bulla suggests a cholesteatoma or tumour since it is not a typical sign of otitis media. The definitive diagnosis between cholesteatoma and neoplasia must be established by histological study, given the similarity of the radiographic findings of these processes, and even of those observed by computed tomography and magnetic resonance.

Cases for **self-assessment**

Case 6.1. Presentation | Explanation

Case 6.2. Presentation | Explanation

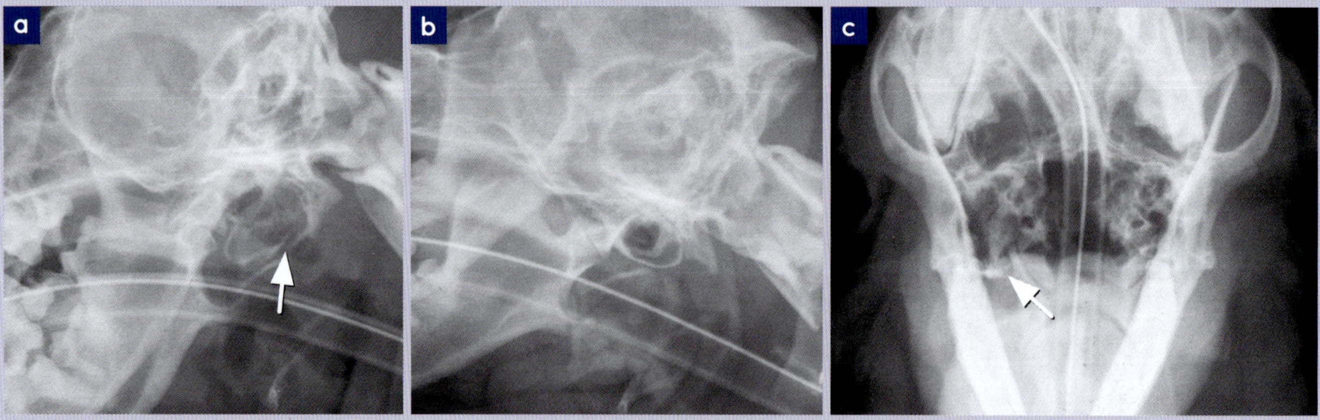

FIGURE 6.56. Enlarged images of the tympanic bullae on a right (a) and left (b) lateral oblique radiograph and a rostrocaudal open-mouth radiograph (c) of the head of a dog with a right middle ear cholesteatoma. This appears as an expansile lesion of the right tympanic bulla, showing enlargement, increased intraluminal opacity and focal wall destruction (arrows).

Most common diagnostic errors 7

The main disadvantages of radiography against other diagnostic imaging techniques are the limited differences of opacity in the image (gas, fat, soft tissues and fluids, mineral and metal) and the superimposition of structures, which often causes a loss of diagnostic information as well as optical effects that may lead to errors in the diagnosis. Diagnostic errors are also frequently caused by apparently anomalous images due to a poor position of the patient when the radiograph was taken, the use of incorrect exposure values, an inappropriate administration of the contrast agent, and by a poor knowledge of the normal anatomical variations of certain structures.

This chapter reviews the most common diagnostic errors divided by anatomical regions and includes a specific reference to those that are typical of digital radiography in the last section. Many of them have already been mentioned in the corresponding chapters of this book.

Note: the text includes references to the figures in this chapter as well as to other figures that have already appeared in previous chapters.

Abdomen

Lack of abdominal fat, wet hair

Very thin (fig. 7.1) or very young (fig. 7.2) animals have very little intra-abdominal fat, which renders identification of abdominal structures more difficult. This image may be mistaken for that caused by ascites, peritonitis or peritoneal carcinomatosis. The image produced by overlying wet hair, for example when a radiograph is taken after an abdominal ultrasound in which gel was applied to enhance the transmission of ultrasonic waves, should not be confused with that of these diseases either.

Underexposure and overexposure

A greatly underexposed abdominal radiograph (taken with very low exposure values) may also give a false appearance of increased and more homogeneous radiopacity than normal, which should not be confused with peritoneal disease. On the other hand, on a highly overexposed abdominal radiograph (taken with very high exposure values), the decrease in radiopacity caused by the technical error may be confused with that caused by a pneumoperitoneum.

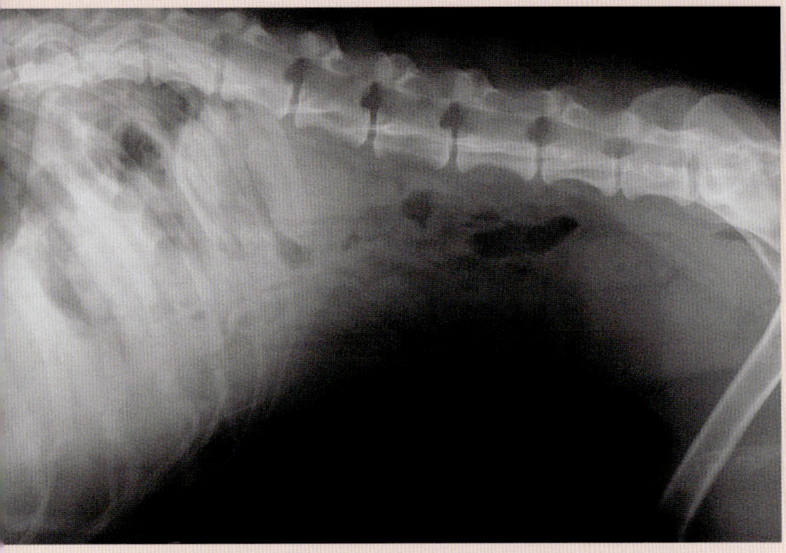

FIGURE 7.1. Lateral radiograph of the abdomen of a very thin, healthy dog. The abdominal organs appear poorly differentiated due to the lack of intraabdominal fat. This could be confused with ascites, peritonitis or peritoneal carcinomatosis. In case of doubt, an ultrasound scan will allow us to establish a precise diagnosis.

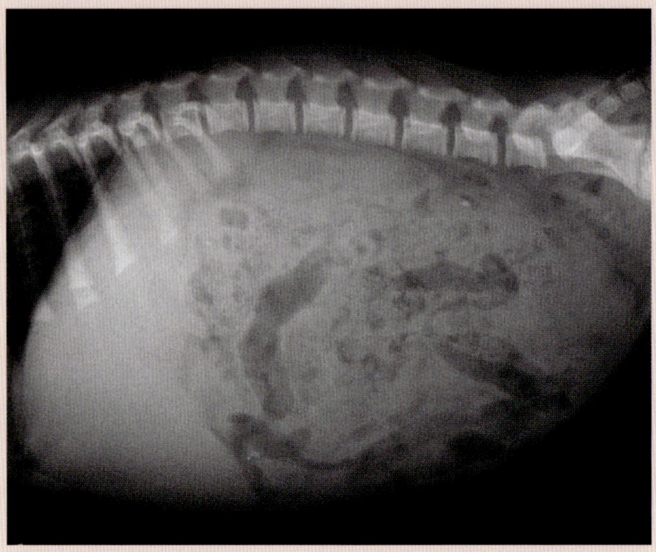

FIGURE 7.2. Lateral radiograph of the abdomen of a healthy young dog. The abdominal organs appear poorly differentiated due to the lack of intraabdominal fat, which is normal in young animals. We should not confuse this image with that caused by ascites, peritonitis or peritoneal carcinomatosis. In case of doubt, an ultrasound scan will allow us to establish a precise diagnosis.

Caudal hepatic border depending on thoracic conformation

The caudal hepatic border is usually seen at the level of or slightly beyond the costal arch on lateral radiographs. In order not to give an incorrect diagnosis of increase or reduction in the size of the liver, it must be borne in mind that, in breeds with a deep and narrow thorax, the whole shadow of the liver may be located in the thoracic cage (false appearance of decrease in size) while, on the other hand, the caudal hepatic border extends beyond the limit of the costal arch to a greater extent in breeds with a wide and shallow thorax (false appearance of increase in size).

Physiological organomegaly in young animals

It should be remembered that young animals display a certain degree of organomegaly in comparison with adult animals. This should be taken into account in the first months of life so as not to make an incorrect diagnose of increase in the size of the abdominal organs.

False impression of splenomegaly

It is also important to highlight that splenomegaly is assessed in function of the thickness of the shadow of the spleen, since its length depends on the position of the tail of the spleen when taking the radiograph. A long shadow with no increase in its thickness does not indicate splenomegaly (fig. 2.38).

Gestation before foetal mineralisation

Before day 45 of pregnancy in the dog and between days 36 and 45 in the cat, the pregnant uterus appears increased in size, but the mineralised foetal structures cannot be differentiated in it (fig. 2.86). We may therefore mistake pregnancy for pathological dilatation of the uterus. Performing an abdominal ultrasound scan will allow us to establish a differential diagnosis.

Superimposition of the prepuce and os penis

The shadow of the prepuce on a ventrodorsal radiograph may be mistaken for the shadow of the bladder or for a mass. Especially on rotated radiographs, the shadows of the prepuce and os penis may create optical effects of superimposition on the hip that may be confused with lesions of the latter.

"Pseudomasses"

Some normal abdominal images may produce a pseudomass effect. Thus, a very distended bladder filled with fluids may be mistaken for masses originated by pathological causes in other organs (fig. 2.64). The fat that accumulates in the falciform ligament of obese cats creates a shadow ventral to the liver that reminds of a mass, although its density, which is lower than that of soft tissues, facilitates its identification as fat (fig. 2.10). The superimposition of the two kidneys on lateral radiographs creates an optical effect since their radiographic densities add up, which may be confused with the presence of a third structure in the area. Another example of pseudomass is the markedly round image that the normal pyloric antrum may have on right lateral radiographs. This is a classical example of a possible diagnostic pitfall, as it may be confused with a mass or with a round foreign body (fig. 7.3).

False thickening of the gastric or intestinal wall

Although this has already been mentioned in the corresponding section of this book, it is important to highlight that one of the most important errors that may be made when assessing an abdominal X-ray is to diagnose a thickening of the gastric (fig. 2.108) or intestinal (fig. 2.125) wall. In the image, it is impossible to distinguish a wall that is really thickened from a normal wall with fluid or mucus adjacent to it, which gives a false impression of increase in thickness. The thickness of the walls of the stomach and intestine must be assessed by ultrasonography.

Increase in the amount of gastric and intestinal fluid/gas

A predominance of fluid (fig. 7.4) or gas (fig. 7.5) content in the small intestine is considered to be indicative of enteritis, but it is important to highlight that these findings alone do not mean there is a disease process. In a similar way, a very dilated stomach filled with gas in a nervous animal may be exclusively due to aerophagia and may not have any pathological significance.

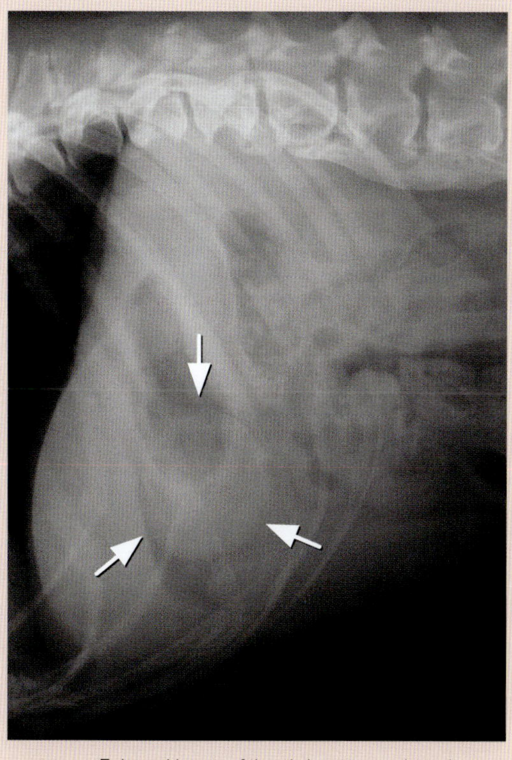

FIGURE 7.3. Enlarged image of the abdomen on a lateral radiograph of a healthy dog. The pyloric antrum (arrows) has a round aspect due to the normal accumulation of fluid/mucus on this view. This image may be confused with a round foreign body or with a mass.

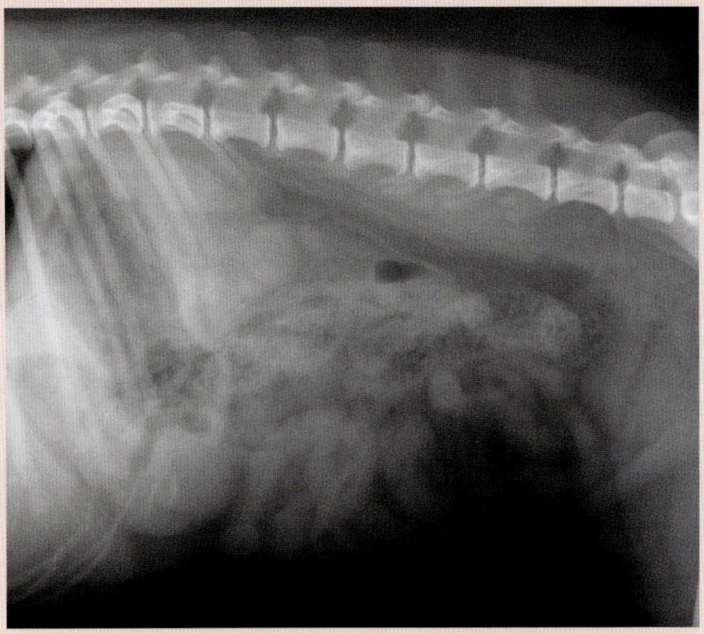

FIGURE 7.4. Lateral radiograph of the abdomen of a healthy dog. In the image, it is possible to observe a marked predominance of fluid content (fluid/mucus) in the small intestine, which is not accompanied by alterations of its diameter. This finding alone does not have any pathological significance, although it sometimes appears associated with processes of enteritis. However, it would be a serious error to establish a diagnosis of enteritis based only on this radiological sign.

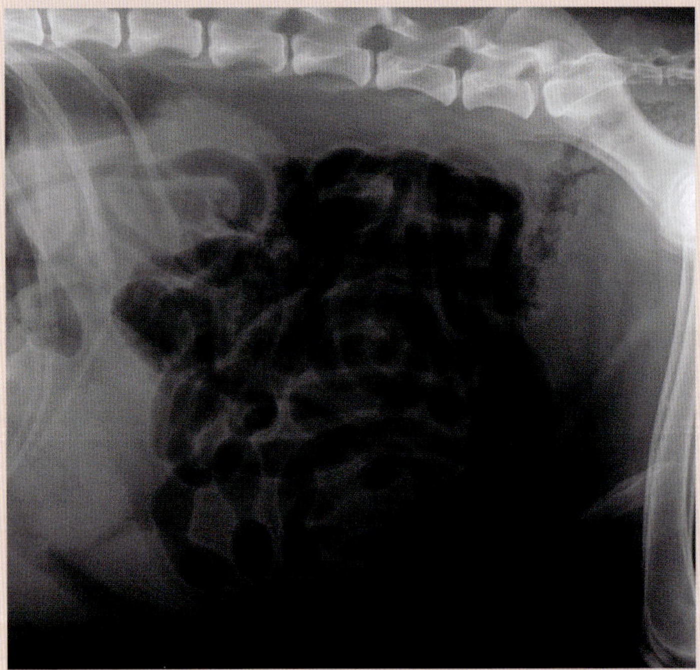

FIGURE 7.5. Lateral radiograph of the abdomen of a healthy dog. In the image, it is possible to observe a marked predominance of gas content in the small intestine, which is not accompanied by alterations of its diameter. This finding alone does not have any pathological significance, although it sometimes appears associated with processes of enteritis. As in the case of a predominance of fluid, it would be a serious error to diagnose enteritis based only on this radiological finding.

Anatomical variations of the gastrointestinal tract in cats

The accumulation of loops of the small intestine in the centre of the abdomen in obese cats is due to the tendency shown by these animals to accumulate fat in the peripheral areas of the abdomen (fig. 2.10), and this finding should therefore not be attributed to pathological causes.

The radiographs of some cats also show a band of fat density in the gastric wall, which is considered an incidental finding with no clinical significance.

Intestinal particularities in dogs

The caecum in dogs often appears dilated, with gas content and a C-shape in the right cranial area of the abdomen on ventrodorsal radiographs (fig. 2.142), and superimposed on the descending colon on lateral radiographs. It is important not to confuse it with a segment of abnormally dilated small intestine so as not to make an incorrect diagnosis of intestinal obstruction.

Some dogs have a longer colon than normal, which is called **redundant colon** and is considered a normal anatomical variation.

Peristaltic waves

A wavy appearance of the wall of the small or large intestine may sometimes be observed. This finding is indicative of an inflammatory or diffuse infiltrative process if it persists on various radiographs taken at different times, but when it is an isolated finding in a radiographic study, it is usually due to the appearance of a peristaltic wave when the radiograph was taken (fig. 7.6).

Inappropriate doses of contrast agent

With regard to contrast techniques, the most frequent cause of diagnostic errors is the administration of an inappropriate dose of contrast medium. For instance, if positive-contrast gastrography is used to evaluate gastric emptying and a lower dose than recommended is administered, the rate of emptying will be slower, while if an excessive dose is administered it will be faster. The results of the test will therefore not be objective.

Patterns of contrast medium accumulation

When carrying out a barium study of the small intestine in small dogs, it is possible to observe out-pouchings in the contrast column as this goes through the duodenum. These are called **pseudoulcers** (fig. 7.7), and are due to the focal accumulation of the contrast medium in areas with lymphatic tissue. In approximately 30 % of cats, it is also possible to observe a peculiar image of the duodenum when administering barium, which is referred to as the **"string of pearls" sign** (fig. 7.8), and is due to strong segmental contractions of the duodenal wall with no pathological significance. This image is similar to the one that the presence of a linear foreign body may cause in any intestinal segment.

Presence of gas bubbles

When retrograde urethrography or positive-contrast cystography are used, it is easy to confuse the image created by the gas bubbles that were introduced when the patient was catheterised with real filling defects caused by calculi or clots (fig. 2.69). These gas bubbles usually have a round morphology, while calculi and clots usually have a more irregular shape and distribution.

Contrast diffusion

Finally, on retrograde urethrograms in males, it is possible to observe the passage of a small amount of contrast medium to the prostatic ducts. This finding does not have any pathological significance, unless it is accompanied by a focal accumulation of contrast material in cavities or cystic areas.

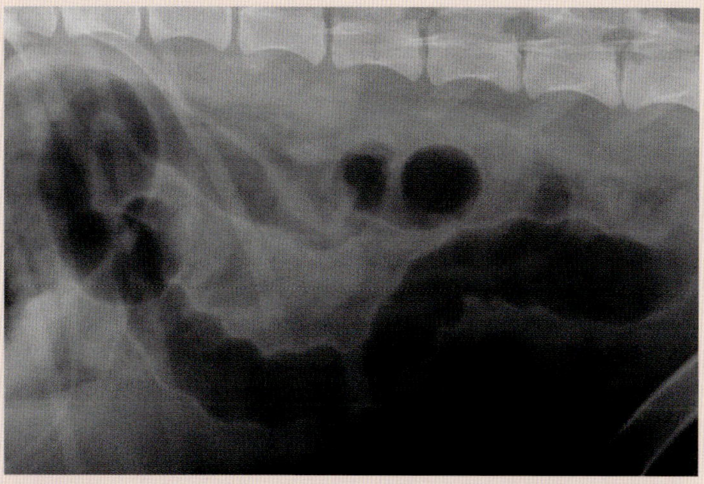

FIGURE 7.6. Enlarged image of the abdomen on a lateral radiograph of a healthy dog. The wavy appearance of the large intestinal wall may be due to an inflammatory process, but it may also be due to normal peristalsis. The persistence of this image on serial radiographs is considered indicative of a disease.

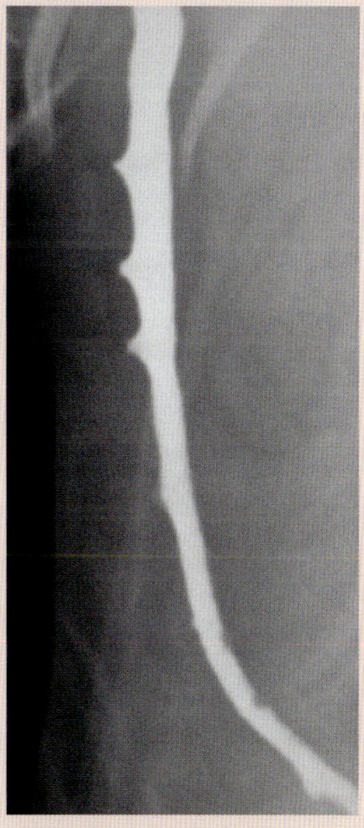

FIGURE 7.7. Enlarged image of the duodenum 20 minutes after administering barium by oral route to a healthy dog. The out-pouchings that appear on the lateral aspect of the contrast column are due to the presence of normal lymphatic tissue in the duodenal wall. This image may be confused with ulcers, which is why it is referred to as pseudoulcers.

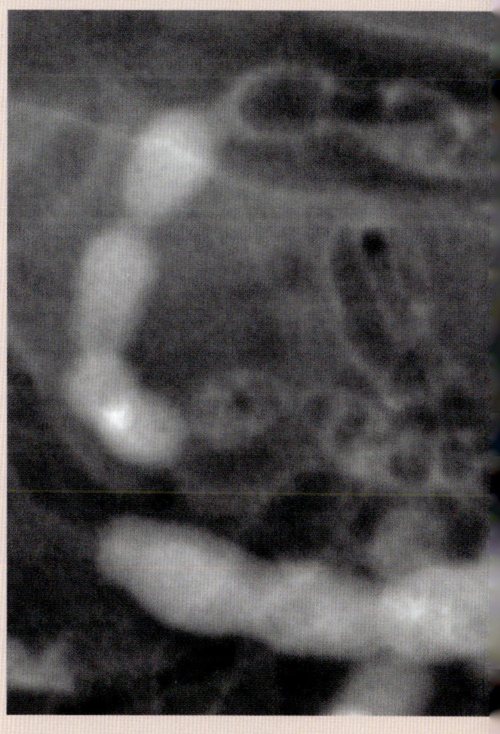

FIGURE 7.8. Enlarged image of the duodenum 30 minutes after administering barium by oral route to a healthy cat. The wavy appearance of the duodenal wall is due to normal peristaltic contractions and is termed "string of pearls" sign. It may be confused with the image of a linear foreign body.

Neck and thorax

Confusion of the hyoid apparatus with foreign bodies

When the presence of a foreign body in the neck is suspected, the bones that form the hyoid apparatus should not be confused with foreign bodies in the pharynx. If a real foreign body is detected on a lateral radiograph, its exact location should always be confirmed by taking a ventrodorsal radiograph.

Cricopharyngeal sphincter

When administering a contrast agent by oral route and evaluating its passage from the orophraynx to the oesophagus, it is important not to confuse the image of the cranial oesophageal sphincter (cricopharyngeal sphincter) with a filling defect or "mass effect" due to pathological causes.

Cutaneous nodules and nipples

Cutaneous nodules may have a similar image to nodular lesions in the lung. The same may sometimes occur when nipples are superimposed (fig. 7.9) on rotated radiographs. In case of doubt, the thoracic wall should be examined thoroughly and a small amount of barium should be applied on the cutaneous lesion or nipple to repeat the radiograph.

Calcification associated with age

Calcification of the costochondral junctions associated with age, which has no clinical significance, should not be confused with aggressive bone lesions (fig. 3.10). On ventrodorsal radiographs, these calcifications may create a false effect of calcified nodular lesions in the lung (fig. 7.10).

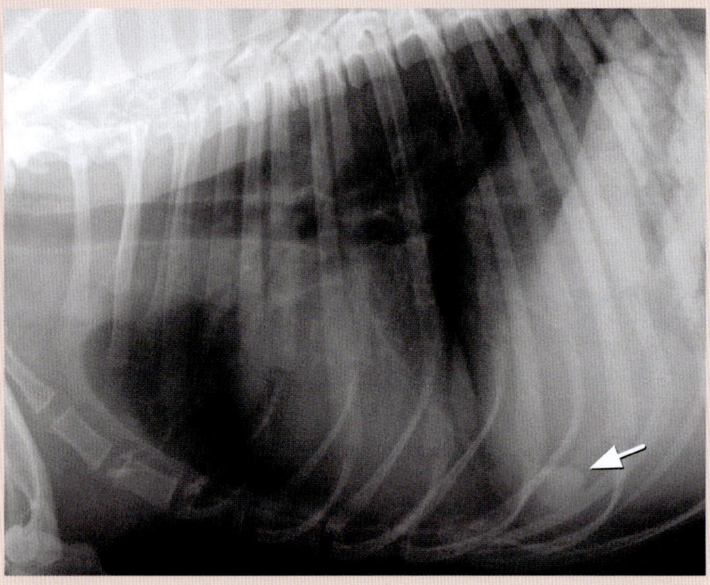

FIGURE 7.9. Lateral radiograph of the thorax of a healthy dog. The arrow indicates a hyperplastic nipple, which, due to the rotated position of the thorax, is superimposed on the ventral area of the shadow of the liver and may be mistaken for a calculus in the gallbladder or for a nodular lesion in the lung.

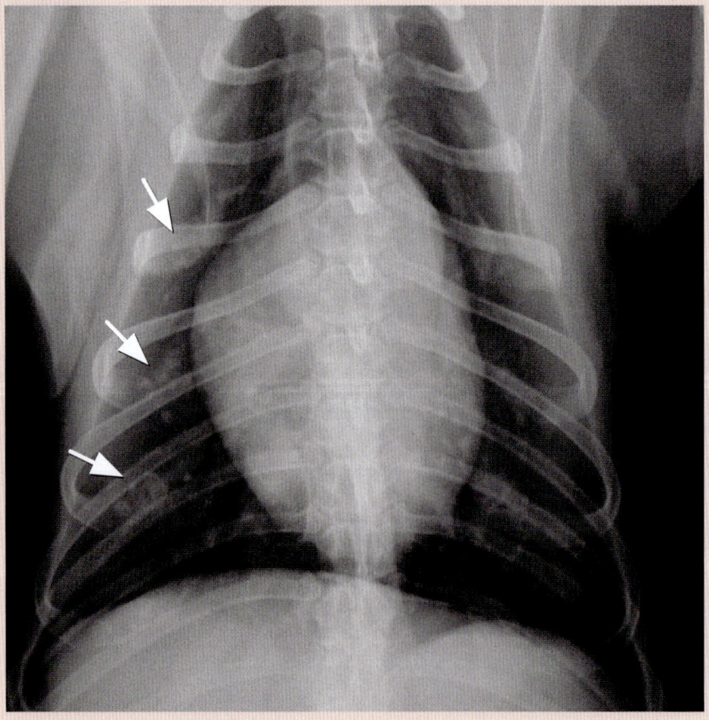

FIGURE 7.10. Ventrodorsal radiograph of the thorax of a healthy dog. The arrows show calcifications of the right costochondral junctions. These should not be confused with aggressive bone lesions or calcified nodular lesions in the lung.

Folds of skin

The folds of skin that form when the patient is placed on the cassette may create well-defined shadows of soft-tissue density surrounded by gas, which should not be confused with diseases (fig. 3.1c).

Rib curvature and costal cartilage calcification

Chondrodystrophic breeds sometimes show a peculiar curvature of the ribs and costal cartilages towards the inside of the cavity, in the area proximal to the costochondral junction. This creates shadows of soft-tissue density that may be similar to a pleural or pulmonary lesion (fig. 3.7).

Costal cartilages may appear partially calcified in cats, which may produce a false impression of a fracture (fig. 3.66).

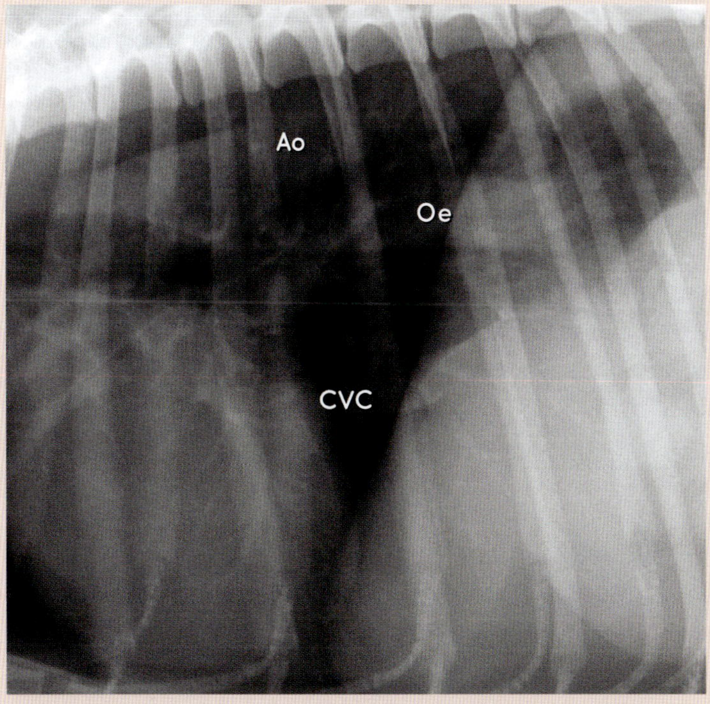

FIGURE 7.11. Left lateral radiograph of the thorax of a healthy dog. It is possible to observe a band of soft-tissue density in the caudodorsal area of the thorax, between the aorta (Ao) and the caudal vena cava (CVC). This shadow is due to the retention of fluid or mucus in the caudal area of the thoracic oesophagus (Oe), and is not considered pathological unless it persists on serial radiographs.

False alterations of the trachea

Minimal variations in the diameter of the trachea between inspiration and expiration are physiological. The rotation of the thorax at the moment when a lateral radiograph is taken may cause the oesophagus and/or muscles and the trachea to be superimposed, thus creating a false image of tracheal collapse. This type of image may also be caused by the so-called redundancy of the dorsal tracheal membrane, or by contraction or invagination of the membrane (fig. 3.24). The thoracic trachea may have a slightly wavy course if the radiograph is taken with the patient's head or neck in an incorrect position. In addition, a false dorsal displacement of the trachea may appear when the radiograph is taken with the median plane of the thoracic cavity inclined on the cassette (fig. 3.4) (this is corrected by placing a positioning block that elevates the sternum). In obese animals, it is possible to observe a right displacement of the trachea on ventrodorsal radiographs, caused by the excessive accumulation of fat in the mediastinum, not by pathological causes. In order not to make an incorrect diagnosis of tracheal hypoplasia, it is important to remember that the diameter of the trachea is proportionally smaller in brachycephalic breeds, especially in the Bulldog (fig. 3.26).

False alterations of the oesophagus

The presence of minimal accumulations of gas in the oesophageal lumen is not considered pathological (fig. 3.28), unless it persists over time. The accumulation of a small amount of fluid/mucus in the distal area of the thoracic oesophagus (fig. 7.11), just before going through the oesophageal hiatus of the diaphragm, is also considered physiological. This finding is more frequent on left lateral radiographs than on the right lateral ones. When barium is administered, the temporary retention of a small amount of contrast medium between the folds of the oesophageal wall is not considered significant, but if it persists over time it would be considered indicative of oesophagitis. We should also remember that the oesophagus may appear moderately dilated in anaesthetised animals (fig. 3.30), so as not to make an incorrect diagnosis of pathological dilatation in these cases.

Mediastinum in brachycephalic breeds and obese animals

In brachycephalic breeds, the shadow of the mediastinum is wider compared with other breeds. In obese animals the mediastinum may also appear enlarged, which could be similar to the image of a mediastinal mass or effusion, especially on ventrodorsal and dorsoventral radiographs. On lateral radiographs, fat may cause a more or less noticeable elevation of the cardiac silhouette (fig.3.61).

False impression of cardiomegaly

A false impression of cardiomegaly may be given by rotated radiographs (they show evident increased cardiosternal contact —fig. 3.4—) and expiratory radiographs (the small volume of the lung gives a false impression of increased cardiac size —fig. 7.12—). We should also remember that in old cats, the heart tends to be in greater contact with the sternum due to the progressive elongation of the aorta. This could be confused with an increase in the width of the cardiac silhouette (fig. 3.76). The cardiac silhouette should not be assessed on ventrodorsal and dorsoventral radiographs when the thorax is in rotated position, since it may result in incorrect diagnoses of increased right or left heart size, depending on the side to which the patient has been rotated (fig. 3.5). The accumulation of fat in the pericardial space that may appear in obese animals may also create a false image of increased cardiac size.

The organomegaly observed in young animals also affects the heart.

Thymus

The thymus is observed until approximately 6 months of age and should not be confused with pleural or pulmonary lesions (fig. 3.62).

Coronary vessels

A serious diagnostic error is to mistake the pulmonary vessels that overlap the heart for coronary vessels (fig. 7.13). These latter have the same radiopacity as the myocardium, so they cannot be differentiated on a radiograph with no contrast.

False pleural effusion

Various normal structures may be mistaken for a pleural effusion on a radiograph. In cats, it is normal to observe a minimal retraction of the dorsocaudal border of the caudal pulmonary lobes (fig. 3.6), while the same finding would be indicative of a mild pleural effusion in dogs. Thickening or calcification of the pleura with no pathological significance may also be mistaken for mild pleural effusion (fig. 3.56).

False pulmonary alterations

The costal cartilages may have the appearance of interlobar fissures, although they can be differentiated since the cartilage is straighter and its junction with the rib can be identified.

Folds of skin may cause an artefact known as **pseudopneumothorax**, which is termed this way because it produces a marked difference of radiopacity between the areas lateral and medial to the fold of skin, resulting in a very dark lateral area (fig. 3.52). This may be mistaken for a pulmonary retraction due to the presence of gas in the pleural space.

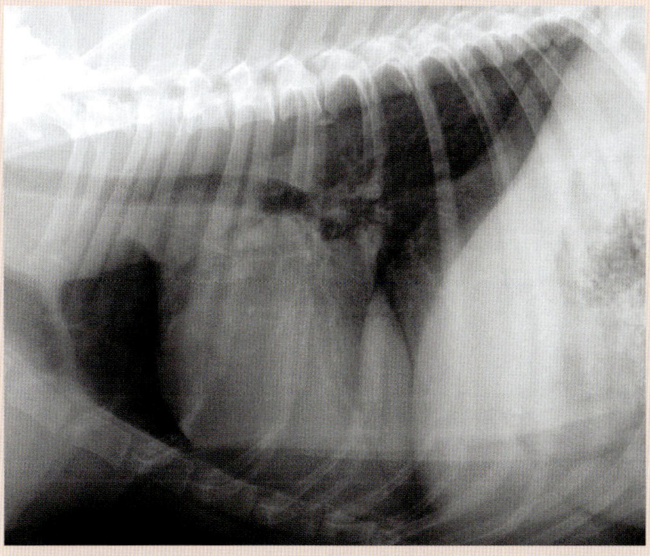

FIGURE 7.12. Lateral radiograph of the thorax of a healthy dog. The radiograph was taken in expiration, which causes a false appearance of cardiomegaly due to the smaller volume of the lung and superimposed shadow of the diaphragm and cardiac silhouette.

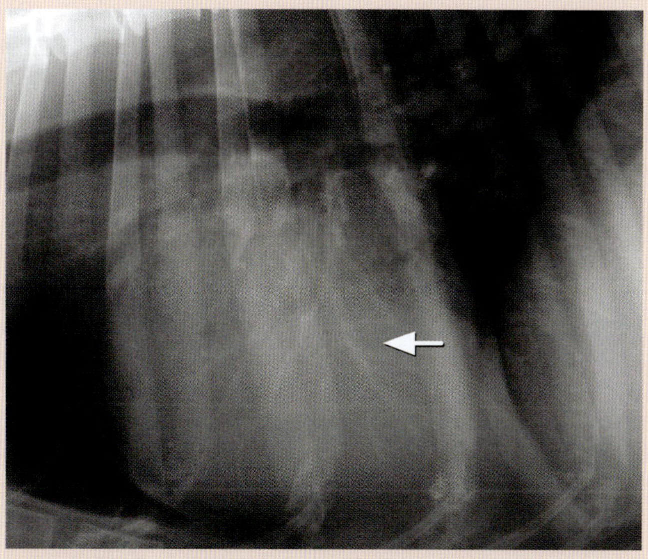

FIGURE 7.13. Enlarged image of a lateral radiograph of the thorax of a healthy dog. Mistaking the pulmonary vessels (arrow), which appear superimposed on the cardiac silhouette, for coronary vessels is a serious diagnostic error. Coronary vessels have the same radiopacity as the cardiac wall and therefore cannot be identified on a plain radiograph.

The radiopacity of the lung may appear falsely increased in obese animals (because of the summation with the density of the subcutaneous fat and limitation of the degree of pulmonary expansion due to the presence of fat in the mediastinum) on underexposed or expiratory radiographs (fig. 1.46b), which should not be confused with a real interstitial pattern due to pathological causes. If a conventional radiograph is overexposed (fig. 1.46a), a false reduction of pulmonary radiopacity is observed, which should not be confused with emphysema or pulmonary hypovascularisation.

The appearance of signs of atelectasis in the lower part of the lung is a usual finding in animals that have remained in lateral recumbency for a long period of time, especially if they have been anaesthetised. The alveolar pattern caused by atelectasis can be differentiated from that caused by oedema, pneumonia or haemorrhage, because a displacement of the mediastinal structures to the side where the atelectasic lung is located will appear on ventrodorsal and dorsoventral radiographs (fig. 3.131).

The superimposed pulmonary vessels and ribs may create shadows of greater radiopacity that are similar to nodular lesions in the lung. It is also possible to confuse the transversal shadows of those vessels that run parallel to the X-ray beam with nodules, in which case we should evaluate the adjacent vascular structures to determine whether the diameter of the shadows corresponds or not with that of the vessels in the area (fig. 7.14). Pleural and pulmonary calcifications (fig 3.56) are usually small and it is difficult to mistake them for pulmonary metastases, as these are very rarely calcified. The presence of calcified sludge in the gallbladder may be confused with areas of pleural or pulmonary calcification, or with pulmonary nodules (fig. 7.15). The location of the gallbladder on the two projections allows differentiation and in case of doubt, an abdominal ultrasound examination may be performed. The shadow of the gastric fundus on left lateral radiographs may also be mistaken for a lesion in the dorsocaudal area of the thorax (fig. 7.16).

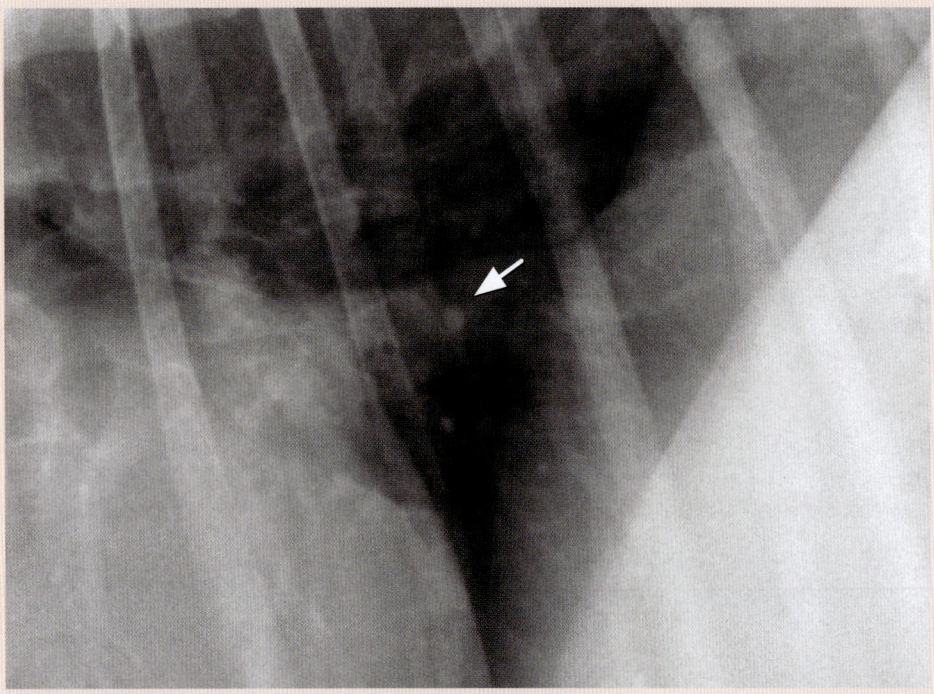

FIGURE 7.14. Enlarged image of a lateral radiograph of the thorax of a healthy dog. The arrow indicates the transverse image of a normal pulmonary vessel, which could be confused with a pulmonary nodular lesion. In order not to make an incorrect diagnosis, we must check whether other vessels in the area have a similar diameter. In case of doubt, a more precise diagnosis may be established with the help of computed tomography.

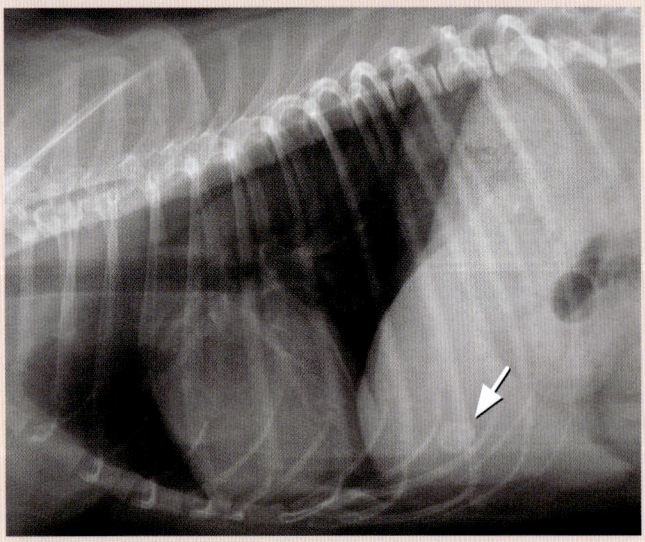

FIGURE 7.15. Lateral radiograph of the thorax of a healthy dog. The arrow shows a calculus/gallbladder sludge, which may be mistaken for a calcified nodular lesion in the lung.

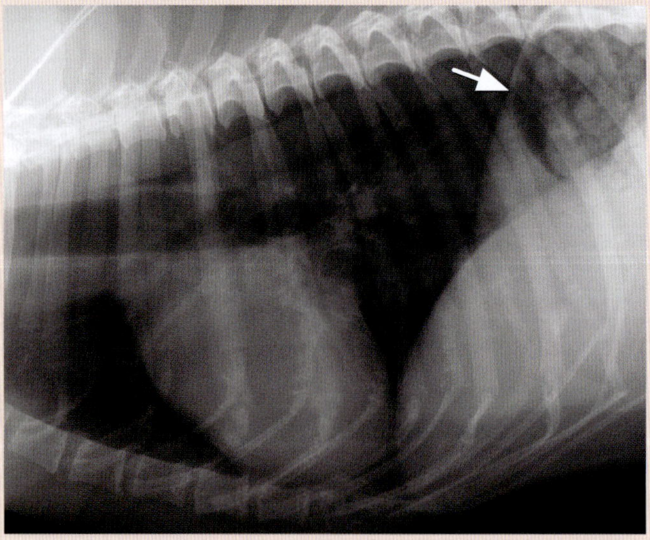

FIGURE 7.16. Left lateral radiograph of the thorax of a healthy dog. The arrow indicates the image of the normal gastric fundus (with gas and food content), which shows an apparently more cranial position on the left lateral view than on the right lateral view. This image may be mistaken for a pulmonary lesion.

Appendicular skeleton

Radiographic technique

An error that is often made when evaluating the appendicular skeleton is not to take two orthogonal projections, since some lesions are evident in only one of them (e.g. fractures with little displacement, joint subluxations) (fig. 7.17).

Overexposure of the radiograph may lead to an incorrect diagnosis of osteopaenia, as the bone appears less radiopaque in the image.

Age and breed

Growth lines in young animals should not be mistaken for fractures (fig. 7.18) and it is therefore recommended to use an atlas with radiographic images of animals throughout their development in case of doubt. It should be remembered that large-breed dogs may have slightly irregular metaphyseal margins, which may be confused with a periosteal reaction or with osteolysis. It is also important to be familiar with the peculiar morphology of bones in chondrodystrophic breeds (e.g. Basset Hound).

Incorrect positioning of the patient

The most frequent cause of diagnostic errors in the assessment of the appendicular skeleton is the incorrect positioning of the patient when taking the radiograph. This is especially significant in the examination of some joints such as the coxofemoral joint, as its image is greatly altered by minimal rotations of the pelvis. When this joint is rotated to one side, it is possible

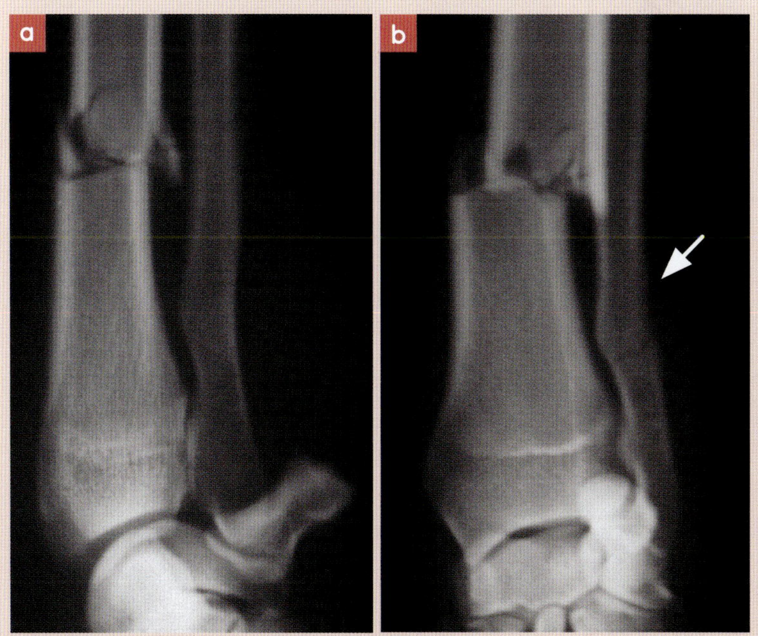

FIGURE 7.17. Enlarged images in mediolateral (a) and craniocaudal (b) projection of the radius and ulna of a dog with a fracture of both bones. The fracture of the ulna (arrow) is not visible on the mediolateral view and would therefore not be diagnosed if this radiograph alone were taken.

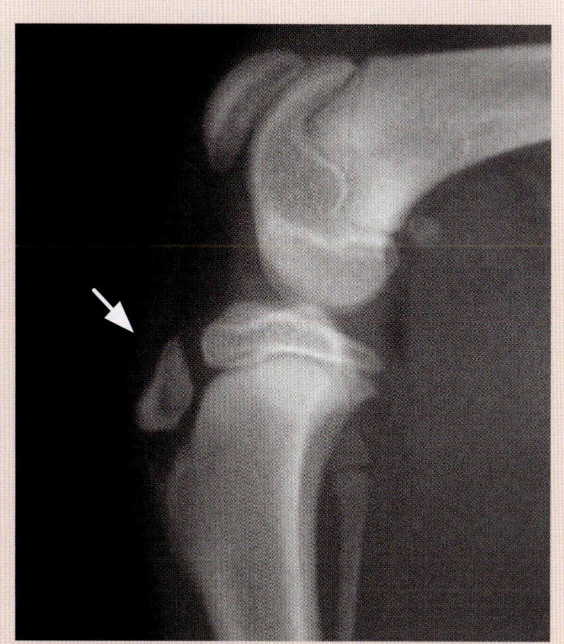

FIGURE 7.18. Mediolateral radiograph of the tibia of an 11-week-old, healthy dog. The growth plate of the tibial tuberosity (arrow) appears separated from the metaphysis until 6-8 months of age, which could be confused with an avulsion fracture of the tuberosity.

to see it in the image because the obturator foramen of the same side appears smaller and the shadow of the wing of the contralateral ilium appears narrower. In these conditions, reduced acetabular coverage (false increase of the joint space) on the side to which the pelvis is rotated, and greater acetabular coverage (false reduction of the joint space) in the contralateral joint will be observed (fig. 7.19). The position of the femurs will also affect the width of the joint space, which means that for a proper assessment of the joint, the femurs must remain parallel, with the patellas aligned with the trochlear groove.

The integrity of the sacroiliac joints is not assessed properly when the pelvis is rotated, since one of the joints will appear falsely enlarged, which could be confused with a luxation or subluxation.

Clavicle and sesamoid bones

Two important anatomical variations among those that may lead to diagnostic errors are vestigial clavicles (fig. 7.20) and some sesamoid bones that do not appear in a constant manner in dogs. Vestigial clavicles appear as small structures with mineral opacity medial to the head of the humerus. The sesamoid bone in the tendon of origin of the supinator muscle sometimes appears on radiographs of the elbow joint (fig. 4.72), craniolateral to the head of the radius. A sesamoid bone may also be observed in some cases on the lateral plantar aspect of the tarsometatarsal joint or in it. Sesamoid bones may also appear in the iliopubic ligament, and these are located cranial to the pubic eminence of the pelvis on lateral radiographs.

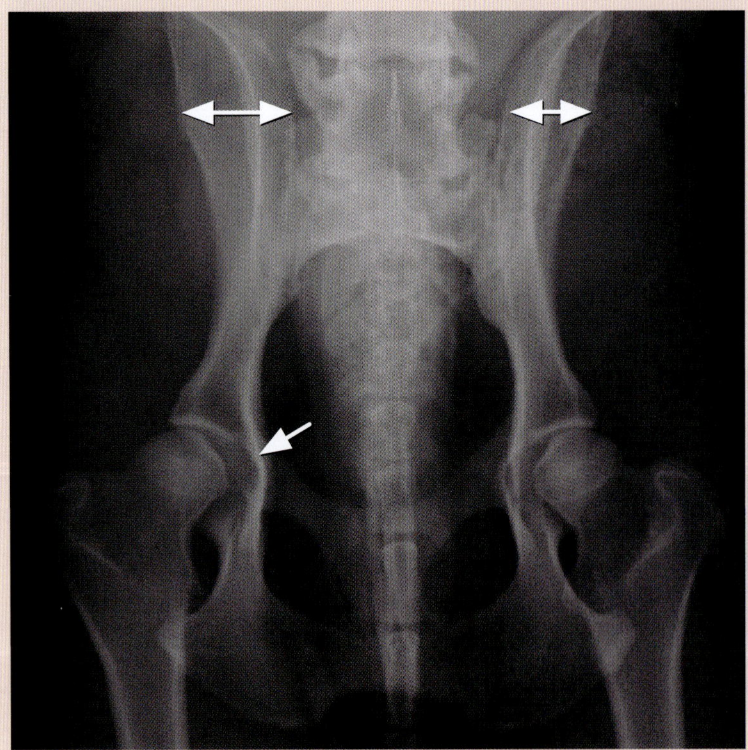

FIGURE 7.19. Ventrodorsal radiograph of the hip of a dog with a mild degree of hip luxation due to dysplasia. We can detect that the pelvis is rotated to the right side because the obturator foramen appears smaller and the shadow of the wing of the ilium is narrower. Due to this rotation, the right hip joint space (arrow) appears falsely increased, while in the left hip joint, the acetabular coverage is falsely increased.

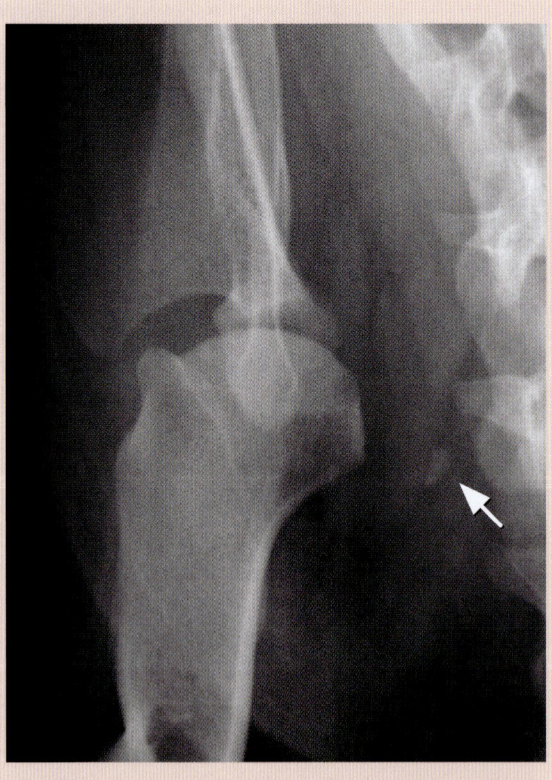

FIGURE 7.20. Caudocranial radiograph of the scapulohumeral joint of a healthy dog. The arrow shows the vestigial clavicle, which is sometimes observed in dogs. It is bilateral and should not be mistaken for a pathological calcification of the soft tissues of the area.

Spine

Incorrect positioning of the patient

The main source of diagnostic errors in the assessment of the spine is the incorrect positioning of the patient when taking a radiograph. If no radiolucent positioning blocks are used to elevate the cervical and lumbar spines, these remain curved towards the cassette/X-ray table, causing an evident narrowing of the intervertebral disc spaces (fig. 7.21). Even if the position of the spine is correct, only the intervertebral disc spaces that are most centred in the image should be evaluated, since the X-ray beam penetrates through them more obliquely as these spaces are farther away from its centre, thus creating a false narrowing in the image.

In order for the median plane of the spine to be parallel to the cassette, it is necessary to place radiolucent positioning blocks between the limbs or under them. If this is not done, the spine remains rotated and the transverse processes of each side appear separated in the image (fig. 5.2a). The most ventral ones may easily be confused with spondylosis deformans.

Overexposure and underexposure

Overexposure or underexposure of the radiograph may cause a false alteration of the radiopacity of the vertebrae, which we may be confused with osteopaenia o sclerosis.

Superimposed structures

The superimposition of the large bowel containing gas or faeces on the sacrum or pelvis may create an image similar to that of lines of fracture in these structures.

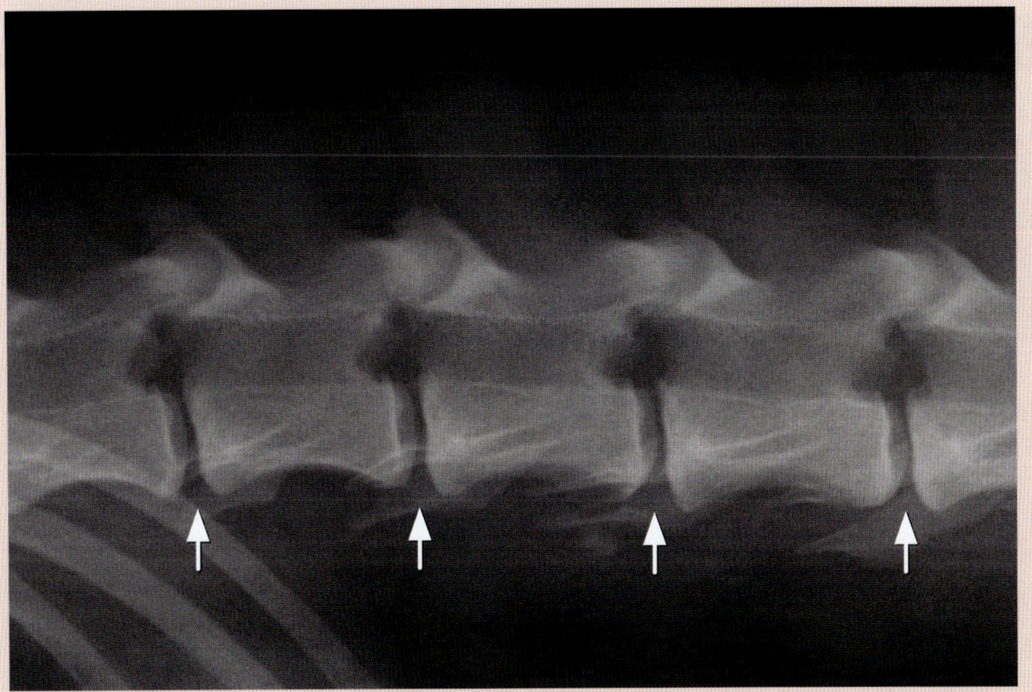

FIGURE 7.21. Enlarged image of the lumbar spine on a lateral radiograph of a healthy dog. When an area of the spine (cervical or lumbar) is curved towards the cassette/X-ray table, a false narrowing of the intervertebral disc spaces (arrows) will be observed on the radiograph. This defect is corrected by placing a radiolucent positioning block under the spine to ensure its axis is parallel to the cassette. In this image, the transverse processes of each vertebra appear at a different height, which indicates that the spine is rotated on its longitudinal axis (this can be corrected by placing a radiolucent positioning block between the limbs). The most ventral transverse processes may be confused with spondylosis deformans.

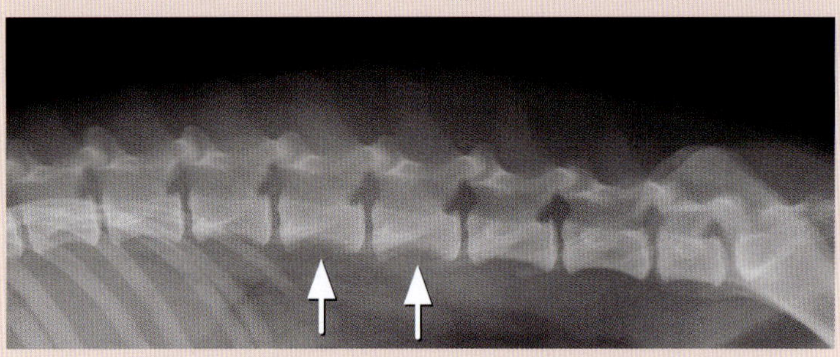

FIGURE 7.22. Lateral radiograph of the lumbar spine of a healthy dog. The ventral margin of the vertebral body of L3 and L4 (arrows) appears less defined due to the insertion of the crura of the diaphragm. This finding is more evident in large breed dogs.

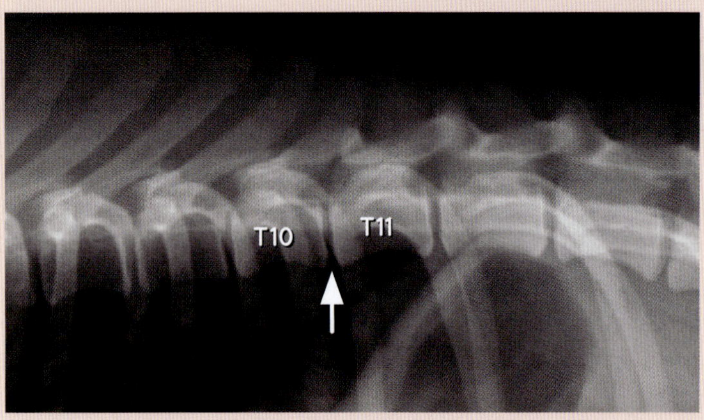

FIGURE 7.23. Enlarged image of the thoracic spine on a lateral radiograph of a healthy dog. A mild narrowing of the T10-T11 intervertebral disc space (arrow) can be seen when compared with the others. This is considered a normal anatomical variation.

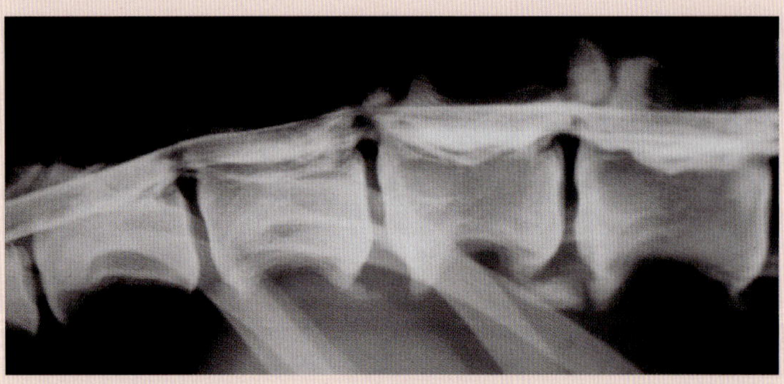

FIGURE 7.24. Enlarged image of the thoracolumbar area of the spine on a lateral radiograph of a dog that has received an injection of an iodinated contrast agent in the subarachnoid space for a myelogram, and in the extradural space by mistake, which creates irregularities in the margin of the contrast columns.

Normal anatomical variations

Some normal anatomical variations that may be mistaken for diseases are: the lack of definition of the ventral margin of the body of L3 and L4, due to the insertion of the crura of the diaphragm (fig 7.22) (more evident in large breed dogs); the narrowing of the T10-T11 intervertebral disc space, as it is an anticlinal space (fig 7.23); and the presence of haemal processes at the ends of the coccygeal vertebrae, which may be confused with spondylosis deformans.

Contrast medium in extradural space

If the contrast medium is introduced by mistake in the epidural space instead of in the subarachnoid space when performing a myelogram, the contrast columns will have a very irregular morphology (fig. 7.24) and making a precise diagnosis will thus be more difficult.

Head

Incorrect positioning of the patient

Most of the interpretation errors made when evaluating radiographs of a patient's head are due to a poor positioning of the patient. In this region, it is essential not to rotate the skull, especially on dorsoventral and ventrodorsal radiographs (fig. 7.25), since the symmetry or lack of symmetry of the structures is a key element on which the diagnosis of many diseases of this anatomical region is based.

On ventrodorsal open-mouth radiographs, the superimposition of the tongue should be avoided, since it may create a false image of mass in the nasal cavity (fig. 7.26).

Rostrocaudal tangential radiographs may provide images of a false increase in radiopacity of the frontal sinuses due to a poor positioning of the patient, or to the actual morphology of the sinuses and nasal bone depending on the breed (fig. 7.27).

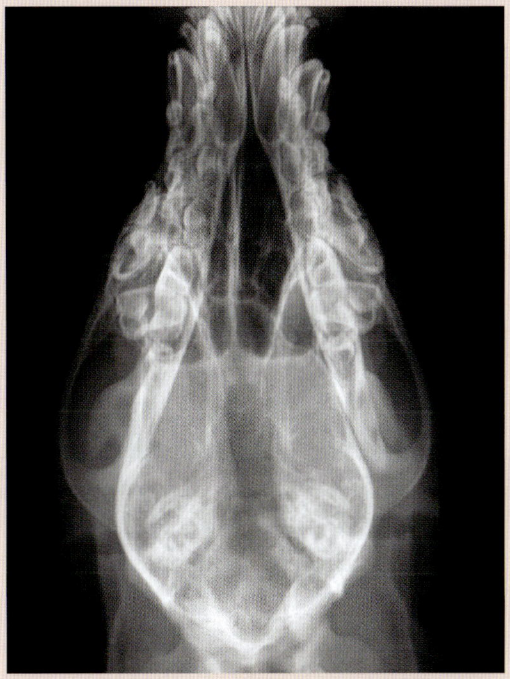

FIGURE 7.25. Dorsoventral radiograph of the head of a healthy young dog (superimposed deciduous and permanent teeth are observed). The rotation of the head increases the summation effect of the right mandibular body and nasal cavity of the same side, which hinders the correct assessment of this region of the skull.

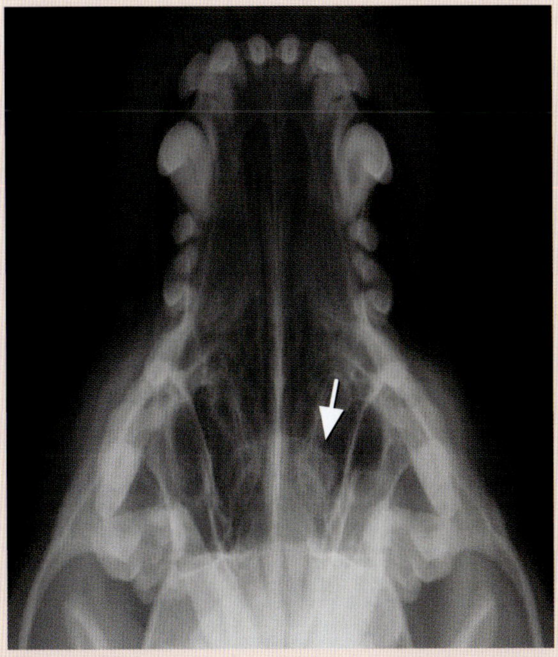

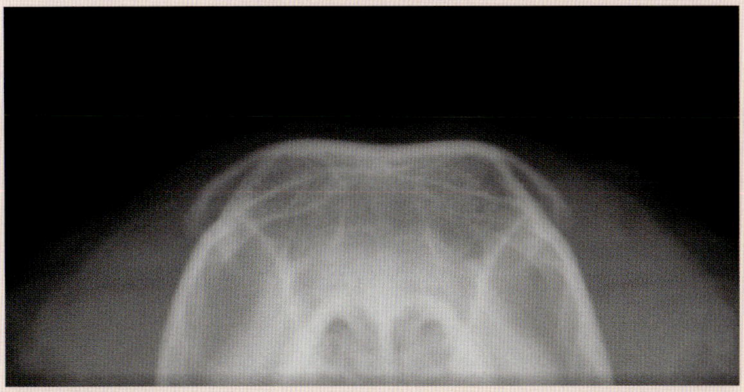

FIGURE 7.27. Rostrocaudal tangential radiograph of the frontal sinuses of a healthy dog. The incorrect positioning of the patient results in the X-ray beam penetrating through the cranial vault and frontal sinuses. The images of both structures add up, which results in a false image of increased radiopacity of the sinuses.

FIGURE 7.26. Ventrodorsal open-mouth radiograph of a healthy dog. The superimposition of the tongue (arrow) creates a false image of mass in the caudal area of the left nasal cavity.

Digital imaging

One of the great advantages of digital radiology is that it has a high contrast resolution compared with conventional radiology. The veterinary surgeon who acquires digital radiology equipment for the first time therefore has to get used to "a new way of observing radiographs". Some diagnostic errors can be made during this transition period.

Greater definition of the elements of the lung

In digital radiography, the blood vessels of the lung are very well-defined, which may lead to an incorrect diagnosis of vascular congestion. In some healthy animals, the bronchial walls may also be identified in the medial area of the lung, a finding that would be considered as indicative of a thickening of the bronchial walls, the presence of peribronchial infiltrates or calcification on a conventional radiograph.

Higher pulmonary radiopacity

The lung generally appears less transparent on a digital radiograph (fig. 1.29), which could be confused with a pathological interstitial pattern. In addition, on a digital radiograph, minimal degrees of lung displacement caused by mediastinal fat or by being in a lateral recumbent position may become more evident and may be similar to a pleural or mediastinal effusion.

Higher tissue contrast

The higher contrast between soft tissues and fat may lead to this latter being mistaken for free peritoneal gas on a digital radiograph of the abdomen. An incor-rect diagnosis of pneumoperitoneum may thus be established.

The trabeculae of bones may also appear better defined, which should not be interpreted as a pathological change in the bone marrow.

Overexposure

On highly overexposed digital radiographs, black areas with a loss of image information may appear in the affected area, and are not possible to recover with post-processing tools (fig. 7.28). When these areas appear in the lung, we may mistake them for pulmonary bullae while if they appear in the bone, they may be similar to areas of osteolysis.

Metallic implants

The appearance of an artefact around metallic implants placed in the bone has already been described. It is observed as radiolucent bands around these implants, and may be confused with a sign of mobility or rejection of the material (fig. 7.29). This artefact has already been corrected in many of the current machines and is caused by an excessive use of the edge-enhancement tool.

Excessive post-processing

In general, post-processing tools allow the improvement of the image quality, but when overused they may worsen it and lead to errors (fig. 7.30), in many cases due to an overdiagnosis (we see more than what is actually there).

Excessive zooming

A significant advantage of digital radiography is that we can use the zoom tool to greatly enlarge small areas of the image. However, we should not overuse this tool as we run the risk of losing the global view of the image, which in many cases is essential to establish a correct diagnosis.

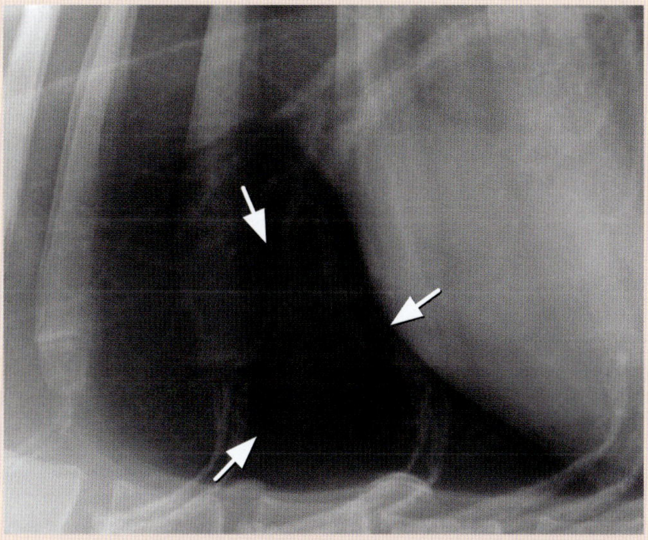

FIGURE 7.28. Enlarged image of the cranioventral area of the thorax of a healthy dog. The arrows indicate an overexposed area of the image (digital), which could be mistaken for an area of hypovascularisation or a pulmonary bulla.

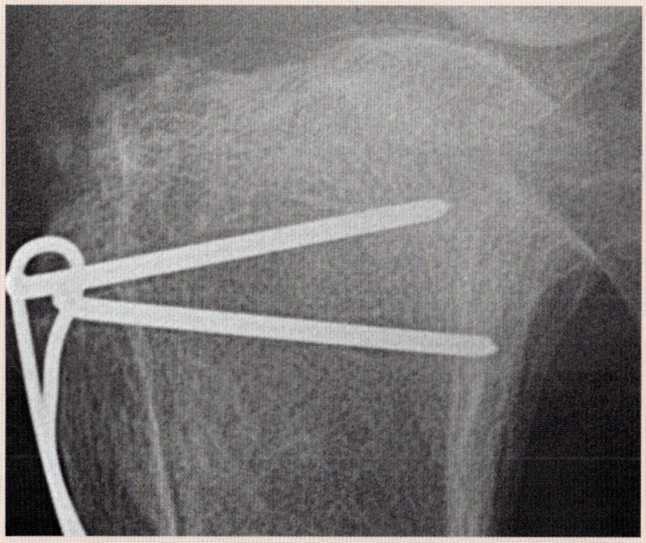

FIGURE 7.29. Enlarged image of the tibia on a mediolateral radiograph of a dog after the placement of pins and a cerclage wire. When the edge-enhancement tool is overused in digital radiography, radiolucent halos may appear around metal implants, which could be mistaken for a sign of rejection or mobility of the material.

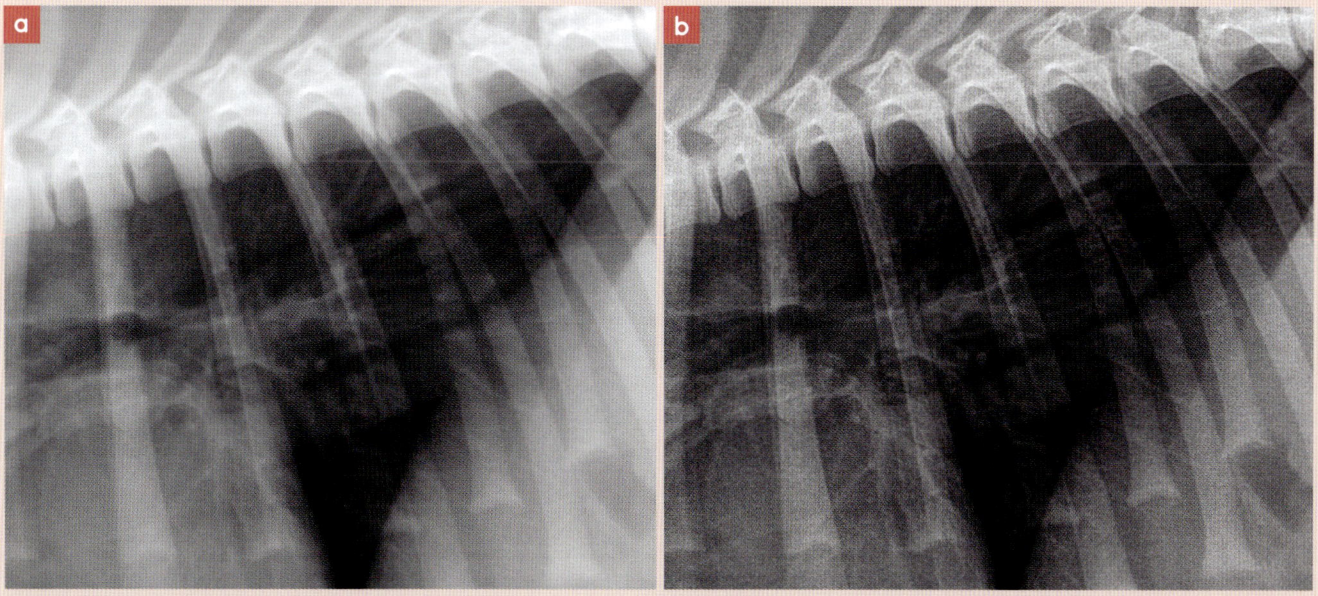

FIGURE 7.30. Enlarged images of the caudodorsal area of a healthy dog. One of them shows the properly processed digital radiograph (a), while the other shows the same image after overuse of the edge enhancement tool (b), which highlights the image of the vessels, bronchial walls and even the lung parenchyma excessively. The overuse of post-processing tools in digital radiology usually leads to diagnostic errors.

Cases for **self-assessment**

Case 7.1.

Presentation

Explanation

Case 7.2.

Presentation

Explanation

Recommended reading list

Chapter 1. Basic principles of radiology

Armbrust, L.J. Comparing types of digital capture. *Vet Clin North Am Small Anim Pract*, 2009; 39(4):677-88.

Armbrust, L.J. PACS and image storage. *Vet Clin North Am Small Anim Pract*, 2009; 39(4):711-8.

Baines, E., Holloway, A. Principles of radiological interpretation. En: Holloway, A., McConnell, F. (eds). *BSAVA Manual of Canine and Feline Radiography and Radiology*. British Small Animal Veterinary Association, Gloucester, 2019; pp. 47-73.

Borrego, P. El procesado de las imágenes. Calidad de la imagen radiográfica. Radiación dispersa. En: Azpeitia, J., Puig, J., Soler, R. (eds). *Manual para Técnico Superior en Imagen para el Diagnóstico y Medicina Nuclear*. Editorial Médica Panamericana, Madrid, 2016; pp. 65-74.

Bushong, S.C. *Manual de radiología para técnicos. Física, biología y protección radiológica*. 11.ª ed. Elsevier España SLU, Barcelona. 2018.

Caine, A. Practical approach to digital radiography. *In Practice*, 2009; 31:334-339.

Caine, A., Dennis, R. Principles of radiography. En: Holloway, A., McConnell, F. (eds). *BSAVA Manual of Canine and Feline Radiography and Radiology*. British Small Animal Veterinary Association, Gloucester, 2019; pp. 21-46.

Consejo de Seguridad Nuclear. *Dosis de radiación*. Consejo de Seguridad Nuclear, Madrid, 2010. https://www.csn.es/documents/10182/914805/Dosis%20de%20radiación

Consejo de Seguridad Nuclear. *La protección radiológica en el medio sanitario*. Consejo de Seguridad Nuclear, Madrid, 2012. https://www.csn.es/documents/10182/914805/La+protección+radiológica+en+el+medio+sanitario

Consejo de Seguridad Nuclear. *Protección radiológica*. Consejo de Seguridad Nuclear, Madrid, 2012. https://www.csn.es/documents/10182/914805/Protección%20radiológica

Coulson, A., Lewis, N. *An Atlas of Interpretative Radiographic Anatomy of the Dog & Cat*. Blackwell Science Ltd, Oxford, 2002.

Dennis, R. Physics and equipment. En: Holloway, A., McConnell, F. (eds). *BSAVA Manual of Canine and Feline Radiography and Radiology*. British Small Animal Veterinary Association, Gloucester. 2019, pp. 1-20.

Douglas, S.W., Herrtage, M.E., Williamson, H.D. *Principles of Veterinary radiography*, 4th ed. Baillière Tindall, Eastbourne, 1987.

Drost, W.T. Transitioning to digital radiography. *J Vet Emerg Crit Care (San Antonio)*, 2011;21(2):137-43.

Drost, W.T., Reese, D.J., Hornof, W.J. Digital radiography artifacts. *Vet Radiol Ultrasound*, 2008; 49:S48-S56.

Fadden, S., Roding, T., de Vries, G., et al. Digital imaging and radiographic practice in diagnostic radiography: An overview of current knowledge and practice in Europe. *Radiography*, 2018; 24:137-141.

Jiménez, D.A., Armbrust, L.J., O'Brien, R.T., Biller, D.S. Artifacts in digital radiography. *Vet Radiol Ultrasound*, 2008; 49:321-332.

Lo, W.Y., Puchalski, S.M. Digital image processing. *Vet Radiol Ultrasound*, 2008; 49:S42-S47.

Muhlbauer, M.C., Kneller, S.K. *Radiography of the Dog and Cat: Guide to Making and Interpreting Radiographs,* 1st ed. Wiley-Blackwell, Iowa, 2013.

Pifarré Martínez, X. La producción de rayos X: generadores y tubos. En: Azpeitia, J., Puig, J., Soler, R. (eds). *Manual para Técnico Superior en Imagen para el Diagnóstico y Medicina Nuclear*. Editorial Médica Panamericana, Madrid, 2016; pp. 29-44.

Pifarré Martínez, X. Protección radiológica en instalaciones de radiodiagnóstico y medicina nuclear. En: Azpeitia, J., Puig, J., Soler, R. (eds). *Manual para Técnico Superior en Imagen para el Diagnóstico y Medicina Nuclear*. Editorial Médica Panamericana, Madrid, 2016; pp. 1163-1177.

Pifarré Martínez, X. Rayos X: generalidades. En: Azpeitia, J., Puig, J., Soler, R. (eds). *Manual para Técnico Superior en Imagen para el Diagnóstico y Medicina Nuclear*. Editorial Médica Panamericana, Madrid, 2016; pp. 15-27.

Puchalski, S.M. Image display. *Vet Radiol Ultrasound*, 2008; 49:S9-S13.

Ramos López, M.M., Pedraza Carballo, M.G. Registro de la imagen: películas, pantallas e intensificadores de imagen. En: Azpeitia, J., Puig, J., Soler, R. (eds). *Manual para Técnico Superior en Imagen para el Diagnóstico y Medicina Nuclear*. Editorial Médica Panamericana, Madrid, 2016; pp. 47-63.

Robertson, I.D., Saveraid, T. Hospital, radiology, and picture archiving and communication systems. *Vet Radiol Ultrasound*, 2008; 49:S19-S28.

Robertson, I.D., Thrall, D.E. Digital radiographic imaging. En: Thrall, D.E. (ed). *Veterinary Diagnostic Radiology*, 7th ed. Elsevier, St. Louis, 2018; pp. 23-38.

Spaulding, K.A., Voges, A.K. Radiographic anatomy of the appendicular skeleton. En: Thrall, D.E. (ed). *Veterinary Diagnostic Radiology*, 7th ed. Elsevier, St. Louis, 2018; pp. 306-333.

Thrall, D.E. Introduction to radiographic interpretation. En: Thrall, D.E. (ed). *Veterinary Diagnostic Radiology*, 7th ed. Elsevier, St. Louis, 2018; pp. 110-122.

Thrall, D.E., Widmer. W.R. Radiation protection and physics of diagnostic radiology. En: Thrall, D.E. (ed). *Veterinary Diagnostic Radiology*, 7th ed. Elsevier, St. Louis, 2018; pp. 2-22.

Torres Cabrera, R., España López, M.L. Protección radiológica en exposiciones médicas. En: Azpeitia, J., Puig, J., Soler, R. (eds). *Manual para Técnico Superior en Imagen para el Diagnóstico y Medicina Nuclear.* Editorial Médica Panamericana, Madrid, 2016; pp. 1179-1205.

Voges, A.K., Spaulding, K.A. Radiographic anatomy of the axial skeleton. En: Thrall, D.E. (ed). *Veterinary Diagnostic Radiology*, 7th ed. Elsevier, St. Louis, 2018; pp. 124-136.

Wallack, S. Digital image storage. *Vet Radiol Ultrasound*, 2008; 49:S37-S41.

Wright, M.A., Ballance, D., Robertson, I.D., Poteet, B. Introduction to DICOM for the practicing veterinarian. *Vet Radiol Ultrasound*, 2008; 49:S14-S18.

Chapter 2. Abdomen

Adams, W.M., Sisterman, L.A., Klauer, J.M., Kirby, B.M., Lin, T.L. Association of intestinal disorders in cats with findings of abdominal radiography. *Journal of the American Veterinary Medical Association*, 2010; 236:880-886.

Adin, C.A., Herrgesell, E.J., Nyland, T.G., Hughes, D.M., Gregory, C.R., Kyles, A.E., Cowgill, L.D., Ling, G.V. Antegrade pyelography for suspected ureteral obstruction in cats: 11 cases (1995-2001). *Journal of the Veterinary Medical Association*, 2003; 222:1576-1581.

Agut, A., Sánchez-Valverde, M.A., Lasaosa, J.M., Murciano, J., Molina, F. Use of iohexol as a gastrointestinal contrast medium in the dog. *Veterinary Radiology and Ultrasound*, 1993; 34:171-177.

Agut, A., Sánchez-Valverde, M.A., Torrecillas, F.E., Murciano, J., Laredo, F.G. Use of iohexol as a gastrointestinal contrast medium in the cat. *Veterinary Radiology and Ultrasound*, 1994; 35:164-168.

Allan, F.J., Guilford, W.G., Robertson, I.D., Jones, B.R. Gastric emptying of solid radiopaque markers in healthy dogs. *Veterinary Radiology and Ultrasound*, 1996; 37:336-344.

Armbrust, L. The spleen. En: O'Brien, R., Barr, F. (eds). *BSAVA Manual of Canine and Feline Abdominal Imaging*. British Small Animal Veterinary Association, Gloucester, 2009; pp. 167-176.

Atalan, G., Barr, F.J., Holt, P.E. Comparison of ultrasonographic and radiographic measurements of canine prostatic dimensions. *Veterinary Radiology and Ultrasound*, 1999; 40:408-412.

Azuma, K., Kanemoto, H., Ohno, K., et al. Pneumatosis coli after partial ligation of congenital portosystemic shunt in a dog. *J Vet Med Sci*, 2018; 80(10):1549-1552.

Baines, E.A. The peritoneal cavity. En: O'Brien, R., Barr, F. (eds). *BSAVA Manual of Canine and Feline Abdominal Imaging*. British Small Animal Veterinary Association, Gloucester, 2009; pp. 29-39.

Barr, F., O'Brien, R. Approach to abdominal imaging. En: O'Brien, R., Barr, F. (eds). *BSAVA Manual of Canine and Feline Abdominal Imaging*. British Small Animal Veterinary Association, Gloucester, 2009; pp. 1-4.

Battiato, P., Fernandez, Y., Salgüero, R., et al. Spontaneous emphysematous splenitis: Radiographic and ultrasonographic findings in three Golden Retriever dogs. *Vet Radiol Ultrasound*, 2021; 62(3):309-315.

Bradley, K. The small intestine. En: O'Brien, R., Barr, F. (eds). *BSAVA Manual of Canine and Feline Abdominal Imaging*. British Small Animal Veterinary Association, Gloucester, 2009; pp. 110-131.

Brown, J.C. The urethra. En: Thrall, D.E. (ed). *Textbook of Veterinary Diagnostic Radiology*, 6th ed. Elsevier Saunders, St. Louis, 2013; pp. 744-748.

Brown, J.C. Urethra. En: Thrall, D.E. (ed). *Veterinary Diagnostic Radiology*, 7th ed. Elsevier, St. Louis, 2018; pp. 865-879.

Burk, R.L., Feeney, D.A. *Small Animal Radiology and Ultrasonography. A Diagnostic Atlas and Text*. Elsevier Science, St. Louis, 2003.

Costello, M. The male reproductive system. En: O'Brien, R., Barr, F. (eds). *BSAVA Manual of Canine and Feline Abdominal Imaging*. British Small Animal Veterinary Association, Gloucester, 2009; pp. 237-245.

Dennis, R., Kirberger, R.M., Barr, F., Wrigley, R.H. *Handbook of Small Animal Radiology and Ultrasound*, 2th ed. Churchill Livingstone Elsevier, Edimburg, 2010.

Farrow, C.S. *Diagnóstico por imagen del perro y el gato.* Multimédica ediciones veterinarias, Barcelona, 2005.

Feeney, D.A., Johnston, G.R., Klausner, J.S., Perman, V., Leininger, J.R., Tomlinson, M.J. Canine prostatic disease – comparison of radiographic appearance with morphologic and microbiologic findings: 30 cases (1981-1985). *Journal of the American Veterinary Medical Association*, 1987; 190:1018-1026.

Fisk, A., Allen-Durrance, A. Pneumatosis Coli in a Dog. *J Am Anim Hosp Assoc*, 2019; 55(4):e55401.

Frank, P.M. The peritoneal space. En: Thrall, D.E. (ed). *Textbook of Veterinary Diagnostic Radiology*, 6th ed. Elsevier Saunders, St. Louis, 2013; pp. 659-678.

Frank, P.M. The stomach. En: Thrall, D.E. (ed). *Textbook of Veterinary Diagnostic Radiology*, 6th ed. Elsevier Saunders, St. Louis, 2013; pp. 769-788.

Fraser, J. Abdominal radiography. En: O'Brien, R., Barr, F. (eds). *BSAVA Manual of Canine and Feline Abdominal Imaging*. British Small Animal Veterinary Association, Gloucester, 2009; pp. 4-17.

Frendin, J., Funkquist, B., Hansson, K., Lonnemark M., Carlsten J. Diagnostic imaging of foreign body reactions in dogs with diffuse back pain. *Journal of Small Animal Practice*, 1999; 40:278-285.

Gaschen, L. The large intestine and perianal region. En: O'Brien, R., Barr, F. (eds): *BSAVA Manual of Canine and Feline Abdominal Imaging*. British Small Animal Veterinary Association, Gloucester, 2009; pp. 132-143.

Graham, J.P., Lord, P.F., Harrison, J.M. Quantitative estimation of intestinal dilation as a predictor of obstruction in the dog. *Journal of Small Animal Practice*, 1998; 39:521-524.

Gremillion, C.L., Savage, M., Cohen, E.B. Radiographic findings and clinical factors in dogs with surgically confirmed or presumed colonic torsion. *Vet Radiol Ultrasound*, 2018; 59(3):272-278.

Hammond, G. The female reproductive system. En: O'Brien, R., Barr, F. (eds). *BSAVA Manual of Canine and Feline Abdominal Imaging*. British Small Animal Veterinary Association, Gloucester, 2009; pp. 222-236.

Herrtage, M.E., Dennis, R. Contrast media and techniques. En: Lee, R. (ed). *Manual of Small Animal Diagnostic Imaging*. British Small Animal Veterinary Association, Shurdington, 1995; pp. 147-156.

Holloway, A., O'Brien, R. Perirenal effusion in dogs and cats with acute renal failure. *Veterinary Radiology and Ultrasound*, 2007; 48:574-579.

Hotston-Moore, A. The bladder and urethra. En: O'Brien, R., Barr, F. (eds). *BSAVA Manual of Canine and Feline Abdominal Imaging*. British Small Animal Veterinary Association, Gloucester, 2009; pp. 205-221.

Johnson, K.L., Porter, E.G., Berry, C.R. Analysis of feline splenic radiographic measurements and their correlation to ultrasonographic measurements. *J Feline Med Surg*, 2017; 19(10):985-991.

Kealy, J.K., McAllister, H., Graham, J.P. *Diagnostic Radiology and Ultrasonography of the Dog and Cat*, 5th ed. Saunders Elsevier, St. Louis, 2010.

Kinns, J., Nelson, N. The uterus, ovaries and testes. En: Thrall, D.E. (ed). *Textbook of Veterinary Diagnostic Radiology*, 6th ed. Elsevier Saunders, St. Louis, 2013; pp. 757-768.

Ko, J.J., Mann, F.A. Barium peritonitis in small animals. *J Vet Med Sci*, 2014; 76(5):621-628.

Lamb, C.R. Radiografía de contraste del tracto urinario. *Proceedings del XVII Congreso de AMVAC*, 2000; pp. 105-114.

Lamb, C.R. Resolución de problemas: la masa abdominal. *Proceedings del XVII Congreso de AMVAC*, 2000; pp. 115-118.

Lattimer, J.C., Essman, S.C. The prostate gland. En: Thrall, D.E. (ed). *Textbook of Veterinary Diagnostic Radiology*, 6th ed. Elsevier Saunders, St. Louis, 2013; pp. 749-756.

Lee, S., Yoon, H., Eom, K. Retrospective quantitative assessment of liver size by measurement of radiographic liver area in small-breed dogs. *Am J Vet Res*, 2019; 80(12):1122-1128.

Llabrés-Díaz, F. The retroperitoneum. En: O'Brien, R., Barr, F. (eds). *BSAVA Manual of Canine and Feline Abdominal Imaging*. British Small Animal Veterinary Association, Gloucester, 2009; pp. 40-48.

Marolf, A.J., Park, R.D. The urinary bladder. En: Thrall, D.E. (ed). *Textbook of Veterinary Diagnostic Radiology*, 6th ed. Elsevier Saunders, St. Louis, 2013; pp. 726-743.

Moon, M. Liver and spleen. En: Thrall, D.E. (ed). *Veterinary Diagnostic Radiology*, 7th ed. Elsevier, St. Louis, 2018; pp. 792-822.

Moon, M. The kidneys and ureters. En: O'Brien, R., Barr, F. (eds). *BSAVA Manual of Canine and Feline Abdominal Imaging*. British Small Animal Veterinary Association, Gloucester, 2009; pp. 185-204.

Moon, M. The liver and spleen. En: Thrall, D.E. (ed). *Textbook of Veterinary Diagnostic Radiology*, 6th ed. Elsevier Saunders, St. Louis, 2013; pp. 679-704.

Murdoch, D.B. The abdomen. En: Lee, R. (ed). *Manual of Small Animal Diagnostic Imaging*. British Small Animal Veterinary Association, Shurdington, 1995; pp. 68-94.

Ng, J., Linn, K.A., Shmon, C.L., et al. The left lateral projection is comparable to horizontal beam radiography for identifying experimental small volume pneumoperitoneum in the canine abdomen. *Vet Radiol Ultrasound*, 2020; 61(2):130-136.

Owens, J.M., Biery, D.N. *Radiographic Interpretation for the Small Animal Clinician*, 2nd ed. Williams & Wilkins, Baltimore, 1999.

Penninck, D.G., Feldman, E.C., Nyland, T.G. Radiographic features of canine hyper-adrenocorticism caused by autonomously functioning adrenocortical tumors: 23 cases (1978-1986). *Journal of the American Veterinary Medical Association*, 1988; 192:1604-1608.

Petite, A., Busoni, V., Heinen, M.P., Billen, F., Snaps, F. Radiographic and ultrasonographic findings of emphysematous cistitis in four nondiabetic female dogs. *Veterinary Radiology and Ultrasound*, 2006; 47:90-93.

Riedesel, E.A. Small bowel. En: Thrall, D.E. (ed). *Veterinary Diagnostic Radiology*, 7th ed. Elsevier, St. Louis, 2018; pp. 926-954.

RIEDESEL, E.A. The small bowel. En: THRALL, D.E. (ed). *Textbook of Veterinary Diagnostic Radiology*, 6th ed. Elsevier Saunders, St. Louis, 2013; pp. 789-811.

ROBERTSON, I.D., BURBRIDGE, H.M. Pros and cons of barium-impregnated polyethylene spheres in gastrointestinal disease. *Veterinary Clinics of North America: Small Animal Practice*, 2000; 30:449-465.

SAUNDERS, W.B., TOBIAS, K.M. Pneumoperitoneum in dogs and cats: 39 cases (1983-2002). *Journal of the American Veterinary Medical Association*, 2003; 223:462-468.

SCHWARZ, T. Large bowel. En: THRALL, D.E. (ed). *Veterinary Diagnostic Radiology*, 7th ed. Elsevier, St. Louis, 2018; pp. 955-969.

SCHWARZ, T. The large bowel. En: THRALL, D.E. (ed). *Textbook of Veterinary Diagnostic Radiology*, 6th ed. Elsevier Saunders, St. Louis, 2013; pp. 812-824.

SCHWARZ, T. The liver and gallbladder. En: O'BRIEN, R., BARR, F. (eds). *BSAVA Manual of Canine and Feline Abdominal Imaging*. British Small Animal Veterinary Association, Gloucester, 2009; pp. 144-156.

SCHWARZ, T. Urinary system. En: SCHWARZ, T., SAUNDERS, J. (eds). *Veterinary Computed Tomography*. Wiley-Blackwell, Oxford, 2011; pp. 331-338.

SCHWARZ, T., STÖRK, C.K., MELLOR, D., SULLIVAN, M. Osteopenia and other radiographic signs in canine hyperadrenocorticism. *Journal of Small Animal Practice*, 2000; 41:491-495.

SEILER, G., MAÏ, W. The stomach. En: O'BRIEN, R., BARR, F. (eds). *BSAVA Manual of Canine and Feline Abdominal Imaging*. British Small Animal Veterinary Association, Gloucester, 2009; pp. 87-109.

SEILER, G.S. The kidneys and ureters. En: THRALL, D.E. (ed). *Textbook of Veterinary Diagnostic Radiology*, 6th ed. Elsevier Saunders, St. Louis, 2013; pp. 705-725.

SHARMA, A., THOMPSON, M.S., SCRIVANI, P.V., DYKES, N.L., YEAGER, A.E., FREER, S.R., ERB, H.N. Comparison of radiography and ultrasonography for diagnosing small-intestinal mechanical obstruction in vomiting dogs. *Veterinary Radiology and Ultrasound*, 2011; 52:248-255.

SHIROMA, J.T., GABRIEL, J.K., CARTER, R.L., SCRUGGS, S.L., STUBBS, P.W. Effect of reproductive status on feline renal size. *Veterinary Radiology and Ultrasound*, 1999; 40: 242-245.

STIFFLER, K.S., STEVENSON, M.A., MAHAFFEY, M.B., HOWERTH, E.W., BARSANTI, J.A. Intravesical ureterocele with concurrent renal dysfunction in a dog: a case report and proposed classification system. *Journal of the American Animal Hospital Association*, 2002; 38:33-39.

SUTHERLAND-SMITH, J., JERRAM, R.M., WALKER A.M., WARMAN, C. Ectopic ureters and ureteroceles in dogs: presentation, cause, and diagnosis. *Compendium of Continuing Education for Veterinarians*, 2004; 26:303-316.

THRALL, D.E. Principles of radiographic interpretation of the abdomen. En: THRALL, D.E. (ed). *Textbook of Veterinary Diagnostic Radiology*, 6th ed. Elsevier Saunders, St. Louis, 2013; pp. 650-658.

TREVAIL, T., GUNN-MOORE, D., CARRERA, I., et al. Radiographic diameter of the colon in normal and constipated cats and in cats with megacolon. *Vet Radiol Ultrasound*, 2011; 52(5):516-520.

WANG, K.Y., SAMII, V.F., CHEW, D.J., MCLOUGHLIN, M.A., DIBARTOLA, S.P., MASTY, J., LEHMAN, A.M. Vestibular, vaginal and urethral relationships in spayed and intact normal dogs. *Theriogenology*, 2006; 66:726-35.

WANG, K.Y., SAMII, V.F., CHEW, D.J., MCLOUGHLIN, M.A., DIBARTOLA, S.P., MASTY, J., LEHMAN, A.M. Vestibular, vaginal, and urethral relations in spayed dogs with and without lower urinary tract signs. *Journal of Veterinary Internal Medicine*, 2006; 20:1065-73.

ZONTINE, W., ANDREWS, L. Fatal air embolization as a complication of pneumocystography in two cats. *Journal of the American Veterinary Medical Association*, 1978; 19:8-11.

Chapter 3. Neck and thorax

ABBOTT, J.A. Enfermedad valvular adquirida. En: TILLEY, L.P., SMITH, F.W.K. JR., OYAMA, M.A., SLEEPER, M.M. (eds). *Manual de Cardiología Canina y Felina*, 4.ª ed. Multimédica Ediciones Veterinarias, Barcelona, 2009; pp: 95-118.

ALEXANDER, K. Canine and feline larynx and thachea. En: THRALL, D.E. (ed). *Veterinary Diagnostic Radiology*, 7th ed. Elsevier, St. Louis, 2018; pp. 583-595.

ALEXANDER, K. The pharynx, larynx, and thachea. En: THRALL, D.E. (ed): *Textbook of Veterinary Diagnostic Radiology*, 6th ed. Elsevier Saunders, St. Louis, 2013; pp: 489-499.

BAGARDI, M., MANFREDI, M., ZANI, D.D., et al. Interobserver variability of radiographic methods for the evaluation of left atrial size in dogs. *Vet Radiol Ultrasound*, 2021; 62(2):161-174.

BAHR, R. Canine and feline cardiovascular system. En: THRALL, D.E. (ed). *Veterinary Diagnostic Radiology*, 7th ed. Elsevier, St. Louis, 2018; pp. 684-709.

BAHR, R. The heart and pulmonary vessels. En: THRALL, D.E. (ed): *Textbook of Veterinary Diagnostic Radiology*, 6th ed. Elsevier Saunders, St. Louis, 2013; pp: 585-607.

BAINES, E. The mediastinum. En: SCHWARZ, T., JOHNSON, V. (eds): *BSAVA Manual of Canine and Feline Thoracic Imaging*. British Small Animal Veterinary Association, Gloucester, 2008; pp: 177-199.

BARRETT, L.E., POLLARD, R.E., ZWINGENBERGER, A., et al. Radiographic characterization of primary lung tumors in 74 dogs. *Vet Radiol Ultrasound*, 2014; 55:480-487.

BEGON, D. La radiografía torácica. *Proceedings del XVII Congreso de AMVAC*, 2000; pp: 53-95.

Berent, A.C. Diagnosis and management of nasopharyngeal stenosis. *Vet Clin North Am Small Anim Pract*, 2016; 46(4):677-689.

Bodh, D., Hoque, M., Saxena, A.C., et al. Vertebral scale system to measure heart size in thoracic radiographs of Indian Spitz, Labrador retriever and Mongrel dogs. *Vet World*, 2016; 9(4):371-376.

Bradley, K. Radiology of the thorax. En: Holloway, A., McConnell, J.F. (eds). *BSAVA Manual of Canine and Feline Radiography and Radiology.* A Foundation Manual. British Small Animal Veterinary Association, Gloucester, 2013; pp. 109-175.

Brinkman, E.L., Biller, D., Armbrust, L. The clinical usefulness of the ventrodorsal versus dorsoventral thoracic radiograph in dogs. *Journal of the American Animal Hospital Association*, 2006; 42:440-449.

Buchanan, J.W., Bucheler, J. Vertebral scale system to measure canine heart size in radiographs. *Journal of the American Veterinary Medical Association*, 1995; 206:194-199.

Burk, R.L., Feeney D.A. *Small Animal Radiology and Ultrasonography. A Diagnostic Atlas and Text.* Elsevier Science, St. Louis, 2003.

Coyne, B.E., Fingland, R.B. Hypoplasia of the trachea in dogs: 103 cases (1974-1990). *Journal of the American Veterinary Medical Association*, 1992; 201:768-772.

D'Anjou, M., Schwarz, T. Heart and vessels. En: Schwarz, T., Saunders, J. (eds): *Veterinary Computed Tomography.* Wiley-Blackwell, Oxford, 2011; pp: 229-242.

D'Anjou, M.A., Tidwell, A.S., Hecht, S. Radiographic diagnosis of lung lobe torsion. *Veterinary Radiology and Ultrasound*, 2005; 46:478-484.

Della Maggiore, A. An update on tracheal and airway collapse in dogs. *Vet Clin North Am Small Anim Pract*, 2020; 50(2):419-430.

Dennis, R., Kirberger, R.M., Barr, F., Wrigley, R.H. *Handbook of Small Animal Radiology and Ultrasound*, 2nd ed. Churchill Livingstone Elsevier, Edimburg, 2010.

Diana, A., Guglielmini, C., Pivetta, M., Sanacore, A., Di Tommaso, M., Lord, P.F., Cipone, M. Radiographic features of cardiogenic pulmonary edema in dogs with mitral regurgitation: 61 cases (1998-2007). *Journal of the American Veterinary Medical Association*, 2009; 235:1058-1063.

Duler, L., Visser, L.C., Jackson, K.N., et al. Evaluation of radiographic predictors of left heart enlargement in dogs with known or suspected cardiovascular disease. *Vet Radiol Ultrasound*, 2021; 62(3):271-281.

Farrow, C.S. *Diagnóstico por imagen del perro y el gato.* Multimédica ediciones veterinarias, Barcelona, 2005.

Fasanella, F.J., Shivley, J.M., Wardlaw, J.L., Givaruangsawat, S. Brachycephalic airway obstructive syndrome in dogs: 90 cases (1991-2008). *Journal of the American Veterinary Medical Association*, 2010; 237:1048-1051.

Frame, M, King, A. The pleural space. En: Schwarz, T., Johnson, V. (eds): *BSAVA Manual of Canine and Feline Thoracic Imaging.* British Small Animal Veterinary Association, Gloucester, 2008; pp: 321-339.

Fujita, M., Miura, H., Yasuda, D., Hasegawa, D., Orima, H. Tracheal narrowing secondary to airway obstruction in two cats. *Journal of Small Animal Practice*, 2004; 45:29-31.

Gadbois, J., d'Anjou, M.A., Dunn, M., Alexander, K., Beauregard, G., D'Astous, J., De Carufel, M., Breton, L., Beauchamp, G. Radiographic abnormalities in cats with feline bronchial disease and intra- and interobserver variability in radiographic interpretation: 40 cases (1999-2006). *Journal of the American Veterinary Medical Association*, 2009; 234:367-375.

Gaschen, L. Canine and feline esophagus. En: Thrall, D.E. (ed). *Textbook of Veterinary Diagnostic Radiology*, 7th ed. Elsevier, St. Louis, 2018, pp. 596-617.

Gaschen, L. The canine and feline esophagus. En: Thrall, D.E. (ed): *Textbook of Veterinary Diagnostic Radiology*, 6th ed. Elsevier Saunders, St. Louis, 2013; pp: 500-521.

Hammond, G., Geary, M., Coleman, E., Gunn-Moore, D. Radiographic measurements of the trachea in domestic shorthair and Persian cats. *J Feline Med Surg*, 2011; 13(12):881-884.

Hansson, K., Häggström, J., Kvart, C., Lord, P. Interobserver variability of vertebral heart size measurements in dogs with normal and enlarged hearts. *Veterinary Radiology and Ultrasound*, 2005; 46:122-130.

Hayward, N., Schwarz, T., Weisse, C. The trachea. En: Schwarz, T., Johnson, V. (eds): *BSAVA Manual of Canine and Feline Thoracic Imaging.* British Small Animal Veterinary Association, Gloucester, 2008; pp: 213-227.

Herrtage, M.E., Dennis, R. Contrast media and techniques. En: Lee, R. (ed): *Manual of Small Animal Diagnostic Imaging.* British Small Animal Veterinary Association, Shurdington, 1995; pp: 147-156.

Herrtage, M.E., Dennis, R. The thorax. En: Lee, R. (ed): *Manual of Small Animal Diagnostic Imaging.* British Small Animal Veterinary Association, Shurdington, 1995; pp: 43-67.

Huguet, E.E., Vilaplana Grosso, F., Lamb, W.R., et al. Interpretation of cardiac chamber size on canine thoracic radiographs is limited and may result in the false identification of right-sided cardiomegaly in the presence of severe left-sided cardiomegaly. *Vet Radiol Ultrasound*, 2021, Jul 22.

Jepsen-Grant, K., Pollard, R.E., Johnson, L.R. Vertebral heart scores in eight dog breeds. *Vet Radiol Ultrasound*, 2013; 54(1):3-8.

Johnson, L. Tracheal collapse. Diagnosis and medical and surgical treatment. *Veterinary Clinics of North America: Small Animal Practice*, 2000; 30:1253-1266.

Johnson, L.R. *Cor pulmonale* y tromboembolismo pulmonar. En: Tilley, L.P., Smith, F.W.K. Jr., Oyama, M.A., Sleeper, M.M. (eds). *Manual de Cardiología Canina y Felina*, 4.ª ed. Multimédica Ediciones Veterinarias, Barcelona, 2009; pp: 155-160.

Johnson, L.R., Johnson, E.G., Vernau, W., et al. Bronchoscopy, imaging, and concurrent diseases in dogs with bronchiectasis: (2003-2014). *J Vet Intern Med*, 2016; 30:247-254.

Johnson, V., Hansson, K., Maï, W., Dukes-McEwan, J., Lester, N., Schwarz, T., Chapman, P., Morandi, F. The heart and major vessels. En: Schwarz, T., Johnson, V. (eds): *BSAVA Manual of Canine and Feline Thoracic Imaging*. British Small Animal Veterinary Association, Gloucester, 2008; pp: 86-176.

Kaye, B.M., Boroffka, S.A., Haagsman, A.N., Ter Haar, G. Computed tomographic, radiographic, and endoscopic tracheal dimensions in English bulldogs with grade 1 clinical signs of brachycephalic airway syndrome. *Vet Radiol Ultrasound*, 2015; 56(6):609-616.

Kealy, J.K., McAllister, H., Graham, J.P. *Diagnostic Radiology and Ultrasonography of the Dog and Cat*, 5th ed. Saunders Elsevier, St. Louis, 2010.

Keene, B.W., Atkins, C.E., Bonagura, J.D., et al. ACVIM consensus guidelines for the diagnosis and treatment of myxomatous mitral valve disease in dogs. *J Vet Intern Med*, 2019; 33(3):1127-1140.

Kirberger, R.M., Avner, A. The effect of positioning on the appearance of selected cranial thoracic structures in the dog. *Veterinary Radiology and Ultrasound*, 2006; 47:61-68.

Lam, C., Gavaghan, B.J., Meyers, F.E. Radiographic quantification of left atrial size in dogs with myxomatous mitral valve disease. *J Vet Intern Med*, 2021; 35(2):747-754.

Lamb, C.R., Tyler, M., Boswood, A., Skelly, B.J., Cain, M. Assessment of the value of the vertebral heart scale in the radiographic diagnosis of cardiac disease in dogs. *Veterinary Record*, 2000; 146:687-690.

Lamb, C.R., Wikeley, H., Boswood, A., Pfeiffer, D.U. Use of breed-specific ranges for the vertebral heart scale as an aid to the radiographic diagnosis of cardiac disease in dogs. *Veterinary Record*, 2001; 148:707-711.

Leonard, C.D., Johnson, L.R., Bonadio, C.M., Pollard, R.E. Changes in tracheal dimensions during inspiration and expiration in healthy dogs as detected via computed tomography. *American Journal of Veterinary Research*, 2009; 70:986-991.

Lindl-Bylicki, B.J., Johnson, L.R., Pollard, R.E. Comparison of the radiographic and tracheoscopic appearance of the dorsal tracheal membrane in large and small breed dogs. *Vet Radiol Ultrasound*, 2015; 56(6):602-608.

Llabrés-Díaz, F., Petite, A., Saunders, J., Schwarz, T. The thoracic boundaries. En: Schwarz, T., Johnson, V. (eds): *BSAVA Manual of Canine and Feline Thoracic Imaging*. British Small Animal Veterinary Association, Gloucester, 2008; pp: 340-376.

MacPhail, C.M. Laryngeal disease in dogs and cats: An update. *Vet Clin North Am Small Anim Pract*, 2020; 50(2):295-310.

Macready, D.M., Johnson, L.R., Pollard, R.E. Fluoroscopic and radiographic evaluation of tracheal collapse in dogs: 62 cases (2001-2006). *Journal of the American Veterinary Medical Association*, 2007; 230:1870-1876.

Maï, W. Pleura. En: Schwarz, T., Saunders, J. (eds): *Veterinary Computed Tomography*. Wiley-Blackwell, Oxford, 2011; pp: 279-284.

Maï, W., O'Brien, R., Scrivani, P., Porat-Monseco, Y., Tobin, E., Seiler, G., McConnell, F., Schwarz, T., Zwingenberger, A. The lung parenchyma. En: Schwarz, T., Johnson, V. (eds): *BSAVA Manual of Canine and Feline Thoracic Imaging*. British Small Animal Veterinary Association, Gloucester, 2008; pp: 242-320.

Malcolm, E.L., Visser, L.C., Phillips, K.L., Johnson, L.R. Diagnostic value of vertebral left atrial size as determined from thoracic radiographs for assessment of left atrial size in dogs with myxomatous mitral valve disease. *J Am Vet Med Assoc*, 2018; 253(8):1038-1045.

Mantis, P., Johnson, V., Morandi, F. The bronchial tree. En: Schwarz, T., Johnson, V. (eds): *BSAVA Manual of Canine and Feline Thoracic Imaging*. British Small Animal Veterinary Association, Gloucester, 2008; pp: 228-241.

McConnell, F. Basics of thoracic magnetic resonance imaging. En: Schwarz, T., Johnson, V. (eds): *BSAVA Manual of Canine and Feline Thoracic Imaging*. British Small Animal Veterinary Association, Gloucester, 2008; pp: 71-74.

Mims, H.L., Hancock, R.B., Leib, M.S., Waldron, D.R. Primary tracheal collapse in a cat. *Journal of the American Animal Hospital Association*, 2008; 44:149-153.

Muhlbauer, M.C., Kneller, S.K. *Radiography of the Dog and Cat: Guide to Making and Interpreting Radiographs*. Wiley-Blackwell, Iowa, 2013.

Munro, E.A.C. Thoracic radiology. En: Fuentes, V.L., Swift, S. (eds): *Manual of Small Animal Cardiorespiratory Medicine and Surgery*. British Small Animal Veterinary Association, Shurdington, 1998; pp: 35-51.

Murphy, K.A., Brisson, B.A. Evaluation of lung lobe torsion in Pugs: 7 cases (1991-2004). *Journal of the American Veterinary Medical Association*, 2006; 228:86-90.

Neath, P.J., Brockman, D.J., King, L.G. Lung lobe torsion in dogs: 22 cases (1981-1999). *Journal of the American Veterinary Medical Association*, 2000; 217:1041-1044.

Nemanic, S., London, C.A., Wisner, E.R. Comparison of thoracic radiographs and single breath-hold helical CT for detection of pulmonary nodules in dogs with metastatic neoplasia. *Journal of Veterinary Internal Medicine*, 2006; 20:508-515.

Owens, J.M., Biery D.N. *Radiographic Interpretation for the Small Animal Clinician*, 2nd ed. Williams & Wilkins, Baltimore, 1999.

Petite, A., Kirberger, R. Mediastinum. En: Schwarz, T., Saunders, J. (eds): *Veterinary Computed Tomography*. Wiley-Blackwell, Oxford, 2011; pp: 249-260.

Poteet, B.A. Radiología del corazón. En: Tilley, L.P., Smith, F.W.K. Jr., Oyama, M.A., Sleeper, M.M. (eds): *Manual de Cardiología*

Canina y Felina, 4.ª ed. Multimédica Ediciones Veterinarias, Barcelona, 2009; pp: 23-43.

Puccinelli, C., Citi, S., Vezzosi, T., et al. A radiographic study of breed-specific vertebral heart score and vertebral left atrial size in Chihuahuas. *Vet Radiol Ultrasound*, 2021; 62(1):20-26.

Rubin, J.A., Holt, D.E., Reetz, J.A., Clarke, D.L. Signalment, clinical presentation, concurrent diseases, and diagnostic findings in 28 dogs with dynamic pharyngeal collapse (2008-2013). *J Vet Intern Med*, 2015; 29(3):815-821.

Rudorf, H., Taeymans, O., Johnson, V. Basics of thoracic radiography and radiology. En: Schwarz, T., Johnson, V. (eds): *BSAVA Manual of Canine and Feline Thoracic Imaging*. British Small Animal Veterinary Association, Gloucester, 2008; pp: 1-19.

Samii, V.F. The thoracic wall. En: Thrall, D.E. (ed): *Textbook of Veterinary Diagnostic Radiology*, 6th ed. Elsevier Saunders, St. Louis, 2013; pp: 522-534.

Sánchez Salguero, X., Prandi, D., Llabrés-Díaz, F., et al. A radiographic measurement of left atrial size in dogs. *Ir Vet J*, 2018; 71:25.

Saunders, J., Vignoli, M., Gielen, I. Thoracic boundaries. En: Schwarz, T., Saunders, J. (eds): *Veterinary Computed Tomography*. Wiley-Blackwell, Oxford, 2011; pp: 285-296.

Schwarz, T. Basics of thoracic computed tomography. En: Schwarz, T., Johnson, V. (eds): *BSAVA Manual of Canine and Feline Thoracic Imaging*. British Small Animal Veterinary Association, Gloucester, 2008; pp: 66-70.

Schwarz, T., Johnson, V. Lungs and bronchi. En: Schwarz, T., Saunders, J. (eds): *Veterinary Computed Tomography*. Wiley-Blackwell, Oxford, 2011; pp: 261-277.

Schwarz, T., Saunders, J. Trachea. En: Schwarz, T., Saunders, J. (eds): *Veterinary Computed Tomography*. Wiley-Blackwell, Oxford, 2011; pp: 243-248.

Seiler, G. Thorax. En: Barr, F., Gaschen, L. (eds): *BSAVA Manual of Canine and Feline Ultrasonography*. British Small Animal Veterinary Association, Gloucester, 2011; pp: 29-36.

Seiler, G., Dukes-McEwan, J., Gaschen, L. Basics of thoracic ultrasonography. En: Schwarz, T., Johnson, V. (eds): *BSAVA Manual of Canine and Feline Thoracic Imaging*. British Small Animal Veterinary Association, Gloucester, 2008; pp: 20-65.

Seiler, G., Schwarz, T., Vignoli, M., Rodriguez, D. Computed tomographic features of lung lobe torsion. *Veterinary Radiology and Ultrasound*, 2008; 49:504-8.

Sleeper, M.M., Roland, R., Drobatz, K.J. Use of the vertebral heart scale for differentiation of cardiac and noncardiac causes of respiratory distress in cats: 67 cases (2002-2003). *J Am Vet Med Assoc*, 2013; 242(3):366-371.

Stepien, R.L., Rak, M.B., Blume, L.M. Use of radiographic measurements to diagnose stage B2 preclinical myxomatous mitral valve disease in dogs. *J Am Vet Med Assoc*, 2020; 256(10):1129-1136.

Strikland, K.N. Cardiopatía congénita. En: Tilley, L.P., Smith, F.W.K. Jr., Oyama, M.A., Sleeper, M.M. (eds): *Manual de Cardiología Canina y Felina*, 4.ª ed. Multimédica Ediciones Veterinarias, Barcelona, 2009; pp: 189-209.

Taeymans, O., Schwarz, T. Pharynx, larynx and thyroid gland. En: Schwarz, T., Saunders, J. (eds): *Veterinary Computed Tomography*. Wiley-Blackwell, Oxford, 2011; pp: 175-184.

Thrall, D.E. Canine and feline lung. En: Thrall, D.E. (ed). *Veterinary Diagnostic Radiology*, 7th ed. Elsevier, St. Louis, 2018; pp. 710-734.

Thrall, D.E. Canine and feline mediastinum. En: Thrall, D.E. (ed). *Veterinary Diagnostic Radiology*, 7th ed. Elsevier, St. Louis, 2018; pp. 649-669.

Thrall, D.E. Canine and feline pleural space. En: Thrall, D.E. (ed). *Veterinary Diagnostic Radiology*, 7th ed. Elsevier, St. Louis, 2018; pp. 670-683.

Thrall, D.E. Principles of radiographic interpretation of the thorax. En: Thrall, D.E. (ed): *Textbook of Veterinary Diagnostic Radiology*, 6th ed. Elsevier Saunders, St. Louis, 2013; pp: 474-488.

Thrall, D.E. Principles of radiographic interpretation of the thorax. En: Thrall, D.E. (ed). *Veterinary Diagnostic Radiology*, 7th ed. Elsevier, St. Louis, 2018; pp. 568-582.

Thrall, D.E. The canine and feline lung. En: Thrall, D.E. (ed): *Textbook of Veterinary Diagnostic Radiology*, 6th ed. Elsevier Saunders, St. Louis, 2013; pp: 608-631.

Thrall, D.E. The mediastinum. En: Thrall, D.E. (ed): *Textbook of Veterinary Diagnostic Radiology*, 6th ed. Elsevier Saunders, St. Louis, 2013; pp: 550-570.

Thrall, D.E. The pleural space. En: Thrall, D.E. (ed): *Textbook of Veterinary Diagnostic Radiology*, 6th ed. Elsevier Saunders, St. Louis, 2013; pp: 571-584.

Tobias, A.H., McNiel, E.A. Afecciones pericárdicas y tumores cardiacos. En: Tilley, L.P., Smith, F.W.K. Jr., Oyama, M.A., Sleeper, M.M. (eds): *Manual de Cardiología Canina y Felina*, 4.ª ed. Multimédica Ediciones Veterinarias, Barcelona, 2009; pp: 177-188.

Vezzosi, T., Puccinelli, C., Citi, S., Tognetti, R. Two radiographic methods for assessing left atrial enlargement and cardiac remodeling in dogs with myxomatous mitral valve disease. *J Vet Cardiol*, 2021; 34:55-63.

Vezzosi, T., Puccinelli, C., Tognetti, R., et al. Radiographic vertebral left atrial size: A reference interval study in healthy adult dogs. *Vet Radiol Ultrasound*, 2020; 61(5):507-511.

Wagner, W.M. The oesophagus. En: Schwarz, T., Johnson, V. (eds): *BSAVA Manual of Canine and Feline Thoracic Imaging*. British Small Animal Veterinary Association, Gloucester, 2008; pp: 200-212.

Zekas, L.J., Adams, W.M. Cranial mediastinal cysts in nine cats. *Veterinary Radiology and Ultrasound*, 2002; 43:413-418.

Chapter 4. Appendicular skeleton

ADAMS, G. Radiographic signs of joint disease in dogs and cats. En: THRALL, D.E. (ed): *Textbook of Veterinary Diagnostic Radiology*, 6th ed. Elsevier Saunders, St. Louis, 2013; pp. 319-348.

ALLAN, G., DAVIES, S. Radiographic signs of joint disease in dogs and cats. En: THRALL, D.E. (ed). *Veterinary Diagnostic Radiology*, 7th ed. Elsevier, St. Louis, 2018; pp. 403-433.

ALLAN, G., NICOLL, R. Joints - general. En: BARR, F.J., KIRBERGER, R.M. (eds): *BSAVA Manual of Canine and Feline Musculoskeletal Imaging*. British Small Animal Veterinary Association, Gloucester, 2006; pp. 71-85.

ALLAN, G.S. Radiographic features of feline joint diseases. *Veterinary Clinics of North America: Small Animal Practice*, 2000; 30:281-302.

BARR, F. Long bones - juvenile. En: BARR, F.J., KIRBERGER, R.M. (eds): *BSAVA Manual of Canine and Feline Musculoskeletal Imaging*. British Small Animal Veterinary Association, Gloucester, 2006; pp. 19-31.

BARR, F. Soft tissues. En: BARR, F.J., KIRBERGER, R.M. (eds): *BSAVA Manual of Canine and Feline Musculoskeletal Imaging*. British Small Animal Veterinary Association, Gloucester, 2006; pp. 1-8.

BRINKER, W.O. *Small Animal Fractures*. Michigan State University Press, East Lansing, 1978.

BURK, R.L., FEENEY D.A. *Small Animal Radiology and Ultrasonography. A Diagnostic Atlas and Text*. Elsevier Science, St. Louis, 2003.

BUTTERWORTH, S.J. Long bones - fractures. En: BARR, F.J., KIRBERGER, R.M. (eds): *BSAVA Manual of Canine and Feline Musculoskeletal Imaging*. British Small Animal Veterinary Association, Gloucester, 2006; pp. 49-70.

DAVIES, J.V., LEE, R. The appendicular skeleton. En: LEE, R. (ed): *Manual of Small Animal Diagnostic Imaging*. British Small Animal Veterinary Association, Shurdington, 1995; pp. 95-135.

DECAMP, C.E., JOHNSTON, S.A., DÉJARDIN, L.M., SCHAEFER, S.L. Brinker, *Piermattei and Flo's Handbook of Small Animal Orthopedics and Fracture Repair*, 5th ed. Elsevier, St. Louis, 2016.

DENNIS, R., KIRBERGER, R.M., BARR, F., WRIGLEY, R.H. *Handbook of Small Animal Radiology and Ultrasound*, 2nd ed. Churchill Livingstone Elsevier, Edimburg, 2010.

DENNIS, R., KIRBERGER, R.M., WRIGLEY, R.H., BARR, F.J. *Handbook of Small Animal Radiological Differential Diagnosis*. W.B. Saunders, London, 2001.

EKMAN, S., CARLSON, C.S. The pathophysiology of osteochondrosis. *Veterinary Clinics of North America: Small Animal Practice*, 1998; 28:17-32.

FARROW, C.S. *Diagnóstico por imagen del perro y el gato*. Multimédica ediciones veterinarias, Barcelona, 2005.

FRAZHO, J.K., GRAHAM, J., PECK, J.N., DE HAAN, J.J. Radiographic evaluation of the anconeal process in skeletally inmature dogs. *Veterinary Surgery*, 2010; 39:829-832.

GAVIN, P.R., HOLMES, S.P. Orthopedic. En: GAVIN, P.R., BAGLEY, R.S. (eds): Practical Small Animal MRI. Wiley-Blackwell, Iowa, 2009; pp. 233-272.

HAMMOND, G., MCCONNELL, F. Radiology of the appendicular skeleton. En: HOLLOWAY, A., MCCONNELL, F. (eds). *BSAVA Manual of Canine and Feline Radiography and Radiology. A Foundation Manual*. British Small Animal Veterinary Association, Gloucester, 2013; pp. 240-301.

HENRY, G.A. Fracture healing and complications. En: THRALL, D.E. (ed): *Textbook of Veterinary Diagnostic Radiology*, 6th ed. Elsevier Saunders, St. Louis, 2013; pp. 283-306.

HORNOF, W.J., WIND, A.P., WALLACK, S.T., SCHULTZ, K.S. Canine elbow dysplasia. The early radiographic detection of fragmentation of the coronoid process. *Veterinary Clinics of North America: Small Animal Practice*, 2000; 30:257-266.

INNES, J.F., COSTELLO, M., BARR, F.J., RUDORF, H., BARR, A.R.S. Radiographic progression of osteoarthritis of the canine stifle joint: a prospective study. *Veterinary Radiology and Ultrasound*, 2004; 45:143-148.

JACKSON, L.C., PACCHIANA, P.D. Common complications of fracture repair. *Clinical Techniques in Small Animal Practice*, 2004; 19:168-179.

JACOBSON, L.S., KIRBERGER, R.M. Canine multiple cartilaginous exostoses: unusual manifestations and a review of the literature. *Journal of the American Animal Hospital Association*, 1996; 32:45-51.

JOHNSON, K. Osteomyelitis in dogs and cats. *Journal of the American Veterinary Medical Association*, 1994; 205:1882-1887.

KEALY, J.K., MCALLISTER, H., GRAHAM, J.P. *Diagnostic Radiology and Ultrasonography of the Dog and Cat*, 5th ed. Saunders Elsevier, St. Louis, 2010.

KIRBERGER, R.M. Bones - general. En: BARR, F.J., KIRBERGER, R.M. (eds): *BSAVA Manual of Canine and Feline Musculoskeletal Imaging*. British Small Animal Veterinary Association, Gloucester, 2006; pp. 9-18.

LAFOND, E., BREUR, G.J., AUSTIN, C.C. Breed susceptibility for developmental orthopedic diseases in dogs. *Journal of the American Animal Hospital Association*, 2002; 38:467-77.

MASON, D.R., SCHULTZ, K.S., SAMII, V.F., FUJITA, Y., HORNOF, W.J., HERRGESELL, E.J., LONG, C.D., MORGAN, J.P., KASS, P.H. Sensitivity of radiographic evaluation of radio-ulnar incongruence in the dog in vivo. *Veterinary Surgery*, 2002; 31:125-132.

MCALLISTER, H., TOBIN, E. Long bones - mature. En: BARR, F.J., KIRBERGER, R.M. (eds): *BSAVA Manual of Canine and Feline Musculoskeletal Imaging*. British Small Animal Veterinary Association, Gloucester, 2006; pp. 32-48.

McNicholas, W.T. Jr, Wilkens, B.E., Blevins, W.E., et al. Spontaneous femoral capital physeal fractures in adult cats: 26 cases (1996-2001). *J Am Vet Med Assoc*, 2002; 221(12):1731-1736.

Morgan, J.P. *Radiology of skeletal disease – principles of diagnosis in the dog*. Iowa State University Press, Iowa, 1981.

Nolte, D.M., Fusco, J.V., Peterson, M.E. Incidence of and predisposing factors for nonunion of fractures involving the appendicular skeleton in cats: 18 cases (1998-2002). *Journal of the American Veterinary Medical Association*, 2005; 226:77-82.

Owens, J.M., Biery D.N. *Radiographic Interpretation for the Small Animal Clinician*, 2nd ed. Williams & Wilkins, Baltimore, 1999.

Pollard, R.E., Phillips, K.L. Orthopedic diseases of young and growing dogs and cats. En: Thrall, D.E. (ed). *Veterinary Diagnostic Radiology*, 7th ed. Elsevier, St. Louis, 2018; pp. 348-365.

Pollard, R.E., Wisner, E.R. Orthopedic diseases of young and growing dogs and cats. En: Thrall, D.E. (ed): *Textbook of Veterinary Diagnostic Radiology*, 6th ed. Elsevier Saunders, St. Louis, 2013; pp. 267-282.

Salter, R., Harris, W. Injuries involving the epiphyseal plate. *Journal of Bone and Joint Surgery*, 1963; 45:587-622.

Samii, V., Gielen, I., Ludewig, E., Adams, W.H., Kiefer, I., van Bree, H., Saunders, J. Joints. En: Schwarz, T., Saunders, J. (eds): *Veterinary Computed Tomography*. Wiley-Blackwell, Oxford, 2011; pp. 387-419.

Sande, R. Radiography of orthopedic trauma and fracture repair. *Veterinary Clinics of North America: Small Animal Practice*, 1999; 29:1247-1260.

Schultz, R.M., Wisner, E.R. Long bones. En: Schwarz, T., Saunders, J. (eds): *Veterinary Computed Tomography*. Wiley-Blackwell, Oxford, 2011; pp. 381-386.

Smith, R.N. Appearance of ossification centres in the kitten. *Journal of Small Animal Practice*, 1968; 9:497-511.

Smith, R.N. Fusion of ossification centres in the cat. *Journal of Small Animal Practice*, 1969; 10:523-530.

Sumner-Smith, G. Observations on epiphyseal fusion of the canine appendicular skeleton. *Journal of Small Animal Practice*, 1966; 7:303-312.

Thrall, D.E. Principles of radiographic interpretation of the appendicular skeleton. En: Thrall, D.E. (ed): *Textbook of Veterinary Diagnostic Radiology*, 6th ed. Elsevier Saunders, St. Louis, 2013; pp. 252-266.

Thrall, D.E. Principles of radiographic interpretation of the appendicular skeleton. En: Thrall, D.E. (ed). *Veterinary Diagnostic Radiology*, 7th ed. Elsevier, St. Louis, 2018; pp. 334-247.

Thrall, D.E. Radiographic features of bone tumors and bone infection. En: Thrall, D.E. (ed): *Textbook of Veterinary Diagnostic Radiology*, 6th ed. Elsevier Saunders, St. Louis, 2013; pp. 307-318.

Wrigley, R.H. Malignant versus non-malignant bone disease. *Veterinary Clinics of North America: Small Animal Practice*, 2000; 30:315-347.

Chapter 5. Spine

Bahr, A. The vertebrae. En: Thrall, D.E. (ed). *Textbook of Veterinary Diagnostic Radiology*, 5th ed. Saunders Elsevier, St. Louis, 2007; pp: 179-193.

Begon, D. Radiología en neurología. Proceedings del XVII Congreso de AMVAC, 2000; pp. 43-52.

Burk, R.L., Feeney, D.A. The spine. En: *Small Animal Radiology and Ultrasonography. A Diagnostic Atlas and Text*. Elsevier Science, St. Louis, 2003; pp: 661-713.

Damur-Djuric, N., Steffen, F., Hassig, J.P., Morgan, J.P., Fluckiger, M.A. Lumbosacral transitional vertebrae in dogs: classification, prevalence and association with sacroiliac morphology. *Veterinary Radiology & Ultrasound*, 2006; 47:32-38.

Davies, J.V. Spine-intervertebral disc disease and Wobbler syndrome. En: Barr, F.J., Kirberger, R.M. (eds). *BSAVA Manual of Canine and Feline Musculoskeletal Imaging*. British Small Animal Veterinary Association, 2006; pp: 247-256.

De Risio, L., Thomas, W.B., Sharp, N.J. Degenerative lumbosacral stenosis. *Veterinary Clinics of North America: Small Animal Practice*, 2000; 30:111-132.

Dennis, R., Kirberger, R.M., Barr, F., Wrigley, R.H. Spine. En: *Handbook of Small Animal Radiology and Ultrasound*, 2th ed. Churchill Livingstone Elsevier, Edimburg, 2010; pp: 115-144.

Dewey, C.W., Davies, E., Bouma, J.L. Kyphosis and kyphoscoliosis associated with congenital malformations of the thoracic vertebral bodies in dogs. *Vet Clin North Am Small Anim Pract*, 2016; 46(2):295-306.

Farrow, C.S. La columna vertebral. En: *Diagnóstico por imagen del perro y el gato*. Gráficas IN – Multimédica, Barcelona, 2005.

Fluckiger, M.A., Damur-Djuric, N., Hassig, J.P., Morgan, J.P., Steffen, F. A lumbosacral transitional vertebra in the dog predisposes to cauda equina syndrome. *Veterinary Radiology & Ultrasound*, 2006; 47:39-44.

Gibbons, S.E., Macias, C., de Stefani, G.L., Pinchbeck, G.L., McKee, W.M. The value of oblique versus ventrodorsal myelographic views for lesion lateralization in canine thoracolumbar disc disease. *Journal of Small Animal Practice*, 2006; 47:658-662.

Guevar, J., Penderis, J., Faller, K., et al. Computer-assisted radiographic calculation of spinal curvature in brachycephalic "screw-tailed" dog breeds with congenital thoracic vertebral malformations: reliability and clinical evaluation. *PLoS One,* 2014; 9(9):e106957.

KEALY, J.K., MCALLISTER, H., GRAHAM, J.P. The skull and the vertebral column. En: *Diagnostic Radiology and Ultrasonography of the Dog and Cat,* 5th ed. Saunders Elsevier, St. Louis, 2010; pp. 447-541.

KIRBERGER, R.M. Early diagnostic imaging findings in juvenile dogs with presumed diskospondylitis: 10 cases (2008-2014). *J Am Vet Med Assoc,* 2016; 249(5):539-546.

KIRBERGER, R.M. Spine – general. En: BARR, F.J., KIRBERGER, R.M. (eds). *BSAVA Manual of Canine and Feline Musculoskeletal Imaging.* British Small Animal Veterinary Association., 2006; pp. 220-232.

LAMB, C.R., NICHOLLS, A., TARGETT, M., MANNION, P. Accuracy of survey radiographic diagnosis of intervertebral disc protrusion in dog. *Veterinary Radiology & Ultrasound,* 2002; 43:222-228.

LANG, J. Spine - lumbosacral region and cauda equina syndrome. En: BARR, F.J., KIRBERGER, R.M. (eds). *BSAVA Manual of Canine and Feline Musculoskeletal Imaging.* British Small Animal Veterinary Association, 2006; pp. 257-271.

LEE, R. La columna vertebral. En: LEE, R. (ed). *Manual de diagnóstico por imagen en pequeños animales.* Ediciones S, 1999; pp. 169-182.

LEWIS, N.D., COULSON, A. *An Atlas of Interpretative Radiographic Anatomy of the Dog and Cat.* Blackwell Science, Oxford, 2002.

LLABRÉS DÍAZ, F. Practical contrast radiography 4. Myelography. *In Practice,* 2005; 27:502-510.

MARIONI-HENRY, K., VITE, C.H., NEWTON, L., VAN WINKLE, T.J. Prevalence of diseases of the spinal cord of cats. *Journal of Veterinary Internal Medicine,* 2004; 18: 851-858.

MCEVOY, F.J. Spine – conditions not related to intervertebral disc disease. En: BARR, F.J., KIRBERGER, R.M. (eds): *BSAVA Manual of Canine and Feline Musculoskeletal Imaging.* British Small Animal Veterinary Association, 2006; pp. 233-246.

NEWITT, A., GERMAN, A.J., BARR, F.J. Congenital abnormalities of the feline vertebral column. *Veterinary Radiology & Ultrasound,* 2008; 49:35-41.

ORTEGA, M., GONÇALVES, R., HALEY, A., et al. Spondylosis deformans and diffuse idiopathic skeletal hyperostosis (dish) resulting in adjacent segment disease. *Vet Radiol Ultrasound,* 2012; 53(2):128-34.

OWENS, J.M., BIERY, D.N. Spine. En: *Radiographic Interpretation for the Small Animal Clinician,* 2nd ed. Williams & Wilkins, Baltimore, 1999; pp:. 127-146.

RAMEREZ III, O., THRALL, D.E. A review of imaging techniques for cauda equina syndrome. *Veterinary Radiology & Ultrasound,* 1998; 39:283-296.

RUOFF, C.M., KERWIN, S.C., TAYLOR, A.R. Diagnostic imaging of discospondylitis. *Vet Clin North Am Small Anim Pract,* 2018; 48(1):85-94.

SCHWARZ, T., HOLLOWAY, A. Radiology of the vertebral column. En: HOLLOWAY, A., MCCONNELL, F. (eds). *BSAVA Manual of Canine and Feline Radiography and Radiology.* A Foundation Manual. British Small Animal Veterinary Association, Gloucester, 2013; pp. 355-386.

SCRIVANI, P.V. Myelographic artefacts. *Veterinary Clinics of North America: Small Animal Practice,* 2000; 30:303-314.

SHARP, N.J.H., WHEELER, S.J., COFONE, M. Radiological evaluation of Wobbler syndrome - caudal cervical spondylomyelopathy. *Journal of Small Animal Practice,* 1992; 33:491-499.

SLANINA, M.C. Atlantoaxial instability. *Vet Clin North Am Small Anim Pract,* 2016; 46(2):265-275.

SQUIRES BOS, A., BRISSON, B.A., HOLMBERG, D.L., NYKAMP, S. Use of the ventrodorsal myelographic view to predict lateralization of extruded disk material in small-breed dogs with thoracolumbar intervertebral disk extrusion: 104 cases (2004–2005). *Journal of the American Veterinary Medical Association,* 2007; 230:1860-1865.

WAIBL, H., MAYRHOFER, E., MATIS, U., BRUNNBERG, L., KÖSTLIN, R. *Atlas of Radiographic Anatomy of the Dog.* Parey Verlag, Stuttgart, 2005.

WIDMER, W.R., THRALL, D.E. Canine and feline intervertebral disc disease, myelography and spinal cord disease. En: THRALL, D.E. (ed): *Textbook of Veterinary Diagnostic Radiology,* 5th ed. Saunders Elsevier, St. Louis, 2007; pp. 194-219.

WIDMER, W.R., THRALL, D.E. Canine and feline vertebrae. En: THRALL, D.E. (ed). *Veterinary Diagnostic Radiology,* 7th ed. Elsevier, St. Louis, 2018; pp. 249-270.

Chapter 6. Head

BANNON, K.M. Clinical canine dental radiography. *Vet Clin North Am Small Anim Pract,* 2013; 43(3):507-532.

BENIGNI, L., LAMB, C. Diagnostic imaging of ear disease in the dog and cat. *In Practice,* 2006; 28:122-130.

BISCHOFF, M.G., KNELLER, S.K. Diagnostic imaging of the canine and feline ear. *Veterinary Clinics of North America: Small Animal Practice,* 2004; 34:437-458.

BURK, R.L., FEENEY, D.A. The skull. En: *Small Animal Radiology and Ultrasonography. A Diagnostic Atlas and Text.* Elsevier Science, St. Louis. 2003; pp. 607-660.

COHN, L.A. Canine nasal disease: An update. *Vet Clin North Am Small Anim Pract,* 2020; 50(2):359-374.

DENNIS, R. Radiología del cráneo en pequeños animales. Proceedings del XVII Congreso de AMVAC, 2000; pp. 33-42.

DENNIS, R. Skull – general. En: BARR, F.J., KIRBERGER, R.M. (eds). *BSAVA Manual of Canine and Feline Musculoskeletal*

Imaging. British Small Animal Veterinary Association, 2006; pp. 173-191.

Dennis, R., Kirberger, R.M., Barr, F., Wrigley, R.H. Head and neck. En: *Handbook of Small Animal Radiology and Ultrasound*, 2th ed. Churchill Livingstone Elsevier, Edimburg, 2010; pp. 85-114.

Dickie, A.M., Sullivan, M. The effect of obliquity on the radiographic appearance of the temporomandibular joint in dogs. *Veterinary Radiology & Ultrasound*, 2001; 42:205-217.

Farrow, C.S. Cráneo, encéfalo, ojos y oídos. En: *Diagnóstico por imagen del perro y el gato*. Multimédica ediciones veterinarias, Barcelona, 2005; pp. 201-262.

Forrest, L. The cranial nasal cavities. Canine and feline. En: Thrall, D.E. (ed). *Veterinary Diagnostic Radiology*, 7th ed. Elsevier, St. Louis, 2018; pp. 183-203.

Forrest, L.J. Cranial and nasal cavities: canine and feline. En: Thrall, D.E. (ed). *Textbook of Veterinary Diagnostic Radiology*, 5th ed. Saunders Elsevier, St. Louis, 2007; pp: 119-141.

Guaraglia, C. Canine and feline dental disease. En: Thrall, D.E. (ed). *Veterinary Diagnostic Radiology*, 7th ed. Elsevier, St. Louis, 2018; pp. 153-182.

Hofer, P., Meisen, N., Bartholdi, S., Kaser-Hotz, B. Radiology corner – A new radiographic view of the feline tympanic bulla. *Veterinary Radiology & Ultrasound*, 1995; 36:14-15.

Holloway, A., Avner, A. Radiology of the head. En: Holloway, A., McConnell, F. (eds). *BSAVA Manual of Canine and Feline Radiography and Radiology*. A Foundation Manual. British Small Animal Veterinary Association, Gloucester, 2013; pp. 302-354.

Kealy, J.K., McAllister, H., Graham, J.P. The skull and the vertebral column. En: *Diagnostic Radiology and Ultrasonography of the Dog and Cat*, 5th ed. Saunders Elsevier, St. Louis, 2010; pp. 447-541.

Lamb, C.R. Skull – nasal chambers and frontal sinuses. En: Barr, F.J., Kirberger, R.M. (eds). *BSAVA Manual of Canine and Feline Musculoskeletal Imaging*. British Small Animal Veterinary Association, 2006; pp. 192-205.

Lamb, C.R., Richbell, S., Mantis, P. Radiographic signs in cats with nasal disease. *Journal of Feline Medicine and Surgery*, 2003; 5:227-235.

Lewis, N.D., Coulson, A. *An Atlas of Interpretative Radiographic Anatomy of the Dog and Cat*. Blackwell Science, Oxford, 2002.

Muhlbauer, M.C., Kneller, S.K. *Radiography of the Dog and Cat: Guide to Making and Interpreting Radiographs*. Iowa: John Wiley & Sons, Inc, 2013; pp. 123-274.

Niemiec, B., Gawor, J., Nemec, A., et al. World Small Animal Veterinary Association Global Dental Guidelines. *J Small Anim Pract*, 2020; 61(7):E36-E161.

Owens, J.M., Biery, D.N. Skull. En: *Radiographic Interpretation for the Small Animal Clinician*, 2nd ed. Williams & Wilkins, Baltimore, 1999; pp. 105-126.

Pownder, S., Rose, M., Crawford, J. Radiographic techniques of the nasal cavity and sinuses. *Clinical Techniques in Small Animal Practice*, 2006; 21:46-54.

Risselada, M. Diagnosis and management of cholesteatomas in dogs. *Vet Clin North Am Small Anim Pract*, 2016; 46(4):623-634.

Russo, M., Lamb, C.R., Jakovljevic, S. Distinguishing canine nasal neoplasia and rhinitis by radiography. *Veterinary Radiology & Ultrasound*, 2000; 41:108-124.

San Román, F., Llorens, P. Radiología dental: ese desconocido… ¿Es necesaria? Descubriendo la cavidad oral. Proceedings Formación Continuada. AVEPA, 2014; pp. 41-45.

Saunders, J.H., van Bree, H. Comparison of radiography and computed tomography for the diagnosis of canine nasal aspergillosis. *Veterinary Radiology & Ultrasound*, 2003; 44:414-419.

Steenkamp, G. Skull – teeth. En: Barr, F.J., Kirberger, R.M. (eds). *BSAVA Manual of Canine and Feline Musculoskeletal Imaging*. British Small Animal Veterinary Association, 2006; pp. 206-219.

Thrall, D.E. Basic principles of radiographic interpretation of the axial skeleton. En: Thrall, D.E. (ed). *Veterinary Diagnostic Radiology*, 7th ed. Elsevier, St. Louis, 2018; pp. 137-152.

Waibl, H., Mayrhofer, E., Matis, U., Brunnberg, L., Köstlin, R. *Atlas of Radiographic Anatomy of the Dog*. Parey Verlag, Stuttgart, 2005.

Zacher, A.M., Marretta, S.M. Oral and maxillofacial surgery in dogs and cats. *Vet Clin North Am Small Anim Pract*, 2013;43(3):609-649.

Chapter 7. Most common diagnostic errors

Baines, E.A., Grandage, J., Herrtage, M.E., Baines, S.J. Radiographic definition of the anticlinal vertebra in the dog. *Veterinary Radiology and Ultrasound*, 2009; 50:69-73.

Barr, F., O'Brien, R. Approach to abdominal imaging. En: O'Brien, R., Barr, F. (eds): *BSAVA Manual of Canine and Feline Abdominal Imaging*. British Small Animal Veterinary Association, Gloucester, 2009; pp. 1-4.

Dennis, R., Kirberger, R.M., Barr, F., Wrigley, R.H. *Handbook of Small Animal Radiology and Ultrasound*, 2nd ed. Churchill Livingstone Elsevier, Edimburg, 2010.

Drost, W.T., Reese, D.J., Hornof, W.J. Digital radiography artifacts. *Veterinary Radiology and Ultrasound*, 2008; 49:S48-56.

Kirberger, R.M., Avner, A. The effect of positioning on the appearance of selected cranial thoracic structures in the dog. *Veterinary Radiology and Ultrasound*, 2006; 47:61-68.

Rudorf, H., Taeymans, O., Johnson, V. Basics of thoracic radiography and radiology. En: Schwarz, T., Johnson, V. (eds): *BSAVA Manual of Canine and Feline Thoracic Imaging.* British Small Animal Veterinary Association, Gloucester, 2008; pp. 1-19.

Thrall, D.E. Introduction to radiographic interpretation. En: Thrall, D.E. (ed): *Textbook of Veterinary Diagnostic Radiology*, 6th ed. Elsevier Saunders, St. Louis, 2013; pp. 74-86.

Thrall, D.E. Principles of radiographic interpretation of the abdomen. En: Thrall, D.E. (ed): *Textbook of Veterinary Diagnostic Radiology*, 6th ed. Elsevier Saunders, St. Louis, 2013; pp. 650-658.

Thrall, D.E. Principles of radiographic interpretation of the appendicular skeleton. En: Thrall, D.E. (ed): *Textbook of Veterinary Diagnostic Radiology*, 6th ed. Elsevier Saunders, St. Louis, 2013; pp. 252-266.

Thrall, D.E. Principles of radiographic interpretation of the axial skeleton. En: Thrall, D.E. (ed): *Textbook of Veterinary Diagnostic Radiology*, 6th ed. Elsevier Saunders, St. Louis, 2013; pp. 101-113.

Thrall, D.E. Principles of radiographic interpretation of the thorax. En: Thrall, D.E. (ed): *Textbook of Veterinary Diagnostic Radiology*, 6th ed. Elsevier Saunders, St. Louis, 2013; pp. 474-488.

Thrall, D.E., Robertson, I.D. *Atlas of normal radiographic anatomy and anatomic variants in the dog and cat.* Elsevier-Saunders, St. Louis, 2011.